Physical Therapy Treatment of Common Orthopedic Conditions

Physical Therapy Treatment of Common Orthopedic Conditions

Editors

Neeraj D Baheti PT DPT OCS CSCS
Senior Physical Therapist
UCSF Benioff Children's Hospital Oakland
Sports Medicine Center for Young Athletes
Oakland, California, United States

Moira K Jamati PT MSPT ATC CSCS
Consultant
San Jose, California, United States

Foreword

Robert I Naber

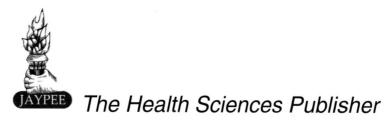

JAYPEE *The Health Sciences Publisher*

New Delhi | London | Philadelphia | Panama

Jaypee Brothers Medical Publishers (P) Ltd

Headquarters

Jaypee Brothers Medical Publishers (P) Ltd
4838/24, Ansari Road, Daryaganj
New Delhi 110 002, India
Phone: +91-11-43574357
Fax: +91-11-43574314
Email: jaypee@jaypeebrothers.com

Overseas Offices

J.P. Medical Ltd
83 Victoria Street, London
SW1H 0HW (UK)
Phone: +44-2031708910
Fax: +02-03-0086180
Email: info@jpmedpub.com

Jaypee-Highlights Medical Publishers Inc
City of Knowledge, Bld. 237, Clayton
Panama City, Panama
Phone: +1 507-301-0496
Fax: +1 507-301-0499
Email: cservice@jphmedical.com

Jaypee Medical Inc.
325 Chestnul Street
Suite 412, Philadelphia, PA 19106, USA
Phone: +1 267-519-9789
Email: support@jpmedus.com

Jaypee Brothers Medical Publishers (P) Ltd
17/1-B Babar Road, Block-B, Shaymali
Mohammadpur, Dhaka-1207
Bangladesh
Mobile: +08801912003485
Email: jaypeedhaka@gmail.com

Jaypee Brothers Medical Publishers (P) Ltd
Bhotahity, Kathmandu
Nepal
Phone: +977-9741283608
Email: kathmandu@jaypeebrothers.com

Website: www.jaypeebrothers.com
Website: www.jaypeedigital.com

Physical Therapy Treatment of Common Orthopedic Conditions

First Edition: **2016**

ISBN 978-93-5250-167-0

Printed at Sanat Printers

Dedications

This book is dedicated to my father and mother, Dr Dwarkadas Baheti and Sudha Baheti. Thank you for always being a source of inspiration to me and for encouraging me to do this project. I love you papa and mummy!

Neeraj D Baheti

I would like to dedicate this work to Edna and Francois Jamati—my parents and my heroes, whose example and support have both inspired and enabled me to pursue my profession with a passion.

Moira K Jamati

Contributors

EDITORS

Neeraj D Baheti PT DPT OCS CSCS
Senior Physical Therapist
UCSF Benioff Children's Hospital Oakland
Sports Medicine Center for Young
Athletes
Oakland, California, United States

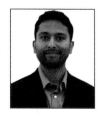

Moira K Jamati PT MSPT ATC CSCS
Consultant
San Jose, California, United States

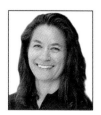

CONTRIBUTING AUTHORS

JH Abbott DPT MScPT PhD FNZCP
Research Associate Professor
Centre for Musculoskeletal Outcomes
Research
Dunedin School of Medicine
University of Otago
Dunedin, New Zealand

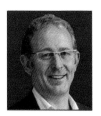

Powell J Bernhardt PT DPT CMTPT COMT
Adjunct Professor
Department of Physical Therapy
Howard University
Washington DC, United States

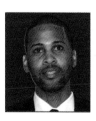

Kristen M Branham PT MPT OCS
Physical Therapist
Physical Therapy and Training Center
Folsom, California, United States

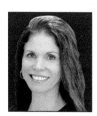

Luis A Feigenbaum PT DPT SCS
ATC LAT CSCS
Associate Professor and Chief of Sports
Physical Therapy
Department of Physical Therapy
University of Miami Miller School of
Medicine, Florida, United States

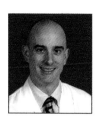

Lisa M Giannone PT MPT
Founder/Owner Active Care
San Francisco, California, United States

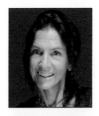

Ross M Nakaji PT MSPT OCS SCS ATC SCSC
Executive Director/Co-Founder
Los Gatos Orthopedic Sports Therapy
Los Gatos, California, United States

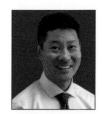

Joseph P Hannon PT DPT SCS CSCS
Sports Physical Therapist
Texas Health Ben Hogan Sports Medicine
Texas, United States

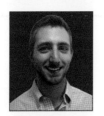

Kris B Porter PT DPT OCS
Director of Orthopedic Residency Program
The Jackson Clinics
Virginia, United States

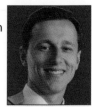

Daniel J Hass PT DPT SCS
Staff Physical Therapist
Cleveland Clinic Sports Health
Garfield Height, Ohio, United States

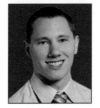

Bill Seringer DPT SCS OCS CSCS
Clinical Supervisor and Physical
Therapist
Stanford Health Care
Redwood City, California, United States

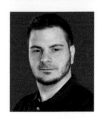

Robert C Manske PT DPT SCS MEd ATC
CSCS
Associate Professor
Department of Physical Therapy
Wichita State University
Wichita, Kansas, United States

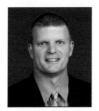

Steven Talajkowski PT MPT OCS Cert MDT
Clinic Director
Physiotherapy Associates
Hayward, California, United States

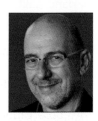

Judy L Matsuoka-Sarina OTR/L CHT
Occupational Therapist III
Good Samaritan Hospital
San Jose, California, United States

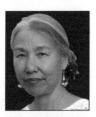

Timothy L Vidale PT DPT
Assistant Professor
Department of Physical Therapy
Howard University
Washington, DC, United States

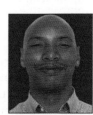

Joseph M Miller PT DSc OCS SCS CSCS
Faculty
Military Physical Therapy
Musculoskeletal Residency
Fort Bragg, North Carolina, United States

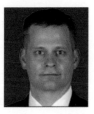

Rachel S Worman PT DPT
Staff Physical Therapist
Folsom Physical Therapy and
Training Center
Folsom, California, United States

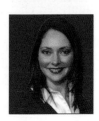

Foreword

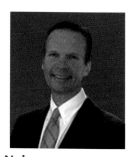

Robert I Naber PT OCS SCS AT C
President and Chief Executive Officer
Physical Therapy of Los Gatos
California, USA

It is a pleasure to write the Foreword for *Physical Therapy Treatment of Common Orthopedic Conditions*. As I read the chapters of this book, I was reminded of the first time I read the Orthopedic and Sports Physical Therapy, 1ˢᵗ edition by Gould and Davies, a book that addressed the diagnoses and problems I was facing each day in the clinic. The chapters were written, not by researchers, but by clinicians—physical therapists—just like me. They turned to the literature to understand their observations, strategy, treatment successes, and failures. All their writings were to share their experience in order to improve our profession and to better help our patients.

Déjà vu! I get that same impression from *Physical Therapy Treatment of Common Orthopedic Conditions*. It presents sixteen chapters on sixteen separate and current topics (medial tibial stress syndrome, plantar fascitis, patello-femoral syndrome, lumbar strain etc.). Some of these diagnoses, such as scapular dyskinesis, were not well known 10 years ago. There are new and innovative treatments applied to classic problems, such as patello-femoral syndrome and lumbar strain. Each chapter is uniformly organized to provide the reader with background information, basic anatomy and mechanics, clinical presentation by the patient, specific clinical examination, and treatments.

Overall, *Physical Therapy Treatment of Common Orthopedic Conditions* does an exceptional job of presenting and sharing this clinical information for orthopedic and sports physical therapists, physicians, chiropractors, occupational therapists, athletic trainers, and students. I admire the effort by editors, Baheti and Jamati, to bring this large body of knowledge together in one place to share with our profession and again to better help our patients.

Preface

The concept for this book evolved from a desire to create a resource for practicing clinicians from which they can draw the best practice and evidence-based physical therapy treatment ideas in addressing the most common musculoskeletal disorders that they confront. Authors with clinical expertise and/or academic focus specific to these orthopedic diagnoses agreed to share their practice approaches, integrated with a review of the most recent research available in the professional literature. The authors represent a diverse group of professionals who work in a wide range of settings—academic, military, hospital-based, and private practice—and who collectively offer a regional and international perspective.

The text is organized based on anatomical regions—upper extremity, spine, and lower extremity, and follows a proximal to distal, cranial to caudal approach. Within each chapter is a brief review of relevant information pertinent to the diagnosis, followed by more detailed development of evaluation and treatment approaches. While complimentary, alternative, and medical or surgical interventions are considered, the emphasis of each chapter, and of the work as a whole, remains on conservative physical therapy intervention.

Authors were encouraged to maximize the number of photos and supporting references throughout their work, to create an ease to follow guidelines for readers from which to draw ideas for intervention, as well as for readers to identify materials for further reference and future study. While the authors hail from many prestigious institutions and organizations, the material they present in this text is theirs, and theirs alone. The opinions they express do not reflect on the organizations with which they are affiliated. Similarly, while this text is expected to be an excellent resource for any clinician treating musculoskeletal dysfunction, many of the techniques presented require advanced training or further certification and should not be attempted by entry level practitioners without the requisite training. This book is not intended to be the sole source of material prior to treatment implementation.

The editors are grateful for the collaboration and contribution of the sixteen different professionals whose work constitutes the sixteen chapters that form this publication.

Neeraj D Baheti

Moira K Jamati

Contents

Section 1

Upper Extremity

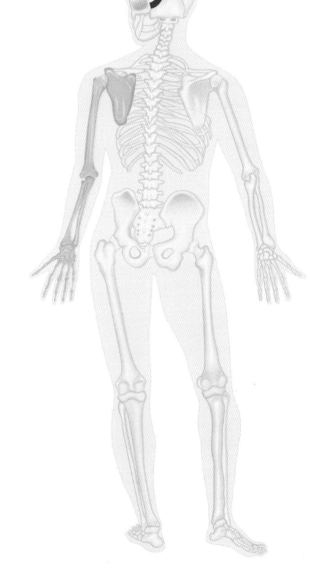

CHAPTERS

CHAPTER 1

Thoracic Outlet Syndrome

Steven Talajkowski

ABSTRACT

Thoracic outlet syndrome (TOS) is a varied pattern of signs and symptoms caused by compression of the upper extremity neurovascular bundle (brachial plexus, subclavian artery and vein) as it travels within the thoracic outlet space. About 5% of patients suffering from TOS present with clear, clinical evidence of the condition. The vast majority of patients suffering from TOS, greater than 90%, will present a little, if any, hard clinical evidence to support the diagnosis. Adding to the clinician's dilemma of definitively identifying TOS is that many patients presenting with the hallmark symptoms have coexisting conditions in the spine or upper extremity. These secondary or primary conditions may have signs and symptoms which present similar to, or overlap with, those caused by TOS. As a result, diagnosis and treatment of TOS can pose a challenge, even to those skilled in treating these patients. This chapter reviews the relevant anatomy, classifications and presentation of TOS. Tools and objective measures unique to TOS, as well as specific exercise protocols are presented in the examination and treatment portions of the chapter. Physical therapy assessment and intervention, which are the focus of this manuscript, provide a viable first line of action in the conservative management of these patients, and can have significant impact on their ability to manage the condition as well as on their quality of life.

◼ INTRODUCTION

Thoracic outlet syndrome (TOS) is a varied pattern of signs and symptoms caused by compression of the upper extremity (UE) neurovascular bundle (brachial plexus, subclavian artery and vein) as it travels within the thoracic outlet space. The thoracic outlet space may be generally visualized as the area starting at the scalene triangle and prescalene space and ending at the lateral border of the pectoralis minor muscle and axilla.[1-4]

Because there are multiple anatomical sites that can cause compression upon different sections of the neurovascular bundle, the presentation of TOS varies, as does its diagnosis and treatment. About 5% of patients suffering from TOS present with clear, clinical evidence (such as bony and/or fibrous tissue anomalies), along with obvious clinical signs (such as UE vascular changes and muscular wasting). However, the vast majority of patients suffering from TOS, greater than 90% will present with little, if any, hard clinical evidence to support the diagnosis.[4-10] Adding to the dilemma of definitively identifying TOS is that some patients presenting with the hallmark symptoms have coexisting conditions in the spine or UE. These secondary or primary conditions may have signs and symptoms which present similar to, or overlap with, those caused by TOS.[11] As a result, diagnosis and treatment of TOS can pose a challenge, even to those skilled in treating these patients.

Thoracic outlet syndrome is a condition often treated conservatively.[7,8,12-21] The physical therapist will play a significant role in the treatment plan of the conservatively-managed TOS patient.[17,22-25] The importance of recognizing the signs and symptoms of TOS early and treating it effectively cannot be overstated. Improper treatment of patients with neurogenic or vascular compression syndromes can delay improvement or possibly worsen the condition.[1,26,27] Development of chronic pain syndromes can make effective treatment more difficult to provide,[28] and delayed intervention for motor deficits can lead to permanent compromises.

Anatomical Review

The thoracic outlet can be thought of as a section in the series of tunnels through which the UE neurovascular bundle (brachial plexus, subclavian artery and vein) travels on its path to the UEs (Fig. 1). Starting medially and moving laterally, the thoracic outlet is the scalene triangle and prescalene space, the costoclavicular space and the retropectoralis space (Fig. 2).[12,29] Some authors differentiate pectoralis minor space compression as a unique entity.[3,30] This condition, considered a subset of TOS, it is referred to as pectoralis minor syndrome (PMS).

The scalene triangle, which contains the brachial plexus and subclavian artery, is formed medially and laterally by the anterior and middle scalene, respectively, and inferiorly by the first rib. The prescalene space, which contains only the subclavian vein, is formed laterally by the anterior scalene, inferiorly by the first rib, superiorly by the clavicle and subclavius muscle, and medially by the costoclavicular ligament.[3,4,31,32] The infraclavicular

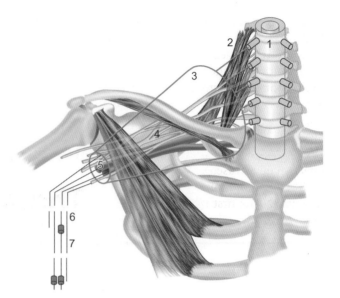

FIG. 2: The overlay shows the relationship of the tunnels to the anatomy of the upper extremity

Source: Reproduced with permission from Peter Edgelow.

or costoclavicular space, which now contains all of the neurovascular bundle, is formed inferiorly by the first rib and superiorly by the clavicle and subclavius muscle. The retropectoralis minor space, which also contains all of the neurovascular bundle, is formed anteriorly by the pectoralis minor muscle, superiorly by the pectoralis minor tendon and coracoid process and posteriorly by the anterolateral third, fourth and fifth ribs.[30,33,34]

Components of the Thoracic Outlet

The anatomic components of the thoracic outlet are summarized in Table 1.

Muscular Components

The attachments of the anterior, medial and posterior scalene muscles originate from the transverse process of

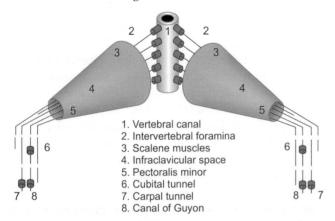

1. Vertebral canal
2. Intervertebral foramina
3. Scalene muscles
4. Infraclavicular space
5. Pectoralis minor
6. Cubital tunnel
7. Carpal tunnel
8. Canal of Guyon

FIG. 1: A graphic representation of the many tunnels the upper extremity nervous system must travel through, starting with the spinal canal and ending at the wrist

Source: Reproduced with permission from Peter Edgelow.

TABLE 1: Muscular, bony, neural and vascular components of the thoracic outlet

Muscular	Bony	Neural	Vascular
• Anterior and middle scalene	• Cervical ribs (when present)	• Brachial plexus	• Subclavian artery
• Subclavius	• First rib		• Subclavian vein
• Pectoralis minor	• Clavicle		

C2 through C7 and travel anteriorly and laterally to attach to the first rib (anterior and middle scalene) and second rib (posterior scalene), with an occasional attachment of the posterior scalene to the third rib.[35] Innervation of this musculature originates from cranial nerves III through VI. The scalene muscles are responsible for lateral flexion of the neck, forward flexion if both muscles are active, and elevation of the upper ribs during respiration.[32] In the case of TOS, it appears the posterior scalene has no direct effect on neurovascular compression.

The subclavius muscle originates at the costochondral junction of the first rib and inserts onto the subclavian groove on the clavicle. Its innervation is from the subclavian nerve. The muscle's action is to depress and stabilize the clavicle.[35]

The pectoralis minor muscle origins are the third, fourth and fifth ribs, and it inserts on the medial and upper surface of the coracoid process. Its innervation is from the medial pectoral nerve. The muscle serves to elevate the ribs and protract the scapula.[35]

Relevance

Abnormal development of the scalene muscles, variations in the scalene triangle space and anomalous fibrous bands can diminish the space through which the brachial plexus and subclavian artery pass.[3] Roos identified thirteen variations of fibromuscular bands in thoracic outlet space.[8,36] Anomalous cases have been reported where parts of the brachial plexus travel around or directly through the anterior or middle scalene.[29,37] The scalene triangle is the shape of an acute triangle with the first rib as the base. The top vertex of the triangle or interscalene angle has been measured from 4° to 22°, with an average of 11.3°.[32] The distance between the anterior and middle scalene at the base of the first rib has been measured between 0 mm and 25 mm, with an average width of ranging from 9 mm to 12 mm.[32,37] There is no predetermined minimum scalene angle, nor width that would require surgical intervention. TOS patients, however, who do have rib resection and/or scalenectomy surgery often have a narrower than average interscalene space.[32,38] The scalene muscles can suffer damage and tissue changes as a result of direct trauma to the neck—caused by a motor vehicle accident (MVA) or fall, for example. A change in muscle fiber types with a conversion of some type II muscle fibers to type I can result from tissue tearing and bleeding in the scalene muscles, which is correlated with signs of deconditioning and weakness, resembling the changes associated with aging.[2,39] Also

associated with traumatic insult is a significant increase fibrous connective tissue, increasing the bulk and decreasing the elasticity of the muscle fibers.[2]

Subclavian muscle involvement in TOS is the result of an uncommon, anomalous muscle, which can attach to the first rib and compromise the costoclavicular space.[40]

Recognition of PMS as a subset of TOS is relatively new. Sanders and Rao comment that although the condition was described by Wright in 1945,[41] it was not until 2005 that they resurrected PMS, following communication with Dr George Thomas of Seattle. Since then Sanders and Rao have observed and documented 75% of neurogenic TOS patients have some involvement of PMS, and in some cases PMS is the only source of compression.[34,42] Of the components of the neurovascular bundle, the brachial plexus lies closest to the pectoralis minor muscle, thus pectoralis minor compression is typically a neurogenic condition.[33] Symptom presentation is typically in the area of the pectoralis minor muscle and the shoulder, and travels distally to the hand. A less common presentation is when PMS symptoms extend only in the neck, face and scapula, with or without headaches.[34]

Bony Components

The first rib is the shortest, broadest and most curved of all the ribs. The second rib is almost twice as long but half as wide as the first. The first rib has a prominent scalene tubercle, formed by the attachment of the anterior scalene, and a shallow groove, formed by the subclavian vein. The first rib attaches to the first thoracic body by a single facet joint. The single vertebral body facet joint attachment occurs with the other atypical ribs (2, 11 and 12). The typical ribs (3–10) have two facet joints, which attach to the vertebral body at the same level as the rib as well as to the vertebral body superior to it.[35]

The clavicle attaches medially to the manubrium and laterally to the acromion. Its role in shoulder movement is multidirectional. In the thoracic outlet, the clavicle is the lateral attachment for the subclavian muscle and is the superior border of the costoclavicular space. It also provides bony protection for the neurovascular bundle.

Relevance

The shape of the first rib can be a predictor of TOS problems. Ribs with a straighter shaft are more often resected than the ribs with a larger curve.[43]

Cervical ribs, when present, are the result of an elongated C7 transverse process. Their size varies from insignificant to, in 30% of cases, almost fully formed. Connection of the cervical rib to the first rib is through fibrous bands, or in some cases, a direct pseudo joint.[3,44,45] Longer cervical ribs are more likely to cause neurogenic or vascular compression and are the main cause of arterial TOS.[44]

Fractures of the medial clavicle can create a bony callus that can in turn compromise the space between the clavicle and first rib, creating impingement on the neurovascular bundle.[7,46,47] The presence of such a callus is usually found in plain X-rays.

Of all the thoracic outlet spaces, the costoclavicular space is the mostly likely to close and cause neural compression during hyperabduction of the arm[29,32,41] or during shoulder abduction combined with external rotation.[48] A depressed or lower shoulder can also be a risk factor for neural compression.[47] The downward movement of the clavicle over the first rib has been described as a "pincer action", compressing the brachial plexus.[19,48] The effect is even greater when the first rib is elevated.[19]

Neural Components

The brachial plexus is responsible for supplying the motor and sensory innervation to the UE and shoulder girdle. Formation of the brachial plexus starts at the anterior (ventral) rami of C5, C6, C7, C8 and T1. In addition, C5 receives a small branch from C4, and T1 a small branch from T2. In some cases, the C4 branch may be less or absent, with a larger contribution from T2. This is referred to as a postfixed plexus. Conversely a prefixed plexus exists when the T2 branch small or absent, and the C4 branch is larger.[49]

The C5 to T1 spinal nerves continue on to create the three trunks of the brachial plexus. The C5 and C6 become the upper trunk at the medial scalene, the C7 becomes the middle trunk, and C8 and T1 form the lower trunk, just posterior to the anterior scalene.

The brachial plexus and subclavian artery pass together through the scalene triangle, while the subclavian vein passes alone through the prescalene space. Anterior to the scalene triangle and prescalene space the brachial plexus further divides into cords and, along with the subclavian artery and vein, moves together through the costoclavicular space and retropectoralis space. The neurovascular bundle continues on to the axilla and medial upper arm, where the brachial plexus splits into its five terminal branches, which are (1) the median, (2) ulnar, (3) radial, (4) musculocutaneous and (5) circumflex (axillary) nerves.

Relevance

As the brachial plexus travels through the scalene triangle, the rami of C5 to T1 are stacked with T1 at the bottom. Because the C8 and T1 spinal nerves are closer in proximity to the first rib, brachial plexus compression syndromes with a more dominate ulnar nerve distribution are more common in neurogenic TOS, and account for 70–90% of cases.[44] This contrasts upper trunk compression, which results in a more radial or median nerve distribution of symptoms.[50]

The postfixed plexus individual is at risk based on the neurologic anatomical relationships: the T1 nerve root emerges below the first rib, increasing the likelihood of a downward pull on the inferior trunk of the brachial plexus, thereby increasing its vulnerability to injury.[12,49,51]

Classifications of Thoracic Outlet Syndrome

The incidence of TOS in the general population appears to vary widely, with authors reporting anywhere from 3 to 80 incidents per 1,000.[52,53] Debate continues in the literature as to whether TOS is overdiagnosed or underdiagnosed.[5,54,55] The disagreement may be attributed to lack of consensus as to the causes or definition of neurogenic TOS.

Table 2 identifies the hallmarks of TOS classification as either neurogenic, arterial or venous.

■ CLINICAL PRESENTATION

For the sake of simplicity, this chapter will discuss a neurogenic thoracic outlet syndrome (NTOS) patient presenting with symptoms in only one extremity. This circumstance allows the clinician to infer normative measures when making comparisons to the uninvolved side. While some patients will report unilateral symptoms, it is also common to have bilateral complaints with one extremity more involved than the other.

Patient intake paperwork should include a body diagram, pain scale and medical history (including past injuries, surgeries, treatments and diagnostic test results). When completing the body diagram, the TOS patient will often fill in the UEs from the neck to the hand. While the arm and hand symptoms may initially appear to encompass the entire UE, symptom distribution can often demonstrate a distinct ulnar nerve pattern, starting from the medial arm and elbow and reaching into the ring and pinky fingers (Fig. 3). Symptoms can spread to the anterior shoulder and chest, as well as into the side

patients may have stopped working completely. Even those who are unable to work will have some need to do family and/or household activities, or to use a computer, tablet or smartphone. It may be helpful to inquire about the level of potentially stressful ADL's the patient is still participating in. Many patients understand the need and value of exercise. However, many TOS patients do not do well with a focus on stretching and strengthening exercise. Even the less severe TOS patient can show an adverse response to certain home exercises, no matter how carefully these programs are presented. It is helpful to know what other exercises the patient is already doing, so as to not conflict with the treatment plan that will be presented to the patient. Included in the questioning is if the patient is participating in aerobic exercise. Some TOS patients will have cut back so much on their activity level that they become extremely sedentary. Static postural positions such as reading, watching television, even without UE movement, can contribute to sustaining the patient's condition.

Objective Examination

The physical or objective examination will be designed to support the diagnosis of TOS. Care must be taken in performing the objective examination. The patient may report that performing simple ADLs such as reaching can aggravate symptoms for days, and even weeks. If this is the case, then care should be taken when asking the patient to move, or when moving the patient, so as not to aggravate their symptoms.

Postural Screen

Observation of sitting posture can start during the subjective examination. A more formal screen, to be done with the patient in standing, can start the objective exam. Posture can be assessed as the therapist wishes; however, some suggestions follow.

Frontal observation

- Shoulder height
- Lateral shifts at shoulder and pelvis
- Lower extremity (LE) weight bearing shifts
- Knee and foot position/alignment.

Sagittal observation

- Position of hips and pelvis forward or back
- Shape of lumbar lordosis, thoracic kyphosis and cervical lordosis

- Anterior versus posterior position of scapular and glenohumeral joint
- Head position.

Posterior observation

- Scapular position with attention to location of medial and inferior boarder
- Lateral and rotational deformities of the spine
- Any other abnormalities that may not have been obvious in other positions.

Hand Temperature

While the testing of hand temperature could be placed in the special tests section of this chapter, it may make sense to perform the test earlier in the exam. More than 50% of TOS patients present with cold and/or asymmetrical hand temperatures. The existence of a cold hand in NTOS is likely related to Raynaud's phenomenon, caused by an adverse reaction of the sympathetic nervous system.[47] This is not to be confused with the arterial blood flow problem found in arterial thoracic outlet syndrome (ATOS). Since the objective examination can aggravate the patient's symptoms, taking hand temperatures now gives the examiner a baseline measurement that can be used later for reassessment.

Hand temperature is easily tested with a noncontact infrared thermometer. The opening at the tip of the thermometer is placed against the distal pad of the second and fifth finger (Fig. 4). Measurements for both

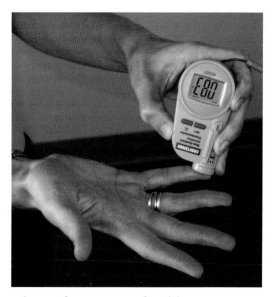

FIG. 4: The use of a noncontact infrared thermometer to measure hand temperature

hands are recorded. A positive test is for the involved hand to be colder than the noninvolved hand and/or to measure a difference between the second and fifth fingers. A difference of greater than 2°F is considered significant.[22] Cold or asymmetrical temperatures are found in about 50% of TOS patients.[69] The patient may not experience cold hands during the evaluation but may report intermittent periods of coldness or asymmetry in hand temperature during the day and related to activity. This should be noted and used by the patient to assess the effectiveness of their home program, as will be described later.

Active Movements

The patient is asked to actively raise the arm into shoulder flexion, abduction and shoulder flexion with the elbow flexed (increasing stress to the ulnar nerve).[12] The hand position is thumb up for each of these maneuvers. When recording UE active range of motion (ROM) in cases of TOS, it is recommended that instead of raising the arm as far as possible, that the patient be instructed to stop active movement at the onset of tension or pulling, commonly felt somewhere along the extremity or up into the neck. A report of increased pain is usually a sign that the patient has moved too far. While there can be cases where pain and tension occur simultaneously, if attention is focused, tension can usually be felt by the patient before an increase in pain. Consideration should be made for a loss of active ROM because of other shoulder pathology. Measurements for both arms are recorded as active ROM to the onset of symptoms.

Cervical active ROM in all planes is tested next. Often rotation and side bending away from the involved side are more limited and/or elicit some reproduction of symptoms into the neck, shoulder and/or extremity in TOS patients. Rotation toward the involved side is usually not painful, or if painful on the same side, then may be related to a cervical condition. Patients with cervical conditions can present in various ways, and their movement patterns should match common cervical conditions. However, it can also be that the patient presents with both TOS and a cervical condition concomitantly.

Special Tests in Standing

Reversible weakness of the adductor pollicis muscle

Assessment of thumb adductor pollicis strength is an important aspect of the examination as well as the treatment program. Herman Kabat introduced the

concept of reversible weakness of the adductor pollicis to Peter Edgelow. Dr Kabat, a neurologist, along with Maggie Knott, a physical therapist, were responsible for developing the proprioceptive neuromuscular facilitation methods still in use today. In Dr Kabat's later years he developed the Kabat protocol treatment methods as an approach to chronic neck, UE, and low back pain.[70] Kabats protocol tested adductor pollicis strength: if thumb strength was asymmetrical, the neck was then stabilized. In the event the weaker thumb tested stronger with neck stabilization, the test was positive for reversible weakness.

Assessment of thumb adductor pollicis strength has been modified by Peter Edgelow.[12,22,23] Instead of using a manual muscle test done by the practitioner, as proposed by Kabat, thumb strength can be quantified by using a device named the "thumbometer" (Fig. 5). This device also allows the patient to do a self-assessment.

The patient is directed to hold the hand flat and palm up, with the fingers slightly extended. Edgelow uses the example of holding the hand open as if feeding a horse a sugar cube. The squeeze bottle end of the thumbometer is placed deep into the thenar web space and the patient is instructed to squeeze the bottle with maximum effort while still keeping the palm open and the fingers and thumb extended (Fig. 5). Both hands are tested. If the

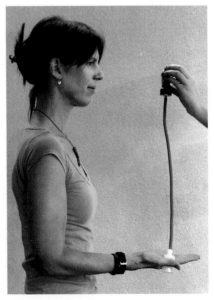

FIG. 5: Using the thumbometer to test for reversible weakness of the thumb. The thumbometer is made using the gauge of a manual blood pressure cuff and a small plastic squeeze bottle (such as one used for eyedrops) linked together by a length of rubber tubing

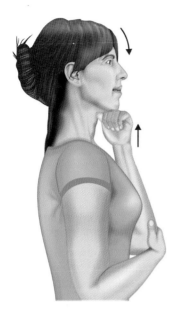

FIG. 6: The "thinker pose"
Source: Reproduced with permission from Peter Edgelow.

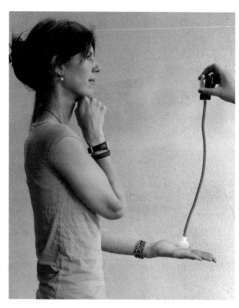

FIG. 7: Using the thinker pose and thumbometer to test for reversible weakness of the thumb adductor pollicis

test shows one hand is weaker than the other, the patient is instructed to perform the thinker pose (Figs 6 and 7), using the stronger hand to align and stabilize the neck. The term "thinker pose" was coined by Edgelow and inspired by the Rodin sculpture *The Thinker*. Pressure between the fist and chin is light. The chin moves down slightly with the movement to facilitate activation of the deep neck flexors and to stabilize and align the neck. The weak thumb is tested again using the thumbometer (Fig. 7). If the weak thumb becomes stronger, the test is positive for reversible weakness of the thumb and has been coined, by Edgelow, as a positive Kabat sign.[22]

A positive Kabat sign is weakness of the thumb adductor that can be reversed or improved through improved alignment of the neck and facilitation of the anterior stabilizers of the cervical spine. If thumb strength is improved through alignment and facilitation of the cervical stabilizers, it can also be made weak as a result of poor posture and a poorly stabilized neck. This concept will become a pillar of treatment, understanding that measureable weakness of the thumb is only one indicator of nerve compression.

In his studies, Dr Kabat also found that wrist flexion could also be used for testing. This can be useful in cases where there is thumb pathology that would interfere with applying the test. However, the patient cannot self-assess wrist flexion strength.

Elevated Arm Stress Test

The elevated arm stress test (EAST), or Roos test, is a common diagnostic clinical test. The test, as described by Roos, instructs the patient to hold the shoulder in 90° of abduction, external rotation and elbow flexion then open and close the hands for 3 minutes.[8] A positive test is the patient report of pain and/or paresthesia, or an inability to hold the position due to pain or fatigue. Peter Edgelow recommends using a modified EAST without opening and closing the hand.[22] The modification of this test may be necessary for more acute or severe TOS patients, so as not to aggravate their symptoms. The test is stopped once arm fatigue sets in.

EAST with Pulse Oximetry

The addition of a finger pulse oximeter can be added to the EAST. Clinically there have been observations showing a reduction of peripheral oxygen saturation (SpO_2) blood levels with TOS patients during the modified EAST test. SpO_2 level can drop 5–10% below the normal 98% level. This procedure has been used by Braun and shown a similar drop in SpO_2 levels when testing TOS patients.[47,70-72] The pulse oximeter can be placed on the thumb if the test is done with opening and closing the hand.

Adson's Test

Pulse obliterating tests, such as the Adson's test, though still commonly used, have not proven selective enough, especially with the neurogenic TOS patients who will not have an arterial blockage. The test often provides positive results in normal subjects.[57,65] The test may be somewhat more useful in cases of ATOS.[59]

Supine Tests

Neural mobility and sensitivity

With the patient lying supine, upper and lower neural mobility and sensitivity will be assessed passively. Description of nerve tension and mobility testing is described in detail in works by David Butler and Michael Shacklock.[19,72]

Typically neural testing for the TOS patient is simplified and brief. Care should be taken during testing, as the nervous system is likely sensitive and irritated and may be directly aggravated by the testing movements. Loss of nerve mobility may be displayed sooner than expected. Often a skilled physical therapist can feel guarding or tension before the patient reports it. Provocative neural testing is usually avoided unless the patient has low irritability or full passive ROM.

Peter Edgelow uses straight leg raise (SLR) testing as another way to assess sensitivity of the nervous system.[23] When comparing SLR measurements one leg may test lower than the other. The lower leg is commonly on the same side as the involved UE. During the SLR test, tension can sometimes be felt in the neck or extremity. Consideration should be made for patients with lumbar conditions or known cases of sciatica.

A simplified UE neural dynamic test is to abduct the arm to the feeling of tension, back off slightly and then add in wrist and finger extension, again stopping at the onset of tension or guarding. The test is recorded by the arm and hand position measured in degrees goniometrically. An ulnar nerve bias to the test can start in the same direction, then add elbow flexion and wrist extension, with the hand moving toward the patient's head. Maneuvers to alleviate UE symptoms (e.g. elevating the scapula) are useful for assessment, as well as for showing the patient the effects of proximal movements of the shoulder on distal symptoms.

Palpation

Palpation includes the following areas: the scalene triangle, the pectoralis minor muscle, the medial arm near the axilla and the cubital and carpal tunnels. Sensitivity to palpation over the scalenes has been shown to be a diagnostic feature found in 95% of neurogenic TOS patients.[69] The patient may report either localized tenderness or pain but also the reproduction of distal UE symptoms. Palpation is performed bilaterally to compare the involved side with the uninvolved side. Tinel's test can be done at the supraclavicular space and the cubital, carpal and Guyton's canals.

Shoulder Mobility

Shoulder clearing tests should be performed carefully, if at all, with patients with obvious TOS symptoms or altered neurodynamics. If appropriate, common tests such as the subacromial impingement test, the apprehension test (for capsular instability), biceps tendon tests (to determine tendon irritability) can be performed. Positive shoulder test can exist either alongside or independently of TOS.

Differential Diagnostic Testing

Spurling's Test

The Spurling's test is effectively used to test for cervical nerve root pain. The test places the head in side bending and extension, which causes a closing down of the foramina on same side, pinching the nerve root increasing symptoms on that same side.[73] In contrast, with the TOS patient, often side bending toward the affected side can lessen arm symptoms due to a slacking of the brachial plexus.[22]

EAST in Non-TOS Patients

Holding the arms in the EAST position may offer relief to the patient with cervical nerve root irritability. This is consistent with a C5 nerve root problem, where the patient will hold the arm overhead to relieve symptoms.[74] Patients having shoulder pathology will often show signs and symptoms more localized to the shoulder area, as expected with that condition. Patients with ulnar nerve neuritis may experience arm and hand pain related to the position of sustained elbow flexion.

Cervical Traction

Cervical traction does not typically lessen TOS symptoms and may actually increase symptoms in TOS patients. This is likely due to increasing tension on a sensitive nervous system. Patients that do respond positively to cervical traction may have a cervical problem. In some cases, a patient may have both TOS and a cervical condition and respond both positively and negatively to cervical traction. In these cases, it should be determined if cervical traction can be applied in a way that helps relieve or abolish cervical symptoms, without aggravating the patient's TOS symptoms.

Tinel's Test

The common tests for median, ulnar and radial nerve sensitivity are the Tinel's test for the median nerve at the carpal tunnel, and ulnar nerve at the cubital tunnel. Typically signs and symptoms of these peripheral nerve conditions are specific to the distribution pattern of the nerve involved, and less encompassing than those of TOS. Positive findings for distal nerve compression syndromes may not rule out TOS and instead may be part of the double crush syndrome. The prevalence of this double crush syndrome is unclear with studies reporting 44% of patients having both carpal tunnel syndrome and TOS, with others reporting cubital tunnel and TOS in 10% of cases.[11]

Pectoralis Minor Test

The pectoralis minor test, described by Thompson, helps determine the involvement of the pectoralis minor muscle in UE symptoms.[30] The technique involves palpating the pectoralis minor muscle at the infraclavicular subcoracoid space. With the pectoralis major muscle, relaxed palpation should reproduce UE symptoms. With the pectoralis major muscle tensed, (the patient pushes out against the hand of the therapist), the tense muscle blocks pressure to the pectoralis minor beneath it, and UE symptoms are lessened or absent.[30]

■ PHYSICAL THERAPY TREATMENT

While a small number of TOS patients have clear anatomical and physical findings requiring surgery, the general consensus advocates a conservative approach to TOS treatment. This is particularly true for the majority of patients who present with limited clinical findings.

Physical therapy treatment in the literature generally relies on a program of UE and cervical ROM exercises and strengthening, with specific focus on core, scapular and rotator cuff strengthening.[17] Stretching is directed toward the muscles bordering the thoracic outlet space such as the scalenes or pectoralis minor muscle. Nerve mobilization techniques as described by Butler, Elvey and Shacklock are also popular.[19,27,72] Patient education typically focuses on the anatomy of the thoracic outlet area, as well as postural training and ergonomic assessment. The author cautions that overly strenuous TOS treatment programs may provoke the patient. Pain is to be avoided, and progression of treatment is to be based upon subjective and objective improvement.

Edgelow Neurovascular Entrapment Syndrome Treatment

The Edgelow Neurovascular Entrapment Syndrome Treatment (ENVEST) program was developed by physical therapist Peter Edgelow and forms the basis of the treatment techniques in this chapter.[12,22,23,66,75,76] The guiding principles of the ENVEST exercise program are summarized in Table 3. The program has eight specific goals and seven distinct categories of exercise, but the success of these measures is grounded in assessment—of not only the clinician, but also the patient.

Assessment and Patient Self-assessment

One of the basic principles of the ENVEST program is assessment of objective measurements by the clinician and self-assessment by the patient. This assessment provides the therapist and patient information needed to progress or alter the treatment program.

During the objective examination, a number of measurements were taken. These measurements reveal some of the consequences of TOS. Limited ROM in the shoulder, cervical spine and SLR can indicate decreased neural mobility, increased sensitivity to movement, or compression of the nervous system. A cold hand can be a sign of sympathetic sensitivity expressed through a Raynaud's phenomenon. Weakness in the thumb can be the result of poor motor control of the cervical spine and

TABLE 3: The ABCs of the Edgelow Neurovascular Entrapment Syndrome Treatment (ENVEST) program

A (activate)	B (breathing)	C (cardiovascular)
Activate the core stabilizers of the spine using the thinker pose and using pressure biofeedback to retrain the deep neck flexors	Focus on diaphragmatic breathing during ENVEST program exercises and carry through to daily activities	Restore cardiovascular fitness with a goal of walking 20 minutes/four times a day without aggravating symptoms

postural dysfunction. Any or all of these measurements may be found to be positive and relevant in the patient with TOS. The effects of TOS can be listed under objective information as just noted, or subjective reports such as pain, numbness tingling, heaviness or fatigue. Subjective information cannot be measured directly. Not only can objective information such as UE and cervical active ROM, hand temperature, and thumb strength be easily measured, clinicians can teach their patients to do the same. This enables patients to do their own pretreatment and post-treatment check of objective measures. Physical therapists routinely use this tactic to determine the efficacy of specific interventions, and modify treatment parameters to optimize patient response.

The patient is asked to measure the relevant objective measures (e.g. ROM, temperature, strength) before starting their exercises and again at the end of the exercise. The expected response is to see an improvement in one or all of those measures. When objective measures improve, the patient is given a green light, and the patient directed to progress to the next exercise in the ENVEST program. If any of the objective measures worsen, the patient is given a red light, and there is no progression in the program. Instead the exercise that was just completed should be either modified, or further instruction is needed to make sure the patient is doing the exercise properly. In the event that no objective changes are observed, the patient is given a yellow light, and may progress to the next exercise, as long as the patient demonstrates proper technique with the prior exercise.

An exercise session typically lasts for 20 minutes, and if possible, patients will perform the program four times a day. This will coincide with aerobic exercise that will be prescribed four times a day. The patient will need a tool kit to perform the self-assessment and for some of the specialized exercises prescribed in the program (Fig. 8).

Goals of Treatment

1. Calm the nervous system
2. Increase strength and functional stability in the core muscles of the spine, shoulder and trunk
3. Improve cardiovascular conditioning
4. Restore normal movement and mobility of the nervous system
5. Educate the patient in a way that explains the nature of their condition to their level of understanding
6. Educate the patient in the importance of the factors that contribute to their condition including dysfunctional breathing patterns, poor posture, poor

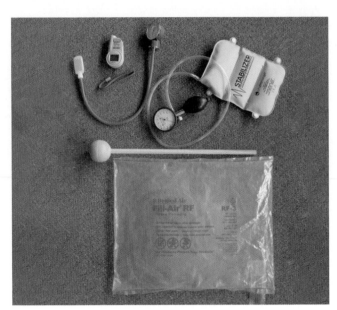

FIG. 8: ENVEST program tool kit. Clockwise from upper left corner thumbometer, noncontact infrared thermometer, Chattanooga Stabilizer™ (spinal stabilization), ball and stick "pinky ball" (2¼ inch solid rubber ball with a ½ by 18 inch wooden dowel), air bag (Fill-Air RF-3)

work habits, and the effects of functional instability and the effects of unmanaged stress
7. Understand the role of emotion and the intellect in the healing process
8. Understand that the patient will be the one most responsible for their recovery.

ENVEST Program Exercises

1. Breathing exercises in supine
2. Seated ball exercises
3. Foam roll exercises and thoracic mobilization
4. Scapular strengthening
5. Neural mobilization
6. Postural training and core strengthening
7. Aerobic conditioning.

(1) Breathing exercises in supine

One of the first goals of ENVEST treatment program is to start to calm the nervous system. By decreasing irritability of the nervous system, the patient can begin to move in ways that do not increase their pain and that, in turn, can lead to a gradual decrease in their symptoms. This is accomplished by providing the patient with an understanding how breathing and posture affect the thoracic outlet space.

The ENVEST program starts with a group of four breathing exercises. The first exercise presents core principals that will be carried forward to all five breathing exercises and through to the rest of the ENVEST program. **Diaphragmatic breathing in supine:** The first exercise will teach the patient: (1) the importance of posture and positioning, breathing, and relaxation, (2) the effects of movement on symptoms—the possibility of movement without increasing pain and (3) the recruitment of core muscles and relaxation of overactive muscles.

The first exercise begins with the patient lying supine. Care should be taken to position the patient in the most comfortable position possible. While the patient could lie flat on the floor (or mat) with the head unsupported (Figs 9 and 10), it would also be common to modify the patient's position to facilitate relaxation. In this modified position, the patient lies with the head on a pillow or pillows and, if necessary, supports the curve of the neck using a rolled towel or cervical roll. The knees are bent in a hook lying position. The arms may remain at the side or rest on the body. Clinical experience has shown that many patients are able to relax the UE and neck more effectively when the arms are supported. This can be done with a cotton T-shirt (Fig. 11) or a mobilization belt (Fig. 12). Adding this UE support can have the effect of relaxing the shoulders, positioning the scapula and clavicle in a more open position, and possibly putting the

brachial plexus in a more favorable resting, non-tension position. Some patients with ulnar nerve irritation at the cubital tunnel may prefer to lie with their elbows more extended.

Breathing is assessed. If a common but dysfunctional upper chest breathing pattern is observed, then a diaphragmatic breathing pattern is introduced. Some patients may not be familiar with this pattern of breathing. Patients who have been involved in music, singing, acting—or other practices such as meditation, yoga or tai chi—will have likely practiced this from of breathing, or at least be familiar with it. The primary intent of diaphragmatic breathing is to limit activation of the scalene muscles used in upper chest breathing. Patients not familiar with diaphragmatic breathing, as well as those in pain, may have difficulty letting go of the upper chest breathing pattern. It is important that the patient be encouraged to successfully demonstrate and practice a diaphragmatic breathing, while realizing it will be difficult to change.

Accompanying diaphragmatic breathing is pelvic movement. As a breath is taken in through the nose, the pelvis is rotated anteriorly (Fig. 9), and during exhalation the breath is expelled through pursed lips while the pelvis is rotated posteriorly (Fig. 10). The breathing is slow and

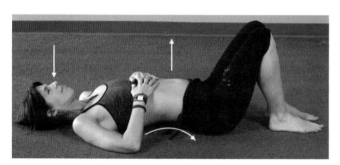

FIG. 9: Diaphragmatic breathing with inhalation

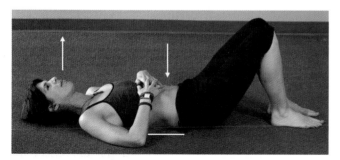

FIG. 10: Diaphragmatic breathing with exhalation

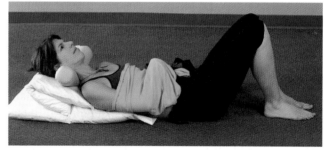

FIG. 11: Positioning patient with T-shirt for upper extremity support, pillows for cervical and thoracic support

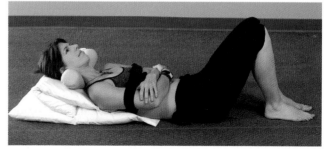

FIG. 12: Positioning patient with strap for upper extremity support, pillows for cervical and thoracic support

controlled, with movement of the pelvis and breathing synchronized. The movement can be compared to that of a large pendulum, which swings back and forth slow and steady as an example of the speed and quality of movement. The pelvic tilt starts at the pelvis. As the pelvis moves anteriorly, the lumbar spine extends (starting at L5–S1). While the spine lengthens, it should be observed that the head moves with slight flexion, while the shoulders and upper body move toward the feet. As the pelvis moves posteriorly during exhalation, the head moves back to neutral and the shoulder and upper body move back toward the head. While this point may seem to be trivial, it is not. Patients may pelvic tilt by arching and flattening primarily the lumbar spine, and the movement of the trunk is mostly directed toward the ceiling and the floor. The result is that little or no movement is seen in the cervical spine, and the head and shoulders will not move. Movement at the middle lumbar segments can be common with patients who lack full lumbar extension at the L5-S1 junction. This overextension of the lumbar spine is an issue often seen later in sitting.

If the patient experiences low back pain when doing pelvic tilts, the amount of tilt can be reduced or eliminated until the patient learns to move the spine correctly. In some cases the air bag, which typically will be added in the fifth exercise, can be added now. The air bag can have the effect of providing cushion between the low back and floor, making it easier to perform the pelvic tilt. After the exercise, the therapist checks objective signs for change, and instructs the patient how to do the same for their home program.

Diaphragmatic breathing with paired lower extremity movements: The upper body position and diaphragmatic breathing pattern are same as in the first exercise. The air bag, if used in the first exercise, is removed and the legs are extended. There are two exercises. In the first, the legs are set slightly apart and kept rested and slightly externally rotated (Fig. 13). Breathing and pelvic tilting are done in the same pattern as the first breathing exercise. In the next exercise, the legs and hips are externally rotated during inhalation (Fig. 14) and then internally rotated position during exhalation (Fig. 15). There are several points on which to focus: with the legs extended there is less pelvic motion available, and the lower back, at rest, is in a more extended position. When exhaling, the patient will exert more effort as they flatten the back. The patient should focus on diaphragmatic breathing and relaxation of the shoulder and neck. When the legs are extended, the body is in a more open and stretched position (as compared to lying with the knees bent), and some TOS patients will

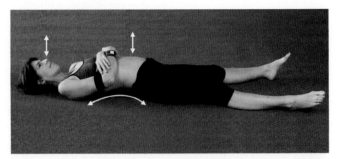

FIG. 13: Diaphragmatic breathing with lower extremity extension

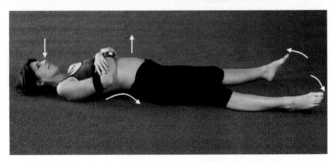

FIG. 14: Diaphragmatic breathing with inhalation and lower extremity extension with external rotation

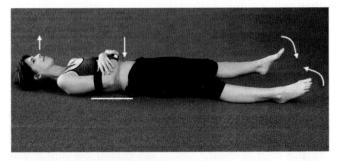

FIG. 15: Diaphragmatic breathing with exhalation and lower extremity extension with internal rotation

report difficulty relaxing. Limiting pelvic motion, focusing on breathing, or placing a pillow under the knees may help. Again, objective signs will be monitored for change.
First rib mobilization using the ball and stick: The ball and stick in this exercise is also referred to by Edgelow as the "pinky ball" because of the pink color of the toy ball used to make the tool. The pinky ball exercise combines the benefits of the breathing exercise with caudal mobilization of the first rib. Since scalene muscle activation elevates the upper ribs, the use of the ball and stick exercise can mobilize the elevated first rib into its normal resting position.

In this exercise, the pinky ball is placed on the posterior section of the first rib, with the stick end of

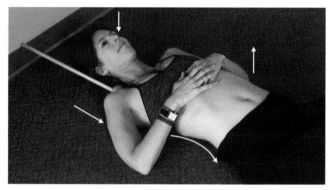

FIG. 16: First rib mobilization using the pinky ball. When performing an anterior pelvic tilt during inhalation, the body moves away from the ball

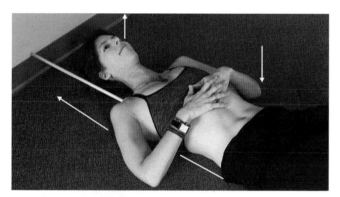

FIG. 17: First rib mobilization using the pinky ball. When performing the posterior pelvic tilt during inhalation, the body moves toward the ball

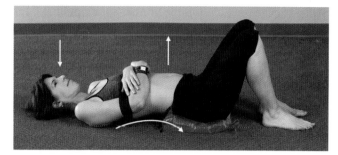

FIG. 18: Air bag in first position

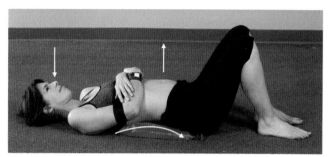

FIG. 19: Air bag in second position

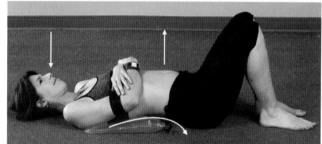

FIG. 20: Air bag in third position

the pinky ball being held against the wall. The ball rests on the floor or pillow, while the side of the ball lightly touches the neck. The stick is angled slightly away so the head remains in alignment. Diaphragmatic breathing and pelvic tilts are performed as described in the first exercise. As the patient tilts the pelvis anteriorly and inhales, the body moves away from the pink ball (Fig. 16). As the patient tilts the pelvic posteriorly and exhales, the body moves toward the ball (Fig. 17). A larger pelvic tilt results in more movement of the body. The patient is instructed to initially use light pressure on the first rib, though the patient's response to the exercise should ultimately determine the amount of pressure used.

Supine breathing with air bag in three positions: This exercise returns to the same position as the first exercise. If the air bag was not used, the air bag is now placed under the hips which is referred to as the first position (Fig. 18), and the patient is instructed to perform the now usual pelvic tilt with diaphragmatic breathing. In the

second position (Fig. 19), the air bag is moved up to the lumbar spine. In the third position (Fig. 20), the patient is instructed to bridge and the bag is placed as far up the back as it will fit beneath the thoracic spine. All of the air bag exercises are done with the same pelvic tilting and breathing as the prior exercises. The intention of these exercises is to increase spinal extension and to open the chest. As with all four supine breathing exercises, objective signs are monitored preactivity and postactivity.

(2) Seated ball exercises

The seated ball exercise integrates the concepts of the stage one exercises while placing the patient in the more functional position of sitting. The patient is instructed to sit on an exercise ball with good posture. The patient may sit slumped, but there may also be an attempt to sit straight by overextending the lumbar spine, pulling back the shoulders and sticking out the chest. This posture is not desirable alignment and results in an overextension of the lumbar spine at the middle segments, overactivation of the spinal extensor muscles, an upward rotation of the rib cage, and a scapular position that cannot be maintained. The patient should be instructed to keep the pelvis rotated anteriorly. To limit overextension of the lower back, the patient is instructed to rotate or pull the lower ribs down slightly, which engages the anterior trunk muscles, creating a more gradual and natural curve of the lumbar-thoracic spine. The shoulders can be raised up and set back, with the scapula sitting in a more neutral position. The thinker pose (Fig. 6) can be done to position the head. Visually, a more aligned spinal posture should be observed. Patients who sit over extended at the lumbar spine may feel that they are leaning forward.

Once good posture is achieved, the patient is instructed to initiate diaphragmatic breathing. The patient now moves the ball in three directions: (1) forward and back (Fig. 21), (2) side-to-side (Fig. 22) and (3) circular rotations (not pictured). Movement is slow, and the pace is dictated by the rate of breathing. The shoulder and hips move together, and the patient can be instructed to imagine balancing a book on the top their head.

Seated ball with pelvic movement: The seated ball with pelvic movement exercise starts the same way as the seated ball exercise. It involves a pelvic tilt, but no added movement of the ball. The patient breathes in, and the pelvis is rotated anteriorly (Fig. 23). The patient exhales, and the pelvis is rotated posteriorly (Fig. 24).

Supine ball exercise: The supine ball exercise starts by stabilizing the neck using the thinker pose (Fig. 25). Patients then walk themselves out and lie back so the head rests on the ball (Fig. 26). Once the head is supported on the ball, the thinker pose can be stopped and the arms placed on the trunk at rest. The patient moves back, exhaling and extending the body over the ball and then

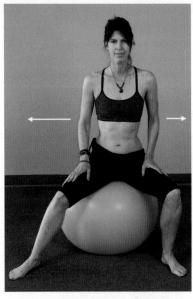

FIG. 22: Seated ball exercises with side-to-side movement

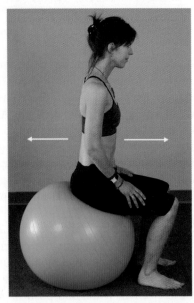

FIG. 21: Seated ball exercise with forward and back movement

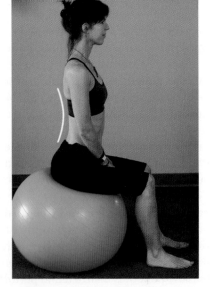

FIG. 23: Seated ball with anterior pelvic tilt

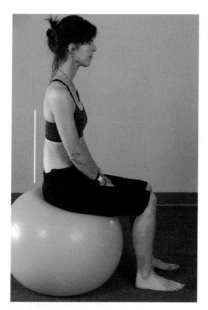

FIG. 24: Seated ball with posterior pelvic tilt

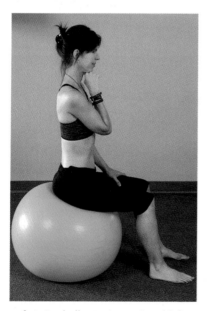

FIG. 25: Start of supine ball exercises using thinker pose

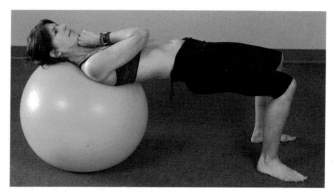

FIG. 26: Supine position with neck stabilized by ball and thinker pose

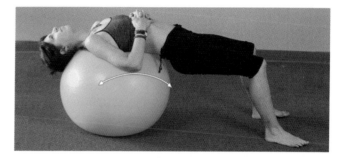

FIG. 27: Diaphragmatic breathing with extension of spine

(3) Foam roll exercises and thoracic mobilization

When performing the first foam roll exercise (in the longitudinal position), the patient lies supine with the spine supported from the occiput to the pelvis. There may be difficulty getting on and off the foam roll. Using the thinker pose to stabilize the neck during the transitional movement can be useful. A towel or small pillow can be placed under the head if lying flat is uncomfortable to the neck. Stretching the arms is not the goal of this exercise so the arms are supported on the body, and often a strap or T-shirt can be used to support the UE (Fig. 28). This supported arms position will help protract the scapula and expose the rib cage, with the specific goal of thoracic spine and rib cage mobilization. Starting the exercise, the patient is centered on the foam roll and slowly inhales through the nose. As the patients begin to exhale they roll the body to one side, moving off the spine and onto the rib cage. As patients return to the starting point, they pause briefly and inhale. The patient starts to exhale and rolls to the opposite side. The patient is instructed to keep the shoulders and hips parallel to the floor—or even keep the shoulders and hips slightly up, following the curve of the back, and not to drop the shoulders (Fig. 28).

moves forward to the starting position while inhaling (Fig. 27). The head stays in contact with the ball. The sequence to end the exercise is done in the reverse order as start. With the head and neck in a neutral, supported position, the neck is stabilized with the thinker pose, and patients walk themselves back up using their legs and a slight flexion at the trunk. The arms are not used to push back to the seated position. Once the patient is again erect, the thinker pose is released.

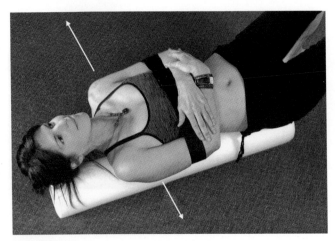

FIG. 28: Diaphragmatic breathing on foam roll, longitudinally with lateral movement. Note the hips and shoulders move together and the body stays horizontal to the floor

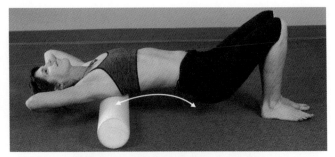

FIG. 29: Thoracic extension with hips off floor

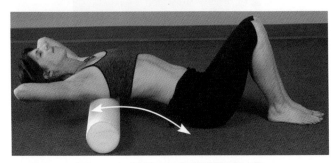

FIG. 30: Thoracic extension with hips on floor

Transverse foam roll exercise: In the transverse position, the patient lies across the foam roll starting at the midscapular level. The head is supported with the hands, and the hips are raised as in a bridge (Fig. 29). The spine is flat or slightly extended. The patient rolls toward the upper thoracic area and then down just past the inferior angle of the scapula. Diaphragmatic breathing is done with the exhalation over the stiff areas of the thoracic spine. An alternative position is to keep the hips on the floor and extend over the roll while exhaling (Fig. 30). The patient scoots up or down to change position on the thoracic spine. Some patients have limited or painful shoulder ROM and may have difficulty using the hands to support the neck.

Pinky ball thoracic mobilization: The patient lies supine with the knees bent. The patient rolls to one side, and the pinky ball is placed on the ribs in the area between the thoracic spinous process and medial border of the scapula (Fig. 31). The patient breathes in, and while rolling back onto the ball, exhales at the same time (Fig. 32). While the maneuver is not intended to painfully reproduce symptoms, this is a mobilization technique and some local discomfort may be experienced. The patient does not have to roll completely onto the ball if painful. Patient comfort is important to successfully maintain a diaphragmatic breathing pattern and relax the neck and upper chest.

Three-inch roller at sacrum and lumbothoracic spine: The patient starts with the 3-inch foam roll at the sacrum. The knees are moved gently side-to-side to loosen the area at the sacroiliac joint (Fig. 33). Next, the 3-inch foam roll is placed at L5–S1 (Fig. 34). The foam roll is gradually

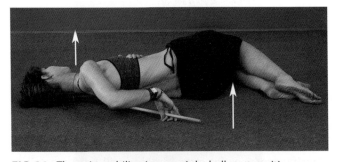

FIG. 31: Thoracic mobilization on pinky ball start position

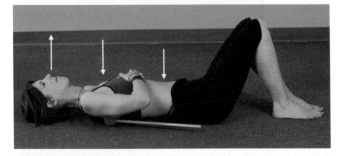

FIG. 32: Thoracic mobilization on pinky ball end position

moved up the lumbar spine to the lower thoracic spine, while several pelvic tilts are performed at each level. The goal of the exercise is mobilization at the stiff segments of the lumbar spine, so hypermobile segments should

56. Jordan SE. Differential diagnosis in patients with possible NTOS. In: Illig KA, Thompson RW, Freischlag JA, Donahue DM, Jordan SE, Edgelow PI (Eds). Thoracic Outlet Syndrome, 1st edition. London: Springer; 2013. pp. 49-60.

57. Sanders RJ, Hammond SL, Rao NM. Thoracic outlet syndrome: a review. Neurologist. 2008;14(6):365-73.

58. Sanders RJ. Anatomy and pathophysiology of ATOS. In: Illig KA, Thompson RW, Freischlag JA, Donahue DM, Jordan SE, Edgelow PI (Eds). Thoracic Outlet Syndrome, 1st edition. London: Springer; 2013. pp. 545-9.

59. Azizzadeh A, Thompson RW. Clinical presentation and patient evaluation in ATOS. In: Illig KA, Thompson RW, Freischlag JA, Donahue DM, Jordan SE, Edgelow PI (Eds). Thoracic Outlet Syndrome, 1st edition. London: Springer; 2013. pp. 551-6.

60. Hooper TL, Denton J, McGalliard MK, Brismee JM, Sizer PS Jr. Thoracic outlet syndrome: a controversial clinical condition. Part 1: anatomy, and clinical examination/diagnosis. J Man Manip Ther. 2010;18(2):74-83.

61. Feinberg RF. Clinical presentation and patient evaluation in VTOS. In: Illig KA, Thompson RW, Freischlag JA, Donahue DM, Jordan SE, Edgelow PI (Eds). Thoracic Outlet Syndrome, 1st edition. London: Springer; 2013. pp. 345-53.

62. Pascarelli EF. NTOS and repetitive trauma disorders. In: Illig KA, Thompson RW, Freischlag JA, Donahue DM, Jordan SE, Edgelow PI (Eds). Thoracic Outlet Syndrome, 1st edition. London: Springer; 2013. pp. 89-92.

63. Doyle AJ, Gillespie DL. VTOS for the primary care team: when to consider the diagnosis. In: Illig KA, Thompson RW, Freischlag JA, Donahue DM, Jordan SE, Edgelow PI (Eds). Thoracic Outlet Syndrome, 1st edition. London: Springer; 2013. pp. 333-8.

64. Urschel HC Jr, Pool JM, Patel AN. Anatomy and pathophysiology of VTOS. In: Illig KA, Thompson RW, Freischlag JA, Donahue DM, Jordan SE, Edgelow PI (Eds). Thoracic Outlet Syndrome, 1st edition. London: Springer; 2013. pp. 339-43.

65. Jordon SE. Clinical presentation of patients with NTOS. In: Illig KA, Thompson RW, Freischlag JA, Donahue DM, Jordan SE, Edgelow PI (Eds). Thoracic Outlet Syndrome, 1st edition. London: Springer; 2013. pp. 41-8.

66. Stralka SW. Thoracic outlet syndrome. In: de las Penas CF, Cleland J, Huijbregts PA (Eds). Neck and Arm Pain Syndromes. Springer; 2011. pp. 141-52.

67. Johansen KH, Illig KA. Conservative (non-operative) treatment of VTOS. In: Illig KA, Thompson RW, Freischlag JA, Donahue DM, Jordan SE, Edgelow PI (Eds). Thoracic Outlet Syndrome, 1st edition. London: Springer; 2013. pp. 395-400.

68. Gelabert HA. Differential diagnosis, decision making, and pathways of care for VTOS. In: Illig KA, Thompson RW, Freischlag JA, Donahue DM, Jordan SE, Edgelow PI (Eds). Thoracic Outlet Syndrome, 1st edition. London: Springer; 2013. pp. 379-90.

69. Thompson RW. Development of consensus-based diganostic criteria for NTOS. In: Illig KA, Thompson RW, Freischlag JA, Donahue DM, Jordan SE, Edgelow PI (Eds). Thoracic Outlet Syndrome, 1st edition. London: Springer; 2013. pp. 143-55.

70. Kabat H. Low Back and Leg Pain from Herniated Cervical Disc, 2nd edition. St. Louis, MO: Warren H Green; 1991.

71. Braun RM, Rechnic M, Shah KN. Pulse oximetry measurements in the evaluation of patients with possible thoracic outlet syndrome. J Hand Surg Am. 2012;37(12):2564-9.

72. Butler D, NOI Group. Neurodynamic Techniques, 1st edition. Orthopedic Physical Therapy Products; 2005.

73. Ghasemi M, Golabchi K, Mousavi SA, Asadi B, Rezvani M, Shaygannejad V, et al. The value of provocative tests in diagnosis of cervical radiculopathy. J Res Med Sci. 2013;18:S35-8.

74. Voorhies RM. Cervical spondylosis: recognition, differential diagnosis, and management. Ochsner J. 2001;32(2):78-84.

75. Edgelow PI. Passive and active rehabilitation after first rib resection. In: Illig KA, Thompson RW, Freischlag JA, Donahue DM, Jordan SE, Edgelow PI (Eds). Thoracic Outlet Syndrome, 1st edition. London: Springer; 2013. pp. 247-52.

76. Illig KA. TOS: the perspective of the patient. In: Illig KA, Thompson RW, Freischlag JA, Donahue DM, Jordan SE, Edgelow PI (Eds). Thoracic Outlet Syndrome, 1st edition. London: Springer; 2013. pp. 635-41.

77. Jull G, Sterling M, Falla D, Treleaven J, O'Leary S. Whiplash, Headache and Neck Pain: Research-Based Directions for Physical Therapies, 1st edition. Edinburgh: Churchill Livingstone, Elsevier; 2008.

78. Matthews CE, George SM, Moore SC, Bowles HR, Blair A, Park Y, et al. Amount of time spent in sedentary behaviors and cause-specific mortality in US adults. Am J Clin Nutr. 2012;95(2):437-45.

79. Dunlop D, Song J, Arnston E, Semanik P, Lee J, Chang R, et al. Sedentary time in U.S. Older adults associated with disability in activities of daily living independent of physical activity. J Phys Act Health. 2014.

80. McLaughlin L, Goldsmith CH, Coleman K. Breathing evaluation and retraining as an adjunct to manual therapy. Man Ther. 2011;16:51-2.

81. Bradley H, Esformes J. Breathing pattern disorders and functional movement. Int J Sports Phys Ther. 2014;9(1):28-39.

82. Sahrmann S. Diagnosis and Treatement of Movement Impairment Syndromes, 1st edition. St. Louis, MO: Mosby; 2002.

83. Hooten MW, Qu W, Townsend CO, Judd JW. Effects of strength vs aerobic exercise on pain severity in adults with fibromyalgia: a randomized equivalence trial. Pain. 2012;153:915-23.

84. Chen YW, Hsieh PL, Chen YC, Hung CH, Cheng JT. Physical exercise induces excess hsp72 expression and delays the development of hyperalgesia and allodynia in painful diabetic neuropathy rats. Anesth Analg. 2013;116(2):482-90.

85. Butler D, Moseley L. Explain Pain, 1st edition. NOI Group Publications; 2003.

86. Streit RS. NTOS symptoms and mobility: a case study on neurogenic thoracic outlet syndrome involving massage therapy. J Bodyw Mov Ther. 2014;18:42-8.

87. Weinberg MA. Chiropractic treatment for NTOS. In: Illig KA, Thompson RW, Freischlag JA, Donahue DM, Jordan SE, Edgelow PI (Eds). Thoracic Outlet Syndrome, 1st edition. London: Springer; 2013. pp. 183-8.

88. Weinberg MA. Ergonomic and postural issues in NTOS. In: Illig KA, Thompson RW, Freischlag JA, Donahue DM, Jordan SE, Edgelow PI (Eds). Thoracic Outlet Syndrome, 1st edition. London: Springer; 2013. pp. 105-10.

89. Kase K, Wallis J, Kase T. Thoracic outlet. Clinical Therapeutic Applications for the Kinesio Taping Method, 2nd edition. Tokyo, Japan: Ken Ikai Co.; 2003. p. 73.

90. Landry G, Moneta G, Taylor L Jr, Edwards J, Porter J. Long-term functional outcome of neurogenic thoracic outlet syndrome in surgically and conservatively treated patients. J Vasc Surg. 2001;33:312-7.

91. Franklin GM. Disability and workman's compensation issues in TOS. In: Illig KA, Thompson RW, Freischlag JA, Donahue DM, Jordan SE, Edgelow PI (Eds). Thoracic Outlet Syndrome, 1st edition. London: Springer; 2013. pp. 669-73.

92. Weiss A, Chang DC. Functional outcome and quality-of-life assessment instruments in TOS. In: Illig KA, Thompson RW, Freischlag JA, Donahue DM, Jordan SE, Edgelow PI (Eds). Thoracic Outlet Syndrome, 1st edition. London: Springer; 2013. pp. 655-62.

93. Dugan MM. Psychosocial factors in NTOS. In: Illig KA, Thompson RW, Freischlag JA, Donahue DM, Jordan SE, Edgelow PI (Eds). Thoracic Outlet Syndrome, 1st edition. London: Springer; 2013. pp. 271-5.

CHAPTER 2

Scapular Dyskinesis

Joseph Hannon

ABSTRACT

Over the past two decades, an increase in attention and understanding has been given to the role of the scapula in upper extremity function. It has become widely accepted that the scapula plays an important role in the proper movement of the shoulder, and that alterations to that movement (scapular dyskinesis) can result in inefficient and potentially painful motion. Scapular dyskinesis has been linked to numerous shoulder pathologies across a variety of patient populations.

When faced with treating a patient with scapular dyskinesis, it is important to complete a thorough examination to help recognize all the potential contributing factors. Once all the contributing factors are realized, a specific treatment plan can be implemented to address these deficits and improve the patients' outcome.

◼ INTRODUCTION

Epidemiology

The primary function of the shoulder joint complex is to help position the elbow and hand in space, allowing the individual to interact with the environment.[1,2] To accomplish this task, the shoulder joint requires both, sufficient mobility to achieve the extremes of motion, and adequate stability to control the extremity through these large motions.

The mobility of the shoulder joint comes from the interaction of the articular surfaces of the humerus, clavicle, scapula and thorax. Together these joints (and pseudo joints) allow for large degrees of freedom. The stability of the shoulder joint comes from the surrounding capsule, labrum, ligaments, muscles and other soft tissue restraints.[2-4] In an active orthopedic patient, the relationship and balance between the stability and mobility becomes extremely important to allow proper pain-free function.

Over the past two decades, an increase in attention and an improved understanding of the role of the scapula in upper extremity function has evolved.[5] It is now widely accepted that the scapula plays an important role in the proper movement of the shoulder, and that alterations to that movement (scapular dyskinesis) can result in inefficient and potentially painful motion.[6] Scapular dyskinesis has been linked to numerous shoulder pathologies across a variety of patient populations, including those patients diagnosed with labral or rotator cuff pathologies.[7,8] Dyskinesis is most commonly seen in athletes performing repetitive overhead motions, specifically in baseball and volleyball players. However, anyone required to perform daily and repetitive overhead motions is likely at an increased risk.[9-11] The actual prevalence of scapular dyskinesis is not known. This is likely because quantifying dyskinesis across examiners is not consistent.

Additionally, dyskinesis is usually found in the presence of additional shoulder complaints and may be missed in the evaluation, or may have been misdiagnosed as a different shoulder pathology. The focus of this chapter will be on the treatment of scapular dyskinesis with or without concurrent glenohumeral (GH) pathology. To better assess and treat this deficit, it is important for the clinician have a thorough understanding of normal scapular kinematics and how to test for faulty scapular mechanics.

Kinematics of Shoulder Girdle

Normal scapular humeral rhythm, that is the proper alignment and motion of the scapula on the humerus, is the key to proper and efficient shoulder function.[12] Centering the humeral head on the glenoid during overhead motion arises from proper scapular positioning, which is a result of the synchronized cocontractions of the muscles controlling the scapula and humerus.

The scapula has no bony articulation with the thorax, and thus the available motion is quite large.[5] Scapular movement (Fig. 1) is typically thought of in three planes of motion: (1) upward and downward rotation, (2) internal and external rotation and (3) anterior and posterior tilting. Upward and downward rotation is the movement of the scapulae around a horizontal axis perpendicular to the plane of the scapulae. Internal and external rotation is rotation of the scapulae around a vertical axis perpendicular to the plane of the scapulae. Lastly, anterior and posterior tilting is movement of the scapulae around an axis along the plane of the scapulae.[12]

The clavicle acts as a strut between the humerus and the more proximal sternum, helping to transfer loads from the distal joints to the more proximal sternum.[1] The complimentary movements of the clavicle include protraction-retraction, elevation-depression and anterior-posterior rotation. With scapular movement of upward and downward translation, clavicular protraction and retraction occur, respectively, to help stabilize the scapulae along the thorax. With shoulder elevation, clavicular elevation, retraction and posterior tilting occur at the acromioclavicular (AC) joint. During this same motion, 31° of posterior clavicular rotation occurs at the sternoclavicular (SC) joint.[12]

The SC and AC joints complement each other's movements. While the SC joint retracts, the AC joint internally rotates, allowing scapular internal and external rotation. The AC joint is primarily responsible for scapular posterior tilting, an important motion during full shoulder flexion.[12]

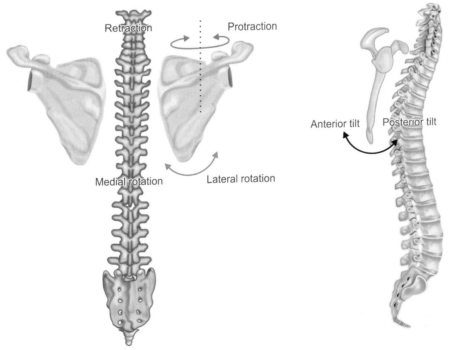

FIG. 1: Scapular kinematics: the three planes of scapular movement[13]
Source: Reproduced with permission from Elsevier.

27

To summarize, shoulder flexion in a healthy shoulder should include scapular elevation, upward rotation, posterior tilting and end range external rotation. During this same motion clavicular elevation, retraction and posterior tilting should occur. The coordinated movement of the scapula, humerus and clavicle is complex. However, having an appreciation and understanding of the required movements (especially during shoulder flexion) is necessary to effectively treat patients with faulty scapular patterning.

CLINICAL PRESENTATION

Scapular dyskinesis (Fig. 2) is most often seen in the overhead athlete, but can be found in any patient presenting with shoulder pain.[9-11] Dyskinesis alone may or may not accompany other findings such as shoulder and neck pain, neural tension and/or shoulder and arm weakness. A common finding that accompanies dyskinesis is shoulder impingement.[15,16] Other diagnoses that commonly present with scapular dyskinesis include labral pathologies, rotator cuff tears, and nerve palsies of the long thoracic and suprascapular nerves.[7,8] Given the likelihood that scapular dyskinesis will not present alone, a proper differential diagnosis including screening for the above pathologies is warranted to help best direct treatment.

Patients with scapular dyskinesis typically complain of an insidious onset of shoulder pain with no specific incident related to the onset of pain. However, as previously mentioned, patients who present with GH

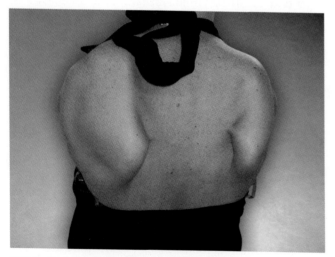

FIG. 2: Patient with bilateral scapular dyskinesis[14]
Source: Reproduced with permission from Elsevier.

joint pathologies (e.g. labral tears), and rotator cuff pathologies, will often also demonstrate dyskinesis.[8,17] In both instances, it is important to take a thorough history and rule in or rule out other possible contributing factors. Patients with scapular dyskinesis may complain of coracoid pain, anterior and posterior shoulder joint pain, referred pain down into the deltoid musculature, and/or periscapular pain.

CLINICAL EXAMINATION

Observation

Observation of the normal resting alignment of the shoulder complex is the starting point of the physical examination, as this is the starting point of shoulder movement. The clinician assesses the scapulae and clavicle for any gross bony abnormalities. Abnormalities may indicate a fracture or dislocation and significantly impact the treatment plan. In some cases, such findings will require a referral to an orthopedic surgeon.

Once assessment of the scapulae and clavicle is complete, the clinician's focus will shift to appreciating the overall appearance of the scapulae. The normal slope of the shoulder is slightly downward in regards to the angle of the upper trapezius (UT). Struyf et al. describe normal scapulothoracic alignment as scapula's medial border sitting approximately 3 inches from the nearest thoracic spinous processes, in approximately 5° of upward rotation, with 30–40° of internal rotation, with 10° of anterior tilt, and sitting with the spine of the scapulae approximately at the level of the second thoracic vertebra.[18] In a patient with long thoracic nerve palsy (affecting the serratus anterior muscle), a resting alignment of scapular winging may be seen. In nerve palsies of the spinal accessory nerve (affecting the trapezius muscle), a resting alignment of scapular protraction and elevation may be seen. The dorsal scapular nerve, which innervates the rhomboids, can also contribute to scapular winging, if compromised. Isolated weakness of any of these muscles is unlikely, except in the case of nerve palsies, with a typical resting alignment being a combination of both of these positions.

In addition to assessing the winging of the scapula, assessment of elevation and depression is warranted. An easy way to assess this is by assessing the location of the root of the spine of the scapulae. A depressed scapulae will be one in which the root of the spine of the scapulae sits below the third thoracic vertebra. Assessing the slope of the shoulders may also be helpful. An increased slope, specifically on the effected side may also indicate a depressed scapula.

Next, the examiner's attention should be directed toward muscular assessment. Any obvious muscle atrophy, specifically in the superior or inferior spinous fossa, could indicate suprascapular nerve pathology and should be examined closely. Comparisons should be made bilaterally and any asymmetries noted.

Consideration should be paid to the resting alignment of the shoulders and cervical spine. A cervical spine alignment of upper cervical extension with lower cervical flexion can coincide with excessive forward shoulders. This can accompany abduction of the scapulae with a thoracic kyphosis. These patients will also tend to present with a shortened resting length of the pectoralis minor. Secondary to its attachment on the coracoid process, the pectoralis minor causes the scapulae to anteriorly tilt.[19,20] This restriction interferes with upward rotation of the scapulae during shoulder flexion,[21] and needs to be corrected to treat scapular dyskinesis.

Range of Motion Assessment

As discussed previously, the shoulder complex allows for large amounts of motion. The motion is a result of the interaction of the GH joint, the scapulothoracic joint, the AC and the SC joints. At the GH joint alone, the shoulder has approximately 100–120° of flexion and abduction, 60–80° of external rotation, 80–90° of internal rotation and between 10–90° of shoulder extension.[2] Assessing both active and passive range of motion (ROM) in all planes of movement is important to determine if any limitations exist. Specifically, assessing the true GH joint motion is important in that deficits in motion through this joint may result in increased motion through the scapulothoracic joint, contributing to dyskinesis.

The examiner must assess the patient's true GH internal rotation ROM (Fig. 3). Measurement of internal rotation is completed in supine. The patient is placed in the supine position, the scapula is blocked by depression of the examiner's hand, and the passive internal rotation range is then measured at 90° of shoulder abduction.[22-24] The clinician must take care to assess isolated GH motion without concurrent scapular motion. Monitoring for movement of the scapula through the coracoid process and body of the scapula is imperative to ensure this. The measurement should be taken when the scapulae begin to move, as this indicates that all the motion through the

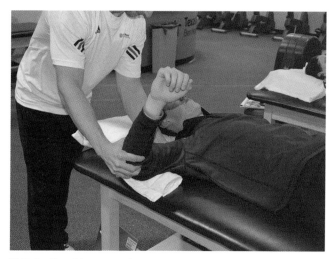

FIG. 3: Shoulder internal rotation range of motion testing

GH joint has been reached. If restrictions in ROM are found, addressing these may be necessary to completely resolve the dyskinesis.

Glenohumeral internal rotation deficit (GIRD) is a common finding in overhead athletes and has been associated with numerous shoulder pathologies.[8,25,26] The true cause of GIRD is likely multifactorial.[22,27] Research has consistently demonstrated that there are likely both soft tissue and bony changes that contribute to this loss of motion found in overhead athletes. Soft tissue changes in both the muscles surrounding the shoulder (for example, the posterior rotator cuff, and the latissimus dorsi) and the posterior capsule and capsular ligament have been implicated in GIRD.[22,27] Bony changes, specifically changes in the degrees of torsion, have also been found to contribute to GIRD.[28] In this instance, the excessive and repetitive rotational stress across the bone as it develops/ creates changes in humerus that result in a decrease in internal rotation.

Additional ROM measures of the shoulder should include passive shoulder external rotation (Fig. 4) and horizontal adduction. To accurately measure GH joint external rotation, the patient is placed in the same position as if measuring internal rotation, and the arm is passively externally rotated until the patient's scapula begins move into the fingers of the examiner.[22-24] To measure horizontal adduction, the patient again should be placed in supine, the lateral scapular border is blocked and the arm is passively brought across their body. The measurement should be taken by placing the center of the goniometer as the AC joint with the stationary arm vertical, and the movement arm following the humerus.[22-24]

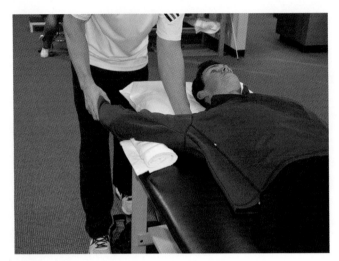

FIG. 4: External rotation shoulder ROM testing

As mentioned above, contributions throughout the kinetic chain should be assessed. In the context of ROM measurements, this should include cervical, thoracic, lumbar and hip. As alluded to earlier, the attachment of the levator scapulae muscle onto the scapula can affect scapular positioning and cervical motion. Forward head posturing can limit cervical motion and potentially result in shortening of the levator scapulae, further altering scapular positioning. While this will likely not be the main focus of the treatment, screening cervical motion may assist in developing the overall treatment plan. Additionally, assessing thoracic flexion and extension will also assist in guiding the intervention. A general screen of thoracic motion can be completed by asking the patient to flex and extend in the seated position. A more detailed segmental motion assessment can be completed in prone, with a posterior-anterior joint assessment. In this instance, having adequate thoracic extension is imperative to allow pain-free shoulder flexion.[29] Research has demonstrated that a decrease in thoracic extension coincides with a decrease in shoulder flexion motion.

Lastly, a brief screen of lumbar and hip ROM should be completed. Performing standing lumbar flexion and extension and noting any abnormalities allows a quick screen of the patient's spinal movement. Hip ROM can be quickly assessed in standing by asking the patient to perform a single-leg stance and rotating fully over the stance leg into internal and external rotation. If gross limitations are noted, placing the patient prone and assessing true internal and external rotation may be warranted. As with all ROM measurements, comparisons should be made bilaterally. Deficits in motion should be noted and corrected as part of the treatment plan.

Strength Assessment

Muscle testing of the scapulothoracic and scapulo-humeral muscles is an important part of the examination process. When examining faulty movement patterns, differentiating between apparent muscle weaknesses versus poor motor control or recruitment patterns is helpful. For instance, if a patient has difficulty performing active scapular retraction correctly, the cause may be faulty movement patterning (e.g. excessive UT recruitment when trying to retract), or the cause may be related to inherent weakness in their scapular retractors.

Proper positioning during muscle testing is important to isolate the correct muscles. Testing of the lower trapezius (LT) and middle trapezius (MT) should be completed in prone. The serratus anterior is tested with the patient in supine. Kendall describes the proper positioning for these tests in detail.[19] In addition to muscle testing of the LT and MT muscles, a quick test of isometric scapular retraction can be performed in sitting. The patient is required to hold a position of scapular retraction for 10–20 seconds, any onset of pain as these muscles fatigue should be noted.[11,30] This could indicate extreme weakness of LT and MT muscles. The wall push-up test can also be used to assess for excessive scapular winging, indicating potential weakness in the serratus anterior muscle.[11] With this test, the patient performs 5–10 wall push-ups while the examiner observes the scapular movement. During this test, winging may not be noted initially, but may appear as the patient fatigues. A second test that can be used for suspected serratus anterior weakness is the sitting hand press-up test (Fig. 5).[31] The patient begins in the seated position

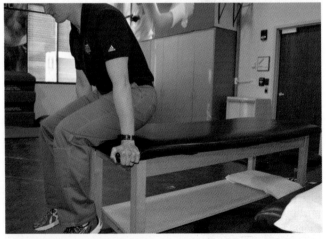

FIG. 5: Seated press-up test

with their hands by their sides. They are instructed to press up and support their body weight through their arms while they maintain their hips at a 90° angle. Assessment of medial border prominence should be made bilaterally.

In addition to testing of the scapulothoracic muscles, muscle testing of the scapulohumeral muscles is also important. Studies have shown that poor posture and misalignment of the scapula at rest can result in apparent weakness of the lateral rotators.[11,32] However, with correction of the scapula position, by cueing scapular retraction and better posture, muscle strength can be normalized. The scapular retraction test can be used if this is suspected. The examiner performs a muscle test of the supraspinatus muscles while the patient sits in their normal resting alignment. The examiner then retests the patients after helping to stabilize the scapulae in the retracted position. A positive test is increased strength and/or a resolution of symptoms in the second position.[12] This is an important finding, as it suggests the correction of the faulty scapulae positioning can improve function and/or decrease pain.[33]

Special Tests

There are a number of special tests that may assist the clinician in correctly diagnosing scapular dyskinesis. In addition to making an accurate diagnosis, these tests may also serve as a tool to measure improvement in the patients' scapular movement. The lateral scapular slide test, as described by Kibler,[34] is part of the examination process. In this test, the distance from the inferior angle of the scapula to the nearest vertebral spinous process is measured (Figs 6A to C). Measurements are performed with the patient in a neutral shoulder position; at 40–45° of coronal plane abduction, with hands resting on hips; and with the shoulder at 90° abduction, with the arms in full internal rotation. A bilateral difference of 1.5 cm should be the threshold for deciding whether scapular symmetry is present.[34]

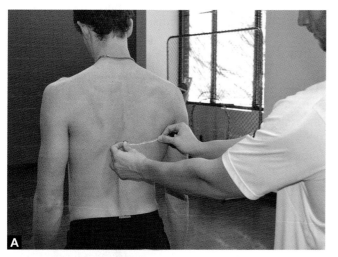

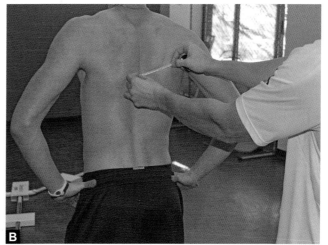

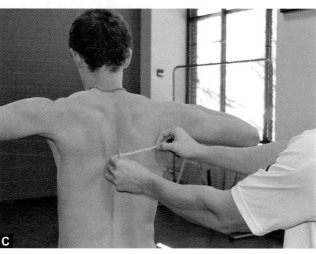

FIGS 6A TO C: The lateral scapular slide test. Measures are recorded from the inferior angle of the each scapula to the nearest spinous process in three defined positions: (A) with the patient's shoulders resting in neutral, (B) with the patient's hands placed on their hips and (C) with the patient's shoulders placed in 90° of abduction and full internal rotation

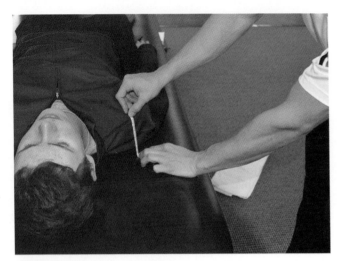

FIG. 7: Pectoralis minor length measurement

A second test that may assist the clinician in both diagnosis and monitoring for improvement is a test of the pectoralis minor length. To assess pectoralis minor length, the patient should be positioned in supine (Fig. 7). The distance from the table to the posterior aspect of the acromion on the affected and unaffected side is measured.[35] A measurement greater than 2.54 cm on the affected side has been suggested to indicate tightness through this muscle.[21] Following the measurement at rest, the clinician assesses whether the shoulder can be lowered to the table with the use of overpressure by stabilizing the contralateral shoulder with one hand while a posterior force is applied to the affected shoulder in an attempt to correct the position of the scapula. This test of pectoralis minor length will indicate whether or not the shortening can be easily corrected with proper scapular

alignment and cueing, or if direct soft tissue work to the pectoralis minor is needed to allow proper scapulae retraction.

In addition to the assessing the static position of the scapulae, thoracic and cervical spine, the effect of dynamic movement on these areas needs to be evaluated. Scapulohumeral rhythm is the synchronized movement of the scapula together with the humerus as the arm is elevated overhead. This relationship allows for the increased motion, while decreasing stress on the articular surfaces and soft tissue. Scapulohumeral rhythm is typically a 2:1 ratio. During the first 60° of shoulder flexion, the movement comes primarily from the humerus. Past this point, the motion becomes a 2:1 relationship between the humerus and the scapula allowing for a complete 180° of motion.[1,36] Observing this movement for alterations in this pattern is imperative. As discussed above, when the humerus is moved into shoulder flexion the scapulae must elevate, upwardly rotate, posteriorly tilt and externally rotate. Identifying irregularities in this pattern is important to better appreciate alterations in muscle firing patterns and/or restrictions in movement.

To test for faulty scapular movements, the scapular dyskinesis test described by Mcclure[37] should be used (Figs 8A and B). In this test, the patient should stand with scapulae exposed and perform active shoulder flexion to end range, then slowly return to the starting position. The therapist should observe the movement of the scapulae for winging, anterior tilting, or any obvious impairment. If no deficits are found, the use of 3- to 5-pound dumbbells may be needed to expose underlying movement faults or muscle weakness.

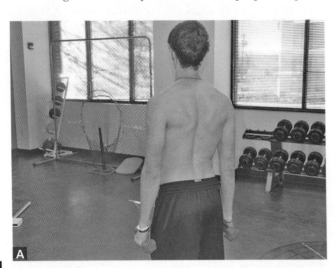 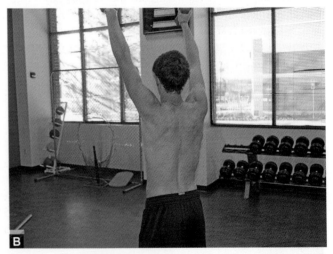

FIGS 8A AND B: Scapular dyskinesis test: (A) starting position and (B) maximum elevation prior to return

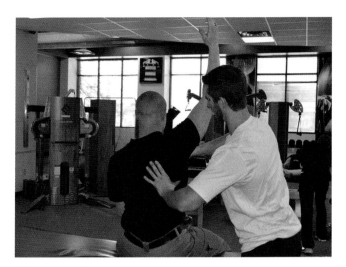

FIG. 9: Scapular assist test

The scapular assist test (Fig. 9) may also be useful during this portion of the examination. The patient performs active shoulder flexion. The therapist monitors for reports of pain as the arm is raised overhead. If pain is noted, the therapist places his or her hand on the medial and inferior border of the scapulae and assists the scapulae into upward rotation. If this abolishes the patient's complaint, then addressing the lack of scapular upward rotation will likely be beneficial. Specifically, patients who present with impingement syndrome have been shown to demonstrate decreases in scapular upward rotation, a decrease in posterior tilting and a decrease in scapular external rotation. As such, a positive finding on this test may help to make the diagnosis of shoulder impingement secondary to scapular dyskinesis.[18] Conversely in a patient with instability, a decrease in upward rotation with an increase in internal rotation is typically found. In this case, simply improving upward rotation with the scapular assist test may not resolve their symptoms.

In addition to the objective measures of the examination, it is important to determine when during the overhead motion the patient complains of pain. For instance, dyskinesis in a thrower who complains of pain during the late cocking phase (maximal abduction with external rotation) may indicate a lack of adequate posterior tilting of the scapulae. However, dyskinesis in a thrower who complains of pain during release (maximal internal rotation with horizontal adduction) may indicate—among other things—excessive scapular abduction with deficits in eccentric control of the scapular adductors and retractors. In addition to complaints of pain, patients with scapular dyskinesis may report weakness through their arm. This may be evident to the patient during activities requiring them to reach out away from their body or lift an object overhead.

Understanding the functional needs of the patient is also important. In a throwing athlete, it is obvious that the patient needs to be able to throw without pain. However, an electrician may need to maintain shoulder flexion at or above 90° while working overhead for extended periods of time. Gathering the full picture of the symptoms and impairments will better help to better guide the treatment.

Differential Diagnosis

Scapular dyskinesis can be missed and can be confused with other conditions. Other pathologies the clinician should consider in the examination and treatment of scapular dyskinesis are:

- Rotator cuff pathology
- Labral pathology
- Thoracic outlet syndrome
- Subacromial impingement
- Internal impingement
- Nerve palsies involving long thoracic nerve, suprascapular nerve, dorsal scapular nerve, or spinal accessory nerve.

▬ PHYSICAL THERAPY TREATMENT

During the rehabilitation of scapular dyskinesis, it is important to address all the potential causative factors. This will allow for restoration joint motion and of muscle imbalances, allowing proper positioning and movement of the scapula.[11] The examination of the patient enables the therapist to decide what factors are potentially contributing (Box 1) to the dyskinesis, and to create a well-designed treatment plan to address each factor.

Box 1: Potential contributing factors to scapular dyskinesis
• Nerve palsies: Long thoracic, dorsal scapular and spinal accessory nerves[38]
• Internal joint derangement: For example, labral tears or rotator cuff pathologies[12]
• Bony factures: Scapular or clavicular fractures[39]
• Hypomobility of the shoulder joint and inflexibility of upper extremity musculature: For example, glenohumeral internal rotation deficit (GIRD) and pectoralis minor muscle tightness[40,41]
• Muscular function: For example, weakness or altered firing of the trapezius and serratus anterior muscles[39,42]
• Kinetic chain: Alterations in lower extremity balance, range of motion (ROM) and neuromuscular control[43]

Box 2: Principles of scapular dyskinesis treatment

- Address posture and flexibility
- Proper progression is key
- Implement the entire kinetic chain
- Modalities help to compliment the treatment, they are not the treatment

There are multiple treatment approaches to the management of scapular dyskinesis, and the efficacy of the approach may vary, depending on the patient. However, there are underlying principles (Box 2) that need to be considered and will help in the design of an appropriate treatment plan. First, addressing flexibility before strength will improve outcomes.[7] Tightness through antagonist muscles can inhibit strength activation in the agonistic muscle. Restrictions in flexibility will also limit the patient's ability to achieve and maintain correct posturing, and as such, this must be where treatment is initiated. Second, proper progression is imperative. Research has demonstrated that scapular muscular activation is improved when activated in functional patterns.[44] However, if the patient lacks the neuromuscular control to activate the appropriate muscle, they will struggle with functional movements. Focus early on during exercise should be on proper scapular retraction.[30,32] Third, trunk muscle strength and use of the kinetic chain must be included. This will assist in restoring coupled scapular muscle forces and help to create proximal stability, allowing the patient to maintain postural control during exercise.[45,46] Additionally, it will allow improved force generation of the posterior musculature—a goal of the

treatment of scapular dyskinesis is facilitation of this musculature. Lastly, modalities should be used sparingly to help assist in the overall treatment plan. They should never be the focus of the treatment plan.

While the above principles will help to guide the treatment, it is important to understand that correcting scapular dyskinesis is not as easy as simply following these principles. Many patients have long-standing postural and flexibility deficits, and altered muscle activation patterns, including UT substitution with inhibition of the LT.[7] Correction will take time and a focused effort on the part of the patient and therapist to correct these impairments.

Flexibility and Mobility

If, during the clinical examination, restrictions in the patient's flexibility were noted, these must be addressed early on. When the patient is in the clinic, they should be put through a stretching routine including hands-on stretches by the physical therapist. In order to mobilize the GH joint into internal rotation, place the patient in the same position described to measure internal rotation in the examination portion of this chapter. The sleeper stretch (Figs 10A and B) and cross body horizontal adduction stretch should be implemented as part of a home program.[27] To perform the sleeper stretch, the patient lies on the involved side with the humerus abducted to 90° and the elbow bent to 90°. They will then use their contralateral hand to push the involved arm down into internal rotation until a stretch is felt on the posterior aspect of the shoulder. The cross body stretch

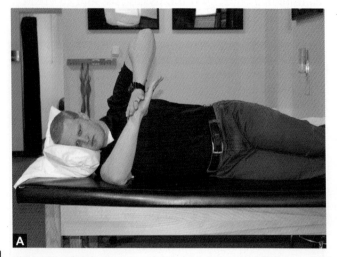
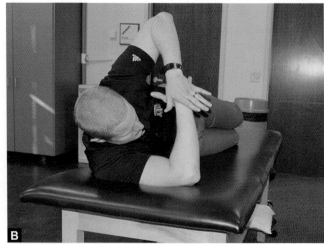

FIGS 10A AND B: Sleeper stretch: (A) front view and (B) coronal view

can be performed in the same position; however, instead of levering the forearm to induce internal rotation, the patient grasps the elbow of the involved arm and lifts it upward, in a horizontal adduction movement across their body. This stretch can be performed in standing as well with the use of a wall. In both instances, it is important to block the ipsilateral scapulae from sliding out.

In addition to limitations in internal rotation, the patient may have demonstrated pectoralis minor shortening. Improving flexibility in this musculature can again be done in the position that was described in the examination section. However, in this instance, overpressure is applied bilaterally, and a sustained stretch is held.[47] The use of a posterior buttress over which to stretch may be needed such as a towel roll or wedge.

If, during the examination, restrictions were found through the thoracic spine and ribs, this will also need to be addressed. The use of posterior to anterior (PA) mobilizations through the thoracic spine may be indicated.[48,49] This can be performed in prone or in a seated position. If the patient can tolerate more aggressive treatment, thoracic manipulations may also be used.

Posture

In addition to the directed physical therapy interventions, proper patient education is imperative. The patient must understand the role their posture is likely playing in their symptoms. This means that constant verbal cueing may be necessary during the treatment session to assist the patient in maintaining proper posture. Additionally, it may be necessary to devise a plan to assist the patient in maintaining better posture throughout the day. For instance, instructing the patient to take a break from their work every hour to perform active thoracic extension and scapular retraction may be a way to assist the patient in maintaining proper posture throughout the day.

Neuromuscular Re-education

Early on in the rehabilitation process, neuromuscular re-education should take precedence over general strengthening or high-level functional exercise. While functional patterns and the use of the kinetic chain are important, this will likely be too difficult for someone with long-standing dyskinesis. The patient must first learn how to properly position their scapulae by recruiting the appropriate musculature, and only then can they be progressed. Increased activation of the LT, MT and serratus anterior muscles, with a decrease in recruitment

of the UT muscle, should be the goal.[50] For patients with long-standing complaints of pain or long-standing movement impairments, this can be very difficult.

The most basic starting position for initiating scapular proprioceptive exercises is sidelying. With the patient in sidelying (unaffected side down), the therapist stands behind the patient, cups the patient's scapula between the web spaces of the clinician's hands, sandwiching the inferior and superior scapular borders (Fig. 11). From this position, the therapist uses manual cues to have the patient elevate and depress their scapula. With a change in hand position (therapist places their hands on the medial and lateral borders), the therapist can cue the patient to retract and protract the scapulae (Fig. 12). When the

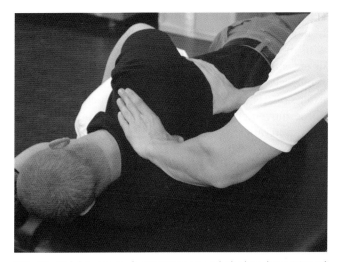

FIG. 11: Sidelying scapular positioning, with the hands positioned superiorly and inferiorly

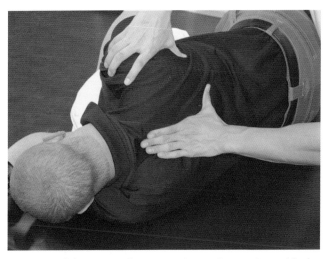

FIG. 12: Sidelying scapular protraction and retraction, with the hands positioned medially and laterally

patient can actively achieve the desired positions, manual resistance can be used to resist movements into these planes and/or perform isometric contraction in each position. While remaining in the sidelying position, the patient can be advanced to more dynamic exercises while still working on activating the appropriate musculature. Sidelying external rotation and sidelying flexion have demonstrated good middle to UT muscle activation ratios. Meaning that while performing these exercises, there is an increase in MT activation with a decrease in UT activation.[50,51]

From the sidelying position, the patient can be transitioned to the prone position. In prone, performing scapular retraction becomes more difficult as gravity plays a bigger role. Having the patient work on pure active scapular retraction (without UT substitution) is a good starting point. Have the patient lay prone with their affected arm off of the table in a dependent, flexed starting position. From here, the patient can be progressed to more challenging exercises like shoulder extension (Fig. 13) and horizontal abduction (Fig. 14). These movements have demonstrated favorable muscle activation ratios.[50,51]

A basic rowing movement performed in prone is not recommended. This is because electromyography (EMG) studies have shown that the prone row does not demonstrate favorable muscle activation ratios of the LT and MT to UT.[50] This is important to note, especially for patients who continue to struggle with appropriate muscle firing. It may be more advantageous to begin with exercises like sidelying external rotation or prone shoulder extension, knowing that there is a higher likelihood of the

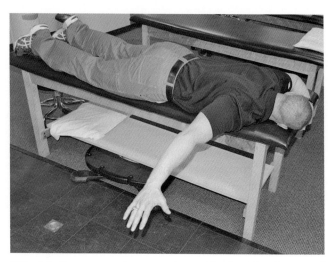

FIG. 14: Prone scapular retraction with shoulder horizontal abduction

patient correctly performing these exercises. In patients who demonstrate good scapular retraction patterns, the row may be used safely and effectively.[45,46]

The above exercises are all open chain in design and have demonstrated favorable MT and LT to UT ratios, which should be the focus of treatment early on. Additionally, they have placed the patient in a position that allows them to succeed. By minimizing the impact of gravity and starting with basic scapular positioning exercises, the patient should be encouraged by their ability to successfully complete these exercises. Some patients will struggle with these exercises, while others will find them not challenging enough. In either case, these are good exercise choices initially, to help lay the ground work for more dynamic movements.

From these basic open chain exercises, the patient can be progressed to more closed chained movements. Closed chain exercises have demonstrated the ability to help re-establish normal firing patterns of the muscles surrounding the shoulder because they stimulate the normal cocontractions of the scapular stabilizers.[34]

Introductory closed chain exercises that focus on scapular control and positioning. During the low row exercise (Fig. 15), the patient stands facing away from the treatment table and performs shoulder extension with scapular retraction isometrically into the table. This exercise has been shown to elicit favorable EMG activation patterns.[50,51]

In comparison to the open chain exercise, having a stable base in which to place resistance can help facilitate the scapular retractors, and the patient may find this easier than the open chain variation. Progression from

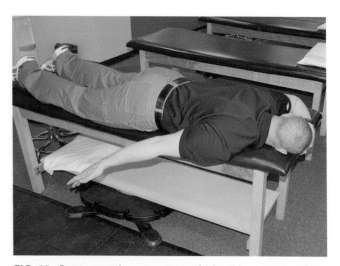

FIG. 13: Prone scapular retraction with shoulder extension from a flexed starting posture

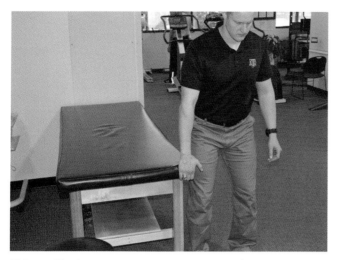

FIG. 15: The low row exercise: Isometric scapular retraction and shoulder extension

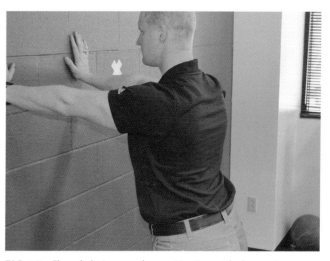

FIG. 17: Closed chain scapular positioning with depression

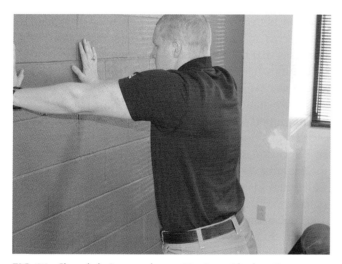

FIG. 16: Closed chain scapular positioning with elevation

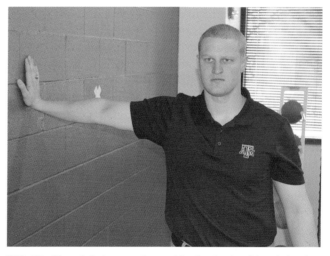

FIG. 18: Closed chain scapular positioning in shoulder abduction

exercises with the patient's hand at their side, to exercises with their hands away from their body should ensue.

Once the patient demonstrates good control with their arm at their side, progression to basic scapular positioning with the arms away from their body is next. The patient stands facing the wall, and is instructed to elevate their shoulders to 90° of flexion, placing their hands on the wall. The patient elevates (Fig. 16), depresses (Fig. 17), protracts, and retracts the scapulae when cued with verbal commands. This can be done in a pattern or with isolated movement repetitions. Additionally, this can be performed only on the involved side alone or bilaterally.

Versions of this exercise can also be done in abduction with involved shoulder nearest to the wall (Fig. 18).[34] If the patient struggles or becomes easily fatigued with simple

active or weight bearing positioning, it is important that they demonstrate improvement before advancing to more dynamic exercises. It is also important to note that these exercises are being performed in approximately 90° of shoulder elevation. Another basic closed chain exercise is the ABCs (Fig. 19) and manual closed chain perturbations. The patient stands facing the wall with involved hand on a small medicine ball. Keeping the palm open, the elbow extended, the patient performs an isometric protraction into the ball.

Maintaining this positioning, the patient begins to spell the alphabet with the ball. A variation of this exercise involves manual perturbations. The patient begins in the same position as the ABC exercise; however, instead of actively moving through the letters, they are required to

37

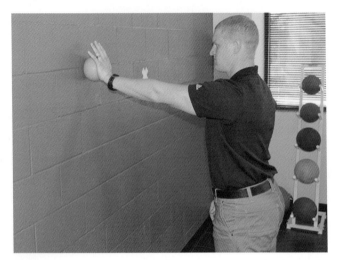

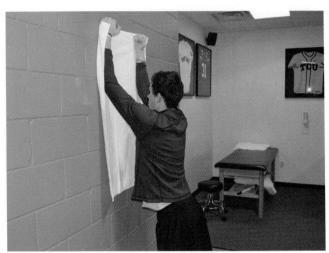

FIG. 19: Closed chain scapular positioning with the ABC's exercise

FIG. 20: Wall slide exercise: Isometric scapular protraction with concurrent shoulder flexion and shrug

stabilize their hand while the therapist provides manual perturbations through the humerus and forearm. Like the basic scapular positioning exercises, this can be performed in flexion and abduction. Changes in the variables such as ball size, size of the perturbations and length of the exercise can be adjusted to achieve the correct intensity.

The above exercises, both open and closed chained focus on proper scapular positioning. For healthy individuals, this will seem simple. However, keep in mind that these patients may have had improper movement and activation patterns for years: patients like these often find simply trying to retract their scapulae can be a challenging task. The therapist may need to help the patient facilitate the movement to help them learn how to move properly. This may include manual assistance into retraction during exercise, or it may mean trying to facilitate the musculature with the use of manual cueing—or in some cases, electrical stimulation. For patients having a difficult time with proper scapular positioning, the use of a biofeedback device may be indicated. Research has demonstrated the biofeedback can be effective in improving scapular muscle activation patterns in patients with dyskinesis.[52]

Strengthening

Once the patient demonstrates an adequate ability to control their scapulae during the preceding exercises, more advanced and dynamic exercises can be initiated. The proper progression of exercise should be such that the patient is placed in a position to succeed while ensuring

that the patient is continually challenged in a manner that serves to create neuromuscular adaptation. Basic exercises that have the patient actively move their upper extremity while maintaining correct scapular mechanics would be next in the progression.

Active standing shoulder flexion with cueing should be attempted to assess if the patient can now maintain proper positioning. The same should be assessed in scaption and abduction. If this is still challenging for the patient, despite manual and verbal cues, the use of wall slides (Fig. 20) as described by Sarhmann may be helpful.[21] During this exercise, the patient faces the wall and places the ulnar side of the forearms on the wall so that the elbows are at shoulder height.

From here the patient is cued to perform scapular protraction while pushing into the wall through the forearms. Maintaining this isometric protraction, the patient actively slides their hands up the wall. When the elbows pass shoulder height, the patient should be cued to elevate the shoulders (shrug). The combination of protraction and shoulder elevation with the hands overhead will help to recruit the serratus anterior and UT muscles, respectively. In this case, recruitment of the UT with the hands overhead will help to elevate the scapulae. While maintaining the protracted position, the patient slides their hands back down the wall to the starting position.

A variation of this exercise to increase recruitment the LT may also be used. The performance of this exercise is the same as above; however, at maximal shoulder elevation the patient is cued to activate their LT muscle by removing their hands from the wall. To do this, the patient should focus on retracting and posteriorly tilting their scapulae, and not simply performing end range shoulder flexion.

Now that the patient has entered the strengthening phase of the rehabilitation, resistance can be added, assuming the patient can continue to demonstrate adequate scapular control. Resistance in this case can be in the form of dumbbells or resistance bands. Both types of resistance are useful in the treatment of scapular dyskinesis. While dumbbells will allow for more degrees of freedom, the band resistance will act as a counterforce to the correct scapular movement, and may make it easier for the patient to recruit the correct musculature.

Resistance bands can be used to encourage scapular retraction. Exercise selection should begin with the arms at the side: examples include rows (Fig. 21) and external rotation walkouts (Fig. 22). These movements should be relatively easy for the patient to maintain proper scapular positioning, based on successful completion of preparatory exercises. Nonetheless, the therapist may need to assess scapular positioning by feeling the medial border of the scapular to ensure proper positioning. When the patient can perform these exercises with good scapular positioning and without excessive fatigue, a progression to more dynamic and eventually overhead movement is warranted.

Full body movements (incorporating the kinetic chain) are integrated next into the rehabilitation process. For example, the use of a Bodyblade® (Figs 23A to C) in overhead athletes helps to create dynamic stabilization about the shoulder joint while at the same time promoting stability through the trunk. Performing this exercise

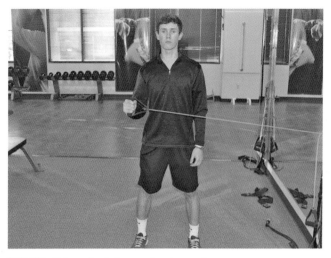

FIG. 22: External rotation walkout exercise

through active shoulder movements like a baseball pitch or tennis serve requires exceptional stabilization and is a good way to challenge the patient while replicating a functional movement.

It may be necessary to return to some of the basic strengthening exercises like the Throwers Ten (Appendix A) or band resistance exercises and modify them to be more dynamic and incorporate more of the kinetic chain.[53] For instance, the lawnmower exercise (Figs 24A to E) has high EMG activity for the LT and MT muscles and places the patient in a position to succeed by allowing full scapular protraction prior to retraction. This initial protraction places the scapular retractors on stretch, making recruitment of these muscles easier. A progression of this exercise from finishing with the arm at the side to eventually finishing with the arm overhead is a simple yet effective way to encourage correct scapular movement in the overhead position and is an example of incorporating more full body motion into the movement. The position of the patient can then be changed to have them start in a contralateral single leg stance and mimic the throwing or serving motion during the lawnmower exercise. This will help to recreate the actual feeling of throwing or serving while continuing to focus on scapular control.

In a similar manner, the shoulder extension (Figs 25A and B) exercise can be initiated in varying degrees of trunk and hip flexion. As the patient begins the shoulder extension movement, they will also go into trunk and hip extension, helping to facilitate this movement. Not only does this make the movement more functional and dynamic, but it is also has been shown to actually facilitate correct scapular muscle activation.[51]

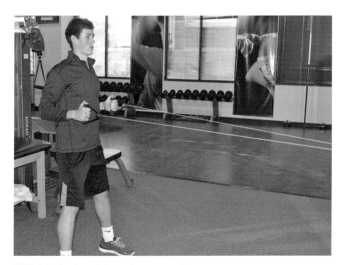

FIG. 21: End position of row exercise

39

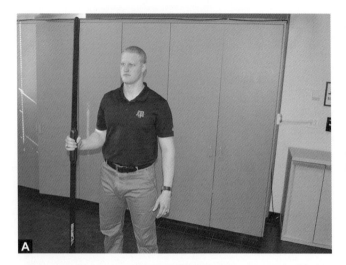

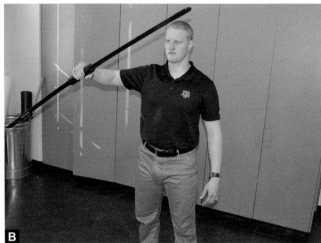

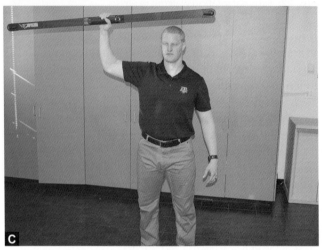

FIGS 23A TO C: Bodyblade® exercises performed (A) in neutral at the patient's side, (B) in abduction and (C) in combined abduction and ER

This principle can be applied in the same manner to the "W" exercise (a combination of scapular retraction, shoulder extension and external rotation), as shown in Figure 26, and to external rotation-extension exercise, as shown in Figure 27. While it is tempting to be as functional as possible with during treatment, these advanced exercises can only be initiated once the patient demonstrates good control.

Taping and Bracing

The use of tape has been suggested to assist the patient during the rehabilitation process. There is a growing body of research examining the effects of taping on scapular dyskinesis. In some cases, taping has been shown to be effective in the treatment of scapular dyskinesis.[54] Kinematic changes were found following the application of scapular taping to baseball players with impingement syndrome.[54] Additional studies have demonstrated a decrease in UT activation with an increase in LT activation during overhead motions.[54-56] However, many of the studies that examined the effects of taping on shoulder pain are inconsistent. A variety of tapes are used including Kinesio® Tex tape and Leukotape®. Kinesio® tape is growing in popularity and is typically used to facilitate or inhibit the muscles to which it is applied. In addition to Kinesio® tape, Leukotape® is sometimes used to facilitate or inhibit muscle firing. However, little standardization across the literature makes its efficacy difficult to determine. In addition to variety in tape and taping technique, most studies have had very small sample sizes. Research is unclear on the effects of taping on scapular dyskinesis. However, the effects of taping other joints of the body have been shown to enhance proprioception and the use of tape with this in mind may still be warranted.[55]

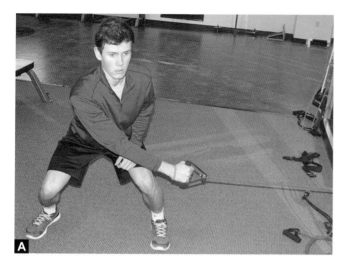

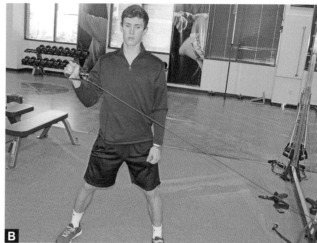

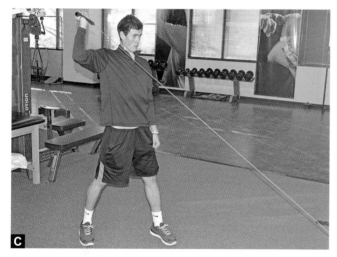

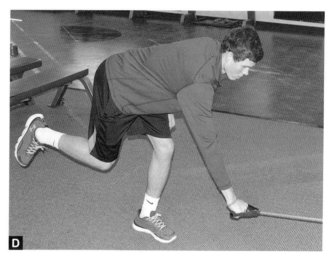

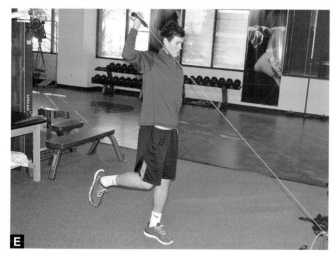

FIGS 24A TO E: Lawnmower exercise: (A) starting position, (B) ending position for basic lawnmower, (C) ending position for overhead lawnmower, (D) starting position for single limb lawnmower and (E) ending position for single limb overhead lawnmower

Anecdotally, the use of scapular taping has been reported to be a useful tool in the treatment of dyskinesis. If the therapist chooses to implement taping into the treatment, this should be done early in the rehabilitation process. It may be helpful to assist with postural correction by acting as feedback to encourage proper positioning

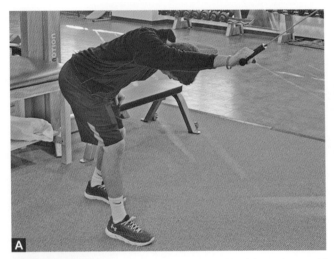 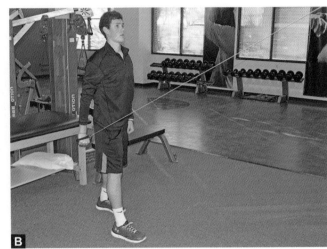

FIGS 25A AND B: Shoulder extension exercise: (A) starting position and (B) ending position

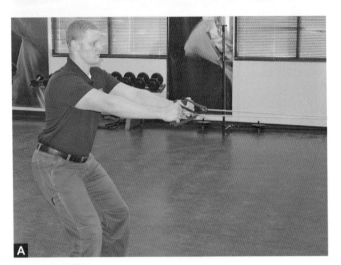 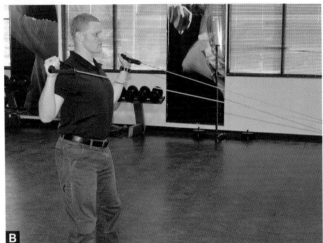

FIGS 26A AND B: The W exercise (A) starting position, and (B) ending position

during the day. It may also be helpful during the early phases of neuromuscular re-education as a source of proprioceptive input to the patient. Lastly, taping may be used to help inhibit UT activation in a patient with a tonic UT muscle firing that is inhibiting LT activation.

In some instances, the use of a posture apparatus may be warranted. There are a variety of devices available including Intelliskin™, which is an example of a posture shirt. There are also figure eight braces available that are designed to assist with improving posture. In either case, the key is that the patient is constantly encouraged to maintain correct posturing.[57] Like taping, there is a continued need for further research to fully support the use of bracing and posture garments. However, also like taping, there are anecdotal reports of improvement with the use of bracing.

In conclusion, the use of taping and bracing may be helpful in the treatment of dyskinesis and should be used as a tool to help augment the rehabilitation process. Neither should be the primary focus of the treatment.

Modalities

Neuromuscular electrical stimulation (NMES) has also been suggested in the treatment of scapular dyskinesis.[58] The application of NMES in this instance is to enhance the recruitment of the scapular retractors during exercise. This may be useful in patients who initially struggle with contracting the appropriate musculature. Research in this area is, again, lacking. If a patient is struggling with scapular positioning, it may be helpful to trial NMES to demonstrate to the patient what it feels like to activate the

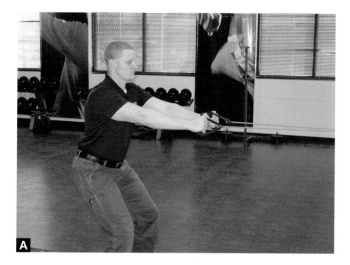

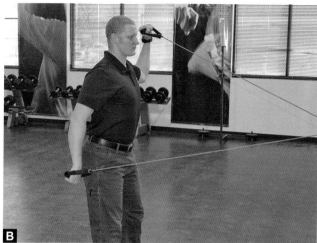

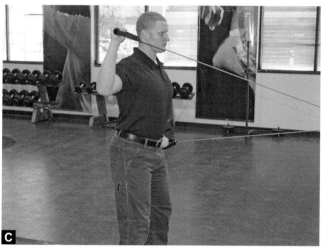

FIGS 27A TO C: The external rotation-extension exercise: (A) starting position, (B) right arm extended and left arm flexed, and (C) right arm flexed and left arm extended

correct musculature. Similarly, biofeedback in the form of EMG is often used clinically for the same reasons, and has proven useful, as mentioned earlier, in identifying exercises that create the greatest activation of targeted musculature.

Medical Intervention and Surgery

Despite physical therapy intervention and the use of bracing and taping to try and augment patient progress, some patients do not improve satisfactorily. In these instances, a more aggressive intervention may be warranted. Initial treatment may be in the form of corticosteroid injections to relieve pain.[34,39] If patients do not demonstrate significant improvement from conservative treatment and corticosteroid injections, surgery may be warranted.[34,39] In these circumstances, surgery is usually indicated to correct other underlying structural pathology. In the instance of a patient who presents with dyskinesis in addition to a labral or rotator cuff pathology, that may mean surgical debridement or repair of the injured tissue.[16,34,39] In a patient who presents with dyskinesis and bursitis, this may mean debridement of the subacromial, subscapular or subcoracoid bursa.[59-61] In rare cases, when the bony articulation between the scapulae and thorax is altered due to a tumor or change in the bony morphology, a scapulectomy may be performed allowing for better articulation of the scapulae on the thoracic cage and facilitating improved scapular alignment.

■ CONCLUSION

Scapular dyskinesis is a challenging diagnosis to treat successfully. Despite a large body of research on the activation of scapular musculature, there is little research demonstrating actual changes in position, motion, or dyskinesis following treatment. However, research does indicate that the implementation of scapular exercises improves patient outcomes. This is especially true when these scapular exercises incorporate the use of the entire kinetic chain.

When faced with treating a patient with scapular dyskinesis, it is important to complete a thorough examination to understand all the contributing factors. Once all the contributing factors are realized, a specific treatment plan can be implemented to address these deficits and improve the patient's outcome. When developing the treatment plan, the guiding principles are, in order of priority: (1) first addressing posture and flexibility, (2) proper progressing increasingly demanding activities, (3) implementing activities that incorporate the entire kinetic chain and (4) modalities may help to compliment the treatment, but in isolation modalities are not the treatment. With these guidelines in mind, and with the understanding that treatment should be individualized to each patient's deficits, the likelihood of a successful outcome greatly increases. While further research is needed in the area of scapular dyskinesis as a means to better understand the pathology and appropriate treatment, it is clear at this time that physical therapy interventions aimed at improving scapular muscle activation, improves patient outcomes and should be the treatment of choice in this patient population.

■ REFERENCES

1. Terry GC, Chopp TM. Functional anatomy of the shoulder. J Athl Train. 2000;35:248-55.
2. Dutton M. The Response of Biological Tissue to Stress. In: Brown M, Davis K, Eds, Orthopaedic Examination, Evaluation, and Intervention, McGraw-Hill, New York, 2004;87-100.
3. Lippitt S, Matsen F. Mechanisms of glenohumeral joint stability. Clin Orthop Relat Res. 1993;(291):20-8.
4. Veeger HE, van Der Helm FC. Shoulder function: the perfect compromise between mobility and stability. J Biomech. 2007;40:2119-29.
5. Paine R, Voight ML. The role of the scapula. Int J Sports Phys Ther. 2013;8:617-29.
6. Voight ML, Thomson BC. The role of the scapula in the rehabilitation of shoulder injuries. J Athl Train. 2000;35:364-72.
7. Kibler WB, Ludewig PM, McClure PW, Michener LA, Bak K, Sciascia AD. Clinical implications of scapular dyskinesis in shoulder injury: the 2013 consensus statement from the 'scapular summit'. Br J Sports Med. 2013;47:877-85.
8. Burkhart SS, Morgan CD, Kibler WB. The disabled throwing shoulder: spectrum of pathology Part III: The SICK scapula, scapular dyskinesis, the kinetic chain, and rehabilitation. Arthroscopy. 2003;19:641-61.
9. Ebaugh DD, McClure PW, Karduna AR. Effects of shoulder muscle fatigue caused by repetitive overhead activities on scapulothoracic and glenohumeral kinematics. J Electromyogr Kinesiol. 2006;16:224-35.
10. Burkhart SS, Morgan CD, Kibler WB. Shoulder injuries in overhead athletes: the "dead arm" revisited. Clin Sports Med. 2000;19:125-58.
11. Kibler WB, McMullen J. Scapular dyskinesis and its relation to shoulder pain. J Am Acad Orthop Surg. 2003;11:142-51.
12. Kibler WB, Sciascia A. Current concepts: scapular dyskinesis. Br J Sports Med. 2010;44:300-5.
13. De Baets L, Jaspers E, Desloovere K, Van Deun S. A systematic review of 3D scapular kinematics and muscle activity during elevation in stroke subjects and controls. J Electromyogr Kinesiol. 2013;23:3-13.
14. Seitz AL, McClure PW, Lynch SS, Ketchum JM, Michener LA. Effects of scapular dyskinesis and scapular assistance test on subacromial space during static arm elevation. J Shoulder Elbow Surg. 2012;21:631-40.
15. Cools AM, Witvrouw EE, Mahieu NN, Danneels LA. Isokinetic scapular muscle performance in overhead athletes with and without impingement symptoms. J Athl Train. 2005;40:104-10.
16. Ludewig PM, Reynolds JF. The association of scapular kinematics and glenohumeral joint pathologies. J Orthop Sports Phys Ther. 2009;39:90-104.
17. Myers JB, Laudner KG, Pasquale MR, Bradley JP, Lephart SM. Scapular position and orientation in throwing athletes. Am J Sports Med. 2005;33:263-71.
18. Struyf F, Nijs J, Baeyens JP, Mottram S, Meeusen R. Scapular positioning and movement in unimpaired shoulders, shoulder impingement syndrome, and glenohumeral instability. Scand J Med Sci Sports. 2011;21:352-8.
19. Kendall FP, McCreary EK, Provance PG. Muscles: Testing and Function. Baltimore: Williams & Wilkins; 1993.
20. Host HH. Scapular taping in the treatment of anterior shoulder impingement. Phys Ther. 1995;75:803-11.
21. Sahrmann SA. Diagnosis and Treatment of Movement Impairment Syndromes. St. Louis: Mosby; 2002.
22. Wilk KE, Reinold MM, Macrina CL, Porterfield R, Devine KM, Suarez K, et al. Glenohumeral internal rotation measurements differ depending on stabilization techniques. Sports Health. 2009;1:131-6.
23. Shanley E, Rauh MJ, Michener LA, Ellenbecker TS, Garrison JC, Thigpen CA. Shoulder range of motion measures as risk factors for shoulder and elbow injuries in high school softball and baseball players. Am J Sports Med. 2011;39:1997-2006.
24. Garrison JC, Arnold A, Macko MJ, Conway JE. Baseball players diagnosed with ulnar collateral ligament tears demonstrate decreased balance compared to healthy controls. J Orthop Sports Phys Ther. 2013;43:752-8.
25. Burkhart SS, Morgan CD, Kibler WB. The disabled throwing shoulder: spectrum of pathology. Part I. Arthroscopy. 2003;19:404-20.
26. Burkhart SS, Morgan CD, Kibler WB. The disabled throwing shoulder: spectrum of pathology. Part II. Arthroscopy. 2003;19:531-9.
27. Wilk KE, Hooks TR, Macrina LC. The modified sleeper stretch and modified cross-body stretch to increase shoulder internal rotation range of motion in the overhead throwing athlete. J Orthop Sports Phys Ther. 2013;43:891-4.
28. Oyama S, Hibberd EE, Myers JB. Changes in humeral torsion and shoulder rotation range of motion in high school baseball players over a 1-year period. Clin Biomech. 2013;28:268-72.
29. Nagarajan M, Vijayakumar P. Functional thoracic hyperkyphosis model for chronic subacromial impingement syndrome: an insight on evidence based "treat the cause" concept—a case study and literature review. J Back Musculoskelet Rehabil. 2013;26:227-42.
30. Kibler WB, Sciascia A, Dome D. Evaluation of apparent and absolute supraspinatus strength in patients with shoulder injury using the scapular retraction test. Am J Sports Med. 2006;34:1643-7.
31. Hong J, Barnes MJ, Leddon CE, Van Ryssegem G, Alamar B. Reliability of the sitting hand press-up test for identifying and quantifying the level of

scapular medial border posterior displacement in overhead athletes. Int J Sports Phys Ther. 2011;6:306-11.

32. Tate AR, McClure PW, Kareha S, Irwin D. Effect of scapular reposition test on the shoulder impingement symptoms and elevation strength in overhead athletes. J Orthop Sports Phys Ther. 2008;38:4-11.

33. Merolla G, De Santis E, Campi F, Paladini P, Procellini G. Supraspinatus and infraspinatus weakness in overhead athletes with scapular dyskinesis: strength assessment before and after restoration of scapular musculature balance. Musculoskelet Surg. 2012;94:119-25.

34. Kibler WB. The role of the scapula in athletic shoulder function. Am J Sports Med. 1998;26:325-37.

35. Lewis JS, Valentine RE. The pectoralis minor length test: a study of the intra-rater reliability and diagnostic accuracy in subjects with and without shoulder symptoms. BMC Musculoskelet Disord. 2007;8:64.

36. Bagg SD, Forrest WJ. A biomechanical analysis of scapular rotation during arm abduction in the scapular plane. Am J Phys Med Rehabil. 1988;67:238-45.

37. McClure PW, Michener LA, Sennett BJ, Karduna AR. Direct 3-dimensional measurements of scapular kinematics during dynamic movements in vivo. J Shoulder Elbow Surg. 2001;10:269-77.

38. Kuhn JE, Plancher KD, Hawkins RJ. Scapular winging. J Am Acad Orthop Surg. 1995;3:319-25.

39. Kibler WB, Sciascia A, Wilkes T. Scapular dyskinesis and its relation to shoulder injury. J Am Acad Orthop Surg. 2012;20:364-72.

40. Kibler WB, Sciascia A, Thomas SJ. Glenohumeral internal rotation deficit: pathogenesis and response to acute throwing. Sports Med Arthrosc. 2012;20:34-8.

41. Borstad JD, Ludewig PM. The effect of long versus short pectoralis minor resting length on scapular kinematics in healthy individuals. J Orthop Sports Phys Ther. 2005;35:227-38.

42. Kibler WB, Ludewig PM, McClure P, Uhl TL, Sciascia A. Scapula summit 2009: introduction. July 16, 2009, Lexington, Kentucky. J Orthop Sports Phys Ther. 2009;39:A1-A13.

43. Sciascia A, Thigpen C, Namdari S, Baldwin K. Kinetic chain abnormalities in the athletic shoulder. Sports Med Arthrosc. 2012;20:16-21.

44. De May K, Danneels L, Cagnie B. Are kinetic chain rowing exercises relevant in shoulder and trunk injury prevention training? Br J Sports Med. 2011;45:320-1.

45. Sciascia AD, Cromwell R. Kinetic chain rehabilitation: a theoretical framework. Rehabil Res Pract. 2012; 2012:853037.

46. McMullen J, Uhl TL. A kinetic chain approach for shoulder rehabilitation. J Athl Train. 2000;35:329-37.

47. Williams JG, Laudner KG, McLoda T. The acute effects of two passive stretch maneuvers on pectoralis minor length and scapular kinematics among collegiate swimmers. Int J Sports Phys Ther. 2013;8:25-33.

48. Liebler EJ, Tufano-Coors L, Douris P, Makofsky HW, McKenna R, Michels C, et al. The effect of thoracic spine mobilization on lower trapezius strength testing. J Man Manip Ther. 2001;9:207-12.

49. Strunce JB, Walker MJ, Boyles RE, Young BA. The immediate effects of thoracic spine and rib manipulation on subjects with primary complaints of shoulder pain. J Man Manip Ther. 2009;17:230-6.

50. Cools AM, Dewitte V, Lanszweert F, Notebaert D, Roets A, Soetens B, et al. Rehabilitation of scapular muscle balance: which exercises to prescribe? Am J Sports Med. 2007;35:1744-51.

51. Kibler WB, Sciascia AD, Uhl TL, Tambay N, Cunningham T. Electromyographic analysis of specific exercises for scapular control in early phases of shoulder rehabilitation. Am J Sports Med. 2008;36:1789-98.

52. Huang HY, Lin JJ, Guo YL, Wang WT, Chen YJ. EMG biofeedback effectiveness to alter muscle activity pattern and scapular kinematics in subjects with and without shoulder impingement. J Electromyogr Kinesiol. 2013;23:267-74.

53. Wilk KE, Yenchak AJ, Arrigo CA, Andrews JR. The Advanced Throwers Ten Exercise Program: a new exercise series for enhanced dynamic shoulder control in the overhead throwing athlete. Phys Sportsmed. 2011;39:90-7.

54. Hsu YH, Chen WY, Lin HC, Wang WT, Shih YF. The effects of taping on scapular kinematics and muscle performance in baseball players with shoulder impingement syndrome. J Electromyogr Kinesiol. 2009;19:1092-9.

55. Selkowitz DM, Chaney C, Stuckey SJ, Vlad G. The effects of scapular taping on the surface electromyographic signal amplitude of shoulder girdle muscles during upper extremity elevation in individuals with suspected shoulder impingement syndrome. J Orthop Sports Phys Ther. 2007;37:694-702.

56. Smith M, Sparkes V, Busse M, Enright S. Upper and lower trapezius muscle activity in subjects with subacromial impingement symptoms: is there imbalance and can taping change it? Phys Ther Sport. 2009; 10:45-50.

57. Cipriani DJ, Yu TS, Lyssanova O. Perceived influence of a compression, posture-cueing shirt on cyclists' ride experience and post-ride recovery. J Chiropr Med. 2014;13:21-7.

58. Kaya E, Zinnuroglu M, Tugcu I. Kinesio taping compared to physical therapy modalities for the treatment of shoulder impingement syndrome. Clin Rheumatol. 2011;30:201-7.

59. Manske RC, Reiman MP, Stovak ML. Nonoperative and operative management of snapping scapula. Am J Sports Med. 2004;32:1554-65.

60. Conduah AH, Baker CL 3rd, Baker CL Jr. Clinical management of scapulothoracic bursitis and the snapping scapula. Sports Health. 2010;2:147-55.

61. Warth RJ, Spiegl UJ, Millett PJ. Scapulothoracic bursitis and snapping scapula syndrome: a critical review of current evidence. Am J Sports Med. 2015;43:236-45.

CHAPTER 3

Rotator Cuff Impingement

Bill Seringer

ABSTRACT

Shoulder pain is quite common. Studies report the prevalence may be as high at 70–260 per 1,000 cases, with rotator cuff impingement representing 30–65% of these cases. In the United States, the direct cost for treatment of shoulder related issues was greater than 7 billion dollars in 2000. In 2003, approximately 13.7 million people were affected with shoulder pain, requiring medical care, and it is second only to low back pain in its prevalence. There are many options to treat rotator cuff impingement operatively and nonoperatively including but not limited to manual therapy, exercise, corticosteroid injections, surgery, nonsteroidal anti-inflammatory drugs, and activity modification to name a few.

This chapter will focus on the examination, and emphasize treatment of the shoulder with advanced evidenced-based techniques which the clinician can immediately use in the clinic. Provided, will be a progressive sequence and clinical algorithm to treat the shoulder from the early irritable phases to the late athletic phases of rehabilitation. The chapter will also provide insight into how to utilize a combination of clinical reasoning and the best evidence to determine the most efficacious manual therapy techniques to maximize outcomes.

INTRODUCTION

Rehabilitation of rotator cuff (RTC) impingement is both complex, and multifaceted, with relatively high success rates from the combination of exercise and manual therapy. With the limited gains appreciated from surgery, it appears that physical therapy provides the best recourse.

Epidemiology

Shoulder pain is quite common. Studies report the prevalence may be as high as 70–260 per 1,000 cases, with RTC impingement representing 30–65% of these cases.[1] In the United States, the direct cost for treatment of shoulder related issues was greater than 7 billion dollars in 2000.[2]

In 2003, approximately 13.7 million people were affected with shoulder pain requiring medical care, and shoulder pain is second only to low back pain in its prevalence.[3] There are many operative and nonoperative options to treat RTC impingement, including but not limited to manual therapy, exercise, corticosteroid injections, surgery, nonsteroidal anti-inflammatory drugs, and activity modification. Multiple studies have looked at the cost as well as the success, comparing physical therapy to surgical interventions. Many of these studies, including multiple randomized control trial (RCT) studies, have found that exercise, and exercise with manual therapy, when compared to surgery at up to 2½ years follow-up, demonstrate little to no difference with respect to pain, function, and overall satisfaction. From an outcomes standpoint, there is a positive shift toward rehabilitation with respect to management of shoulder impingement.[4-7]

Anatomical Review

As far back as 1867, Jarjavay first noted the disorder of subacromial bursitis and in 1875 Hamilton described the acromion as a source of pain in the shoulder. Even today with advanced imaging and understanding, the shoulder's anatomy (Fig. 1) remains somewhat controversial as a primary source of insult. In 1972, Neer popularized the term impingement syndrome, in response to his understanding that the RTC was being impinged upon by the anterior third of the acromion, the acromioclavicular (AC) joint, and the coracohumeral ligament. Neer suggested performing an anterior acromioplasty, focusing on the undersurface of the acromion, thus decompressing the subacromial space. The subacromial space is defined by the humeral head inferiorly, the anterior edge and undersurface of the anterior third of the acromion, the coracohumeral ligament and the AC joint superiorly.[8] The distance between the acromion and the humeral head, as seen on radiographs, is approximately 10-15 mm. This subacromial space is thought to be encroached on, for varying reasons. The humeral head has been reported as translating 1–3 mm in a superior direction during the first 30–60° of active elevation. This is likely due to the force vector of the deltoid acting on the humerus.[9-13] Between 60° and 120° of elevation the acromial undersurface of the RTC tendons are in close proximity, with the greatest amount of contact area prevalent to type III acromions.[14] The subacromial bursa is a redundant sac, which lies in this space. It functions to allow gliding, and decreases friction

between the two layers of tissue. Although it is diagnosed commonly, bursitis is a diagnosis that rarely occurs on its own. It is thought to be secondary to other pathologic processes. It has been noted that with impingement, chronic inflammatory cells are present in the subacromial bursa, but not the coracohumeral ligament. Free nerve endings also exist in the subacromial bursa, suggesting pain emanating from this region could be linked to the free nerve endings exposed in this region.[4] Both extrinsic and intrinsic factors can lead to narrowing of the subacromial space and aggravation of the subacromial contents. Intrinsic factors include: muscle weakness,[15,16] muscular fatigue,[14,17-19] overuse, and degenerative tendinopathy. Extrinsic factors include: glenohumeral (GH) instability, AC joint degeneration, impingement by the coracohumeral ligament, as well as coracoid impingement, Os Acromiale and acromial morphology.[10] Many terms are utilized with respect to the impingement type syndromes: RTC impingement, subacromial impingement, subacromial impingement syndrome, RTC syndrome, impingement, and impingement syndrome are representative of the abundance of terms used to classify this often misdiagnosed presentation. These terms will be used synonymously throughout this chapter.

CLINICAL PRESENTATION

Rotator cuff impingement has distinct characteristics, which distinguish it from other diagnoses. With RTC impingement, the pain is often referred to the lateral deltoid, a region which rarely, if ever, has pain of a nontraumatic nature of its own (Figs 2A and B).[20] Patients will usually point to a specific region located along the lateral aspect of the deltoid near the insertion. They will typically draw a line from the lateral aspect of the acromion down toward the deltoid insertion with slightly diffuse characteristics. In a study by Stackhouse et al.,[19] all 17 patients demonstrated pain with the administration of a hypertonic solution into the subacromial space. More interestingly, though, 3 out of 17 patients exhibited pain in the distal arm extending as far as the hand (Figs 3A and B).

Differential Diagnosis

In the shoulder region, the clinician must be aware of the potential confounding diagnoses that exist relative to RTC and the many potential sources of pain in the GH region. Some of the key diagnoses to consider include AC joint pain, bicipital tendinitis or tendinosis, cervical pathology

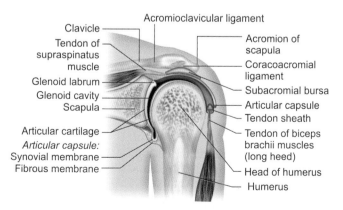

FIG. 1: Shoulder joint
Source: Reproduced from Connexion website via Wikimedia Commons.

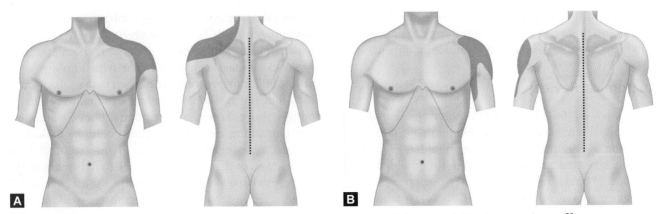

FIGS 2A AND B: Distribution of pain after irritation of—(A) Acromioclavicular (AC) joint; and (B) Subacromial space[20]
Source: Reprinted with permission from Elsevier.

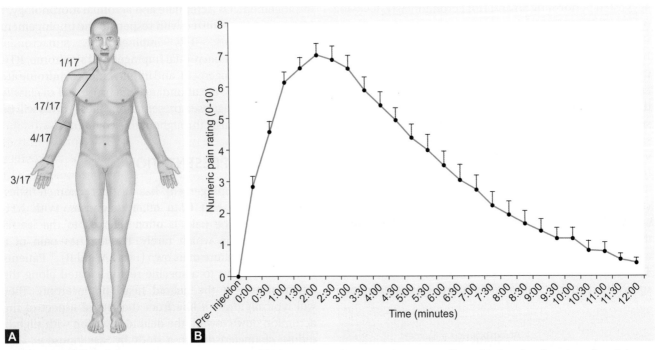

FIGS 3A AND B: (A) Diagram shows the distribution of pain after the subacromial injection of hypertonic saline (number of participants with pain in region/number of total participants). The pain had a dull/diffuse quality, and all participants experienced symptoms in the anterior/lateral upper arm region; (B) Summary plot shows numeric pain ratings (mean standard error) across time for all participants after injection of hypertonic saline into the subacromial space[19]
Source: Reprinted with permission from Elsevier.

including radicular pain, C5-C6 apophyseal joint disease[7] RTC tear, and a labral tear. *Cervical Radiculopathy and Cervical Sprain and Strain* chapters in this book describe these conditions in further detail. Table 1 can be utilized as a guide to differentiate between RTC impingement from other shoulder and scapular pathologies. RTC impingement is differentiated from AC joint pain by the location of the pain. AC joint pain is felt deep in the AC joint, and is aggravated by maneuvers that compress the AC joint. AC joint pain occasionally radiates superiorly into the cervical region and upper trapezius.

CLINICAL EXAMINATION

Evaluation of the shoulder is complicated by the amount of motion, function, and tissue pathology that are characteristic of this region. There are many components to a shoulder examination. The clinician must clear the cervical spine, as well as the neurological regions distally. Neural tension may play a role in this evaluation. In a clinical prediction rule for cervical radiculopathy, Upper Limb Tension Test-1 (ULTT) was the most predictive for radicular symptoms.[21-25] However, when testing for neural tension, attention must be paid to high amounts of false positives, which are created with ULTT in normal subjects between 44° and 54° of elbow extension.[22,23] Once the cervical spine has been cleared, observation of shoulder range of motion (ROM) can occur while looking at the scapula for any aberrant motions. The hands-on-hips position can be utilized for visualizing muscle atrophy in the supraspinatus and infraspinatus regions. The arms may be pressed against the wall to adequately view the scapula under tension. Strength testing should then follow. After strength testing, palpation is performed, including identification the biceps tendon, in the bicipital groove, as a possible secondary generator of pain. The RTC muscles and their insertions should be palpated for any tenderness. The clinician should palpate the numerous muscles that attach from the cervical spine to the shoulder girdle (Figs 4A and B). If appropriate, neurovascular testing should also be performed as a part of the general testing.

The clinician can now commence special testing. There are typically five categories of shoulder special tests. These include impingement tests, RTC pathology—including tendons and tears, labral and biceps pathology, AC joint pathology, and issues relating to GH instability. There are a plethora of tests, which exist for the shoulder (Table 1). In orthopedics, when many tests exist and minimal consensus is conferred in identifying a diagnosis, it usually indicates that the testing procedures are inadequate. However, this does not mean one cannot clinically deduce the dysfunction from the clinical examination. It simply means that one must include all of the data, such as history, screening items, injury mechanism, and understanding of the tests ability to rule in or rule out a diagnosis. Particular emphasis is placed on what findings are indicative of a positive test. For example, pain at the anterior biceps with a Hawkins-Kennedy test is not a positive test for impingement, despite eliciting pain. Such a finding leads the clinician to appreciate there may be a biceps problem which needs further examination. In one study, the accuracy of shoulder impingement testing was shown to be improved by clustering of the Hawkins-Kennedy test, painful arc sign, and infraspinatus strength test. If all three were present, the post-test probability of secondary impingement was 95%.[27] Table 2 provides an evaluation algorithm to garner information about the shoulder region and adequately diagnose shoulder pathology. It is designed to begin the evaluation process and is not comprehensive. Individual patient's variances will guide the clinical evaluation and decision-making.

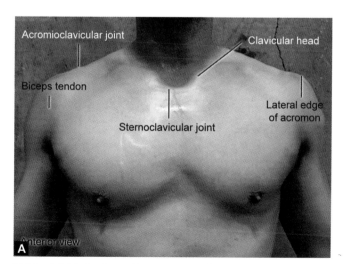

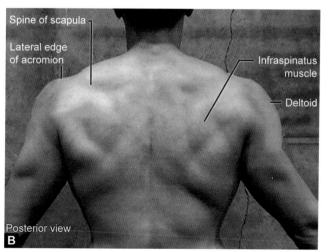

FIGS 4A AND B: General appearance of the shoulder. (A) Anterior; and (B) Posterior[26]
Source: Reprinted with permission from Elsevier.

TABLE 1: Data summary of the 17 articles yielding diagnostic statistics for the 26 special tests included in the shoulder examination algorithm[28]

Special test	Test category	N	Reference standard	Sp	Sn	LR+	LR−
Internal rotation resisted strength test	Screening test	110	Surgical observation	0.96	0.86	0.86	0.13
RTC impingement cluster (3/3)	RTC impingement	552	Surgical observation	NR	NR	10.56	NR
RTC impingement cluster (2/3)	RTC impingement	552	Surgical observation	NR	NR	5.03	NR
External rotation lag sign (Hertel et al.)	RTC (Supra/infraspinatus tear	87	Surgical observation	0.69	0.98	15.50	0.32
External rotation lag sign (Walch et al.)	RTC (Supra/infraspinatus tear	87	Surgical observation	0.98	0.98	34.50	0.02
Dropping-sign	RTC (Infraspinatus) tear	87	Surgical observation	1.00	1.00	0.00	0.00
Hornblower's sign	RTC (Teres minor) tear	87	Surgical observation	0.93	1.00	14.29	0.00
Internal rotation lag sign	RTC (subscapularis) tear	54	Surgical observation	0.96	0.97	24.30	0.03
Apprehension test (Lo et al.)	Anterior instability	46	Radiograph	0.99	0.53	20.20	0.47
Apprehension test (Farber et al.)	Anterior instability	363	Surgical observation	0.96	0.72	53.00	0.47
Anterior release (surprise) test (Lo et al.)	Anterior instability	46	Radiograph	0.99	0.64	8.36	0.37
Anterior release (surprise) test (Gross et al.)	Anterior instability	100	Surgical observation	0.89	0.92	58.60	0.09
Anterior labral tear cluster	Bankart lesion/anterior labral tear	62	MRI	0.85	0.90	6.00	0.12
Jerk test	Posterior instability/labral tear	172	Surgical observation	0.98	0.73	36.50	0.28
Kim test	Posterior instability/labral tear	172	Surgical observation	0.94	0.80	13.30	0.21
Biceps load test I	SLAP lesion	75	Surgical observation	0.97	0.90	30.00	0.10
Biceps load test II	SLAP lesion	127	Surgical observation	0.97	0.90	30.00	0.10
Posterior impingement sign	Articular internal impingement	69	Surgical observation	0.85	0.76	5.00	0.29
Yergason's test (Naredo et al.)	LHB tendinopathy	31	Ultrasonography	0.58	0.74	1.76	0.45
Yergason's test (Holtby et al.)	LHB tendinopathy	50	Surgical observation	0.79	0.43	2.05	0.72
Speed test (Bennett)	LHB tendinopathy	46	Surgical observation	0.14	0.90	1.00	0.71
Speed test (Holtby et al.)	LHB tendinopathy	50	Surgical observation	0.75	0.90	1.28	0.91
Gilcrist palm-up Test (Leroux)	LHB tendinopathy	55	Surgical observation	0.35	0.63	0.97	1.06
Gilcrist palm-up Test (Naredo)	LHB tendinopathy	31	Ultrasonography	0.58	0.74	1.76	0.45
AC joint cluster (3/3)	AC joint lesion	325	AC joint injection	0.97	0.25	8.30	0.77

AC, acromioclavicular; LHB, long head of the biceps; RTC, rotator cuff; SLAP, superior labrum anterior posterior; Sp, specificity; Sn, sensitivity; LR, likelihood ratio

Source: Used with permission of The International Journal of Sports Physical Therapy.

TABLE 2: Shoulder evaluation algorithm to diagnose shoulder pathology

Test/action performed	Test/action performed
Active range of motion (AROM) abduction	AROM forward flexion
Hands-on-hips to observe for muscle atrophy	Scapular mechanics
Resisted forward flexion	Resisted abduction

Continued

Continued

Test/action performed	Test/action performed
Resisted external rotation (ER) 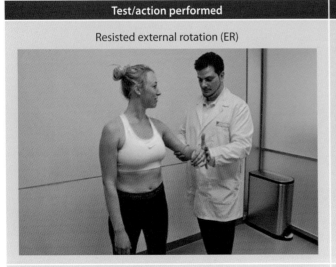	Resisted internal rotation (IR) 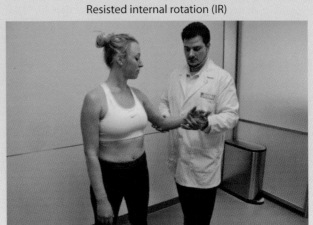
Posterior capsule subluxation position 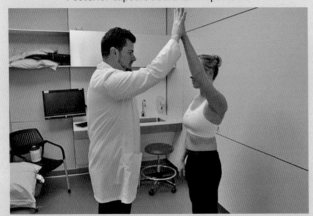	Empty can AROM 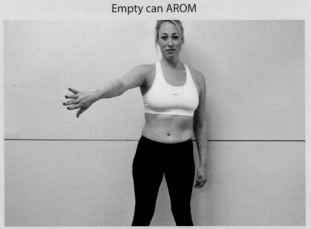
Active Neer test 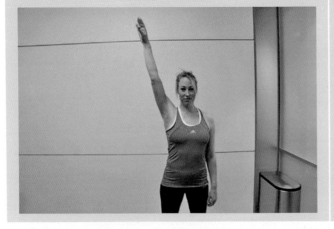	Resisted empty can test 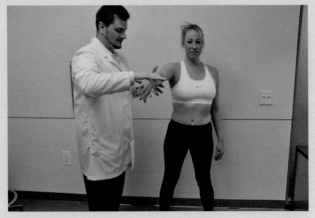

Continued

Continued

Test/action performed	Test/action performed
Sulcus sign	Load-shift test. To the glenoid rim or over for proper evaluation. The movement should be in an anteromedial to posterolateral direction

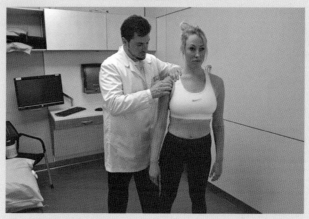

Hawkins-Kennedy test	Coracoid impingement test

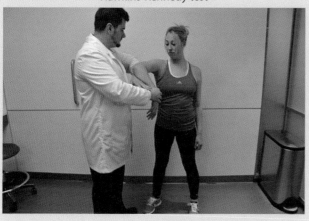
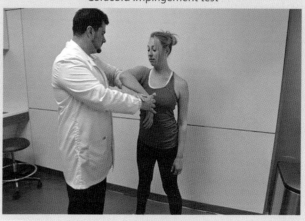

Cross arm abduction with slight IR for AC joint pathology	Yocum test

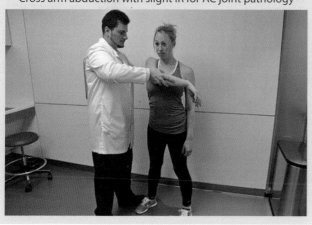
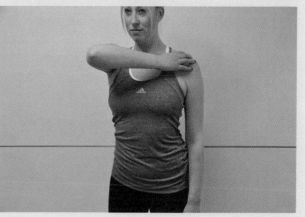

Continued

Test/action performed	Test/action performed
	Belly press test is positive for moderate tears if painful without elbow retraction. However, if the elbow retracts, then the test is a positve for a large tear, and is called Napolean test

Bear-hug test for subscapularis

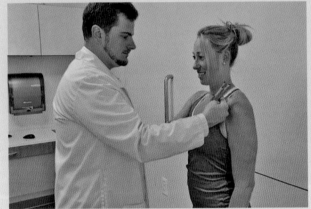

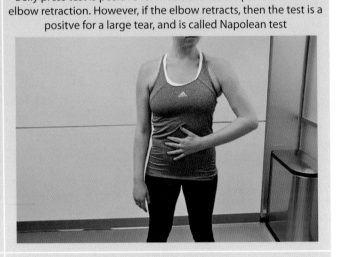

Lift-off test for massive subscapularis tears

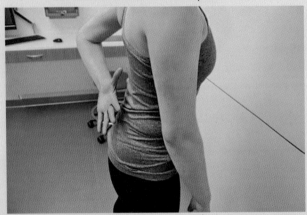

O'Brien's test for biceps labrum

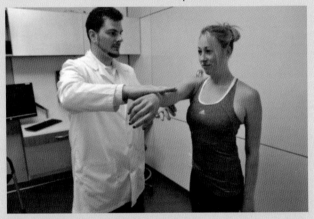

Spurlings test

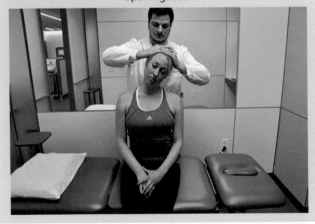

Cervical distraction—can also be done in supine

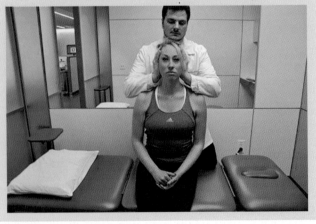

Continued

Continued

Test/action performed	Test/action performed
ULTT	Generalized joint mobility testing in anterior/posterior and superior/inferior direction

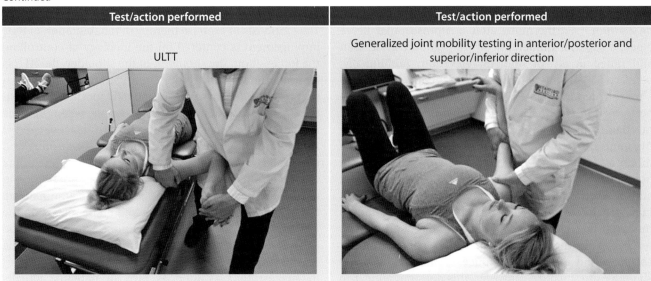

This algorithmic sequence would include ROM testing and measurements in supine. Further special testing of strength testing may be required based on clinical presentation. This algorithm is designed to provide a starting point for evaluation process and with sufficient practice should require less than 10 minutes to complete.

AC, acromioclavicular; ULTT, upper limb tension test

■ PHYSICAL THERAPY TREATMENT

Nonoperative treatment of RTC impingement is equally or more successful as compared to operative treatment.[4-7] This is true when nonoperative treatment regimens include stretching and strengthening exercises.[29] In many cases, success of rehabilitation may be predicted by acromial morphology. In a study by Morrison, 67% of 616 patients had a satisfactory result with nonoperative intervention.[29] In this study, patients with a type I acromion demonstrated 91% success rate. Subjects with a type III acromion demonstrated success 64% of the time. Subjects with a type III acromion, represent the largest percentage of subjects in this study group. However from a results standpoint, the subjects demonstrated similar success with little difference existing between type II and type III acromions. In the general population, type II acromions are most prevalent and demonstrate the acromion's morphologic impact on impingement-like symptoms.[8,14,29] Since Morrison published his study, our understanding of rehabilitation has improved, including improved manual therapy techniques, better understanding of strengthening techniques and principles, and relative ability to differentiate impingement from other pathologies. The author believes that the success rate is likely higher than reported in this study at the present time.

Rotator cuff impingement can be either structural or functional. Most of the structural changes are a result of acromial morphology, degeneration, and/or inflammation of the ligaments or tendons and other soft tissues existing in the subacromial space. These structures are minimally impacted with rehabilitation. Functional issues include muscle weakness, muscular force imbalances, posture, muscle fatigue, and selective hypomobility[30] of the shoulder capsule, potentially due to GH instability. Most rehabilitation techniques are focused on functional issues. The addition of exercise therapy has been shown to be effective in the treatment of these functional issues.[31] The focus of exercise therapy is concentrated on controlling and balancing the forces around the GH and scapulothoracic regions.[15,32,33] Superior migration of the humeral head has long been considered a mechanical factor for degenerative changes in this region, often caused by imbalances of muscular forces.[34,35] When discussing depression of the humeral head, the clinician must consider all of the muscles surrounding the GH and scapulothoracic regions and their interactions with each other. Depression of humeral head has been demonstrated through various means including fluoroscopic assessment and radiographs. Patients with impingement, as well as normal subjects, who demonstrate RTC weakness due to repetitive stress, pain, and/or RTC fatigue, present with superior humeral head migration.[17,36,37] In a study by Chen et al., muscular fatigue to exhaustion increased humeral head excursion by 2.5 mm.[38] Furthermore, after a suprascapular nerve block, a superior humeral head translation can be seen and noted at 60° of humeral elevation. Additionally, between 60° and 90° of flexion, the scapula demonstrates a more anteriorly rotated position.[16] Matsuki et al. have performed *in vivo* measurements and described normal mechanics of the GH joint in healthy subjects.[39] The AC joint also represents significant motions about the thorax and GH region.[40] Posture plays a significant role in functional mechanical issues.[41-44] It is obvious weakness and/or fatigue in the GH and scapulothoracic regions may proliferate negative consequences in relation to humeral mechanics and may potentially drive pain responses in patients. Theoretically, some consider corticosteroid injection to induce a fatiguing effect on shoulder musculature. However, this does not appear to significantly influence strength and therefore testing and strengthening may proceed.[45]

The primary goal of shoulder strengthening is to optimize force couples about the shoulder to control humeral mechanics. The infraspinatus, teres major and minor as well as the latissimus act as humeral head depressors with the supraspinatus exhibiting minimal impact as a humeral depressor functionally.[46] The dynamic stabilizers for neuromuscular control of the shoulder region include the RTC muscles (supraspinatus, infraspinatus, teres minor, and subscapularis) as well as the long head of biceps, which can act as a weak secondary humeral head depressor. Therefore the biceps tendon may act as a pain generator to be noted as secondary to RTC impingement due to its inability to cope with this role. Other secondary stabilizers in the shoulder region are the pectoralis muscles, the teres major, and the latissimus dorsi. The role of these muscles is to produce a combined neuromuscular response to control and stabilize the humeral head. In some studies the combined activation of these muscles serve to provide compression and centering of the humeral head.[30] Finally it is important to control or balance deltoid's biomechanical action on the humeral head through these force couples. To do this, one must be cognizant of how active the deltoids are with shoulder motion. Patients with subacromial impingement demonstrate higher deltoid use than normal subjects at all exercise intensity levels and during active ROM.[47] Patients will also demonstrate a shrug sign, assisting active elevation utilizing the upper trapezius and the levator scapulae muscles to assist with overhead motion.[48,49]

Exercise Therapy

The emphasis of exercise therapy in rehabilitation of RTC impingement is centered on the ideology of controlling the forces about the shoulder. In the shoulder, the RTC is typically the weak link. Pain, injury, trauma, and edema may result in deactivation of regionally specific muscles to the site of the dysfunction.[19] For example, when the knee is injured, the quadriceps muscles are deactivated.[50,51] In the lumbar region, it is common to see atrophy and decreased activation of various muscles including the quadratus lumborum.[52,53] A similar phenomenon occurs in the RTC when the shoulder is traumatized. During rehabilitation, emphasis should be placed on the RTC muscles, specifically on gaining external rotation (ER) strength. Despite having strong evidence for the effectiveness of exercise therapy, research continues to suggest that as little as 50% of patients actually receive exercise therapy as a current practice treatment option.[54] Appropriate exercises for the weakened muscles should be identified during the evaluation. The role of each muscle and the consequences of not maximally activating certain muscles, while inhibiting others, must be properly understood (e.g. activation of deltoid muscle negatively impacts humeral control). If necessary, total arm strengthening should be initiated in the late phases of rehabilitation.[55,56]

One of the more recent issues in the field of physical therapy is the dose-response relationship. Appropriately dosing exercise adequately stresses the targeted muscle group to create muscle overload and the desired physical changes in line with the goals of rehabilitation.[57,58] One such study compared, in a randomized fashion, high dosage interventions with lower dosage interventions (Table 3). When one is considering prescribing an exercise intervention, it is important to appreciate the repetition and intensity required to create overload and thus impact strength, endurance, coordination and circulation in a way that stimulates change at a cellular level adequate to affect mechanics and pain. In this study, high dosage was emphasized, which successfully demonstrated functional improvements in patients with long standing unilateral subacromial pain. Patients performed 720 repetitions with 25–30 minutes of aerobic conditioning.[59] In this study, 10–15 Repetition Maximum and increases in overall volume with 4 days of training versus 3 and 2 days proved a more effective methodology of training. Compared to many rehabilitation programs currently in use today, this would be considered high dosage and high intensity. Resistance exercise is also more likely to be adhered to

TABLE 3: Interventions in two groups, showing difference in dosage[57]

High-dosage	Low-dosage
15–20 minutes aerobic (stationary bike/treadmill)	5–10 minutes global aerobic
4 local exercises 3 sets of 30 repetitions	5 local exercises 2 sets of 10 repetitions
10 minutes aerobic (stationary bike/treadmill)	
4 local exercises 3 sets of 30 repetitions	
10 minutes aerobic (stationary bike/treadmill)	

Source: Reprinted with permission from Østerås and Torstensen; Licensee Bentham Open.

when compared to all-around exercise, with an increased dose-response relationship demonstrating a positive impact on pain.[60-63] High dosages should be emphasized as an effective and efficient treatment alternative.

The progressive nature of these exercises is also an important parameter.[64] All too often the volume of exercise, intensity, and progressive nature are lost due to changes in the patient's pain, exercise compliance, or patient's desire to have more passive modalities performed. Passive modalities have not demonstrated good results.[65] One must stay steadfast with known avenues of treatment effectiveness, despite the potential for patients to report initial apprehension with mild pain, discomfort, and/or muscle fatigue. Researchers emphasize that controlled prescriptions of progressive, periodized resistance exercise negate daily fatigue and its effect on delayed onset muscle soreness. In essence, great emphasis is placed on adequate rest to prevent the negative effects associated with overtraining over the long term.

Specific Exercise Prescription

Moseley and Townsend were some of the first researchers to utilize fine wire electromyography (EMG) to rank order GH and scapulothoracic exercises.[64,66] Since that time, there has been a proliferation of research articles addressing this very topic. Many authors have attempted to quantify exercises that maximally target the muscles surrounding the GH and scapulothoracic regions.[48,67-74] Furthermore, many have specifically attempted to quantify exercises that maximally activate the scapula and scapular stabilizers. Reinold et al. compiled this data

in their study to rank order previous studies and provided a concise overview of exercises to maximally activate in isolation individual muscles.[73,75-79] Listed later in Table 4 is a suggested sequence to treat patients who demonstrate RTC impingement as their primary diagnosis. This sequence utilizes the concepts of progressive resistance exercise, overload, and high dosage strength training. It has been reported in the literature that 0–20% maximum voluntary isometric contraction (MVIC) is considered low muscle activity, 21–40% MVIC is considered moderate muscle activity, and 41–60% MVIC is considered high muscle activity, with greater than 60% MVIC was considered very high muscle activity.[71]

The treatment flow in Table 4 is designed to serve as a guideline and not to supersede clinical judgment. This flow also represents clinical time constraints observed in actual practice, and sequencing may be accelerated or slowed as appropriate.

If the patient's shoulder is highly irritable, specifically: (1) reports high levels of pain ($\geq 7/10$), (2) has consistent night or resting pain, (3) demonstrates high levels of reported disability on standardized self-report outcome tools, (4) pain occurs before end ranges of active or passive movements, and (5) active ROM is significantly less than passive ROM due to pain,[89] then the irritability progression (Table 5) is recommended. For such a patient, the timetable described earlier may have to be deferred by 1–6 weeks, and more independent exercise performance may be appropriate. Minimal pain reduction can be expected in the first few weeks, and in mildly irritated impingement patients, it will likely take 8–12 weeks to see substantial gains with clinical tests and functional shoulder measures.

Table 6 lists additional strengthening exercises that can be performed in the first 8 weeks of rehabilitation, while Table 7 lists sports-specific exercises.

Minimizing Deltoid Activation

It is important, during GH and scapulothoracic exercises, to minimize the contributions of the deltoid and to maximize infraspinatus and teres minor muscle activity, which are considered to have the greatest effect on humeral depression within the GH joint. Initially in rehabilitation, some patients prefer to start with weighted exercises—specifically, athletes, patients with previous history of strength training, or people with a strong desire to get back quickly to their desired sport of activity. In the author's opinion, these patients may be overzealous in shoulder rehabilitation by adding too much weight,

TABLE 4: Suggested treatment flow for patients who demonstrate rotation cuff (RTC) impingement as their primary diagnosis

Treatment week	Technique performed	Clinical pearls	Picture
1 (1–2 sessions)	Prone horizontal extension	Shoulder should be placed in ER to tension the RTC prior to exercise initiation	
	Prone horizontal abduction	Typically this can be the most aggravating of the initial exercises and should be attempted with less motion if pain is elicited as the patient approaches 90°. Shoulder should be placed in ER.	
	Side-lying ER	Elbow must be maintained near the hip, a pillow helps with the proper positioning and the patient must be cued to not allow elbow to slide down the pillow.	

The emphasis of week one should be on beginning strengthening as based on physiological principles this will take the longest time to take effect and based on evidence will be the most important aspect of shoulder rehabilitation.

Week one exercises are initially tolerated by the vast majority of patients, as they do not place undue stress on irritated tissue. If the patient is highly irritable, refer to the irritable section discussed later.

One should not to be overzealous with the introduction of increased weight. Increasing weight too early in the program will overactivate the deltoid and under activate the RTC. A good guideline for the patient is to increase the weight by 1 pound every 2–3 weeks where they can perform a full set with minimal fatigue and perfect technique.

Continued

Continued

Treatment week	Technique performed	Clinical pearls	Picture
2 (2 sessions)	ER with retraction	Maintain palms up and thumbs out as this maximizes ER recruitment. The patient should be cued to maintain elbow at the level of the hips and not to let the elbows drift away from the body. Proper technique is to maintain the elbow bend at 90° throughout. It was a teaching tip I use. May be easier to leave out	
	Robbery[77]	Performed in two steps with shoulders in 90° abduction: 1. 90° shoulder ER from 0° position 2. Scapular retraction. Can be performed with or without spinal flexion/extension	
	Passive range of motion (PROM), AROM and joint mobilizations. These may need to be performed if the clinician determines there are selective capsular hypomobilities.	Flexion	

Continued

Continued

Treatment week	Technique performed	Clinical pearls	Picture
		ER at 45° abduction	
		IR at 45° abduction	
		AROM flexion/extension from 60° to full ROM	
		Grade I–II joint mobilization	

60

Continued

Continued

Treatment week	Technique performed	Clinical pearls	Picture
3 (2 sessions)	Prone abducted row	Patients tend to decrease from 90° of shoulder horizontal abduction lowering their arm. This causes them to begin recruiting middle and lower trapezius to a higher degree when fatigued.	
	Supine serratus press	This exercise is not only a strengthening exercise but also helps with GH AROM	
	PROM	IR in flexion	
	Joint mobilization Grade I–IV	Posterior and lateral glide	

Continued

Continued

Treatment week	Technique performed	Clinical pearls	Picture
		Inferior and lateral glide	
		Anterior-posterior glides	
		Small amplitude flexion mobilizations	
		Caudal glide in full flexion	

Continued

Continued

Treatment week	Technique performed	Clinical pearls	Picture
		Humeral head depression with shoulder abduction	
		Posterior mobilization	

When mobilizing posteriorly, the clinician must ensure the patient's arm is placed in slight adduction with the mobilizing force in the posterior and lateral direction as to not abut the glenoid rim.

Treatment week	Technique performed	Clinical pearls	Picture
	Wand exercises as necessary.	Forward flexion without pillow supporting the scapula	
		ER in 45° abduction	

Continued

Continued

Treatment week	Technique performed	Clinical pearls	Picture
		ER in neutral abduction	
		ER in 90° abduction	
4 (2 sessions)	Standing IR/ER step-outs	Begin with a lighter resistance as the patient will fatigue towards the end of each set with this exercise	

Continued

Continued

Treatment week	Technique performed	Clinical pearls	Picture
	Ball on wall	First time we begin to introduce more functional position of 90° elevation. Rhythmic stabilizations can be utilized as discussed later.	
	Ball clock	This is a progression of ball on wall	
	Rhythmic stabilization in balanced position (This position is defined as 100° of elevation and slight horizontal abduction (scapular plane).[80]	Balanced position allows the arm to maintain stability in the socket whilst utilizing the musculature of the shoulder and RTC to stabilize the shoulder. As reported by Irlenbusch[81] quick rhythmic stabilizations allow for selective type II muscle fiber recruitment not seen in most rehabilitation programs.	

Continued

Continued

Treatment week	Technique performed	Clinical pearls	Picture
	Manual resisted ER		
	Manual resisted scapular protraction		
	Manual resisted scapular retraction		

Depending on multiple factors such as patient progression, exercise capacity, irritability level, muscle endurance and hypertrophy, it may be appropriate to let the patient work independently for weeks at this stage, as the patient has a sufficient program to make strength gains. Muscle physiology dictates that the strength gains demonstrated in the first 4 weeks are mostly neuromuscular in nature and hypertrophy will take up to 12 weeks.

| 5 (0–2 sessions) | May continue manual therapy until unnecessary | | |

Continued

Continued

Treatment week	Technique performed	Clinical pearls	Picture
	Standing IR/ER	Place a towel underneath the arm for maximal muscle contraction. This position is ideal due to the length tension relationship of the muscle, is more comfortable for the patient, and demonstrates improved EMG compared with no towel. Make sure to cue the patient not to allow the arm to drawer anteriorly, as they fatigue, as this increases the activation of the deltoid.	
	ER oscillation[82]	Make sure to cue the patient not to allow the arm to drawer anteriorly as they fatigue, as this increases the activation of the deltoid. This is a muscular endurance-based exercise, and as such should be sustained for 30 seconds minimum during each repetition.	
	Wall walks	Make sure to maintain elbow on wall surface at all times. Perform 4 walks up and 4 down between 6 and 10 times	

Continued

Continued

Treatment week	Technique performed	Clinical pearls	Picture
	Additional table GH and scapulothoracic muscles, as necessary.[70,73,74,83]	Prone forward flexion	
		Prone alphabet Y	
		Prone alphabet T	
		Prone alphabet W	

Continued

Continued

Treatment week	Technique performed	Clinical pearls	Picture
		Prone alphabet I	
6 (0–1 session)	Begin self-stretching program as follows: Sleeper stretch[73,84,85]	The sleeper stretch, once thought to target the posterior capsule, has more recently been demonstrated to primarily stretch the posterior RTC. This is desirable, especially in patients with glenohumeral internal rotation deficit (GIRD) and in overhead athletes (in-season and off-season alike). In-season athletes, particularly baseball pitchers, will lose IR as the season progresses, if not stretching, leading to increased risk of injury.	
	IR towel stretch	Despite the name of this exercise, the combined motions of shoulder extension, adduction and IR are stretched with the hand placed behind the back. Gains in arm reach measured at spinal levels are largely attributable to improvements in shoulder extension and elbow flexion, rather than isolated IR.	

Continued

Continued

Treatment week	Technique performed	Clinical pearls	Picture
	Pectoral stretch[86]	The sequencing to maximally engage the pectoral can be performed in three phases—(1) slight forward lean into the stretch; (2) rotation away from the stretch; (3) slight increase in further forward lean. The patient will be the best judge of the effectiveness of this stretch, once the clinician has provided them with adequate information on the tissues they are attempting to stretch.	
	Caution should be taken during flexibility progression in patients with general laxity, and this progression should not be performed in unstable shoulders.		
7 (0–2 sessions)	Rows[48,71,73,87]	Cue the patient to maintain the knee bent position and not to retract the arms past the midline of the body, rather push the chest out with scapular retraction.	
	Punches[48,71,73,87]	Perform these unilaterally and maintain a good knee bend for a stable base of support.	

Continued

Continued

Treatment week	Technique performed	Clinical pearls	Picture
	Bear Hug[48,71,73,87]	This may be taught in a sequential movement pattern. Training errors include, patients internally rotating their arms, allowing their arms to traverse wide, in turn emphasizing the pectorals and straining the anterior capsular aspects of the shoulder.	
8 (0–1 sessions)	Perform an assessment determining the need for exercise progression, including increased volume and weights. Utilize dynamometry or isokinetic testing to evaluate strength levels.[88] It may be appropriate to discharge, continue current program or allow patient to work independently for 1–4 weeks.		
	Additional higher-level strengthening exercises that can be performed in the first 8 weeks have been presented in Table 6. If return to sports is desired see sports exercise examples below in Table 7.		

IR, internal rotation; ER, external rotation; GH, glenohumeral; AROM, active range of motion; EMG, electromyography

TABLE 5: Suggested treatment flow for patient with highly irritable rotation cuff (RTC) impingement[90]

Treatment week	Technique performed	Clinical pearls
1 (Initial evaluation)	Shoulder shrugs	Emphasis on not anteriorly drawing the shoulder forward as this narrows the subacromial space
	Scapular squeezes	
	Exercises listed above are designed to get the shoulder region moving and to get the patient comfortable and confident in the rehabilitation processes they may experience anxiety and/or fear of failure.	
2 (1–2 sessions)	Begin manual therapy: PROM in flexion, IR/ER at 45° abduction, grade I–II joint mobilization, AROM flexion/extension from 60° to full ROM	
	*May trial tables slides for ROM, limiting discomfort from irritability	
3 (1–2 sessions)	Manual: PROM in flexion, IR, ER at 0-45-90 degrees of abduction, grade I–IV joint mobilization, cross body horizontal abduction, rhythmic stabilization in balanced position slow	
	Robbery	
	Scapular depression[76,77]	
	Lawnmower[76,77]	
	Pendulums, if necessary[91]	
4	May begin regular progression, continue manual, or allow for independent exercise performance.	

IR, internal rotation; ER, external rotation; PROM, passive range of motion; AROM, active range of motion

TABLE 6: Additional higher level exercises which can be performed through first 8 weeks

Exercise	Exercise
Prone 90-90 ER (start) 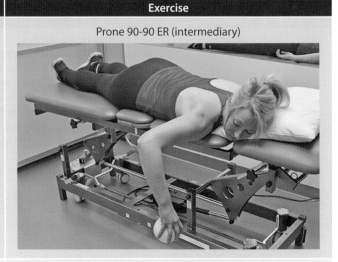	Prone 90-90 ER (intermediary) 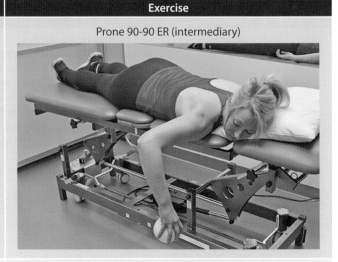
Prone 90-90 ER (finish) 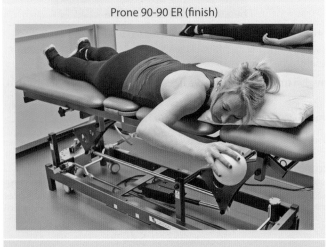	Prone 90-90 ball drop 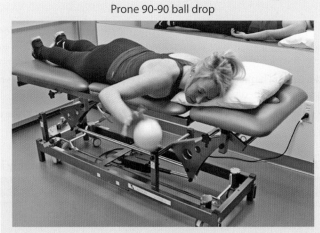
Side-lying Bodyblade® (start) 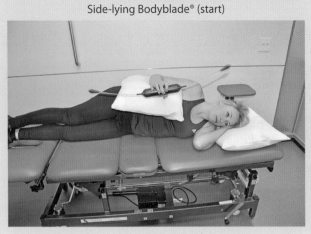	Side-lying Bodyblade® (finish) 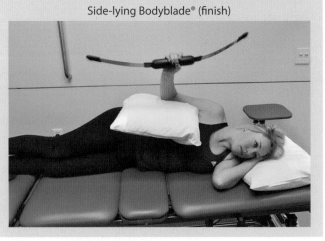

Continued

Continued

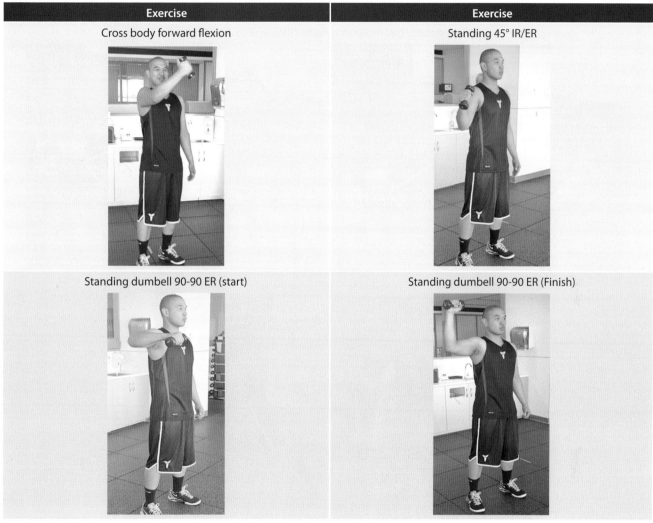

Exercise	Exercise
Cross body forward flexion	Standing 45° IR/ER
Standing dumbell 90-90 ER (start)	Standing dumbell 90-90 ER (Finish)

IR, internal rotation; ER, external rotation.

TABLE 7: Sport-specific exercises. It represents advanced sports related exercise progression unnecessary for basic rehabilitation

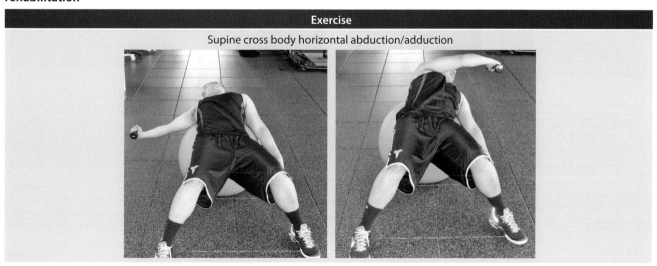

Exercise
Supine cross body horizontal abduction/adduction

Continued

Continued

Exercise

Prone stability ball shoulder dynamic flexion with oscillation

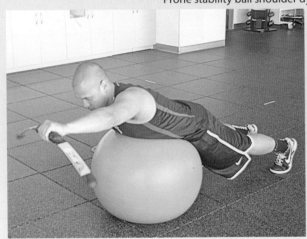 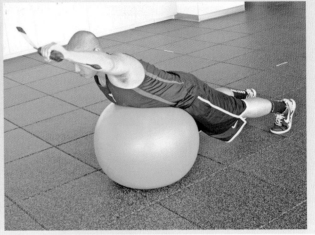

Bodyblade® oscillatory throw

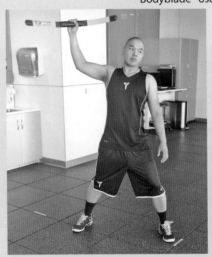 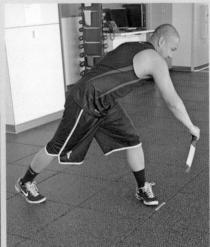

Bilateral dumbell swing

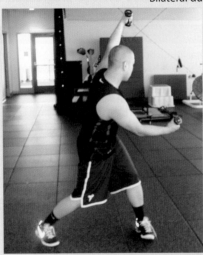 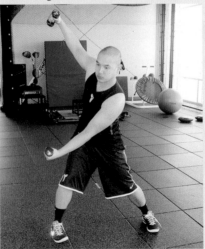

Continued

Continued

Exercise

Prone core dumbell extension

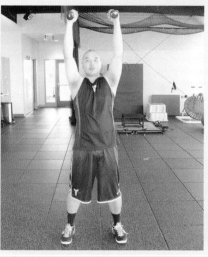 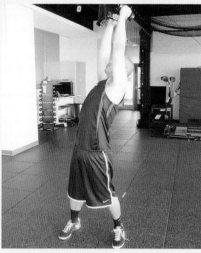

Eccentric overload rebound throw

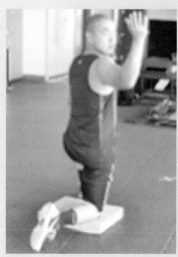 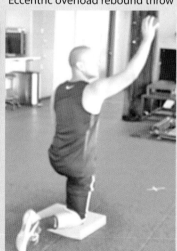 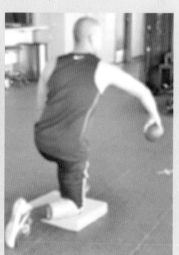

Medicine ball extension push

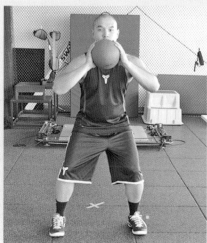 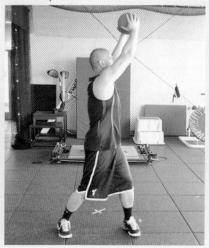

Continued

Continued

Exercise
Concentric/eccentric rebound throw

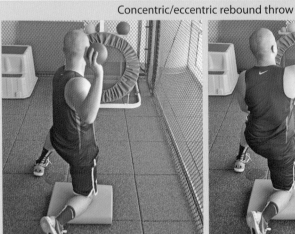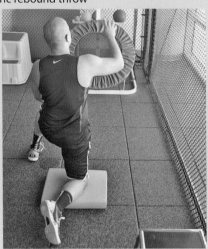

Two hand rebound throw and lateral push press

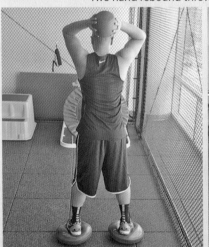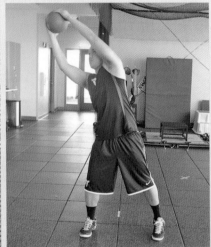

Standing medicine

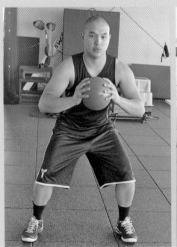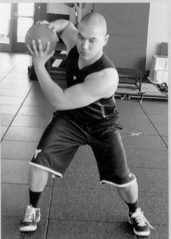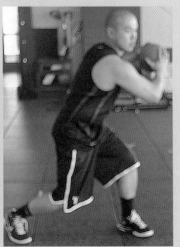

Continued

Continued

Medicine ball ground rebound plyo

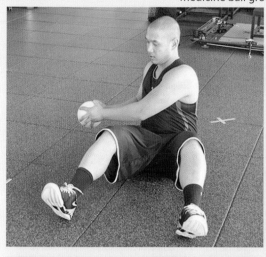 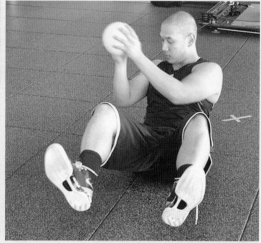

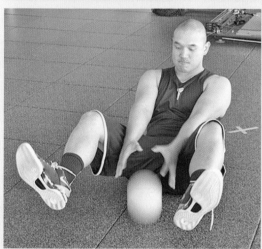 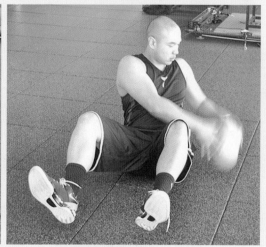

Rapid 90-90 concentric/eccentric rebound ball throw

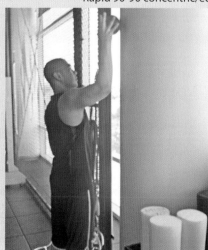 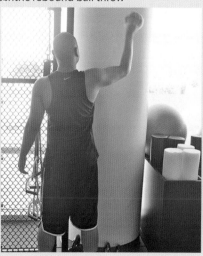

Continued

Continued

Exercise
90-90 concentric eccentric rebound full ball throw

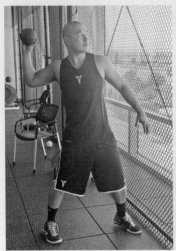 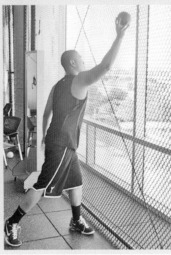 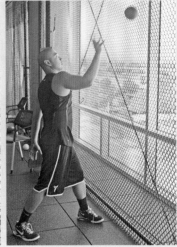

Prone skiers

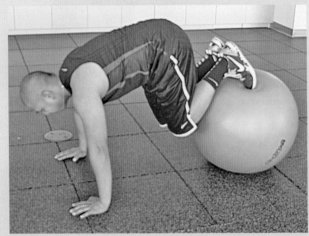 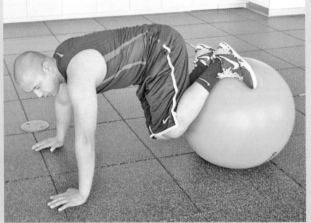

Prone stability ball hip extension

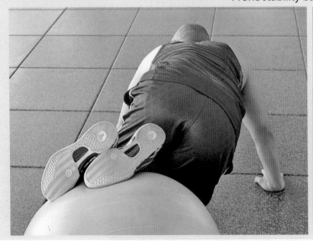 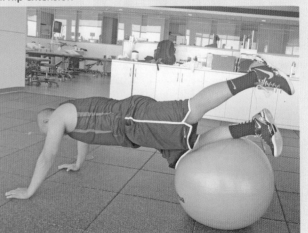

Continued

Continued

Exercise

Side plank with and without arm extension

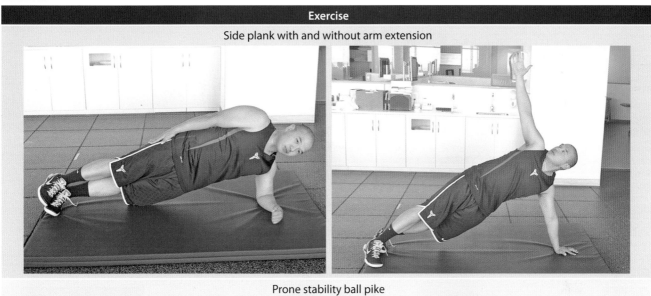

Prone stability ball pike

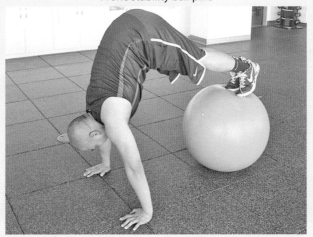

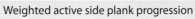
Weighted active side plank progression

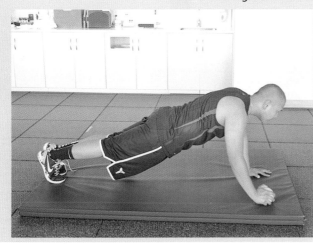 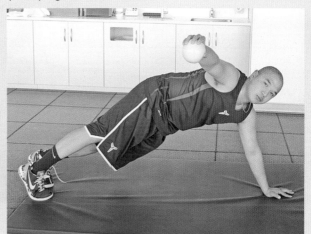

Continued

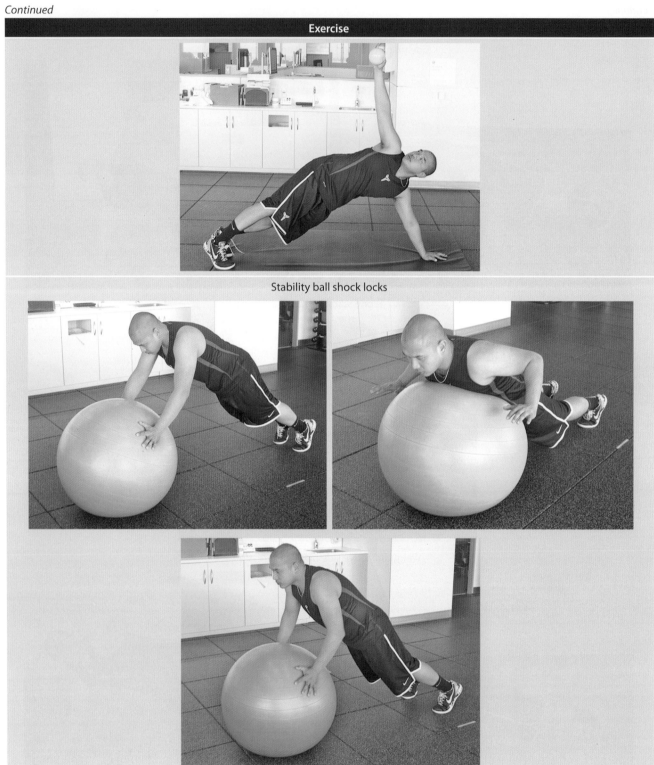

Exercise

Stability ball shock locks

Continued

Continued

Exercise
Stability ball seesaw

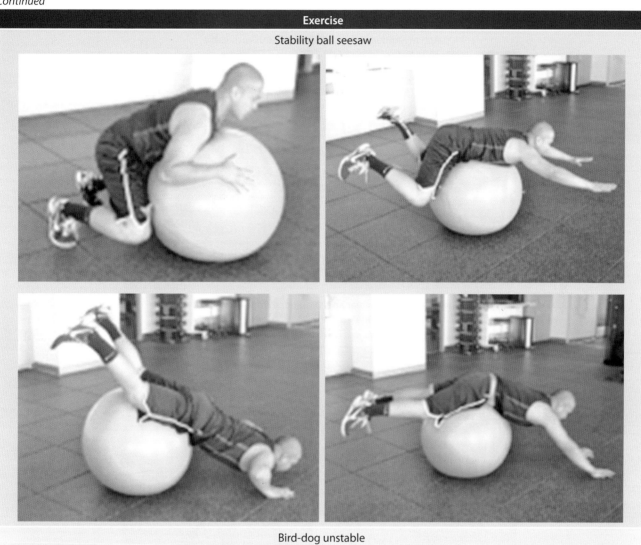

Bird-dog unstable

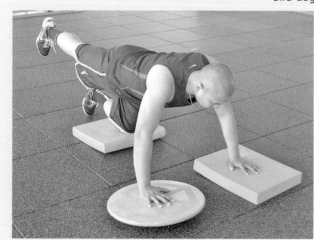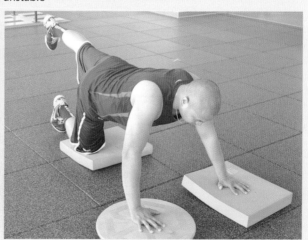

Continued

Continued

Exercise
Active lumbar and shoulder extension with cable

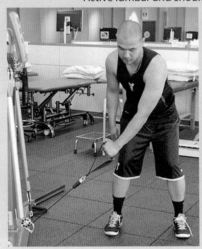 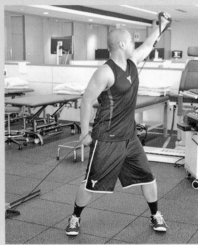

Single leg active lumbar and shoulder extension with cable

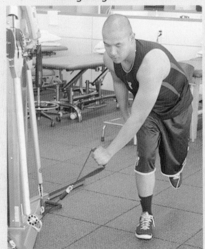 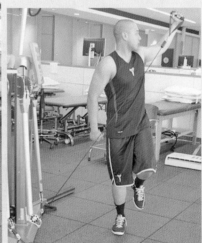

Standing 90-90 ER

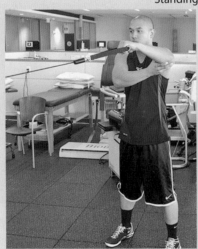 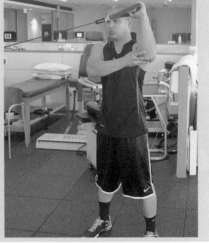

Continued

Continued

Exercise	
Bird-dog with oscillation	Statue of liberty
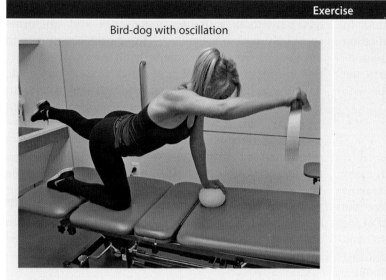	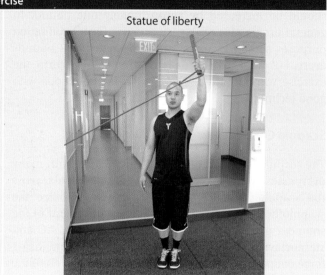

ER, external rotation.

too quickly, resulting in improper muscle activation. It is important to educate the patient regarding the role of the infraspinatus and teres minor musculature and the idea of increasing posterior dominance of the external rotators relative to the internal rotators. The external rotators should be 66–75% as strong as the internal rotators.[92] In healthy subjects, it appears adding weight too quickly underactivates the infraspinatus and overactivates the deltoids. The ideal range that maximally activates the infraspinatus in healthy subjects is approximately 10–40% of MVIC in the early phases of rehabilitation.[93] In another study, similar measurements were taken and exercises were applied to patients who exhibited symptomatic subacromial impingement. Similar findings were appreciated with a 70% load to MVIC ratio subsequently increasing the activation of the deltoids. These two studies, in symptomatic and asymptomatic individuals alike, indicate the ideal MVIC is 40% to maximally activate the external rotators and minimized deltoid activation in early rehabilitation.[47]

In general it is considered good practice to utilize a towel roll in standing and a pillow in side-lying positions to maximize infraspinatus activation and minimize deltoid activation.[74,94] From a biomechanical standpoint, placing the arm in 45° of horizontal abduction places the arm in an optimal length tension relationship allowing for maximal recruitment of the external rotators.[95] This also tends to be a comfortable position for the patient.

Eccentric training

Eccentric training may have a role in assisting with the resolution of RTC impingement. In the presence of symptoms consistent with impingement, there is a strong correlation with tendon degradation.[12,96,97] Eccentric training in the Achilles tendon has been shown to be very effective in treating the morphological and pain-related changes associated with Achilles tendinopathy.[98-106] In one shoulder study, a 12-weeks program of eccentric training, consisting of a muscle contractions which lasted for a greater duration during the eccentric component of the exercise, demonstrated improvements over the control group who performed the exercise at a normal duration of time.[107] Similarly, another 12-weeks study, consisting of eccentric exercise training in combination with scapular control exercises and correction of improper movement patterns, demonstrated effectiveness and a decrease in pain and improvements in overall function.[108] In both these studies, patients were consistently advised to work into pain, which did not exceed 5/10 on a visual analog scale. Concomitantly, pain from eccentric training should not appreciably increase from day-to-day. Furthermore, it should be explained to the patient that discomfort should be limited to muscle soreness, and not impingement-like symptoms (e.g. lateral deltoid pain). Also during the last set of 15 repetitions the patient should feel pain, which exceeds the pain at rest, but again it should not exceed more than 5/10 on the visual analog scale. When no pain is present during the last set of repetitions, the weight should be increased by approximately one pound. In general progressive resistance exercise for rehabilitation purposes should increase at approximately 1–2 pounds every 1–2 weeks if the patient is able to perform the exercise without fatigue through 12–15 repetitions with good technique.

Scapula Control

The scapula is similar to a major interchange with many overpasses. Many muscles connect to the scapula, cross the scapula, and act on the scapula to stabilize the scapulothoracic and GH joints. Proper movement of the shoulder girdle including the scapula, clavicle, AC and sternoclavicular junctions are critical to normalizing force couples, length tension relationships, and enabling the RTC and the surrounding musculature to adequately perform their job. In a study performed on elite junior tennis players, ultrasonographic measurements were taken. The study demonstrated that scapular dyskinesis can play a major role in subacromial space width statically, as well dynamically.[109] Clinically, for patients with subacromial impingement, scapular stabilization programs have been shown to be effective in increasing muscle strength, decreasing muscle fatigue, reducing scapular dyskinesis, improving function and functional outcome scores, and decreasing pain through strengthening and stretching exercises.[76,110-117] Similar to studies addressing the GH musculature fatigue characteristics, there is also research identifying fatigue-type characteristics in the scapular region. Typically these studies demonstrate that the scapula changes its orientation relative to the thorax. When scapular muscles are fatigued, the scapulohumeral rhythm changes and allows for destabilization of the scapula, particularly in the mid-range.[113,118] Fatigue impacts not only the resting position, but also the dynamic position of the scapula. This has negative consequences for muscles that reside around the GH and scapulothoracic regions with respect to length tension relationships, acromion to humeral head distance, and force imbalances. Fatigue may also lead to anteriorly tilted, forward protracted scapular position, progressing to posture related issues and decreased subacromial width.[41,44,113,117,118]

Similar to muscle specificity of the GH joint, there are many exercises to address scapulothoracic muscle weakness. One should be cautious when scapular mechanics are abnormal, as loading during traditional gym based exercises such as shoulder abduction, shoulder forward flexion, and shoulder scaption can perpetuate muscular imbalances and abnormal scapulothoracic mechanics.[119] These exercises appear to downwardly rotate and anteriorly tilt the scapula during the lowering phases of the exercise in symptomatic individuals, thus potentially placing undesirable loads on the shoulder. These exercises should either be avoided altogether—or, if necessary, be performed in the later phases of rehabilitation. For this subset of patients recommended exercises are those that specifically target the scapulothoracic musculature, and place the scapula in optimal positions of retraction, ER, with slight posterior tilting, and clavicular retraction and depression.[72,76,115] When performing retraction based exercises, certain arm and body positions can assist in obtaining these motions.[83]

Neuromuscular Control

Rehabilitation professionals emphasize proper mechanics when performing exercises. With shoulder exercises, proper mechanics emphasize scapular depression, shoulder retraction, and posterior tilting of the scapula during active elevation. These exercises are particularly relevant treating patients with impingement. Conscientious correction of the scapular region has been demonstrated to affect muscle activation, as well as clinically appear to decrease pain.[115] Another technique to consider is EMG biofeedback in patients with subacromial impingement. It has been demonstrated that biofeedback alters the balance of the scapular muscles, particularly during exercise, and has a positive effect on muscle balance ratios.[116] In patients with impingement, the RTC musculature coactivating with the deltoid demonstrate abnormalities during humeral head elevation when compared to controls. This dysfunctional coactivation may lead to encroachment in the subacromial space.[34] In a 10-weeks trial with motor control interventions targeted at correcting alignment and coordination, in combination with optimal shoulder resting position, improvements were noted in pain and function in patients presenting with impingement.[35]

Pain Associated with Concomitant Muscular Spasm and/or Fatigue

One complication associated with RTC impingement is the presence of musculature trigger points along the upper trapezius, levator scapulae, suboccipital, middle trapezius, rhomboids, RTC muscle bellies, and scalene regions. With pain, patients will have a tendency to guard and compensate with abnormal motions. In general, exercise seems to alleviate pain, particularly by reintroducing motion to these regions. Reintroduction of motion decreases trigger points and muscular spasm. Thus a concomitant reduction is appreciated. This added motion early in rehabilitation helps to also minimize the static positions a person may sustain from a neuromuscular standpoint. For instance, performing a shoulder shrug sign each time active forward elevation is performed has deleterious consequences for the shoulder and cervical muscles in this region. This may create an overuse situation for patients, potentially increasing hyperalgesia to the muscles being overused. In particular, the upper trapezius is innervated and is divided among motor and sensory inputs from the accessory nerve and the third and fourth cervical nerves. Patients with neck and shoulder pain demonstrate a change in the activation of the upper trapezius, which is secondary to issues related to the shoulder, such as subacromial impingement. Clinically, when these muscles are first activated, they may create some increased discomfort and delayed onset muscle soreness. However, over a 24-hour period, it appears this discomfort returns to baseline level and there is a shift in the H reflex recruitment curve to the right, indicating higher intensity of stimulation is required in evoking a future pain response. This is thought to occur by a decrease in the number of afferent axons stimulated or via increased presynaptic inhibition. Also of note is a decreased ability of the motor neuron pool to activate—changes are appreciated in the muscle fiber leading to decreased action potential and change in membrane properties.[120] Thus, controlled activation of muscles in the cervical region may be beneficial in controlling pain through the long-term recovery process. These controlled activities contrast the pattern of repetitive overuse of the muscles in this region, which increase the likelihood for trigger points, and muscle pain.

Manual Therapy

When discussing the physical therapy scientific literature, ultrasound, heat therapy, and most passive treatment approaches represent a preponderance of the research. Active treatment including therapeutic exercise as well as manual therapy represent less than 18% of all research performed.[121] Numerous research articles have demonstrated short-term effectiveness of manual interventions, particularly in addition to exercises-based therapies.[122-125] Some of the issues with the research surrounding manual therapy stems from the limited articles in the literature, specificity of the interventions performed, and the generalizations of diagnosis. Desmulues in 2003 reported a need in their systematic review for therapeutic exercise and manual therapy to be more specific and to have more internal validity to allow for better comparison of results. They emphasized the need for studies to focus on specific therapeutic methods, targeted at precise pathologies. In a more recent RCT, patients with chronic rotator cuff disease were followed for 22 weeks, where they were provided manual therapy and home exercises, and compared to a placebo group. In the short-term, it appeared that the manual therapy group appreciated no further benefit compared to the placebo group. However, by the end of the 22 weeks the active group demonstrated a greater improvement in the shoulder pain and disability index than the placebo group. This may indicate that manual therapy treatment effects may propagate over time and have an additive effect for functional gains. However, although not statistically significant, the active group did report greater frequency of successful outcomes at 11 weeks.[126] In another systematic review of shoulder dysfunction, a beneficial effect was appreciated in the short-term when utilizing massage and mobilization with movement (MWM). The combination of soft tissue and joint mobilization were also effective in patients with subacromial impingement, when combined with exercise. High-grade mobilizations were more effective than low-grade mobilizations, based on the Maitland grading scale.[127] In conclusion, it appears certain manual techniques have unique effects for the short term, and maintaining a manual based approach in the short term and midterm, will have long-term functional effects when combined with exercise therapies.[128]

Joint Mobilization Mechanics

It is quite common in clinical practice to see patients with impingement symptoms, and the etiology be mislabeled misidentified as frozen shoulder or adhesive capsulitis. This is no surprise, as studies indicate there is an educational gap from physicians in musculoskeletal evaluation and examination techniques.[129-132] More importantly there is a preponderance of nonspecific physician referrals when it pertains to musculoskeletal related issues.[133] When patients present with shoulder related issues, loss of motion is at the forefront of functional loss. This is particularly troublesome considering the GH joint has the greatest capacity of motion in the human body. This can be mitigated by a multitude of factors including pain, trauma, autoimmune disorders, inflammation, or true loss of motion from capsular shrinkage. In most instances however, the humeral head is unlikely kept centered and encroaches superiorly into glenoid fossa due to contractures globally as in adhesive capsulitis. However in impingement, the result of selective tissue contractures or hypomobilities in the capsular structures around the GH joint are likely responsible for these restrictions. Therefore RTC impingement is often misdiagnosed and seen when one appears to have motion limitations consistent with frozen shoulder; however, with more skilled evaluation it can be more appropriately classified as having impingement or other pathological shoulder symptoms with specific localized contracture decrements in motion. Harryman et al., in a classic study, described the effects of asymmetrically tightening the GH joint. They noted different effects from what is actually appreciated in shoulder kinematics of ball on socket movement (or a convex humeral head, rotating about a concave glenoid fossa). In Harryman's study, translation occurred anteriorly with forward flexion, and posteriorly with extension. Posterior translation was noted with ER and anterior translation was noted with cross body movements. The translation with flexion was considered obligate moving away from the line of tension in the capsule despite opposing normal arthrokinematics.[134] In other studies, joint conformity appears to have more effect when discussing active motions, with capsular restriction affecting more passive related motions. With passive ER, posterior and not anterior humeral head migration was seen.[135] This may be caused by the tension built up from the anterior band of the inferior GH ligament. During AROM, the compression of the humeral head and the force vectors of the RTC muscles as GH stabilizers may offset this translation to protect the capsuloligamentous structures.

When the humeral head begins to glide anteriorly, it creates dynamic ligament tension. As this tension develops from the anterior capsule it results in an ultimate posterior translation and thus a posterior and not anterior stabilizing glide form the clinician is required. This represents a shift from normal arthrokinematics, particularly with active motions. This dynamic ligament tension is likely caused by the interdigitation between the confluences of the RTC with the anterior capsule. With forward flexion, the humeral head translates an average of 9 mm superiorly and 4.4 mm anteriorly, between 20° and 90° of elevation.[136,137]

The rules of concave and convex have been taught for numerous years. These have helped guide our clinical decision-making. Despite evidence suggesting that with static and dynamic positions the variables of roll and glide change, one must be cautious in completely dispensing with these ideologies. The relative size of the humerus in relation to the glenoid rim would indicate that despite small amounts of superior and anterior translation, to accomplish normal mechanics there must be some convex on concave arthrokinematics in play to accommodate such motion, within such a relative small space. To more accurately quantify this, a recent study looked at 3-D/2-D modeling. Results indicated on average the humeral head translated —0.4–3.2 mm with an average of 2.1 mm, with respect to superior migration from neutral to 105° of elevation. From 105° and upward —0.9–2.9 mm in the inferior direction was appreciated. With internal and ER, the humerus rotated between 2° and 26°, with an average of 14°, from the resting position to 60° of elevation, and subsequently internally rotated from —1° to 20° from 75 to full elevation. This provides valuable insight into the complex motion the GH joint undergoes. Overall, the humerus translated superiorly with early forward flexion and then inferiorly in the late phases. With respect to internal and ER, the humerus rotates externally with early forward flexion, and reverses and rotates internally in the late phases of forward flexion.[39] This clearly demonstrates that mobilization techniques need to address restriction as evaluated in the shoulder. Our current understanding is more complex and may not be as simple as once appreciated, and these findings should be considered when applying manual interventions.

Shoulder Joint Mobilization Techniques

Much of the literature on treatment techniques for joint mobilization looks at the capsular structures. The posterior capsule was once thought to represent a significant restraint to normal motion in athletes. It is now understood that this is more than likely shortening of the RTC muscle.[84] Furthermore, if the posterior capsule does restrict motion in shoulder, how it does so, remains in question. Examination of the posterior capsule when held up to light, the tissue is translucent. It can be likened to a tissue, one wipes their nose with. Based on roll and glide principles to gain ER and forward flexion, which are typically the directions most limited in impingement as well as frozen shoulders, one must reconsider the way in which these principles are utilized. Traditionally, based on roll and glide principles, one would mobilize anteriorly to gain ER. An early study first looked at the concept of mobilizing posteriorly to gain ER and forward flexion in frozen shoulders. The participant received a sliding physical therapy manipulation Kaltenborn Grade III, then a Maitland grade 5 under an interscalene brachial plexus block. Excellent results were demonstrated with respect to pain and improvements in all aspects of ROM.[138] A more recent study found similar results with a posterior directed mobilization in adhesive capsulitis. Two groups with adhesive capsulitis were compared. The group with the anterior directed mobilization gained a mean of 3° of improvements, whereas the posteriorly directed mobilization group appreciated 31.3° improvement in ER ROM.[139] Furthermore, it appears that end range joint mobilization is significantly more effective than mid-range mobilization and passive modalities, as indicated by a RCT.[140] One must be careful not to generalize these results, as impingement is a very different etiology from frozen shoulder. It can be assumed that a frozen shoulder may not be selective in its capsular restriction and may actually shrink the entire capsule resulting in decreased anterior translation as well as decreases in the inferior axillary fold.

Overall questions have been raised about the effectiveness of mobilization in patients with shoulder issues. Although a homogenous grouping in one meta-analysis concluded that the addition of joint mobilization was more effective in treating shoulder-related issues when added to exercise, when compared to exercise alone.[141] Assuming for a moment that this simplistic view is true and posterior contracture is present, then there is still a question of magnitude of force and frequency of force to create a change at the capsular level. If the force applied or the frequency applied is too low, no effective change will occur. If the force or frequency is too high, permanent damage of the capsular structures may occur. When joint mobilizations are performed, more than likely, there are short-term transient effects due to the viscoelastic nature of tissues. Also there is the possibility of a change in neural output, which may also affect these positive results in the short term. In one such study, the author looked at the effect of cyclic loading and what magnitude and how intense the loads needed to be to create plastic deformation in capsular tissues. They compared 5N, 20N and 40N of force at the first oscillation, the 600th oscillation, and 1 hour after oscillation. Their findings suggest cyclic loading with 5N of force creates temporary changes in elongation of the capsule. However, no clinical treatment effect appeared

between the first and the 600th cycle.[142] Overall, it would be suggested that higher loads are required and one should gradually build up the oscillations throughout treatment to attain a sub failure change in tissue adaption at the point of the beginning of the linear region. This means sequential oscillations would be required up to the load of final resistance. Initially the goal may be to reduce pain through the use of lower grade joint mobilizations. Conroy et al. demonstrated pain reduction in patients with RTC impingement over a 24-hour period. The effect however was not enough to improve mobility or function.[143] In another trial, MWM was performed with Kinesio Tape™. The idea was that MWM realigns and provides appropriate force throughout the joints range to gain further pain free motion. The assumption with MWM is that subjects will gain motion by assisting with normal mechanics through the use of MWM. Questions arise as to whether MWMs can account for the huge variability in superior/inferior and internal/external changes throughout the range. If so, then this may provide an ideal manual treatment for ROM restrictions. Nonetheless this study demonstrated a positive effect for MWM on patients with a painful shoulder when compared to a supervised exercise program alone.[144] From a more athletic perspective, a recent study looked at posterior shoulder tightness stemming from the posterior shoulder muscles. Multiple authors have suggested that internal rotation (IR) ROM deficits may contribute to impingement like symptoms.[145] Manske et al. in a RCT demonstrated that a cross-body stretch alone or with the addition of joint mobilization in the posterior and anterior directions, both increased IR ROM in the asymptomatic college student.[85] Table 8 provides a list of soft tissue techniques utilized by the author of this chapter.

High Velocity Low Amplitude Thrust Manipulation

Many clinicians avoid spinal manipulation, particularly in acute injuries, because of the perception of tissue damage. They perceive high velocity low amplitude thrust (HVLAT) manipulation as something that can contribute to greater tissue damage. Despite this thinking, spinal manipulation is quite common in clinical practice. The relative risk from manipulation is quite low and the forces are minimal. The precise understanding of the effects of spinal manipulation on symptomology is not entirely understood. There are many proposed effects, including mechanical, neurophysiological, sympathetic nervous system response, motor excitation, changes

TABLE 8: Soft tissue techniques

Soft tissue technique	
Infraspinatus trigger point release	Upper trapezius inferior trigger point release
Tool assisted rhomboid/middle trapezius trigger point release	Tool assisted infrapsinatus trigger point release
Deltoid release (lateral and anterior)	Deltoid release (posterior)

Continued

Continued

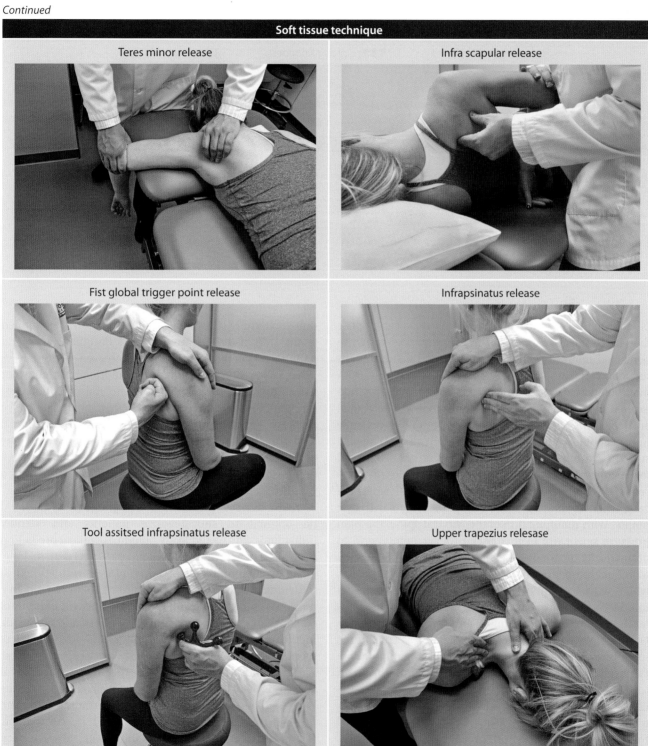

Continued

Continued

Soft tissue technique

T-Bar, 5 prong Knobber

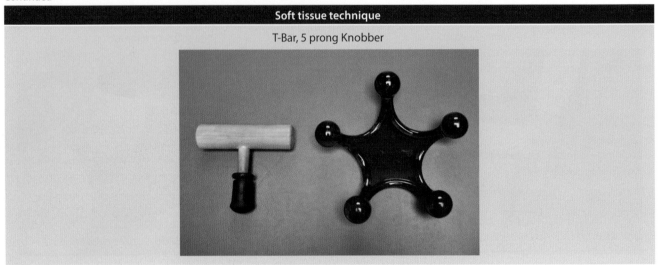

in neuropeptides and so on. It does however appear that mechanical response is in coordination with the perceived neurophysiologic response and a subsequent reduction of pain. One way the pain is reduced from manipulation, is through an increase in neuropeptide expression, which increases neurotensin, oxytocin, and cortisol.[146] Pain from shoulder pathology typically impacts not only the impaired tissue, but also the muscle structures around it. As discussed earlier, the likelihood for increased myofascial trigger points. Pain pressure sensitivity is highly prevalent from the clinical aspects of care, when evaluating and treating for muscular trigger points. With manipulation of the cervical spine, the pain pressure sensitivity in myofascial trigger points tend to dramatically decrease. Cervical manipulation appears to reduce pain pressure sensitivity in upper trapezius, which is a common generator of pain in shoulder injuries.[147] Despite having extremely low relative risk levels, on rare occasions, injury and soreness may occur. On the other hand, thoracic manipulation is considered to be less problematic then cervical spine manipulation. Cervicothoracic (CT) junction manipulation is thought to have a cascading effect, which addresses both the cervical spine and the thoracic regions and clinically has a high neurophysiologic effect. Increasingly, pain elicited from the CT region is more prevalent due to increases in technology-laden avenues of work and lifestyle. This leads to increases in CT joint restriction, with cervical and shoulder related pain in localized to this area.[148,149] The effects of manipulation on pain pressure threshold are not uniquely limited to patients experiencing pain. In one such study, CT junction manipulation was applied to the side of the healthy subject's dominant arm, and pain pressure thresholds were increased bilaterally.[150] When discussing manipulation, one must also consider the comparison of mobilization and manipulation. For example, mobilization of C5-C6 has been shown to increase ER strength of the shoulder musculature.[151] Additionally, it has been proposed that mobilization may be as effective as manipulation.[152] However, studies have demonstrated that HVLAT do appear to be favorable to nonthrust techniques.[153,154]

With respect to HVLAT and impingement, it would be optimal to subcategorize patients and identify individuals who would likely benefit. A clinical prediction rule has been formed to guide ones decision making. Factors which predict short-term success with HVLAT in individuals with shoulder pain are as follows: pain-free motion of shoulder flexion of at least 127°, shoulder IR of 53° at 90° of abduction, negative Neer Test, and not taking medications for their shoulder pain, and symptoms less than 90 days. If all the five criteria are present, success is 100%, and if only three criteria are met probability of success is 89%.[155] One must take caution, as these results have not been validated. It is also important to recognize the short-term effects of manipulation in the thoracic region and its connection to the shoulder girdle. One such study looked at the effects of two specific manipulations, a mid-thoracic and CT junction manipulation. If there was rib tenderness, a manipulation procedure was performed to the third rib. No pain was reported in the shoulder while performing the thoracic manipulations. In the short-term up to 48 hours after manipulation, there was a marked reduction in pain.[156] Multiple articles have looked at manipulations effect on shoulder dysfunction and have found similar results.[157-160] Table 9 provides a list of mobilization techniques utilized by the author of this chapter.

TABLE 9: Mobilization techniques

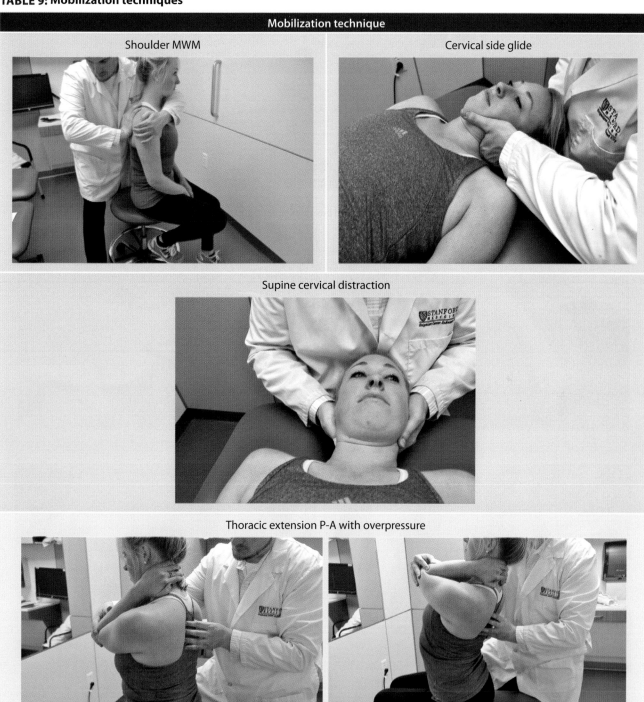

Continued

Continued

Mobilization technique

Thoracic rotation with overpressure

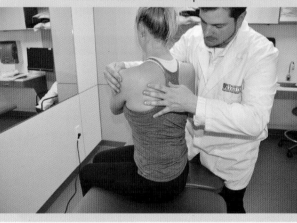

Glenohuemral lateral distraction

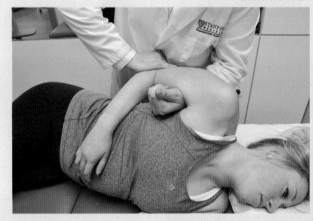
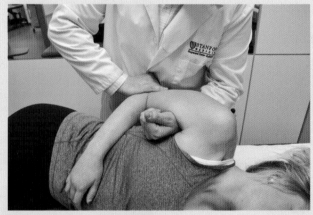

Clavicualr mobilizaiton

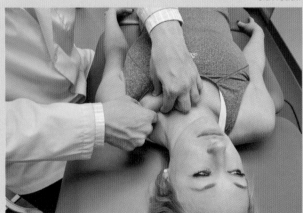
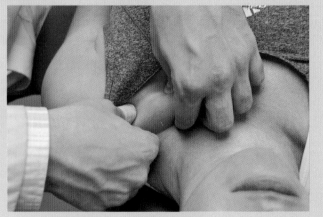

Continued

Continued

Mobilization technique

Inferior clavicualr mobilization

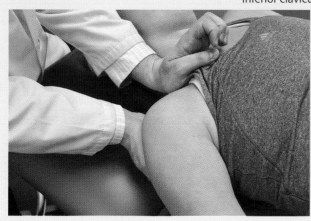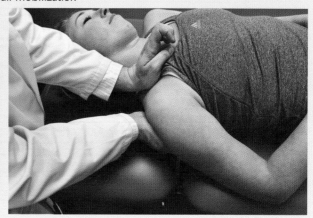

MWM, massage and mobilization with movement; P-A, posterior-to-anterior

Myofascial Trigger Points and Soft Tissue Mobilization

Myofascial trigger points can be defined simply as hypersensitive or hyperirritable regions, which are palpable in taut bands of skeletal muscle. They may be either latent or active.[161] Active trigger points appear during movement and may present spontaneously. Latent trigger points are only present at rest and cause discomfort with compression. In the muscle fiber itself there is thought to be sensitive loci (Nociceptive sensory component), and active loci (motor Components). When these loci are in the vicinity of each other, they form a myofascial trigger point (Fig. 5). Taut band formation is thought to stem from excessive release of intracellular calcium causing uncontrolled shortening and increased cellular metabolism. This impairs circulation, leading to oxygen deprivation and diminished nutrients to the muscular region, leading to energy crisis and taut band. There is also thought to be endplate and muscle spindle related issues with changes in sympathetic activity.[162] Questions exist as to whether taut bands exist. One study measured this with magnetic resonance elastography, which was able to determine asymmetries in muscle tone, which could previously only be appreciated with subjective exam and identification through imaging taut bands of tissue.[163] Bromn et al. studied clinician's ability to diagnose myofascial trigger points with palpation and demonstrated good inter-rater reliability in three different shoulder muscles.[164] Spot tenderness, pain identification, and taut band palpation appears to be the most reliable signs of diagnosing myofascial trigger points. Referred pain and localized twitch response provided the best confirmatory signs.[162] In patients presenting with unilateral subacromial impingement, it has been demonstrated that multiple trigger points exist in the shoulder muscle. Both local and referred pain were present within the multiple trigger points with palpation, as well as pressure sensitivity with increase in hyperalgesia in localized painful areas, and non-painful distally located regions. With greater pain intensity, greater quantities of trigger points were present. It is possible that trigger points are both, a centrally and peripherally mediated sensitization responses.[165] In another study with unilateral shoulder impingement, bilateral shoulder trigger points were present.[166] This may also represent biomechanical changes or central and peripheral sensitization responses.

Myofascial Treatment

The most commonly used form of treatment for trigger points is ischemic compression therapies. This consists of sustaining initially light pressure through the region of trigger points and taut bands. Typically this can be performed by placing the thumb on the taut area and sustaining pressure through the region. Then the pressure is gradually increased through the patient's maximum tolerable range, which will cause mild to moderate discomfort, but should be bearable to the patient. In one such example with shoulder pain, trigger points compressions were performed to the deltoid,

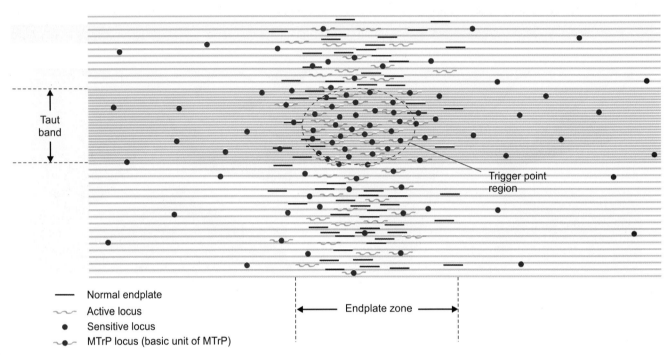

Normal endplate
Active locus
Sensitive locus
MTrP locus (basic unit of MTrP)

Taut band

Trigger point region

Endplate zone

FIG. 5: Sensitive loci and active loci around a myofascial trigger point (MTrP) region. It is hypothesized that a sensitive locus (nociceptor) may be associated with an active locus that is dysfunctional end-plates. Sensitive locus (sensory component) and active locus (motor component) may cause the formation of the basic unit of an MTrP[162]

Source: Reprinted with permission from Elsevier.

supraspinatus, and infraspinatus muscles. Results demonstrated substantial improvements in outcome scores.[167] In another study on office workers with neck and shoulder pain, ischemic compression therapy was performed for 4 weeks and elicited a marked reduction in pain both at 4 weeks and 6 months.[168] When performing ischemic compression, it has been demonstrated that patients with lower pain thresholds should receive lower pressure with longer durations of up to 90 seconds to achieve similar results. When higher pain threshold is recognized as short as 30 seconds may be sufficient to provide pain relief and trigger point sensitivity suppression.[169] To save the clinician's fingers, one may utilize tools to assist with ischemic compression therapy. Initially one may feel they cannot adequately localize trigger points, however with practice, adequate recognition can be felt through the utilization of a tool. To develop this skill, one may utilize their thumb for sensory feedback and then place the end of the tool on the spot found with a thumb.

Similar to ischemic compression therapy, pain pressure threshold may also be reduced through the use of Mulligan's MWM techniques. The utilization of MWM technique demonstrated improvements in ROM, as well as improved pain pressure threshold in the shoulder region in patients presenting with a painful shoulder.[170] The application of soft tissue mobilization and proprioceptive neuromuscular facilitation techniques also demonstrate significant improvements in patients with limited ROM immediately after application, in shoulder disorders.[171] Other therapeutic modalities which are beneficial in patients with myofascial pain are a combination of hot packs and AROM, transcutaneous electrical nerve stimulation and ischemic compression therapy, Gebauer's Stretch and Spray˚ technique, interferential current and myofascial release techniques.[169] Obviously these combinations represent the effectiveness of a multifaceted approach to address myofascial related shoulder pain. Table 10 provides a list of high velocity low amplitude thrust (HVLAT) techniques utilized by the author of this chapter.

Motor Strategies

With respect to motor strategies, pain has an impact on the coordination of movement. In one such study, when

TABLE 10: High velocity low amplitude thrust (HVLAT) manipulation techniques related to the shoulder

Manipulation technique

Prone cork-screw posterio-anterior (PA)

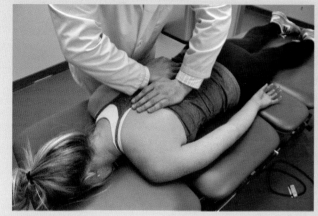 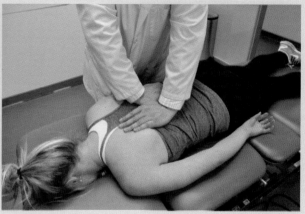

Prone central PA

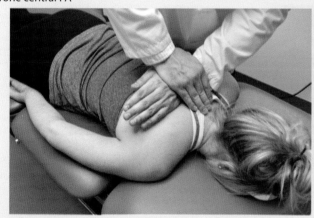 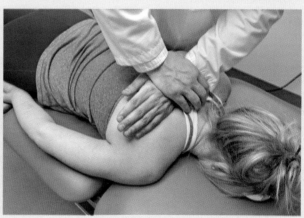

Mid-thoracic (T4-9) HVLA thrust manipulation (step 1–2)

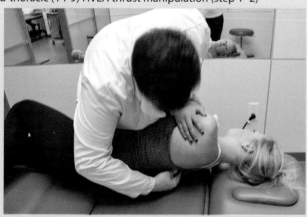 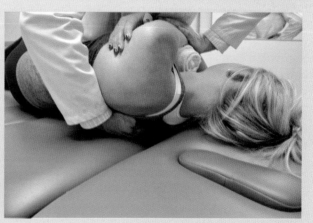

Continued

Continued

Manipulation technique

Mid-thoracic (T4-9) HVLA thrust manipulation (step 3–4)

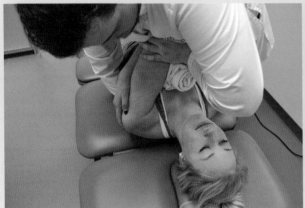
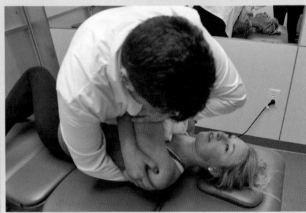

Upper thoracic (T1-3) HVLA thrust manipulation

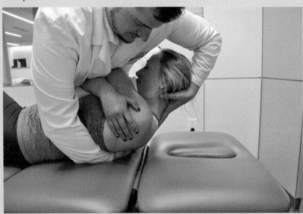

Seated thoracic extension manipulation

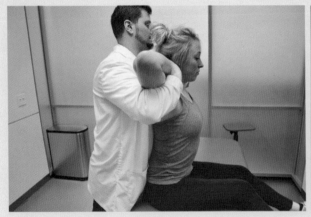
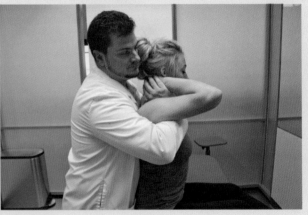

Continued

Continued

Manipulation technique

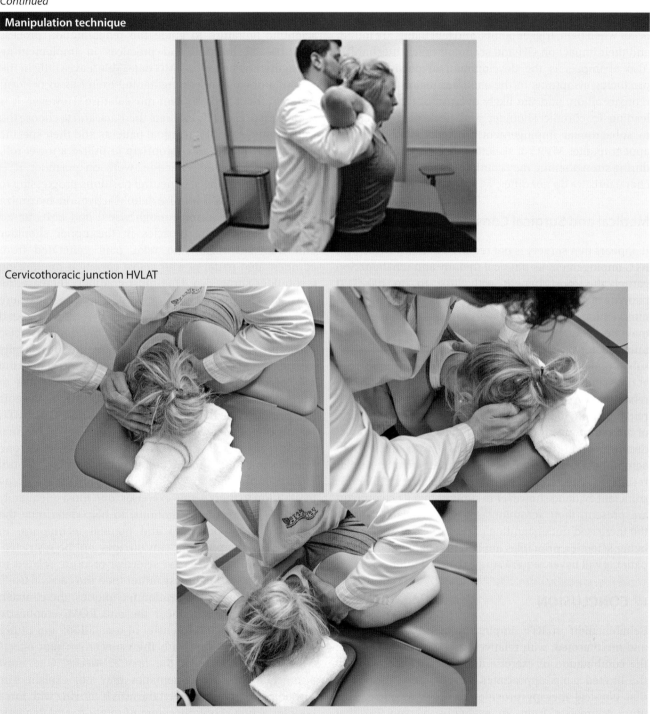

Cervicothoracic junction HVLAT

pain was experimentally created in the upper trapezius, a reorganization and coordination of the upper trapezius muscle was realized during repetitive movements. Furthermore, a decrease in EMG activity occurred in the upper division of the trapezius where the pain was localized, with increased EMG activity on the lower division. Also of note were altered motor strategies in the contralateral side.[172] This could have marked impact when one recognizes the contribution of skeletal muscles response to force couples and the changes which may occur when pain, trigger points, and taut bands are found, and their impact on GH and scapulothoracic mechanics. Also of impact is the development of persistent pain producing symptoms in the shoulder region due to this reorganization, and the likely overuse of these muscles leading to chronic shoulder and neck pain unrelated to subacromial impingement. This does not however appear to alter MVIC of skeletal muscle and normal use during strengthening may continue as muscle contractile characteristics do not differ.[173]

Medical and Surgical Considerations

It appears that surgery is not required in many cases with RTC impingement as physical therapy and rehabilitation garner the most benefit with little to no risk.[29] If patients are unsatisfied with the results of rehabilitation interventions, then further medical management may be required. Options include nonsteroidal anti-inflammatory medications, and injections into the subacromial space with corticosteroids. These options are at times utilized, in severe cases, while in the midst of the rehabilitation process, to allow for pain-free progression of rehabilitation, to ultimately address the underlying cause of the symptoms. If rehabilitation fails then subacromial decompression may be performed, with or without acromioplasty. Bursectomy alone appears to offer similar results to bursectomy with acromioplasty.[174] There is sufficient evidence however to support that if osteophytes are present, then acromioplasty is beneficial.[10] Due to the increased understanding of the issues, as well as the better scientific principles applied to rehabilitation, most patients will never require surgical intervention.

■ CONCLUSION

Rehabilitation of RTC impingement is both complex, and multifaceted, with relatively high success rates from the combination of exercise and manual therapy. With the limited gains appreciated from surgery, it appears that physical therapy provides the best recourse. One must appreciate from an evaluative perspective that although there are a plethora of tests that exist, accurate identification of impingement will drive accurate treatment. Differential diagnosis will be easier if one understands how to accurately rule in and rule pathology, through the use of special testing. Also while testing one must look for symptomology consistent with impingement,

such as lateral deltoid pain. There is also the possibility of proliferation of pain to the distal arm. There is substantial scientific literature to guide the rehabilitation process with best techniques and practices in implementing strengthening based on EMG data. This leaves little in the way of ambiguity on strengthening exercises to perform to target identified problem musculature. However, it is important to critically evaluate this data, and to choose the right strategies with individual patients and their specific deficits in mind. It is appropriate to utilize a towel roll, emphasize scapular retraction, work on posterior RTC strengthening initially, in neutral positions progressing to elevated positions, minimize deltoid activation, maximize neuromuscular control through visual and EMG based feedback, utilize the muscles in the upper shoulder and trapezius regions to relax pain generated from compensated patterns with active elevation minimizing a shoulder shrug sign. One must gradually increase the intensity, and yet overload the muscles to a degree where hypertrophic changes will take place. There is also a need to increase the volume of exercises as traditional exercise programs and medical exercise therapy do not typically provide enough resistance. One must appreciated the role of the scapula, and stabilizing the structures of the GH and scapulothoracic regions as this represents the primary mechanism by which one abolishes RTC impingement related pain. With respect to manual therapy, many styles of techniques work—whether one believes in changes to the tissue, neuromuscular control or just simple placebo. When performing manual therapy in addition to therapeutic exercises, one must adequately diagnose the restricted motions, to help determine the direction of mobilization and manual techniques. In many cases the posterior capsule may not be restricted. Restrictions may either be selective or more related to the posterior RTC tightness rather than the capsule itself. When performing mobilization techniques, the clinician should place the joint near the end ROM, emphasize a higher volume and intensity of oscillation, and utilize over a period of time with the expectation that effects will propagate through the first 22 weeks. One must appreciate that osteokinematics may not explain true physiological motions when the arm is moving with force couples acting about the center of rotation, and dynamic ligament tension affecting the movement. However an understanding of these mechanics can be important at least in isolation. Thoracic and cervical manipulation demonstrates a regional interdependence and can be performed to provide relief of symptoms and normalize mechanics within the thoracic and cervical region. This has a positive effect not only on pain, but on motion in the shoulder region. Myofascial trigger points can impact the upper trapezius to the occipital regions can present major challenges. Muscle activation in this region appears to help through exercise decreasing trigger points. If greater effect is required myofascial therapy is highly effective at decreasing trigger points and hyperalgesia in this region and has a positive impact on RTC impingement. The treatment progression in this chapter provides some insight into how to advance a patient through each phase of rehabilitation, and ultimately to attain a successful outcome for the vast majority of those suffering from RTC impingement.

REFERENCES

1. van der Windt DA, Koes BW, Boeke AJ, Deville W, De Jong BA, Bouter LM. Shoulder disorders in general practice: prognostic indicators of outcome. Br J Gen Pract. 1996;46(410):519-23.

2. Meislin RJ, Sperling JW, Stitik TP. Persistent shoulder pain: epidemiology, pathophysiology, and diagnosis. Am J Orthop (Belle Mead NJ). 2005;34(12):5-9.

3. Harris KD, Deyle GD, Gill NW, Howes RR. Manual physical therapy for injection-confirmed nonacute acromioclavicular joint pain. J Orthop Sports Phys Ther. 2012;42(2):66-80.

4. Brox JI, Gjengedal E, Uppheim G, Bøhmer AS, Brevik JI, Ljunggren AE, et al. Arthroscopic surgery versus supervised exercises in patients with rotator cuff disease (stage II impingement syndrome): a prospective, randomized, controlled study in 125 patients with a 2½-year follow-up. J Shoulder Elbow Surg. 1999;8(2):102-11.

5. Crawshaw DP, Helliwell PS, Hensor EM, Hay EM, Aldous SJ, Conaghan PG. Exercise therapy after corticosteroid injection for moderate to severe shoulder pain: large pragmatic randomised trial. BMJ. 2010;340:c3037.

6. Haahr JP, Ostergaard S, Dalsgaard J, Norup K, Frost P, Lausen S, et al. Exercises versus arthroscopic decompression in patients with subacromial impingement: a randomised, controlled study in 90 cases with a one year follow up. Ann Rheum Dis. 2005;64(5):760-4.

7. Jowett S, Crawshaw DP, Helliwell PS, Hensor EM, Hay EM, Conaghan PG. Cost-effectiveness of exercise therapy after corticosteroid injection for moderate to severe shoulder pain due to subacromial impingement syndrome: a trial-based analysis. Rheumatology (Oxford). 2013;52(8):1485-91.

8. Neer CS. Anterior acromioplasty for the chronic impingement syndrome in the shoulder: a preliminary report. J Bone Joint Surg Am. 1972;54(1):41-50.

9. Bigliani LU, Codd TP, Connor PM, Levine WN, Littlefield MA, Hershon SJ. Shoulder motion and laxity in the professional baseball player. Am J Sports Med. 1997;25(5):609-13.

10. Bigliani LU, Levine WN. Subacromial impingement syndrome. J Bone Joint Surg Am. 1997;79(12):1854-68.

11. Michener LA, McClure PW, Karduna AR. Anatomical and biomechanical mechanisms of subacromial impingement syndrome. Clin Biomech (Bristol, Avon). 2003;18(5):369-79.

12. Uhthoff HK, Trudel G, Himori K. Relevance of pathology and basic research to the surgeon treating rotator cuff disease. J Orthop Sci. 2003;8(3):449-56.

13. Umer M, Qadir I, Azam M. Subacromial impingement syndrome. Orthop Rev (Pavia). 2012;4(2):e18.

14. Flatow EL, Soslowsky LJ, Ticker JB, Pawluk RJ, Hepler M, Ark J, et al. Excursion of the rotator cuff under the acromion. Patterns of subacromial contact. Am J Sports Med. 1994;22(6):779-88.

15. Reddy AS, Mohr KJ, Pink MM, Jobe FW. Electromyographic analysis of the deltoid and rotator cuff muscles in persons with subacromial impingement. J Shoulder Elbow Surg. 2000;9(6):519-23.

16. San Juan JG, Kosek P, Karduna AR. Humeral head translation after a suprascapular nerve block. J Appl Biomech. 2013;29(4):371-9.

17. Chopp JN, O'Neill JM, Hurley K, Dickerson CR. Superior humeral head migration occurs after a protocol designed to fatigue the rotator cuff: a radiographic analysis. J Shoulder Elbow Surg. 2010;19(8):1137-44.

18. Saccol MF, Gracitelli GC, da Silva RT, Laurino CF, Fleury AM, Andrade Mdos S, et al. Shoulder functional ratio in elite junior tennis players. Phys Ther Sport. 2010;11(1):8-11.

19. Stackhouse SK, Eisennagel A, Eisennagel J, Lenker H, Sweitzer BA, McClure PW. Experimental pain inhibits infraspinatus activation during isometric external rotation. J Shoulder Elbow Surg. 2013;22(4):478-84.

20. Gerber C, Galantay RV, Hersche O. The pattern of pain produced by irritation of the acromioclavicular joint and the subacromial space. J Shoulder Elbow Surg. 1998;7(4):352-5.

21. Childs JD, Cleland JA. Development and application of clinical prediction rules to improve decision making in physical therapist practice. Phys Ther. 2006;86(1):122-31.

22. Davis DS, Anderson IB, Carson MG, Elkins CL, Stuckey LB. Upper limb neural tension and seated slump tests: the false positive rate among healthy young adults without cervical or lumbar symptoms. J Man Manip Ther. 2008;16(3):136-41.

23. Nee RJ, Jull GA, Vicenzino B, Coppieters MW. The validity of upper-limb neurodynamic tests for detecting peripheral neuropathic pain. J Orthop Sports Phys Ther. 2012;42(5):413-24.

24. Wainner RS, Fritz JM, Irrgang JJ, Boninger ML, Delitto A, Allison S. Reliability and diagnostic accuracy of the clinical examination and patient self-report measures for cervical radiculopathy. Spine (Phila Pa 1976). 2003;28(1):52-62.

25. Waldrop MA. Diagnosis and treatment of cervical radiculopathy using a clinical prediction rule and a multimodal intervention approach: a case series. J Orthop Sports Phys Ther. 2006;36(3):152-9.

26. Greenberg DL. Evaluation and treatment of shoulder pain. Med Clin North Am. 2014;98(3):487-504.

27. Park HB, Yokota A, Gill HS, El Rassi G, McFarland EG. Diagnostic accuracy of clinical tests for the different degrees of subacromial impingement syndrome. J Bone Joint Surg Am. 2005;87(7):1446-55.

28. Biederwolf NE. A proposed evidence-based shoulder special testing examination algorithm: clinical utility based on a systematic review of the literature. Int J Sports Phys Ther. 2013;8(4):427-40.

29. Morrison DS, Frogameni AD, Woodworth P. Non-operative treatment of subacromial impingement syndrome. J Bone Joint Surg Am. 1997;79(5):732-7.

30. Wilk KE, Arrigo CA, Andrews JR. Current concepts: the stabilizing structures of the glenohumeral joint. J Orthop Sports Phys Ther. 1997;25(6):364-79.

31. Hanratty CE, McVeigh JG, Kerr DP, Basford JR, Finch MB, Pendleton A, et al. The effectiveness of physiotherapy exercises in subacromial impingement syndrome: a systematic review and meta-analysis. Semin Arthritis Rheum. 2012;42(3):297-316.

32. Ludewig PM, Braman JP. Shoulder impingement: biomechanical considerations in rehabilitation. Man Ther. 2011;16(1):33-9.

33. Ludewig PM, Cook TM. Translations of the humerus in persons with shoulder impingement symptoms. J Orthop Sports Phys Ther. 2002;32(6):248-59.

34. Myers JB, Hwang JH, Pasquale MR, Blackburn JT, Lephart SM. Rotator cuff coactivation ratios in participants with subacromial impingement syndrome. J Sci Med Sport. 2009;12(6):603-8.

35. Worsley P, Warner M, Mottram S, Gadola S, Veeger HE, Hermens H, et al. Motor control retraining exercises for shoulder impingement: effects on function, muscle activation, and biomechanics in young adults. J Shoulder Elbow Surg. 2013;22(4):e11-9.

36. Royer PJ, Kane EJ, Parks KE, Morrow JC, Moravec RR, Christie DS, et al. Fluoroscopic assessment of rotator cuff fatigue on glenohumeral arthrokinematics in shoulder impingement syndrome. J Shoulder Elbow Surg. 2009;18(6):968-75.

37. Teyhen DS, Miller JM, Middag TR, Kane EJ. Rotator cuff fatigue and glenohumeral kinematics in participants without shoulder dysfunction. J Athl Train. 2008;43(4):352-8.

38. Chen SK, Simonian PT, Wickiewicz TL, Otis JC, Warren RF. Radiographic evaluation of glenohumeral kinematics: a muscle fatigue model. J Shoulder Elbow Surg. 1999;8(1):49-52.

39. Matsuki K, Matsuki KO, Yamaguchi S, Ochiai N, Sasho T, Sugaya H, et al. Dynamic in vivo glenohumeral kinematics during scapular plane abduction in healthy shoulders. J Orthop Sports Phys Ther. 2012;42(2):96-104.

40. Teece RM, Lunden JB, Lloyd AS, Kaiser AP, Cieminski CJ, Ludewig PM. Three-dimensional acromioclavicular joint motions during elevation of the arm. J Orthop Sports Phys Ther. 2008;38(4):181-90.

41. Finley MA, Lee RY. Effect of sitting posture on 3-dimensional scapular kinematics measured by skin-mounted electromagnetic tracking sensors. Arch Phys Med Rehabil. 2003;84(4):563-8.

42. Kalra N, Seitz AL, Boardman ND, Michener LA. Effect of posture on acromiohumeral distance with arm elevation in subjects with and without rotator cuff disease using ultrasonography. J Orthop Sports Phys Ther. 2010;40(10):633-40.

43. Kebaetse M, McClure P, Pratt NA. Thoracic position effect on shoulder range of motion, strength, and three-dimensional scapular kinematics. Arch Phys Med Rehabil. 1999;80(8):945-50.

44. Lewis JS, Wright C, Green A. Subacromial impingement syndrome: the effect of changing posture on shoulder range of movement. J Orthop Sports Phys Ther. 2005;35(2):72-87.

45. Farshad M, Jundt-Ecker M, Sutter R, Schubert M, Gerber C. Does subacromial injection of a local anesthetic influence strength in healthy shoulders?: a double-blinded, placebo-controlled study. J Bone Joint Surg Am. 2012;94(19):1751-5.

46. Halder AM, Zhao KD, Odriscoll SW, Morrey BF, An KN. Dynamic contributions to superior shoulder stability. J Orthop Res. 2001;19(2):206-12.

47. Clisby EF, Bitter NL, Sandow MJ, Jones MA, Magarey ME, Jaberzadeh S. Relative contributions of the infraspinatus and deltoid during external rotation in patients with symptomatic subacromial impingement. J Shoulder Elbow Surg. 2008;17(1):87S-92S.

48. Escamilla RF, Andrews JR. Shoulder muscle recruitment patterns and related biomechanics during upper extremity sports. Sports Med. 2009;39(7):569-90.

49. Escamilla RF, Barrentine SW, Fleisig GS, Zheng N, Takada Y, Kingsley D, et al. Pitching biomechanics as a pitcher approaches muscular fatigue during a simulated baseball game. Am J Sports Med. 2007;35(1):23-33.

50. Hopkins JT, Ingersoll CD, Krause BA, Edwards JE, Cordova ML. Effect of knee joint effusion on quadriceps and soleus motoneuron pool excitability. Med Sci Sports Exerc. 2001;33(1):123-6.

51. Palmieri-Smith RM, Villwock M, Downie B, Hecht G, Zernicke R. Pain and effusion and quadriceps activation and strength. J Athl Train. 2013;48(2):186-91.

52. Fortin M, Macedo LG. Multifidus and paraspinal muscle group cross-sectional areas of patients with low back pain and control patients: a systematic review with a focus on blinding. Phys Ther. 2013;93(7):873-88.

53. Ploumis A, Michailidis N, Christodoulou P, Kalaitzoglou I, Gouvas G, Beris A. Ipsilateral atrophy of paraspinal and psoas muscle in unilateral back pain patients with monosegmental degenerative disc disease. Br J Radiol. 2011;84(1004):709-13.

54. Ylinen J, Vuorenmaa M, Paloneva J, Kiviranta I, Kautiainen H, Oikari M, et al. Exercise therapy is evidence-based treatment of shoulder impingement syndrome. Current practice or recommendation only. Eur J Phys Rehabil Med. 2013;49(4):499-505.

55. Davies GJ, Ellenbecker TS. Documentation enhances understanding of shoulder function. Biomechanics. 1999:6;47-55.

56. Davies GJ, Ellenbecker TS. Focused exercise aids shoulder hypomobility. Biomechanics. 1999:6;77-81.

57. Nicola F, Catherine S. Dose-response relationship of resistance training in older adults: a meta-analysis. Br J Sports Med. 2011;45(3):233-4.

58. Steib S, Schoene D, Pfeifer K. Dose-response relationship of resistance training in older adults: a meta-analysis. Med Sci Sports Exerc. 2010;42(5):902-14.

59. Osteras H, Torstensen TA. The dose-response effect of medical exercise therapy on impairment in patients with unilateral longstanding subacromial pain. Open Orthop J. 2010;4:1-6.

60. Andersen LL, Jorgensen MB, Blangsted AK, Pedersen MT, Hansen EA, Sjogaard G. A randomized controlled intervention trial to relieve and prevent neck/shoulder pain. Med Sci Sports Exerc. 2008;40(6):983-90.

61. Kell RT, Risi AD, Barden JM. The response of persons with chronic nonspecific low back pain to three different volumes of periodized musculoskeletal rehabilitation. J Strength Cond Res. 2011;25(4):1052-64.

62. Kristensen J, Franklyn-Miller A. Resistance training in musculoskeletal rehabilitation: a systematic review. Br J Sports Med. 2012;46(10):719-26.

63. Pedersen MT, Andersen LL, Jorgensen MB, Sogaard K, Sjogaard G. Effect of specific resistance training on musculoskeletal pain symptoms: dose-response relationship. J Strength Cond Res. 2013;27(1):229-35.

64. Townsend H, Jobe FW, Pink M, Perry J. Electromyographic analysis of the glenohumeral muscles during a baseball rehabilitation program. Am J Sports Med. 1991;19(3):264-72.

65. Koes BW, van Tulder MW, Ostelo R, Kim Burton A, Waddell G. Clinical guidelines for the management of low back pain in primary care: an international comparison. Spine (Phila Pa 1976). 2001;26(22):2504-13; discussion 2513-4.

66. Moseley JB, Jobe FW, Pink M, Perry J, Tibone J. EMG analysis of the scapular muscles during a shoulder rehabilitation program. Am J Sports Med. 1992;20(2):128-34.

67. Blackburn T, McLeod W, White B, Wofford L. EMG Analysis of Posterior Rotator Cuff Exercises. Athletic Training. 1990;25(1):40-5.

68. David G, Magarey ME, Jones MA, Dvir Z, Turker KS, Sharpe M. EMG and strength correlates of selected shoulder muscles during rotations of the glenohumeral joint. Clin Biomech (Bristol, Avon). 2000;15(2):95-102.

69. Decker MJ, Tokish JM, Ellis HB, Torry MR, Hawkins RJ. Subscapularis muscle activity during selected rehabilitation exercises. Am J Sports Med. 2003;31(1):126-34.

70. Ekstrom RA, Donatelli RA, Soderberg GL. Surface electromyographic analysis of exercises for the trapezius and serratus anterior muscles. J Orthop Sports Phys Ther. 2003;33(5):247-58.

71. Escamilla RF, Yamashiro K, Paulos L, Andrews JR. Shoulder muscle activity and function in common shoulder rehabilitation exercises. Sports Med. 2009;39(8):663-85.

72. Lear LJ, Gross MT. An electromyographical analysis of the scapular stabilizing synergists during a push-up progression. J Orthop Sports Phys Ther. 1998;28(3):146-57.

73. Reinold MM, Escamilla RF, Wilk KE. Current concepts in the scientific and clinical rationale behind exercises for glenohumeral and scapulothoracic musculature. J Orthop Sports Phys Ther. 2009;39(2):105-17.

74. Reinold MM, Wilk KE, Fleisig GS, Zheng N, Barrentine SW, Chmielewski T, et al. Electromyographic analysis of the rotator cuff and deltoid musculature during common shoulder external rotation exercises. J Orthop Sports Phys Ther. 2004;34(7):385-94.

75. De Mey K, Danneels L, Cagnie B, Cools AM. Scapular muscle rehabilitation exercises in overhead athletes with impingement symptoms: effect of a 6-week training program on muscle recruitment and functional outcome. Am J Sports Med. 2012;40(8):1906-15.

76. Kibler WB, Ludewig PM, McClure P, Uhl TL, Sciascia A. Scapular Summit 2009: introduction. July 16, 2009, Lexington, Kentucky. J Orthop Sports Phys Ther. 2009;39(11):A1-A13.

77. Kibler WB, Sciascia AD, Uhl TL, Tambay N, Cunningham T. Electromyographic analysis of specific exercises for scapular control in early phases of shoulder rehabilitation. Am J Sports Med. 2008;36(9):1789-98.

78. Lee S, Lee D, Park J. The effect of hand position changes on electromyographic activity of shoulder stabilizers during push-up plus exercise on stable and unstable surfaces. J Phys Ther Sci. 2013;25(8):981-4.

79. Maenhout A, Van Praet K, Pizzi L, Van Herzeele M, Cools A. Electromyographic analysis of knee push up plus variations: what is the influence of the kinetic chain on scapular muscle activity? Br J Sports Med. 2010;44(14):1010-5.

80. Ghodadra NS, Provencher MT, Verma NN, Wilk KE, Romeo AA. Open, mini-open, and all-arthroscopic rotator cuff repair surgery: indications and implications for rehabilitation. J Orthop Sports Phys Ther. 2009;39(2):81-9.

81. Irlenbusch U, Gansen HK. Muscle biopsy investigations on neuromuscular insufficiency of the rotator cuff: a contribution to the functional impingement of the shoulder joint. J Shoulder Elbow Surg. 2003;12(5):422-6.

82. Arora S, Button DC, Basset FA, Behm DG. The effect of double versus single oscillating exercise devices on trunk and limb muscle activation. Int J Sports Phys Ther. 2013;8(4):370-80.

83. Oyama S, Myers JB, Wassinger CA, Lephart SM. Three-dimensional scapular and clavicular kinematics and scapular muscle activity during retraction exercises. J Orthop Sports Phys Ther. 2010;40(3):169-79.

84. Manske R, Wilk KE, Davies G, Ellenbecker T, Reinold M. Glenohumeral motion deficits: friend or foe? Int J Sports Phys Ther. 2013;8(5):537-53.

85. Manske RC, Meschke M, Porter A, Smith B, Reiman M. A randomized controlled single-blinded comparison of stretching versus stretching and joint mobilization for posterior shoulder tightness measured by internal rotation motion loss. Sports Health. 2010;2(2):94-100.

86. Borstad JD, Ludewig PM. The effect of long versus short pectoralis minor resting length on scapular kinematics in healthy individuals. J Orthop Sports Phys Ther. 2005;35(4):227-38.

87. Escamilla RF, Hooks TR, Wilk KE. Optimal management of shoulder impingement syndrome. Open Access J Sports Med. 2014;5:13-24.

88. Ellenbecker TS, Davies GJ. The application of isokinetics in testing and rehabilitation of the shoulder complex. J Athl Train. 2000;35(3):338-50.

89. Kelley MJ, Shaffer MA, Kuhn JE, Michener LA, Seitz AL, Uhl TL, et al. Shoulder pain and mobility deficits: adhesive capsulitis. J Orthop Sports Phys Ther. 2013;43(5):A1-31.

90. Kelley MJ, McClure PW, Leggin BG. Frozen shoulder: evidence and a proposed model guiding rehabilitation. J Orthop Sports Phys Ther. 2009;39(2):135-48.

91. Long JL, Ruberte Thiele RA, Skendzel JG, et al. Activation of the shoulder musculature during pendulum exercises and light activities. J Orthop Sports Phys Ther. 2010;40(4):230-7.

92. Wilk KE, Meister K, Andrews JR. Current concepts in the rehabilitation of the overhead throwing athlete. Am J Sports Med. 2002;30(1):136-51.

93. Bitter NL, Clisby EF, Jones MA, Magarey ME, Jaberzadeh S, Sandow MJ. Relative contributions of infraspinatus and deltoid during external rotation in healthy shoulders. J Shoulder Elbow Surg. 2007;16(5):563-8.

94. Graichen H, Hinterwimmer S, von Eisenhart-Rothe R, Vogl T, Englmeier KH, Eckstein F. Effect of abducting and adducting muscle activity on glenohumeral translation, scapular kinematics and subacromial space width in vivo. J Biomech. 2005;38(4):755-60.

95. Kelly BT, Kadrmas WR, Speer KP. The manual muscle examination for rotator cuff strength. An electromyographic investigation. Am J Sports Med. 1996;24(5):581-8.

96. Hegedus EJ, Cook C, Brennan M, Wyland D, Garrison JC, Driesner D. Vascularity and tendon pathology in the rotator cuff: a review of literature and implications for rehabilitation and surgery. Br J Sports Med. 2010;44(12):838-47.

97. Tempelhof S, Rupp S, Seil R. Age-related prevalence of rotator cuff tears in asymptomatic shoulders. J Shoulder Elbow Surg. 1999;8(4):296-9.

98. Alfredson H, Ohberg L, Forsgren S. Is vasculo-neural ingrowth the cause of pain in chronic Achilles tendinosis? An investigation using ultrasonography and colour Doppler, immunohistochemistry, and diagnostic injections. Knee Surg Sports Traumatol Arthrosc. 2003;11(5):334-8.

99. Alfredson H, Pietila T, Jonsson P, Lorentzon R. Heavy-load eccentric calf muscle training for the treatment of chronic Achilles tendinosis. Am J Sports Med. 1998;26(3):360-6.

100. Allison GT, Purdam C. Eccentric loading for Achilles tendinopathy--strengthening or stretching? Br J Sports Med. 2009;43(4):276-9.

101. Arya S, Kulig K. Tendinopathy alters mechanical and material properties of the Achilles tendon. J Appl Physiol. 2010;108(3):670-5.

102. Fahlstrom M, Jonsson P, Lorentzon R, Alfredson H. Chronic Achilles tendon pain treated with eccentric calf-muscle training. Knee Surg Sports Traumatol Arthrosc. 2003;11(5):327-33.

103. Grigg NL, Wearing SC, Smeathers JE. Eccentric calf muscle exercise produces a greater acute reduction in Achilles tendon thickness than concentric exercise. Br J Sports Med. 2009;43(4):280-3.

104. Langberg H, Ellingsgaard H, Madsen T, Jansson J, Magnusson SP, Aagaard P, et al. Eccentric rehabilitation exercise increases peritendinous type I collagen synthesis in humans with Achilles tendinosis. Scand J Med Sci Sports. 2007;17(1):61-6.

105. Mahieu NN, McNair P, Cools A, D'Haen C, Vandermeulen K, Witvrouw E. Effect of eccentric training on the plantar flexor muscle-tendon tissue properties. Med Sci Sports Exerc. 2008;40(1):117-23.

106. Norregaard J, Larsen CC, Bieler T, Langberg H. Eccentric exercise in treatment of Achilles tendinopathy. Scand J Med Sci Sports. 2007;17(2):133-8.

107. Maenhout AG, Mahieu NN, De Muynck M, De Wilde LF, Cools AM. Does adding heavy load eccentric training to rehabilitation of patients with unilateral subacromial impingement result in better outcome? A randomized, clinical trial. Knee Surg Sports Traumatol Arthrosc. 2013; 21(5):1158-67.

108. Bernhardsson S, Klintberg IH, Wendt GK. Evaluation of an exercise concept focusing on eccentric strength training of the rotator cuff for patients with subacromial impingement syndrome. Clin Rehabil. 2011;25(1):69-78.

109. Silva RT, Hartmann LG, Laurino CF, Bilo JP. Clinical and ultrasonographic correlation between scapular dyskinesia and subacromial space measurement among junior elite tennis players. Br J Sports Med. 2010; 44(6):407-10.

110. Baskurt Z, Baskurt F, Gelecek N, Ozkan MH. The effectiveness of scapular stabilization exercise in the patients with subacromial impingement syndrome. J Back Musculoskelet Rehabil. 2011;24(3):173-9.

111. Cools AM, Dewitte V, Lanszweert F, Notebaert D, Roets A, Soetens B, et al. Rehabilitation of scapular muscle balance: which exercises to prescribe? Am J Sports Med. 2007;35(10):1744-51.

112. Cools AM, Johansson FR, Cambier DC, Velde AV, Palmans T, Witvrouw EE. Descriptive profile of scapulothoracic position, strength and flexibility variables in adolescent elite tennis players. Br J Sports Med. 2010;44(9): 678-84.

113. Cools AM, Struyf F, De Mey K, Maenhout A, Castelein B, Cagnie B. Rehabilitation of scapular dyskinesis: from the office worker to the elite overhead athlete. Br J Sports Med. 2014;48(8):692-7.

114. Cools AM, Witvrouw EE, De Clercq GA, Danneels LA, Willems TM, Cambier DC, et al. Scapular muscle recruitment pattern: electromyographic response of the trapezius muscle to sudden shoulder movement before and after a fatiguing exercise. J Orthop Sports Phys Ther. 2002;32(5):221-9.

115. De Mey K, Danneels LA, Cagnie B, Huyghe L, Seyns E, Cools AM. Conscious correction of scapular orientation in overhead athletes performing selected shoulder rehabilitation exercises: the effect on trapezius muscle activation measured by surface electromyography. J Orthop Sports Phys Ther. 2013; 43(1):3-10.

116. Huang HY, Lin JJ, Guo YL, Wang WT, Chen YJ. EMG biofeedback effectiveness to alter muscle activity pattern and scapular kinematics in subjects with and without shoulder impingement. J Electromyogr Kinesiol. 2013;23(1):267-74.

117. Solem-Bertoft E, Thuomas KA, Westerberg CE. The influence of scapular retraction and protraction on the width of the subacromial space. An MRI study. Clin Orthop Relat Res. 1993(296):99-103.

118. McQuade KJ, Dawson J, Smidt GL. Scapulothoracic muscle fatigue associated with alterations in scapulohumeral rhythm kinematics during maximum resistive shoulder elevation. J Orthop Sports Phys Ther. 1998;28(2):74-80.

119. Camci E, Duzgun I, Hayran M, Baltaci G, Karaduman A. Scapular kinematics during shoulder elevation performed with and without elastic resistance in men without shoulder pathologies. J Orthop Sports Phys Ther. 2013;43(10):735-43.

120. Vangsgaard S, Norgaard LT, Flaskager BK, Sogaard K, Taylor JL, Madeleine P. Eccentric exercise inhibits the H reflex in the middle part of the trapezius muscle. Eur J Appl Physiol. 2013;113(1):77-87.

121. Desmeules F, Cote CH, Fremont P. Therapeutic exercise and orthopedic manual therapy for impingement syndrome: a systematic review. Clin J Sport Med. 2003;13(3):176-82.

122. Bang MD, Deyle GD. Comparison of supervised exercise with and without manual physical therapy for patients with shoulder impingement syndrome. J Orthop Sports Phys Ther. 2000;30(3):126-37.

123. Senbursa G, Baltaci G, Atay A. Comparison of conservative treatment with and without manual physical therapy for patients with shoulder impingement syndrome: a prospective, randomized clinical trial. Knee Surg Sports Traumatol Arthrosc. 2007;15(7):915-21.

124. Senbursa G, Baltaci G, Atay OA. The effectiveness of manual therapy in supraspinatus tendinopathy. Acta Orthop Traumatol Turc. 2011;45(3):162-7.

125. Tate AR, McClure PW, Young IA, Salvatori R, Michener LA. Comprehensive impairment-based exercise and manual therapy intervention for patients with subacromial impingement syndrome: a case series. J Orthop Sports Phys Ther. 2010;40(8):474-93.

126. Bennell K, Wee E, Coburn S, Green S, Harris A, Staples M, et al. Efficacy of standardised manual therapy and home exercise programme for chronic rotator cuff disease: randomised placebo controlled trial. BMJ. 2010;340:c2756.

127. Ho CY, Sole G, Munn J. The effectiveness of manual therapy in the management of musculoskeletal disorders of the shoulder: a systematic review. Man Ther. 2009;14(5):463-74.

128. Gebremariam L, Hay EM, van der Sande R, Rinkel WD, Koes BW, Huisstede BM. Subacromial impingement syndrome--effectiveness of physiotherapy and manual therapy. Br J Sports Med. 2014;48(16):1202-8.

129. Callahan DJ. The adequacy of medical school education in musculoskeletal medicine. J Bone Joint Surg Am. 1999;81(10):1501-2.

130. Childs JD, Whitman JM, Sizer PS, Pugia ML, Flynn TW, Delitto A. A description of physical therapists' knowledge in managing musculoskeletal conditions. BMC Musculoskelet Disord. 2005;6:32.

131. Freedman KB, Bernstein J. The adequacy of medical school education in musculoskeletal medicine. J Bone Joint Surg Am. 1998;80(10):1421-7.

132. Freedman KB, Bernstein J. Educational deficiencies in musculoskeletal medicine. J Bone Joint Surg Am. 2002;84-A(4):604-8.

133. Davenport TE, Watts HG, Kulig K, Resnik C. Current status and correlates of physicians' referral diagnoses for physical therapy. J Orthop Sports Phys Ther. 2005;35(9):572-9.

134. Harryman DT, Sidles JA, Clark JM, McQuade KJ, Gibb TD, Matsen FA. Translation of the humeral head on the glenoid with passive glenohumeral motion. J Bone Joint Surg Am. 1990;72(9):1334-43.

135. Karduna AR, Williams GR, Williams JL, Iannotti JP. Kinematics of the glenohumeral joint: influences of muscle forces, ligamentous constraints, and articular geometry. J Orthop Res. 1996;14(6):986-93.

136. Wuelker N, Brewe F, Sperveslage C. Passive glenohumeral joint stabilization: a biomechanical study. J Shoulder Elbow Surg. 1994;3(3):129-34.

137. Wuelker N, Schmotzer H, Thren K, Korell M. Translation of the glenohumeral joint with simulated active elevation. Clin Orthop Relat Res. 1994;(309):193-200.

138. Roubal PJ, Dobritt D, Placzek JD. Glenohumeral gliding manipulation following interscalene brachial plexus block in patients with adhesive capsulitis. J Orthop Sports Phys Ther. 1996;24(2):66-77.

139. Johnson AJ, Godges JJ, Zimmerman GJ, Ounanian LL. The effect of anterior versus posterior glide joint mobilization on external rotation range of motion in patients with shoulder adhesive capsulitis. J Orthop Sports Phys Ther. 2007;37(3):88-99.

140. Yang JL, Jan MH, Chang CW, Lin JJ. Effectiveness of the end-range mobilization and scapular mobilization approach in a subgroup of subjects with frozen shoulder syndrome: a randomized control trial. Man Ther. 2012;17(1):47-52.

141. Brudvig TJ, Kulkarni H, Shah S. The effect of therapeutic exercise and mobilization on patients with shoulder dysfunction: a systematic review with meta-analysis. J Orthop Sports Phys Ther. 2011;41(10):734-48.

142. Muraki T, Yamamoto N, Berglund LJ, Sperling JW, Steinmann SP, Cofield RH, et al. The effect of cyclic loading simulating oscillatory joint mobilization on the posterior capsule of the glenohumeral joint: a cadaveric study. J Orthop Sports Phys Ther. 2011;41(5):311-8.

143. Conroy DE, Hayes KW. The effect of joint mobilization as a component of comprehensive treatment for primary shoulder impingement syndrome. J Orthop Sports Phys Ther. 1998;28(1):3-14.

144. Djordjevic OC, Vukicevic D, Katunac L, Jovic S. Mobilization with movement and kinesiotaping compared with a supervised exercise program for painful shoulder: results of a clinical trial. J Manipulative Physiol Ther. 2012;35(6):454-63.

145. Myers JB, Laudner KG, Pasquale MR, Bradley JP, Lephart SM. Glenohumeral range of motion deficits and posterior shoulder tightness in throwers with pathologic internal impingement. Am J Sports Med. 2006;34(3):385-91.

146. Plaza-Manzano G, Molina F, Lomas-Vega R, Martinez-Amat A, Achalandabaso A, Hita-Contreras F. Changes in biochemical markers of pain perception and stress response after spinal manipulation. J Orthop Sports Phys Ther. 2014;44(4):231-9.

147. Ruiz-Saez M, Fernandez-de-las-Penas C, Blanco CR, Martinez-Segura R, Garcia-Leon R. Changes in pressure pain sensitivity in latent myofascial trigger points in the upper trapezius muscle after a cervical spine manipulation in pain-free subjects. J Manipulative Physiol Ther. 2007;30(8):578-83.

148. Norlander S, Aste-Norlander U, Nordgren B, Sahlstedt B. Mobility in the cervico-thoracic motion segment: an indicative factor of musculo-skeletal neck-shoulder pain. Scand J Rehabil Med. 1996;28(4):183-92.

149. Norlander S, Gustavsson BA, Lindell J, Nordgren B. Reduced mobility in the cervico-thoracic motion segment--a risk factor for musculoskeletal neck-shoulder pain: a two-year prospective follow-up study. Scand J Rehabil Med. 1997;29(3):167-74.

150. Fernandez-de-Las-Penas C, Alonso-Blanco C, Cleland JA, Rodriguez-Blanco C, Alburquerque-Sendin F. Changes in pressure pain thresholds over C5-C6 zygapophyseal joint after a cervicothoracic junction manipulation in healthy subjects. J Manipulative Physiol Ther. 2008;31(5):332-7.

151. Wang SS, Meadows J. Immediate and carryover changes of C5-6 joint mobilization on shoulder external rotator muscle strength. J Manipulative Physiol Ther. 2010;33(2):102-8.

152. Gross A, Miller J, D'Sylva J, Burnie SJ, Goldsmith CH, Graham N, et al. Manipulation or mobilisation for neck pain: a Cochrane Review. Man Ther. 2010;15(4):315-33.

153. Cleland JA, Glynn P, Whitman JM, Eberhart SL, MacDonald C, Childs JD. Short-term effects of thrust versus nonthrust mobilization/manipulation directed at the thoracic spine in patients with neck pain: a randomized clinical trial. Phys Ther. 2007;87(4):431-40.

154. Dunning JR, Cleland JA, Waldrop MA, Arnot CF, Young IA, Turner M, et al. Upper cervical and upper thoracic thrust manipulation versus nonthrust mobilization in patients with mechanical neck pain: a multicenter randomized clinical trial. J Orthop Sports Phys Ther. 2012;42(1):5-18.

155. Mintken PE, Cleland JA, Carpenter KJ, Bieniek ML, Keirns M, Whitman JM. Some factors predict successful short-term outcomes in individuals with shoulder pain receiving cervicothoracic manipulation: a single-arm trial. Phys Ther. 2010;90(1):26-42.

156. Boyles RE, Ritland BM, Miracle BM, Barclay DM, Faul MS, Moore JH, et al. The short-term effects of thoracic spine thrust manipulation on patients with shoulder impingement syndrome. Man Ther. 2009;14(4):375-80.

157. Bergman GJ, Winters JC, Groenier KH, Meyboom-de Jong B, Postema K, van der Heijden GJ. Manipulative therapy in addition to usual care for patients with shoulder complaints: results of physical examination outcomes in a randomized controlled trial. J Manipulative Physiol Ther. 2010;33(2):96-101.

158. Bergman GJ, Winters JC, Groenier KH, Pool JJ, Meyboom-de Jong B, Postema K, et al. Manipulative therapy in addition to usual medical care for patients with shoulder dysfunction and pain: a randomized, controlled trial. Ann Intern Med. 2004;141(6):432-9.

159. Muth S, Barbe MF, Lauer R, McClure PW. The effects of thoracic spine manipulation in subjects with signs of rotator cuff tendinopathy. J Orthop Sports Phys Ther. 2012;42(12):1005-16.

160. Strunce JB, Walker MJ, Boyles RE, Young BA. The immediate effects of thoracic spine and rib manipulation on subjects with primary complaints of shoulder pain. J Man Manip Ther. 2009;17(4):230-6.

161. Travell JG, Simons DG. Myofascial Pain and Dysfunction: The Trigger Point Manual. Baltimore: Williams & Wilkins; 1983.

162. Hong CZ, Simons DG. Pathophysiologic and electrophysiologic mechanisms of myofascial trigger points. Arch Phys Med Rehabil. 1998;79(7): 863-72.

163. Chen Q, Bensamoun S, Basford JR, Thompson JM, An KN. Identification and quantification of myofascial taut bands with magnetic resonance elastography. Arch Phys Med Rehabil. 2007;88(12):1658-61.

164. Bron C, Franssen J, Wensing M, Oostendorp RA. Interrater reliability of palpation of myofascial trigger points in three shoulder muscles. J Man Manip Ther. 2007;15(4):203-15.

165. Hidalgo-Lozano A, Fernandez-de-las-Penas C, Alonso-Blanco C, Ge HY, Arendt-Nielsen L, Arroyo-Morales M. Muscle trigger points and pressure pain hyperalgesia in the shoulder muscles in patients with unilateral shoulder impingement: a blinded, controlled study. Exp Brain Res. 2010;202(4):915-25.

166. Alburquerque-Sendin F, Camargo PR, Vieira A, Salvini TF. Bilateral myofascial trigger points and pressure pain thresholds in the shoulder muscles in patients with unilateral shoulder impingement syndrome: a blinded, controlled study. Clin J Pain. 2013;29(6):478-86.

167. Hains G, Descarreaux M, Hains F. Chronic shoulder pain of myofascial origin: a randomized clinical trial using ischemic compression therapy. J Manipulative Physiol Ther. 2010;33(5):362-9.

168. Cagnie B, Dewitte V, Coppieters I, Van Oosterwijck J, Cools A, Danneels L. Effect of ischemic compression on trigger points in the neck and shoulder muscles in office workers: a cohort study. J Manipulative Physiol Ther. 2013;36(8):482-9.

169. Hou CR, Tsai LC, Cheng KF, Chung KC, Hong CZ. Immediate effects of various physical therapeutic modalities on cervical myofascial pain and trigger-point sensitivity. Arch Phys Med Rehabil. 2002;83(10):1406-14.

170. Teys P, Bisset L, Vicenzino B. The initial effects of a Mulligan's mobilization with movement technique on range of movement and pressure pain threshold in pain-limited shoulders. Man Ther. 2008;13(1):37-42.

171. Godges JJ, Mattson-Bell M, Thorpe D, Shah D. The immediate effects of soft tissue mobilization with proprioceptive neuromuscular facilitation on glenohumeral external rotation and overhead reach. J Orthop Sports Phys Ther. 2003;33(12):713-8.

172. Falla D, Farina D, Graven-Nielsen T. Experimental muscle pain results in reorganization of coordination among trapezius muscle subdivisions during repetitive shoulder flexion. Exp Brain Res. 2007;178(3):385-93.

173. Myburgh C, Hartvigsen J, Aagaard P, Holsgaard-Larsen A. Skeletal muscle contractility, self-reported pain and tissue sensitivity in females with neck/shoulder pain and upper Trapezius myofascial trigger points-a randomized intervention study. Chiropr Man Therap. 2012;20(1):36.

174. Donigan JA, Wolf BR. Arthroscopic subacromial decompression: acromioplasty versus bursectomy alone--does it really matter? A systematic review. Iowa Ortho J. 2011;31:121-6.

CHAPTER 4

Glenohumeral Instability

Robert C Manske

ABSTRACT

The glenohumeral (GH) joint sacrifices stability for extreme mobility, allowing more motion than any joint in the human body via rotation and three translational degrees of freedom. GH instability is a relatively common shoulder condition that runs the gamut from symptomatic physiologic laxity to complete dislocation. GH instability results from the inability to maintain the humeral head centered on the glenoid fossa. This inherent lack of stability at the GH joint is due to the reliance on soft tissue dynamic and static stabilizers and a lack of bony congruency. A very large humeral head and shallow glenoid fossa create minimal bony contact throughout full range of shoulder motion.

The orthopedic patient with shoulder instability is a very challenging patient. Relatively high incidence rates of subsequent redislocations and chronic GH instability have placed the utmost importance on accurate immediate diagnosis and treatment of this potentially disabling condition. An accurate diagnosis depends on a full understanding of the condition, mechanism of injury and clinical signs and symptoms associated with instability. Due to the instability, unique stress is placed upon capsular and ligamentous structures that further exacerbate this condition. Through a delicate balance of rest, applied stress and loads, nonoperative treatment can yield successful outcomes. However, successful outcomes require a well-structured and designed rehabilitation program that addresses each of the phases that an injured patient will navigate. Emphasis should be placed on normalizing GH motion, restoring both rotator cuff and scapulothoracic strength, enhancing proprioception, neuromuscular control and dynamic stability.

▌ INTRODUCTION

Glenohumeral (GH) instability is a relatively common shoulder condition that runs the gamut from symptomatic physiologic laxity to complete dislocation.[1] In other words, the GH instability results from the inability to maintain the humeral head centered on the glenoid fossa. The GH joint sacrifices stability for extreme mobility. This inherent lack of stability at the GH joint is due to the reliance on soft tissue dynamic and static stabilizers and a lack of bony congruency. A very large humeral head and shallow glenoid fossa create minimal bony contact throughout full range of shoulder motion. Its ball-and-socket configuration provides the shoulder with more mobility than any other joint in the human body, allowing rotation and three translational degrees of freedom.[2]

Epidemiology

The overall incidence of shoulder primary dislocations reported in the literature differs, depending on the studies cited and patient population studied. In one of the more recent large scale studies, Liavaag et al. reported that the overall incidence of acute shoulder dislocations was 56.3/100,000 persons-years.[3] This rate was much higher than the few previous studies of shoulder dislocation incidence in the general population, which reported a range of 11.2–23.9/100,000 person-years.[4-7]

Anatomy

The glenoid labrum and the capsuloligamentous complex are integral to maintaining GH stability. The glenoid labrum provides about 50% of the overall depth of the glenoid fossa and is reported to double the depth of the fossa when it is present.[8] The use of coordinated shoulder muscle activity that compresses the humeral head into the glenoid and allows concentric rotation of the humeral head on the glenoid is termed concavity-compression. Studies indicate that resection of the labrum can reduce the effectiveness of the concavity compression by 20%, and injury to the labrum is thought to disturb negative intra-articular pressure gradient contributing to shoulder instability.[9-13] The GH capsule has several locations of dense collagen tissue that help contribute to static shoulder stability. The anterior portion of the GH ligament and capsule has three thickenings consisting of the superior, middle and inferior GH ligaments. The capsule is thickest and strongest at the anterior inferior GH ligament complex (Fig. 1).[14]

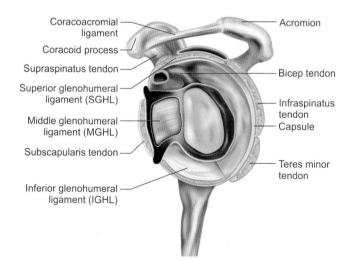

FIG. 1: Glenohumeral (GH) ligaments and the rotator cuff stabilizers of the GH joint[15]

Source: Reproduced with permission from Elsevier.

CLINICAL PRESENTATION

The shoulder patient's clinical presentation depends on the type of GH instability present: anterior, posterior or multidirectional.

Anterior Shoulder Instability

A physical therapist in a clinical setting will rarely see someone who presents with a dislocated shoulder; however a physical therapist present at the sight of injury may see this commonly (e.g. a sports physical therapist covering an event). By far the most common form of GH instability is an anterior dislocation accounting for more than 90% of all shoulder dislocations.[16] Rates of anterior dislocation are increased for men, contact athletes and those who are enlisted in the military.[17] The mechanism of injury for this pathology is a tackle in American football, or when the patient has the shoulder in 90° of abduction and external rotation and another player makes contact with the arm forcing it into further external rotation. The acutely dislocated shoulder will present with some degree of deformity. With an anterior dislocation, the deltoid will appear to be flattened due to the inferior located position of the humeral head, which now rests under the coracoid process.[18] A patient with a shoulder dislocation will also present with an inability to move the arm and severe pain until it is in a reduced position. In most instances, a dislocation will most likely occur in the anterior or anterior-inferior direction. Due to this, the dislocated shoulder is more easily detectable; however in the patient with a subluxing shoulder this may be more subtle and often overlooked. The patient with a subluxing shoulder may present with a history of slipping or clicking sensations without any known trauma.

Posterior Shoulder Instability

As anteriorly directed instability is most common, posterior dislocations or instability are fairly rare. Posterior shoulder instability has an incidence between 2% and 12% in all cases of shoulder instability.[19] Despite this rareness, they will be seen on a regular basis, especially in a clinic that treats a great deal of shoulder patients. Athletes that have their shoulders in flexed position with elbows locked while blocking or vaulting, often sustain this injury, e.g. gymnasts or American football linemen. Additional mechanisms include those who have fallen on an outstretched hand with the arm flexed forward creating a large posterior directed force through the kinetic chain. Lastly this injury is seen in swimmers, who actually may dislocate posteriorly due to generalized ligament laxity from swimming. Athletes typically develop posterior shoulder instability secondary to repetitive, sport-specific motions, which inflict microtraumatic stress to the posterior capsulolabral complex.[20] This same pattern of recurrent microtrauma predisposes the athlete to capsular attenuation and posterior labral tears.[21,22]

Multidirectional Shoulder Instability

The hardest group of orthopedic shoulder instability patients to treat may be those with multidirectional instability (MDI). In the author's experience, these are some of the same patients that have been described in other forms of instability such as gymnasts, swimmers and occasionally tennis players and baseball and softball players. This unique group creates a challenge to the therapist as they typically already are predisposed to instability, due to generalized ligamentous and capsular laxity.[23] Additionally, these patients are often adamant about continuing sports or recreational activities, which continue to create instability issues due to their repetitive nature.

▌ CLINICAL EXAMINATION

History

As with any orthopedic condition, the medical history will provide the foundation for an accurate diagnosis. It is important to note the degree of instability and the direction. The physical therapist must ask the following questions as they examine the patient:

- Does the shoulder feel as though it is slipping out partially or completely?
- Was the injury traumatic—requiring medical personnel to relocate or did it relocation occur spontaneously?
- Is this the first occurrence of this slipping sensation, or has it occurred on multiple occasions?
- What position was the arm in when it subluxed or dislocated?
- Which direction was the dislocation—inferior, anterior, posterior?

A clinical pearl that can be helpful during rehabilitation of an orthopedic patient with shoulder instability is to ensure that the direction, or type of instability, has been correctly established. Although this sounds like a simple task, it is easy to be misled by the history and the physical examination in an acutely injured shoulder. One would assume that the patient would know exactly which direction the shoulder went out, but that is not always the case. Probably due to the excitement, adrenalin and or shock associated with the severity of the injury the patient is not always a fantastic historian.

Postural Assessment

The clinical examination for any orthopedic patient with suspected instability should be done in a consistent manner. To begin with, the therapist should examine the entire patient, looking for subtle hints that relate to instability. An example of one such subtlety would be the identification of a prominent posterior lateral acromion when observing the patient from behind in a relaxed posture. Ordinarily, an inferior force would need to be applied to the humerus to elicit a positive sulcus sign, but in the example noted here, the sulcus is present at rest. Postural assessment continues with the observation of the amount of forward head, shoulder alignment, and overall scapular position. Next, overall symmetry and contour of the shoulder should be examined. Clear signs of discoloration, atrophy, edema or swelling should be noted. As weakness of scapular stabilizers may also contribute to instability, it is important to assess scapular winging or tipping.[24]

Palpation

Palpation should occur around all important structures in the shoulder, however at times the shoulder may be generally sore throughout and not in any one specific area. If the shoulder was recently dislocated there may be isolated tenderness to palpation of the anterior joint line near the deltopectoral groove.

Strength Testing

Strength of the shoulder should be examined with particular emphasis on the rotator cuff and scapular muscles. Controversy exists how much strength loss occurs following shoulder instability. Edouard et al. examined 37 patients with unilateral recurrent anterior post-traumatic shoulder dislocations, with 11 healthy nonathletic subjects. There was an association between instability and external and internal rotator cuff strength side-to-side differences. Both, peak torque, and external to internal rotators strength ratios were lower on the pathologic side.[25] However, more recently Jan et al. performed strength testing of bilateral shoulders in 102 male patients suffering from shoulder instability following trauma-related anterior or anterior-inferior dislocations. After several shoulder dislocations, there was a nonsignificant difference in the external and internal rotator strength ratio, comparing injured to uninjured side.[26] Wilk et al. recommend external rotators to internal rotators strength ratio of 66–76% or higher at 180 degrees per second, and external rotators to abductors ratio of 67–75% or higher at 180 degrees per second in professional baseball players.[27,28]

Neurological Testing

Neurologic testing is important, as a common finding with those following anterior dislocation is transient axillary nerve palsy.[29] Hertel et al. have described a test for axillary nerve palsy in which the examiner grasps the patients wrist and pulls the arm into near full extension.[30] The examiner asks the patient to maintain that position while he releases the wrist. The inability to maintain the shoulder extension position is considered a positive test. Light touch, pressure and sharp dull sensations can be examined and compared bilaterally. Additionally, if neurologic compromise is suspected, deep tendon reflexes for the biceps, triceps and brachioradialis should be tested.

Neurovascular Testing

Neurovascular status is especially important for the patient with acute dislocation or chronic instability to rule out other causes of symptoms such as thoracic outlet syndrome. Neurovascular signs include Adson maneuver,[31,32] Costoclavicular Test,[31] Halstead maneuver,[33] and Roos Test.[31,34] These tests have been discussed in detail, in the "Thoracic Outlet Syndrome" chapter, in this text.

Range of Motion Testing

Range of motion (ROM) will be assessed, and the patient may experience pain near end ROM but especially at the end of abduction and external rotation. ROM should be assessed for elevation in forward flexion, elevation in the scapular plane and in abduction. Following an acute dislocation or with a symptomatic patient, it is best to perform internal and external rotation measurements with the shoulder in neutral. If the patient is able to tolerate it, then internal and external rotation ROM should be measured in a more functional position—shoulder in 90 degrees of abduction and 90 degrees of external rotation. Caution should be used in this position as it is a common position in which the GH joint is anteriorly dislocated.

Special Instability Tests

Shoulder stability tests should be used with all orthopedic patients thought to present with shoulder instability, as the tests may be used to evaluate the extent and direction of the instability. There are two main test categories that are used and recommended: (1) humeral head translation tests, and (2) provocation tests.[35]

Humeral Head Translation Tests

Humeral head translation tests document the amount of passive translation of the humeral head relative to the glenoid fossa. Careful passive movements are applied via directional stresses to the proximal humerus by the evaluator. Inferior, anterior and posterior are the three directions of humeral head translations that are assessed. An inferior humeral head translation is also known as the sulcus sign. Using a three-dimensional tracking device, Harryman et al. measured the amount of humeral head inferior translation and found an average of 10 mm of displacement.[36] To perform the sulcus test, the patient should preferably be in the seated position with arms in neutral adduction and relaxed. The examiner will grasp the distal aspect of the patient's humerus using a firm but unassuming grip with one hand, while several brief, relatively rapid downward pulls are exerted to the humerus in an inferior direction. When a visible sulcus can be seen, the patient has MDI (Fig. 2).[37] By virtue of this sulcus, the excessive translation in the inferior direction indicates a forthcoming pattern of excessive translation in an anterior or posterior direction, or in both anterior and posterior directions.

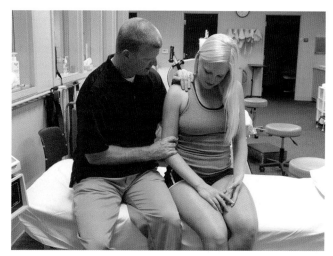

FIG. 2: Sulcus test for multidirectional instability

Anterior and posterior translation tests can be performed in either supine or sitting position. Harryman et al. have shown in vivo, in healthy uninjured subjects, that the humeral head should translate a mean of 7.8 mm anterior and an almost equal amount of 7.9 mm in the posterior direction, which equates to nearly a 1:1 ratio of anterior to posterior translation.[36] The seated tests for humeral translations are commonly called load and shift tests. The author's preferred method is in sitting with the patient's arm relaxed in their lap. The examiner firmly grasps the proximal humeral head with the index and middle finger anteriorly and the thumb posteriorly. The fingers should remain flat as to not pinch the soft tissues on the anterior surface of the humeral head. The stabilizing hand should hold the shoulder with fingers draped anteriorly onto the anterior acromion and coracoid process as to not impede movement of the humeral head. The stabilizing hand forearm should lay flat along the scapula on the posterior shoulder for optimal stabilization to occur. It should also be noted that the translational force provided must be along the line of the GH joint, with an anteromedial and posterolateral direction due to the 30 degrees anteversion of the glenoid (Fig. 3). Anterior and posterior translations can be graded on a classification system designed by Altchek and Dines.[38] In a grade I translation, the humeral head does not move up and over the glenoid rim and will spontaneously return to the neutral position with removal of the load. A grade II translation represents translation of the humeral head up and over the glenoid rim, with spontaneous return on removal of stress. A presence of a grade II translation without symptoms does not indicate instability, but represents ligamentous laxity of the joint. The grade III translation will involve translation of the humeral head over the glenoid rim without relocation upon removal of the force. This will probably not be seen in a clinic but is commonly seen during arthroscopy, when the patient is under anesthesia.

Provocation Tests

The anterior apprehension test was originally described by Rowe and Zarins as a test for overt anterior instability.[39] The patient is placed in supine position, relaxed with the scapula stabilized on the table. The examiner stands along the patient's affected shoulder and abducts the arm to the 90 degrees of shoulder abduction and 90 degrees of elbow flexion (90/90 position). The examiner slowly rotates the shoulder posteriorly, looking for a sign of patient apprehension (Fig. 4). This look of concern or feeling of apprehension by the patient is considered a positive test. This test will create apprehension when positive—it may or may not, also, create pain.

The Jobe's subluxation relocation test can be used to test for anterior microinstability or for internal impingement.[40] This test is done in the same manner as the apprehension test. However at the end of range of abduction and external rotation, the patient with a positive test will complain of pain. If the pain is anterior, the examiner applies a posterior directed force on the humeral head (Fig. 5). If the posterior stress relieves the pain, then the test is positive for anterior microinstability. A person with primary impingement will not demonstrate a change in pain with relocation component of this test.[40-42]

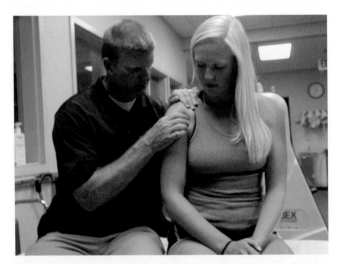

FIG. 3: Anterior and posterior load and shift test

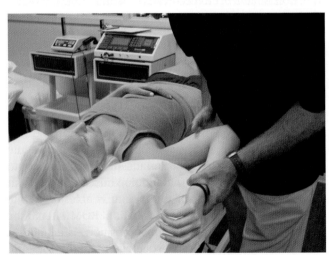

FIG. 4: Apprehension test performed with overpressure at 90° of abduction and external rotation

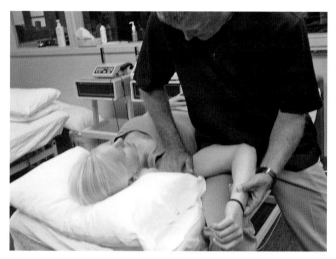

FIG. 5: Jobe's subluxation relocation test

If the patient complains of posterior shoulder pain with the subluxation component of the subluxation relocation test, but pain is relieved by the relocation maneuver, posterior internal impingement is probably the cause of symptoms.

Differential Diagnosis

There are numerous shoulder conditions that can mimic GH instability. Any injury to the shoulder that creates pain or inflammation can create a loss of GH dynamic stability. Even seemingly minor conditions, such as subacromial impingement or small rotator cuff tear, will create disequilibrium in the dynamic function of the shoulder girdle. Rotator cuff and scapulothoracic musculature must function in concert to coordinate normal, nonpathologic motion at the shoulder. The injury-induced weakness brought on by impingement or muscle strains can exacerbate the already lax shoulder, which depends on the rotator cuff for dynamic stability. Additionally conditions such as labral tears (superior labrum anterior to posterior, Bankart, and reverse Bankart) can contribute to GH instability during functional activities resulting in the sensation of instability. Injury to the acromioclavicular (AC) joint must be ruled out, as it can create its own instability challenges. However, this injury typically follows trauma to the top of the shoulder such as falling directly on the ipsilateral shoulder. This injury has an entirely different pain pattern that is localized to the AC joint, and is easily distinguished from GH instability. Other shoulder conditions such as shoulder fractures (humeral, clavicular, or scapular), adhesive capsulitis and/or bursitis rarely create a sensation of GH instability.

Furthermore, remote pathology can create symptoms that can be mistaken for GH instability (e.g. cervical radiculopathy and thoracic outlet syndrome).

PHYSICAL THERAPY TREATMENT

The treatment of an orthopedic patient with instability will depend on the degree and type of instability present. Treatment of acute dislocations following immediate surgery or other postsurgical treatment methods for instability is obviously different than nonoperative management. The focus of this chapter will be on the nonoperative management of general instability, as specific postoperative surgical protocols are beyond the scope of this text. The various nuances of each directional instability will be discussed, followed by a detailed description of nonoperative management, applicable to all forms of instability. However, the nonoperative treatment must be classified and treated in two manners: traumatic versus atraumatic.

Nonoperative Treatment of Directional Instabilities

Anterior Instability

The success of nonoperative care appears to be less in younger patients. Hovelius et al. have demonstrated a diminishing rate of recurrent dislocation as ones age increases. A young patient in their 20's has a recurrence rate of approximately 60%, while a 30–40 years-old patient's risk of recurrence decreases greatly to only 20%.[43-45] Typically treatment following a dislocation entails immobilization in a sling and early controlled ROM exercises. Early rehabilitation following a dislocation revolves around decreasing pain and the inflammatory response, restoring ROM and achieving dynamic shoulder control through use of rotator cuff and scapular stabilizers. Because of the Bankart lesion or Hill Sach's lesion that often occurs with a dislocated shoulder, a brief time of immobilization in a sling is necessary. Times for immobilization range from 2 weeks to 4 weeks. Historically, the shoulder is placed in a sling with the arm held in internal rotation across the body. Itoi et al. have described placing the arm in slight external rotation due to a better coaptation to the glenoid rim with the torn Bankart lesion.[46] Although this novel concept worked well in Itoi's hands, it has not yet become the accepted standard in clinical practice. A rehabilitation program for a patient with anterior instability is presented in Table 1.

TABLE 1: Nonoperative anterior shoulder dislocation or subluxation rehabilitation program

The physical therapy rehabilitation for an anterior shoulder dislocation or subluxation will vary in length depending on factors such as:
- Degree of shoulder instability or laxity
- Acute versus chronic condition
- Length of time immobilized
- Strength and ROM status
- Performance and activity demands.

The rehabilitation program is outlined in three phases. It is possible to overlap phases (Phase I-II, Phase II-III) depending on the progress of each individual. In all exercises during Phase I and Phase II, caution to avoid undue stress on the anterior joint capsule is required as dynamic joint stability is being restored. An isokinetic strength and endurance test may be scheduled during the latter part of Phase II. The focus in Phase III is on progressive isotonic and isokinetic exercises in preparation for returning to the prior activity level (work, recreational activity, sports, etc.)

Phase I
1. Apply modalities as needed (e.g. heat, ice, electrotherapy).
2. Perform ROM exercises (passive, active-assistive, active) as tolerated. For shoulder abduction and external rotation, avoid stress to the anterior joint capsule by positioning the shoulder in the scapular plane (approximately 20–30° forward of the coronal plane). Shoulder hyperextension is contraindicated.
3. Shoulder stretch: Posterior cuff and posterior capsule stretch (if and as needed).
4. Joint mobilization (posterior glides if and as needed).
5. Active shoulder internal and external rotation exercises with surgical or rubber tubing. Arm positioned at side with elbow flexed at 90°. Avoid excessive stress to the anterior joint capsule by limiting external rotation to no greater than 45° (as tolerated). If this causes discomfort, isometric exercises may be performed instead. Adjust the shoulder position to allow a pain-free muscle contraction to occur.
6. Add supraspinatus exercise in the scapular plane, if adequate ROM is available (0–90°).
7. Active shoulder flexion exercise through available pain/symptom free ROM.
8. Active shoulder abduction exercise to 90°. Maintain shoulder in the scapular plane to avoid stress on the anterior joint capsule.
9. Shoulder extension exercise: Lying prone or standing (bent at the waist), with the shoulder dangling in a flexed position. Avoid the shoulder extended position by preventing arm movement beyond the frontal plane of the body. This will decrease excessive stress to the anterior joint capsule.
10. Shoulder shrug exercise: Avoid traction in the GH joint between repetitions by not allowing the arms to drop completely. This will avoid an excessive inferior glide of the humeral head.
11. Active horizontal adduction exercise: Perform supine with the starting position in the scapular plane.
12. Active shoulder internal and external rotation: Progress to free-weights.
    i. Shoulder internal rotation: Perform in side-lying. Elevate or support the lateral chest wall (pillow, bolster, wedge, etc.) to decrease the joint compression on the involved shoulder.
    ii. Shoulder external rotation: Lie on the uninvolved side. Avoid excessive stress to the anterior joint capsule by limiting movement to no greater than 45–50° of external rotation.
13. Add forearm strengthening exercises (elbow, forearm, and wrist).

Phase II
1. Continue posterior cuff and posterior capsule stretch, joint mobilization, and ROM exercises, as needed.
2. Continue shoulder strengthening with surgical tubing and/or free-weights. Emphasize eccentric phase of contraction.
3. Add arm ergometer for endurance exercise (maintain elbow anterior to frontal plane throughout entire stroke).
4. Add push-ups. Maintain proper alignment of the shoulders and elbows at the starting position. Caution is applied during the descent phase of the push-up to avoid excessive stress to the anterior capsule. Do not lower the body beyond the elbows. Begin with wall push-ups. As strength improves progress to floor push-ups (modified hands and knees, or military hands and feet) as tolerated.
5. Isokinetic test: Perform isokinetic strength and endurance test for the following suggested patterns—shoulder internal and external rotation (arm at side), abduction and adduction, and flexion/extension as tolerated. To perform this test, prerequisite strength requirements of the rotator cuff are 5–10 lbs for external rotation, and 15–20 lbs for internal rotation. The shoulder should be pain-free and have no significant amount of swelling.
6. Add isokinetic strengthening and endurance exercises (high speeds—200+ degrees/second) for shoulder internal and external rotation with arm at side. Maintain shoulder in 15–20° of flexion and limit external rotation to 45–50° to avoid excessive stress to the anterior joint capsule.
7. Add total body conditioning with emphasis on strength and endurance, include flexibility exercises as needed.

Continued

Continued

Phase III

1. Continue posterior cuff and posterior capsule stretching, as needed.
2. Continue to emphasize the eccentric phase in strengthening the rotator cuff.
3. Continue to progress isotonic and isokinetic exercises. For shoulder internal and external rotation, gradually increase the stress to the anterior joint capsule by positioning the upper extremity at 45° of shoulder abduction and then 80–90°. Continue to exercise in the functional shoulder position specific to the sport as tolerated.
4. Add isokinetic exercises for shoulder flexion and extension, abduction and adduction, and horizontal abduction and adduction. Take precautions in avoiding excessive stress to the anterior joint capsule.
5. Add chin-ups.
6. Continue arm ergometer for endurance.
7. Add military press (arms maintain position anterior to frontal plane throughout movement).
8. Isokinetic test: The second isokinetic test is administered for shoulder internal and external rotation, abduction and adduction, and flexion and extension. For shoulder internal/external rotation, the shoulder may be tested in the functional position (80–90° of abduction). Test results should demonstrate at least 80% strength and endurance (as compared to the uninvolved side) before proceeding with exercises specific to the activity setting.
9. Continue total body conditioning program with emphasis on the shoulder (rotator cuff).
10. Skill mastery: Begin practicing skills specific to the activity (e.g. work, recreational activity, sport). For example, throwing athletes (e.g. pitchers) may proceed to an interval throwing program.

ROM, range of motion; GH, glenohumeral

Posterior Instability Nonoperative Treatment

Following isolated posterior dislocation of the GH joint, it seems logical to work on dynamically stabilizing the anterior cuff and shoulder muscles. However, strengthening both anterior and posterior cuff muscle groups will improve the concavity compression effect of the rotator cuff, thus enhancing dynamic stability.[9] Exercises in the provocative position of having arms outstretched into forward flexion with adduction or extremes of internal rotation are contraindicated during early management (first 2–4 weeks), as these positions place the patients with posterior shoulder instability at risk. Additionally, avoiding a position that creates posterior shear loads, such as those when starting a bench press movement should be avoided early on in rehabilitation. Early closed kinetic chain (CKC) exercises, attempted in first 2–4 weeks postacute injury, might also cause a problem with posterior instability patients as they place the arm near the position of symptomatic instability. A rehabilitation protocol for a patient with posterior shoulder instability is seen in Table 2.

Multidirectional Instability Nonoperative Treatment

The patient with MDI is the one who needs dynamic stability of both the anterior and posterior cuff muscles and scapular stabilizers. All of these groups of muscles must work in unison to provide a balance of stability and control for rehabilitation to be successful. Additionally, even more critical in those with MDI, treatment should include focus on proprioception and neuromuscular control drills and exercises.

Phases of Rehabilitation

Traumatic Shoulder Instability

Treatment of the first time traumatic GH dislocator will be different from that of a patient with atraumatic instability. A gradually graded advancement of ROM and exercise progression will be required, based on degree of acute injury.

Acute phase

In the acute phase, the patient will be in significant amounts of pain and present with protective muscle spasm and guarding as the shoulder will be in a very irritable state. The extremity will be held alongside the body in internal rotation with guarded movements at best. Goals of the initial acute phase of treatment will be to protect the injured, healing capsular and labral structures, to reestablish pain-free ROM, to decrease pain, inflammation, and muscle spasm, to delay muscle atrophy and to reestablish voluntary muscle activity.

TABLE 2: Posterior shoulder subluxation or dislocation rehabilitation program

The physical therapy rehabilitation for posterior shoulder instability will vary in length depending on factors such as:
- Degree of shoulder instability or laxity
- Acute versus chronic condition
- Length of time immobilized
- Strength and ROM status
- Performance and activity demands.

The rehabilitation program is outlined in three phases. It is possible to overlap phases (Phase I-II, Phase II-III) depending on the progress of each individual. In all exercises during Phase I and Phase II, caution must be applied in placing undue stress on the posterior joint capsule as dynamic joint stability is restored. An isokinetic strength and endurance test may be scheduled during the latter part of Phase II. The focus in Phase III is on progressive isotonic and isokinetic exercises in preparation for returning to the prior activity level (e.g. work, recreational activity, sports).

Phase I

1. Apply modalities as needed (e.g. heat, ice, electrotherapy).
2. Perform ROM exercises (passive, active-assistive) for flexion, abduction, horizontal abduction, external rotation, and internal rotation (if and as needed).
3. Shoulder stretch—anterior cuff and anterior capsule stretch (if and as needed).
4. Joint mobilization (e.g. emphasis on anterior glides) as needed.
5. Active external rotation may be performed from 0° rotation to full external rotation. Arm is positioned at side with elbow flexed at 90°. Use surgical or rubber tubing for resistance. If pain persists, isometric exercises may be added. As strength improves, progress to using free-weights, lying prone with arm abducted to 90° or side-lying with arm at side.
   i. Prone: Perform the combined movements of horizontal abduction followed by external, rotation to protect the posterior joint capsule.
   ii. Side-lying: Limit the degrees of internal rotation to protect the posterior joint capsule.
6. Add active internal rotation performed from full external rotation to 0° rotation using surgical or rubber tubing. Limiting the degrees of internal rotation is necessary to avoid excessive stress to the posterior joint capsule. If there is pain with active movements, strength can be maintained by performing an isometric contraction. The shoulder position may be adjusted to allow a pain-free muscle contraction to occur.
7. Add supraspinatus exercise, if adequate ROM is available (0–90°). Shoulder is positioned in the scapular plane approximately 20–30° forward of the coronal plane.
8. Active shoulder flexion exercise through available asymptomatic ROM.
9. Active shoulder abduction exercise to 90°.
10. Shoulder shrug exercise: Avoid traction in the GH joint between repetitions by not allowing the arms to drop completely. This will avoid an excessive inferior glide of the humeral head.
11. Active horizontal abduction exercise (posterior deltoid) in prone position. Avoid excessive stress to the posterior capsule by limiting movement from 45° of horizontal adduction to full horizontal abduction.
12. Add forearm-strengthening exercises (elbow, wrist).

Phase II

1. Continue anterior cuff and capsule stretch, joint mobilization, and ROM exercises, as necessary.
2. Continue shoulder strengthening (emphasis on rotator cuff and posterior deltoid) with surgical tubing and/or free-weights. Emphasis may be placed on the eccentric phase of contraction in strengthening the rotator cuff.
3. Add arm ergometer for endurance exercise.
4. Add push-ups. Movement should be pain-free with emphasis on protecting the posterior joint capsule. Caution is applied during the ascent phase of the push-up to avoid excessive stress to the posterior capsule. Do not raise the body beyond the scapular plane. Begin with wall push-ups. As strength improves, progress to floor push-ups (modified hands and knees, or military hands and feet) as tolerated by patient.
5. Isokinetic test: Perform isokinetic strength and endurance test for the following suggested movement patterns—shoulder internal and external rotation (arm at side), horizontal abduction, and abduction and adduction. To perform this test, prerequisite strength requirements of the rotator cuff are 5–10 lbs for external rotation and 15–20 lbs for internal rotation. The shoulder should be pain-free and have no significant amount of swelling.

Continued

Continued

6. Active shoulder internal rotation, using free weights, may be added performed supine with the arm positioned at the side.

7. Horizontal abduction may be performed through an increased range (starting position at 90° of horizontal adduction, as tolerated).

8. Add total body conditioning with emphasis on strength and endurance. Include flexibility exercises as needed.

Phase III

1. Continue anterior capsule stretching (if and as needed).

2. Continue to emphasize the eccentric phase in strengthening the rotator cuff.

3. Continue arm ergometer training.

4. Add military press. Press the weight directly over or behind the head.

5. Add isokinetic strengthening and endurance exercises (high speeds—200+ degrees/second) for shoulder internal and external rotation with the arm at the side.

6. Isokinetic strengthening for horizontal abduction and adduction may be added. Shoulder flexion and extension and abduction and adduction may be added as needed.

7. Isokinetic Test: The second isokinetic test for shoulder internal and external rotation, horizontal abduction and adduction and abduction and adduction is administered. For shoulder internal and external rotation, the shoulder may be tested in the functional position (80–90° of abduction). Test results for internal and external rotation and horizontal abduction should demonstrate at least 80% strength and endurance (as compared to the uninvolved side) before proceeding with exercises specific to the activity setting.

8. Continue total body conditioning program with emphasis on the shoulder (rotator cuff, posterior deltoid).

9. Skill mastery: Begin practicing skills specific to the activity (e.g. work, recreational activity, sport). For example, throwing athletes (e.g. pitchers) may proceed to an interval throwing program.

ROM, range of motion; GH, glenohumeral

In most cases, sling immobilization is used up to 2–4 weeks, depending on physician preference and patient symptoms. During this time gentle passive ROM can be started in a protected range, as tolerated by the patient. It should be stressed that passive motion is done, this early, to promote healing by enhancing collagen organization, stimulating joint mechanoreceptors and decreasing pain through neuromuscular modulation. It is not done to aggressively gain more motion, and significant stretching of capsular structures should be avoided. Exercises such as pendulums and cane exercises for short arcs of internal (Fig. 6) and external rotation are used.

Numerous studies have shown that subjects with shoulder laxity and instability have been shown to have altered kinematics and firing patterns of the rotator cuff.[47-51] These studies demonstrate the importance of early and persistent rotator cuff and scapular strengthening exercises in this at risk population. Early strengthening exercises will consist mainly of gentle submaximal isometric contractions of the rotator cuff (Fig. 7) and scapular muscles (Fig. 8). These can be done carefully in the supine or side-lying position. In the early phase, these isometrics are done to recruit rotator cuff and scapular muscles and to delay muscle atrophy, not to achieve hypertrophy. Rhythmic stabilization isometric exercises can be performed in a submaximal manner, to the patient's tolerance. These exercises can be started with the arm at the side, progressing to the arm in scapular

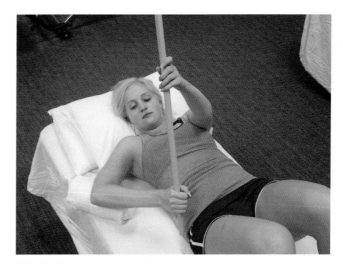

FIG. 6: Cane internal rotation exercise

plane at 45° (Fig. 9) and eventually to the balance position at approximately 100° of flexion (Fig. 10).[52]

As long as the patient does not have isolated posterior instability, CKC weight shifts can be initiated with partial weight bearing (Fig. 11). These exercises create a cocontraction of the scapular and cuff muscles while creating a compressive effect by virtue of the weight-bearing component.

The author recommends judicious use of pain control modalities to be used at this time. Cold therapy,

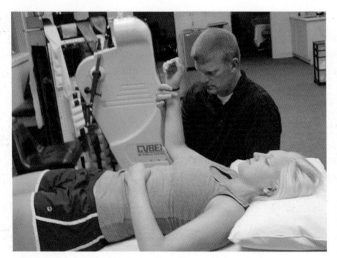

FIG. 7: Submaximal isometrics for the rotator cuff with the arm slightly abducted

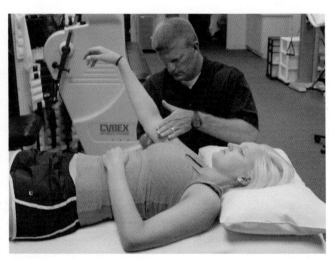

FIG. 9: Submaximal isometrics in scapular plane at 45 degrees of scaption

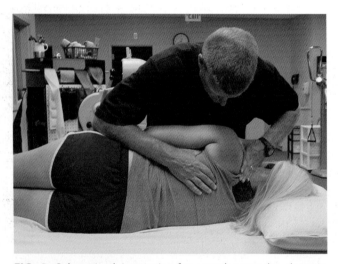

FIG. 8: Submaximal isometrics for scapular muscles done in side-lying

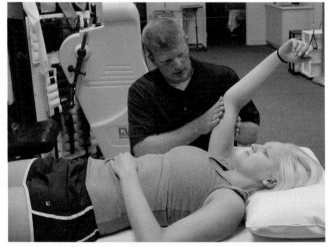

FIG. 10: Submaximal isometrics in balanced position

high-voltage electrical stimulation and transcutaneous electrical nerve stimulation electrical modalities may be useful to decrease perceived pain. These should be used early to reduce inflammation, create relaxation and reduce muscle spasm and guarding.

Intermediate phase

Goals of the intermediate phase include regaining and improving muscle strength, normalization of shoulder motion and arthrokinematics, enhancing dynamic stabilization of cuff and scapular muscles, and improving neuromuscular control of the shoulder for upper extremity activities.

Although not yet aggressive, passive ROM should be progressed at this time. Motion should be advanced to patient's tolerance with the goal at the end of this phase being attainment of full, pain-free ROM. A clinical pearl is not to rush, but rather to help expedite motion. Careful monitoring of motion progression is appropriate. Clinicians may worry about limitation of motions early and push the patient too aggressively, too early. Provided motion is advancing, aggressive stretching is not necessary. A slow progressive increase is appropriate following this type of injury. However, loss of motion, or stagnant motion that is not full, is also a concern and is a point of discussion that should be taken up with referring

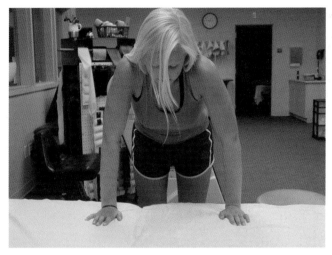

FIG. 11: Partial weight bearing closed kinetic chain (CKC) weight shifts performed over examination table

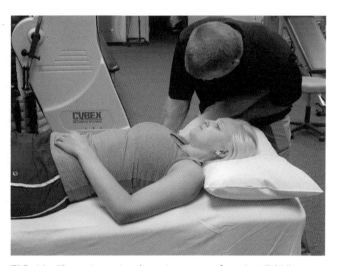

FIG. 13: Therapist-assisted passive range of motion (ROM)

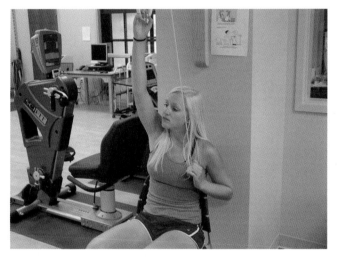

FIG. 12: Passive pulley to gain elevation range of motion (ROM)

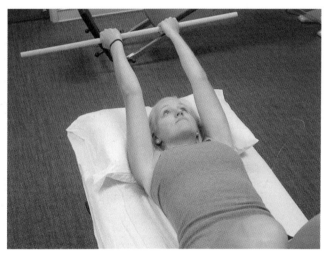

FIG. 14: Self-stretching with cane into flexion

physician as soon as possible. Realistically, completely full motion may not be attained prior to 8–12 weeks. Pulley exercises (Fig. 12) and continued therapist-assisted passive ROM (Fig. 13) are still appropriate at this time. Self-stretching with cane into flexion (Fig. 14) and abduction as well as internal and external rotation cane exercises are also approved. End range of abduction and external rotation (Fig. 15) are usually attained last.

In the intermediate phase, patient pain and spasm should be reduced or absent. Isometric exercises can be progressed to isotonic exercises in limited arcs through a protected ROM. The goal is to enhance dynamic strength through the rotator cuff and scapulothoracic muscles of the shoulder. Isotonic exercises for these muscles groups

can begin in side-lying positions similar to those used for isometric exercises in the acute phase. Resistance can begin with progressive manual resistance advancing to titrated weights or bands. These isotonic exercises should be started initially with the elbow at the side, progressing to scapular plane, and eventually to prone or seated and standing positions.

The importance of the scapular plane is worth further discussion in the context of optimizing targeted muscle activation. The supraspinatus has the ability to generate more abduction torque in the scapular plane with the shoulder in neutral rotation or either slight internal or external rotation.[53,54] A common exercise to perform in this phase to increase rotator cuff strength is elevation in

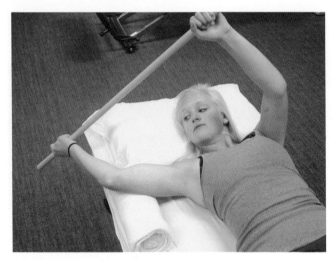

FIG. 15: Self-stretching with cane into end range abduction and external rotation

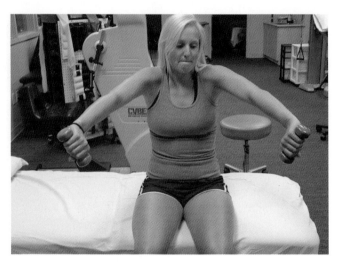

FIG. 17: Empty can scapular plane elevation

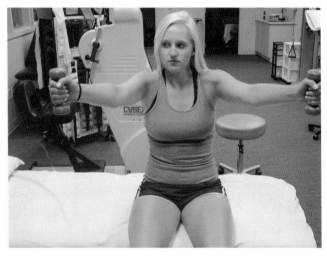

FIG. 16: Full can scapular plane elevation

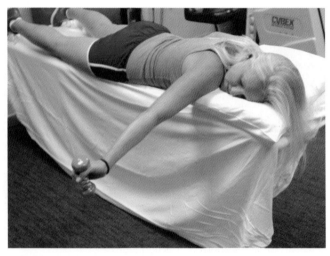

FIG. 18: Prone full can elevation

the scapular plane with the shoulder in internal rotation or the "empty can", which was first described by Jobe and Moynes.[55] Due to the relative risk of iatrogenic impingement from the internally rotated position, others have suggested the same exercise with external rotation of the humerus or the "full can" position.[56-59] When comparing supraspinatus and deltoid activity during full can (Fig. 16), empty can (Fig. 17) and prone full can (Fig. 18), Reinold et al. found that all exercises provided similar supraspinatus muscle activity ranging from 62% to 67% of maximum voluntary isometric contraction.[59] Furthermore, the "full can" position demonstrated significantly lower amounts of deltoid activity than the other two. In patients with instability this

is important to note, as increased deltoid activity could create harmful superior or posterior sheer forces during elevation exercises. Exercises that create relatively high supraspinatus and concomitant high deltoid activity (empty can and prone full can) may be more detrimental than an exercise with relatively high supraspinatus and relatively lower deltoid activity (full can). Following a dislocation, the subscapularis is an important dynamic stabilizer. The subscapularis provides GH compression, internal rotation and anterior stability to the shoulder. Subscapularis activity may allow more torque generation at 0° of abduction.[54] When performing internal rotation strengthening at 0° abduction, other larger muscles may come active (Fig. 19). These include other internal

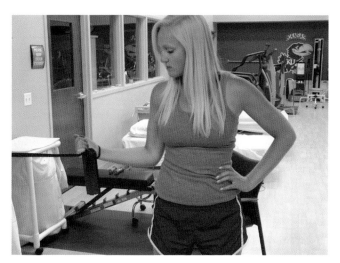

FIG. 19: Shoulder internal rotation strengthening at 0° of abduction

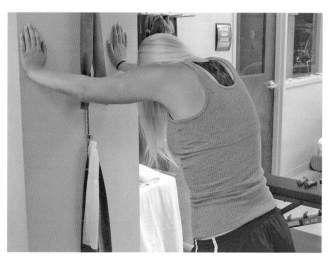

FIG. 21: Standing scapular exercises via wall push-ups with plus

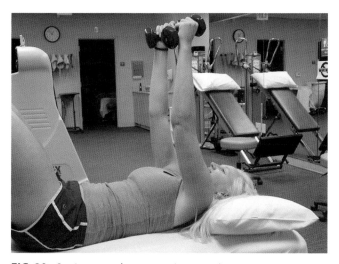

FIG. 20: Supine scapular protraction exercise

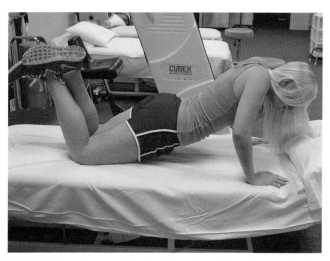

FIG. 22: Scapular strengthening via push-ups from knees with plus

shoulder rotators, such as the pectoralis major, latissimus dorsi and the teres major.[60] Decker has reported that internal rotation at 90° of abduction produced less pectoralis major muscle activity than with the arm at the side in 0° of abduction.[60] Therefore, one may choose to train the internal rotators, when tolerated at higher levels of motion (such as 90° abduction), to better isolate the subscapularis, while minimizing activity of the pectoralis major muscle.

Once the patient exhibits adequate scapular strength, supine scapular protraction exercise can be performed (Fig. 20). CKC exercises can also be added to include a wall drills (Fig. 21) to push-ups, beginning on knees (Fig. 22), progressing to standard push-up position (Fig. 23). Proprioceptive neuromuscular facilitation drills are a neurophysiologic approach to therapeutic exercises that can be used during all phases of shoulder rehabilitation to address multiple and different impairments and functional losses.[61] Proprioceptive facilitation drills can begin in a submaximal manner in this phase.

Advanced strengthening phase

Goals of the advanced strengthening phase are to improve strength, power and muscle endurance, to improve neuromuscular control, to enhance dynamic rotator cuff and scapular stabilizer strength, and to prepare the patient for eventual return to prior level of activity. To achieve these advanced goals, pain should be under control and ROM should be normalized. If these are not achieved, more progressive means to control pain and

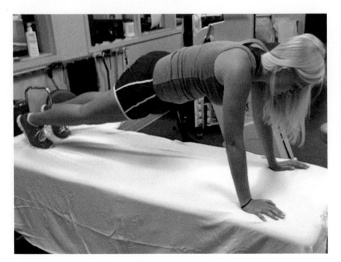

FIG. 23: Scapular strengthening via standard push-ups with plus

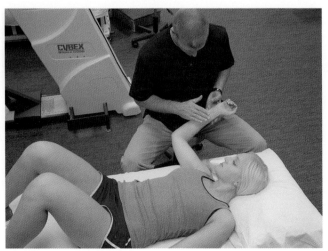

FIG. 24: Advanced cuff strengthening at 90/90 position with manual resistance

normalize ROM may be required. These could include consistent use of modalities and or injections for pain relief, and higher-grade joint mobilizations or dynamic splinting for increasing ROM.

In this phase, advanced shoulder specific, rotator cuff, and scapular muscle strengthening exercises can be performed. A continuation of previous exercises should be performed, although higher repetitions and increased loads may be required to continue to stimulate a strengthening response. The patient should be able to initiate more general weight training exercises, such as latissimus pull downs, and bench press. Caution should be used and modifications to these exercises should be implemented based on directional instability. Latissimus pull downs should be performed anterior to the frontal plane in front of the head and to stop motion just shy of full extension to decrease stress on anterior capsule of GH joint.[62] Additionally, bench press motions should not allow upper arms to break the frontal plane in patients with damage to the anterior capsule. This can be done by using Smith Machine™ with motion stops or placing a rolled towel on chest to limit how far bar drops.[62] These precautions should remain in place until the 9–12 month to allow full remodeling and complete healing of soft tissues. A gradual progression of increasing stress to the GH capsule should be allowed when returning to more traditional ranges of motion during more provocative exercises such as standard shoulder press, latissimus pull downs and bench press. A return of symptoms with these more traditional

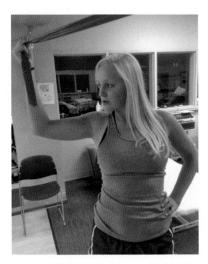

FIG. 25: Advanced cuff strengthening at 90/90 with Theraband®

exercises may necessitate a longer precautionary time frame of even greater than 1 year.

Resistance exercises can be performed in more challenging positions, such as 90 degrees of abduction and 90 degrees of external rotation position while standing. These exercises can be done with manual resistance from therapist (Fig. 24) or use of commercial Theraband® (Fig. 25). These can be done to end ROM to enhance overhead dynamic stabilization of the rotator cuff and scapular stabilizers. Finally, the patient may begin easy plyometric exercises. These should always be started with two hands (Fig. 26), close to the body with lighter weights, progressing to heavier weights and eventually to a single arm (Fig. 27).

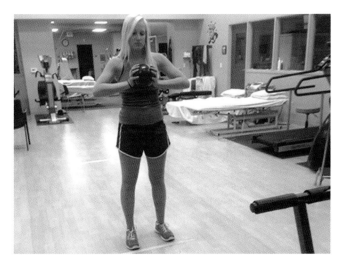

FIG. 26: Two-handed chest pass plyometric exercises

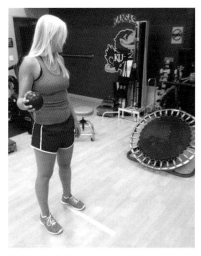

FIG. 27: Single-handed plyometric exercises

Return to activity phase

The return to activity phase demands maintenance of full strength, power and endurance, and progressively increasing level of ability to fully return the patient to their prior status.

Depending on the patient's goals, some orthopedic patients may not require progressing into the return to activity phase. If the patient does not require powerful movements, they may stop at the advanced strengthening phase. However, if the patient desires to return to recreational or competitive sports, then a return to activity phase is a requirement.

All patients will continue to perform exercises as listed in the advanced strengthening phase of treatment.

Athletes will require advanced strength and endurance exercises, including plyometric exercises, proprioceptive neuromuscular control drills and isotonic strengthening that is more sport-specific. An additional requirement of the return to activity phase is some form of interval training program. These programs are developed to slowly and gradually return endurance and confidence in the extremity through simulated gradual sports activities. Interval programs should be chosen based on the patient's unique desires, skills and ultimate goals for return to activity. These interval programs should be initiated well in advance of the desired competitive start date of the patient's specific sport. All too often the patient wants to participate in an upcoming game 1 month from the start of an interval throwing program. Unrealistic expectations should be addressed immediately.

Atraumatic Multidirectional Instability

The patient with atraumatic instability is one that may have MDI. This patient potentially has recurrent subluxation or dislocations due either to congenital looseness or to repetitive activities that have created a looseness of the shoulder capsular and ligamentous structures. Regardless of the cause, the patient probably has multiple factors contributing to this instability. Examples include shallow glenoid fossa, weakness of GH and scapulothoracic muscles, excessive capsular redundancy, laxity due to increased proportion of elastin in soft tissues and decreased collagen density.[63] Due to these factors, rehabilitation of this patient may be very complicated and difficult.

Treatment for the atraumatic shoulder instability patient requires normalizing motion, increasing muscular strength and endurance, restoring proprioception, dynamic stability and neuromuscular control. As the patient progresses, more work, activity or sport-specific drills can be emphasized to prepare for a gradual return to full unrestricted activities as needed.

Acute phase

With atraumatic instability, the acute phase occurs immediately after the most recent subluxation, dislocation or re-exacerbation that has created the symptoms in question. Goals of the initial acute phase of treatment will be to protect the injured structures, to reestablish pain-free ROM, to decrease pain, inflammation, and muscle spasm, to delay muscle atrophy and to reestablish voluntary muscle activity. Severity of symptoms will depend on the amount of energy dissipated during the most recent injury, and the state of irritability of the surrounding soft tissues. With atraumatic instability, symptoms may be minimal or severe. Patients with atraumatic instability will rarely need to be placed in a sling for immobilization. During this acute phase, gentle passive ROM and active-assisted ROM can be initiated in a protected range, as tolerated by the patient. Exercises such as pendulums and cane exercises for short arcs of internal and external rotation are used to normalize motion until it has returned to full. In most instances, with some relative rest from offending activities, the shoulder will soon become less irritable and motion can be regained quickly. Rotational motion should be progressed starting with the arm at the side at 0° of abduction to 30°, 45° and finally 90° of abduction.

When compared to healthy subjects, athletes with generalized joint laxity have been shown to demonstrate altered motor patterns with increased subscapularis activity during internal rotation exercises, and decreased supraspinatus and subscapularis activity during external rotation exercises.[47,64] Early strengthening exercises will consist mainly of gentle submaximal isometric contractions of the rotator cuff (Fig. 7) and scapular muscles (Fig. 8). These can be done carefully in the supine or side-lying position. In the early phase, these isometrics are done to recruit rotator cuff and scapular muscles and to inhibit atrophy, not to achieve hypertrophy. Rhythmic stabilization isometric exercises can be performed in a submaximal manner to the patient's tolerance. These exercises can be started with the arm at the side progressing to the arm in scapular plane at 45° (Fig. 9) and eventually to the balanced position at around 100° of flexion (Fig. 10).

As long as the patient does not have isolated posterior instability, CKC weight shifts can be initiated early with partial weight-bearing. These exercises create a cocontraction of the scapular and rotator cuff muscles while creating a compressive effect by virtue of the weight-bearing component approximating the GH joint. All of the exercises discussed so far are to be performed below 90° of elevation to begin with, as this ROM is much easier tolerated by most patients with shoulder instability.

Judicious use of pain control modalities may be used at this time. Cold therapy, high-voltage electrical stimulating and transcutaneous electrical nerve stimulation electrical modalities may be useful to decrease perceived pain. These should be used early to reduce inflammation, create relaxation and reduce muscle spasm and guarding.

Intermediate phase

Goals for the intermediate phase include enhancing functional dynamic stability of the rotator cuff and scapular muscles, reestablishing normal arthrokinematics patterns of the GH joint, reestablishing neuromuscular control, improving muscular strength, endurance and obtaining full ROM.

If ROM is not full at this point, more aggressive means should be taken to restore normal GH motion. Motion should be progressed to patient's tolerance and the goal of the end of this phase should be attainment of full unrestricted ROM. Full and unrestricted motion should be attained prior to 8–12 weeks. As long as the patient is able to tolerate, active ROM and end range stretching may be needed to facilitate full recovery. End range of abduction and external rotation movements are usually attained last.

Isometric exercises can be progressed to isotonic exercises in limited arcs through a protected ROM. The goal is to enhance dynamic strength of the rotator cuff and scapulothoracic muscles of the shoulder. Isotonic exercises for these muscles groups can begin in side-lying positions similar to those used for isometric exercises in the acute phase. Resistance can begin with progressive manual resistance, by the therapist, progressing to titrated weights or bands. These exercises should be started initially with the elbow at the side, progressing to scapular plane and eventually prone, seated, and standing positions. It is essential to strengthen the posterior cuff muscles, which include the infraspinatus and teres minor, as they provide GH compression and resist both superior and anterior shear forces on the humeral head.[65] External rotation with tubing in several different positions has proven to demonstrate high infraspinatus and teres minor electromyographic activity. Exercises can be performed in side-lying,[58,66,67] and/or in standing.[58,68] Isotonic exercises with light dumbbells can include full can scaption and prone external rotation, performed in either 0°, 45° or 90° of abduction.[58,66-68]

Exercises with these smaller muscle groups should be done with lower weights and higher repetitions initially, to help improve neuromuscular control of the rotator cuff and scapular muscles for dynamic joint stability. A clinical pearl is to place a towel roll under the axilla while performing external rotation exercises with the arm at the side. This has several positive implications. First, it provides a more comfortable position because it allows lower capsular strains as it puts the GH joint closer to the loose packed position. Secondly, it places the rotator cuff and scapular muscles in a more optimal length tension relationship. Third, it allows for an increased amount of arterial blood flow to the supraspinatus by decreasing the "wringing out" effect seen with the arm completely at the side. Lastly, 20–25% more electromyographic activity is found in this position as compared to that with the arm at the side without a towel.[58]

Proper scapulothoracic balance is important for scapulohumeral movements during all motions of the shoulder. Disruption of normal scapular muscle-firing patterns due to pain, fatigue and/or weakness may lead to shoulder injury or persistent symptoms. Strengthening the serratus anterior helps to maintain the normal scapulohumeral rhythm, as it assists the upper and lower trapezius with protracting as well as upwardly rotating the scapula. Collectively these muscles upwardly rotate, posterior tilt and externally rotate the scapula.[69,70] Several exercises have been proven to stimulate high serratus anterior activity including D1 and D2 diagonal proprioceptive neuromuscular facilitation pattern flexion and D2 diagonal pattern extension, scapular protraction, supine upward scapular punch, military press, push-up plus and GH internal and external rotation at 90° abduction.[71-75]

If the patient exhibits adequate scapular strength, CKC exercises can also be progressed to include a progression of standing wall drills, advancing to prone push-ups beginning on knees, then to standard push-up position. During any of the push-up type activities, serratus anterior activity appears to be greatest when full scapular protraction occurs after the elbows are fully extended in the "push-up plus" position.[69] During push-up type exercises, the lowest muscle activity is seen in the wall push-up plus, while moderated activity is seen while on the knees, and high activity during standard pushups.[69,71] The highest serratus anterior activity may actually occur when push-ups are done with the feet elevated which demonstrates elevated activity when gravitational challenges increase (Fig. 28).[76] Closed kinetic chain exercises can be further progressed using advanced techniques in the next phase.

Advanced strengthening phase

Goals of the advanced strengthening phase are to improve and enhance strength, power and muscle endurance of the rotator cuff and scapulothoracic muscles, to improve neuromuscular control, to enhance dynamic rotator cuff and scapular stabilizer strength, and to prepare the patient for eventual return to activity. To achieve these advanced goals, pain should be under control and ROM

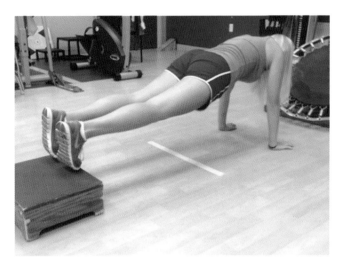

FIG. 28: Push-ups with feet elevated

should be normalized. If these are not achieved more aggressive means to control pain and normalize ROM may be required.

More advanced shoulder specific, rotator cuff, and scapular strengthening exercises can be performed. A continuation of previous exercises should be performed although higher repetitions and increased loads may be required to continue to stimulate a strengthening response. The patient should be able to start to initiate more general weight training exercises such as latissimus pull downs and bench press. Caution should be used and the same modifications to these exercises should be implemented as were described with the traumatic instability patient.

Resistance exercises can be performed in a more challenging position such as the 90/90 position while standing. These exercises can be done with manual resistance from therapist or use of commercial tubing. These can be done to end ROM to enhance overhead dynamic stabilization of the rotator cuff and scapular stabilizers.

Closed kinetic chain exercises are advanced to be performed with perturbations or on unstable surface to maximally challenge the patient. Weight shifts and push-ups on a ball or BOSU® will challenge the patient's dynamic control of the entire upper extremity.

Finally, the patient may begin easy plyometric exercises. These should always be started with two hands, close to the body with lighter weights, progressing to heavier weights and eventually to a single arm. Specific two-handed exercises include the chest pass, overhead throw, and alternating side-to-side throw using low

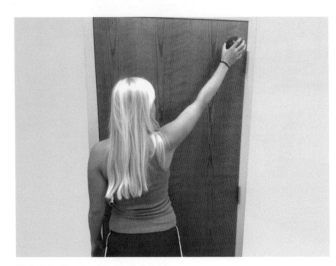

FIG. 29: Single-arm wall dribbles

weighted balls to begin. Once these are tolerated wall dribbles (Fig. 29) can begin as a single arm exercise progressing to the baseball style throw in the 90/90 position with a light weighted ball.

Return to activity phase

The return to activity phase asks for maintenance of full strength, power and endurance and progressively increasing level of ability to fully return the patient to prior status.

If a return to activity phase is needed all patients will continue to perform exercises as listed in the advanced strengthening phase of treatment. Athletes will require more aggressive strength and endurance exercises including plyometric exercises; proprioceptive neuromuscular control drills and isotonic strengthening that are more sport-specific. An additional requirement of the return to activity phase is some form of interval program. These programs are developed to slowly and gradually return endurance and confidence in the extremity through simulated gradual sports activities. Interval programs should be chosen based on patients unique desires and skills, and ultimate goals for return to activity. These interval programs should be initiated well prior to the desired competitive start date of the patient's specific sport.

Return to Play Criteria Following Glenohumeral Instability

It seems self-evident that following the return to activity phase, one should be ready for competition. Clear

decisions must be made regarding each athlete's ability to return to competitive activity based on the individual. However, there is a lack of consensus in the literature as to what constitutes objective return to play criteria. Following an episode of GH instability, an athlete may have both physical and psychological impairments that will render them unable to compete at a full level. Author's guidelines for return to sport include 90% strength of prime shoulder movers, shoulder internal rotators and external rotators. Full active and passive ROM are a prerequisite. Upper extremity functional tests may be performed and scores within 90% of bilateral symmetry or norms should be attained. Depending on shoulder dominance, normative values rather than a side-to-side comparison may be more helpful. For example, using the single arm shot put test on the rehabilitated nondominant arm will not generally yield the same results as the uninjured dominant arm. In a swimmer, who uses both shoulders symmetrically, bilateral symmetry and previously determined norms may be completely appropriate. Several tests for a relatively athletic population would include the seated shot put test, which can be done with either both arms (Fig. 30),[77,78] or a single-arm (Fig. 31).[79-81] During the single arm seated shot put test, using a 5.9 lb ball, patients are in either a chair or sitting with back against the wall. The nonthrowing arm is placed across the chest. These positions are used to minimize trunk or legs from participating in the throw. Participants are asked to "put" the ball using arm motion resembling the standard shot put in track and field. Measurements are taken from front of chair or wall to where the ball first strikes the ground. Test-retest reliability for this functional test has shown to have intraclass correlation coefficients (ICCs) of 0.99 for

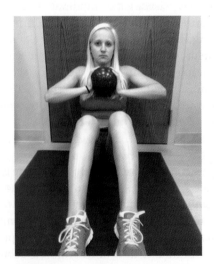

FIG. 30: Seated shot-put test with both hands

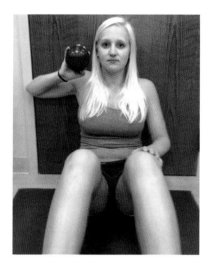

FIG. 31: Seated single-arm shot-put test

the dominant arm and ICCs of 0.97 for the nondominant arm.[79] Additionally, minimal detectable changes have been found to be 17 inches for the dominant arm and 18 inches for the nondominant arm.[79] Minimal detectable change is the minimum amount of change in a patient's test score that ensures that the change is not the result of measurement error and is clinically significant. The reader is referred to Reiman and Manske for detailed descriptions of other upper extremity power functional testing methods.[82]

Glenohumeral Bracing

Patients returning to contact or collision sports such as hockey, football, or rugby may be required to wear a shoulder stability brace for the initiation of return to sports participation. Limited evidence exists for effectiveness of shoulder bracing on injury recurrence rates and motion restrictions. Sawa reports no injury recurrence after GH subluxation or dislocation in hockey players following bracing and a rehabilitation program.[83] Bracing used in the Sawa study permitted variable restriction of shoulder abduction, allowing controlled movement within safe ROM. Both DeCarlo[84] and Weise[85] examined the effect of shoulder braces on limiting active and passive ROM following exercise. In both studies, the braces did exhibit a loosening effect following use, however despite the loosening, neither allowed the shoulder to obtain the vulnerable position of 90° of abduction and full external rotation.

Surgical Considerations

Historically, literally hundreds of procedures have been performed for the surgical treatment of shoulder instability. Many of the older procedures such as the Putti-Platt and Magnusen Stack procedures have been abandoned due to postoperative complications such as persistent motion loss. Open Bankart repairs, which aim to stabilize torn or loose labrum and capsular tissues associated with traumatic dislocations, have mostly now evolved to arthroscopic procedures. Additionally, selective capsular plication procedures are now commonly performed arthroscopically with better cosmetics and less postoperative pain.

■ CONCLUSION

The orthopedic patient with shoulder instability is a very challenging patient. Relatively high incidence rates of subsequent redislocations and chronic GH instability have placed the utmost importance on accurate immediate diagnosis and treatment of this potentially disabling condition. An accurate diagnosis depends on a full understanding of the condition, mechanism of injury and clinical signs and symptoms associated with instability. Due to the instability, unique stress is placed upon capsular and ligamentous structures that further exacerbate this condition. Through a delicate balance of rest, applied stress and loads, nonoperative treatment can yield successful outcomes. However, successful outcomes require a well-structured and designed rehabilitation program that addresses each of the phases that an injured patient will navigate. Emphasis should be placed on normalizing GH motion, restoring both rotator cuff and scapulothoracic strength, enhancing proprioception, neuromuscular control and dynamic stability.

Due to the complexity of the GH joint and capsule, we are scratching the surface of our understanding of this joint. Future research directed toward optimal placement and position of immobilization following acute dislocation may ultimately improve conservative outcomes. Additionally, better understanding of what criteria can be evaluated to determine which acutely injured patient may perform best with conservative or surgical care will help determine most expedient and appropriate treatment. Advanced surgical techniques to tighten loose and/or torn caspulolabral tissue will improve overall functional outcomes.

REFERENCES

1. Matsen F, Harryman D, Sidles J. Mechanics of glenohumeral instability. Clin Sports Med. 1991;10(4):783-8.

2. Curl LA, Warren RF. Glenohumeral Joint stability: selective cutting studies on the static capsular restraints. Clin Orthop. 1996;330:54-65.

3. Liavaag S, Svenningsen S, Reikerås O, et al. The epidemiology of shoulder dislocations in Oslo: The epidemiology of shoulder dislocations in Oslo. Scand J Med Sci Sports. 2011;21(6):e334-40.

4. Simonet WT, Melton LJ III, Cofield RH, Ilstrup DM. Incidence of anterior shoulder dislocation in Olmsted County, Minnesota. Clin Orthop. 1984;186:186-91.

5. Krøner K, Lind T, Jensen J. The epidemiology of shoulder dislocations. Arch Orthop Trauma Surg. 1989;108(5):288-90.

6. Nordqvist A, Petersson C. Incidence and causes of shoulder girdle injuries in an urban population. J Shoulder Elbow Surg. 1995;4(5):107-12.

7. Zacchilli MA. Epidemiology of shoulder dislocations presenting to emergency departments in the United States. J Bone Jt Surg Am. 2010;92(3):542.

8. Howell SM, Galinat BJ. The glenoid-labral socket: a constrained articular surface. Clin Orthop. 1989;243:122-5.

9. Lippitt SB, Vanderhooft JE, Harris SL, Sidles JA, Harryman DT, Matsen FA. Glenohumeral stability from concavity-compression: a quantitative analysis. J Shoulder Elbow Surg. 1993;2(1):27-35.

10. Poppen NK, Walker PS. Normal and abnormal motion of the shoulder. J Bone Joint Surg Am. 1976;58(2):195-201.

11. Howell SM, Galinat BJ, Renzi AJ, Marone PJ. Normal and abnormal mechanics of the glenohumeral joint in the horizontal plane. J Bone Jt Surg Am. 1988;70(2):227-32.

12. Blasier RB, Guldberg RE, Rothman ED. Anterior shoulder stability: contributions of rotator cuff forces and the capsular ligaments in a cadaver model. J Shoulder Elbow Surg. 1992;1(3):140-50.

13. Karduna AR, Williams GR, Iannotti JP, Williams JL. Kinematics of the glenohumeral joint: influences of muscle forces, ligamentous constraints, and articular geometry. J Orthop Res. 1996;14(6):986-93.

14. Gohlke F, Essigkrug B, Schmitz F. The pattern of the collagen fiber bundles of the capsule of the glenohumeral joint. J Shoulder Elbow Surg. 1994;3(3):111-28.

15. Brotzman S, Manske RC. Clinical Orthopaedic Rehabilitation: An Evidence-based Approach, 3rd edition. Philadelphia, PA: Elsevier, Mosby; 2011.

16. Dumont GD, Russell RD, Robertson WJ. Anterior shoulder instability: a review of pathoanatomy, diagnosis and treatment. Curr Rev Musculoskelet Med. 2011;4(4):200-7.

17. Owens BD. Incidence of shoulder dislocation in the United States military: demographic considerations from a high-risk population. J Bone Jt Surg Am. 2009;91(4):791.

18. Arnheim D. Modern principles of athletic training. St. Louis, MO: Mosby; 1985. [online] Available from http://www.abebooks.com/Modern-Principles-Athletic-Training-Arnheim-Daniel/9547903314/bd. [Accessed October, 2014].

19. Antoniou J, Harryman DT. Posterior instability. Orthop Clin North Am. 2001;32(3):463-73.

20. Bradley JP, Baker CL, Kline AJ, Armfield DR, Chhabra A. Arthroscopic capsulolabral reconstruction for posterior instability of the shoulder a prospective study of 100 shoulders. Am J Sports Med. 2006;34(7):1061-71.

21. Fronek J, Warren RF, Bowen M. Posterior subluxation of the glenohumeral joint. J Bone Joint Surg Am. 1989;71(2):205-16.

22. Hawkins RJ, Koppert G, Johnston G. Recurrent posterior instability (subluxation) of the shoulder. J Bone Joint Surg Am. 1984;66(2):169-74.

23. Zarins B, Rowe C. Current concepts in the diagnosis and treatment of shoulder instability in athletes. Med Sci Sports Exerc. 1984;16(5):444-8.

24. Davies GJ, Dickoff-Hoffman S. Neuromuscular testing and rehabilitation of the shoulder complex. J Orthop Sports Phys Ther. 1993;18(2):449-58.

25. Edouard P. Rotator cuff strength in recurrent anterior shoulder instability. J Bone Jt Surg Am. 2011;93(8):759.

26. Jan J, Benkalfate T, Rochcongar P. The impact of recurrent dislocation on shoulder rotator muscle balance (a prospective study of 102 male patients). Ann Phys Rehabil Med. 2012;55(6):404-14.

27. Wilk KE, Andrews JR, Arrigo CA, Keirns MA, Erber DJ. The strength characteristics of internal and external rotator muscles in professional baseball pitchers. Am J Sports Med. 1993;21(1):61-6.

28. Wilk KE, Andrews JR, Arrigo CA. The abductor and adductor strength characteristics of professional baseball pitchers. Am J Sports Med. 1995;23(3):307-11.

29. Yeap JS, Lee DJ, Fazir M, Kareem BA, Yeap JK. Nerve injuries in anterior shoulder dislocations. Med J Malays. 2004;59(4):450-4.

30. Hertel R, Lambert SM, Ballmer FT. The deltoid extension lag sign for diagnosis and grading of axillary nerve palsy. J Shoulder Elbow Surg. 1998;7(2):97-9.

31. Watson LA, Pizzari T, Balster S. Thoracic outlet syndrome part 1: Clinical manifestations, differentiation and treatment pathways. Man Ther. 2009;14(6):586-95.

32. Adson AW, Coffey JR. Cervical rib: a method of anterior approach for relief of symptoms by division of the scalenus anticus. Ann Surg. 1927;85(6):839.

33. Magee DJ. Orthopedic physical assessment. St. Louis, Missouri: Elsevier Health Sciences; 2013.

34. Roos DB. Congenital anomalies associated with thoracic outlet syndrome: anatomy, symptoms, diagnosis, and treatment. Am J Surg. 1976;132(6):771-8.

35. Manske R, Ellenbecker T. Current concepts in shoulder examination of the overhead athlete. Int J Sports Phys Ther. 2013;8(5):554-78.

36. Harryman DT, Sidles JA, Harris SL, Matsen FA. Laxity of the normal glenohumeral joint: a quantitative in vivo assessment. J Shoulder Elbow Surg. 1992;1(2):66-76.

37. McFarland E, Torpey B, Curl L. Evaluation of shoulder laxity. Sports Med. 1996;22(4):264-72.

38. Altchek D, Dines D. The surgical treatment of anterior instability: selective capsular repair. Oper Tech Sports Med. 1993;1:292-5.

39. Rowe C, Zarins B. Recurrent transient subluxation of the shoulder. J Bone Jt Surg Am. 1981;63:863-72.

40. Kvitne R, Jobe F. The diagnosis and treatment of anterior instability in the throwing athlete. Clin Orthop. 1993;291:107-123.

41. Jobe F, Kvitne R, Giangarra C. Shoulder pain in the overhead or throwing athlete: the relationship of anterior instability and rotator cuff impingement. Orthop Rev. 1989;18:963-75.

42. Speer KP, Hannafin JA, Altchek DW, Warren RF. An evaluation of the shoulder relocation test. Am J Sports Med. 1994;22(2):177-83.

43. Hovelius L. Anterior dislocation of the shoulder in teen-agers and young adults. Five-year prognosis. J Bone Joint Surg Am. 1987;69(3):393-9.

44. Hovelius L, Augustini B, Fredin H. Primary anterior dislocation of the shoulder in young patients. A ten-year prospective study. J Bone Jt Surg Am. 1996;78(11):1677-84.

45. Hovelius L, Nilsson J-Å, Nordqvist A. Increased mortality after anterior shoulder dislocation: 255 patients aged 12–40 years followed for 25 years. Acta Orthop. 2007;78(6):822-6.

46. Itoi E, Hatakeyama Y, Sato T, Kido T, Minagawa H, Yamamoto N. Immobilization in external rotation after shoulder dislocation reduces the risk of recurrence. A randomized controlled trial. J Bone Joint Surg Am. 2007;89(10):2124-31.

47. Broström L-A, Kronberg M, Nemeth G. Muscle activity during shoulder dislocation. Acta Orthop. 1989;60(6):639-41.

48. Labriola JE, Jolly JT, McMahon PJ, Debski RE. Active stability of the glenohumeral joint decreases in the apprehension position. Clin Biomech. 2004;19(8):801-9.

49. Labriola JE, Lee TQ, Debski RE, McMahon PJ. Stability and instability of the glenohumeral joint: the role of shoulder muscles. J Shoulder Elbow Surg. 2005;14(1):S32-8.

50. Matias R, Pascoal AG. The unstable shoulder in arm elevation: a three-dimensional and electromyographic study in subjects with glenohumeral instability. Clin Biomech. 2006;21:S52-8.

51. Santos MJ, Belangero WD, Almeida GL. The effect of joint instability on latency and recruitment order of the shoulder muscles. J Electromyogr Kinesiol. 2007;17(2):167-75.

52. Wilk KE, Crockett H, Andrews JR. Rehabilitation after rotator cuff surgery. Tech Shoulder Elbow Surg. 2000;1:128-44.

53. Liu J, Hughes RE, Smutz WP, Niebur G, Nan-An K. Roles of deltoid and rotator cuff muscles in shoulder elevation. Clin Biomech. 1997;12(1):32-8.

54. Otis J, Jiang C, Wickiewicz T, Warren R, Santner T. Changes in the moment arms of the rotator cuff and deltoid muscles with abduction and rotation. J Bone Jt Surg Am. 1994;76:667-76.

55. Jobe F, Moynes D. Delineation of diagnostic criteria and a rehabilitation program for rotator cuff injuries. Am J Sports Med. 1982;10:336-9.

56. Itoi E, Kido T, Sano A, Urayama M, Sato K. Which is more useful, the "full can test" or the "empty can test," in detecting the torn supraspinatus tendon? Am J Sports Med. 1999;27(1):65-8.

57. Kelly BT, Kadrmas WR, Speer KP. The manual muscle examination for rotator cuff strength an electromyographic investigation. Am J Sports Med. 1996;24(5):581-8.

58. Reinold M. Electromyographic analysis of the rotator cuff and deltoid musculature during common shoulder external rotation exercises. J Orthop Sports Phys Ther. 2004;34(7):385-94.

59. Reinold MM, Macrina LC, Wilk KE, Fleisig GS, Dun S, Barrentine SW, et al. Electromyographic analysis of the supraspinatus and deltoid muscles during 3 common rehabilitation exercises. J Athl Train. 2007;42(4):464-9.

60. Decker MJ, Tokish JM, Ellis HB, Torry MR, Hawkins RJ. Subscapularis muscle activity during selected rehabilitation exercises. Am J Sports Med. 2003;31(1):126-34.

61. Wilk KE, Reinold M, Andrews JR. Proprioceptive neuromuscular facilitation for the shoulder. In: Greenfield BH (Ed). The Athletes Shoulder, 2nd edition. St. Louis, MO: Churchill Livingstone; 2009.

62. Durall C, Manske R, Davies GJ. Avoiding shoulder injury from resistance training. Strength Cond J. 2001;23(5):10-8.

63. Rodeo SA, Suzuki K, Yamauchi M, Bhargava M, Warren RF. Analysis of collagen and elastic fibers in shoulder capsule in patients with shoulder instability. Am J Sports Med. 1998;26(5):634-43.

64. Kronberg M, Broström LA, Németh G. Differences in shoulder muscle activity between patients with generalized joint laxity and normal controls. Clin Orthop. 1991;269:181-92.

65. Sharkey NA, Marder RA. The rotator cuff opposes superior translation of the humeral head. Am. J Sports Med. 1995;23(3):270-5.

66. Ballantyne BT, O'Hare SJ, Paschall JL, Pavia-Smith MM, Pitz AM, Gillon JF, et al. Electromyographic activity of selected shoulder muscles in commonly used therapeutic exercises. Phys Ther. 1993;73(10):668-77.

67. Townsend H, Jobe FW, Pink M, Perry J. Electromyographic analysis of the glenohumeral muscles during a baseball rehabilitation program. Am J Sports Med. 1991;19(3):264-72.

68. Greenfield BH, Donatelli R, Wooden MJ, Wilkes J. Isokinetic evaluation of shoulder rotational strength between the plane of scapula and the frontal plane. Am J Sports Med. 1990;18(2):124-8.

69. Ludewig PM, Hoff MS, Osowski EE, Meschke SA, Rundquist PJ. Relative balance of serratus anterior and upper trapezius muscle activity during push-up exercises. Am J Sports Med. 2004;32(2):484-93.

70. McClure PW, Michener LA, Sennett BJ, Karduna AR. Direct 3-dimensional measurement of scapular kinematics during dynamic movements in vivo. J Should Elbow Surg. 2001;10(3):269-77.

71. Decker MJ, Hintermeister RA, Faber KJ, Hawkins RJ. Serratus anterior muscle activity during selected rehabilitation exercises. Am J Sports Med. 1999;27(6):784-91.

72. Ekstrom R, Donatelli R, Soderberg GL. Surface electromyographic analysis of exercises for the trapezius and serratus anterior muscles. J Orthop Sports Phys Ther. 2003;33(5):247-58.

73. Hintermeister RA, Lange GW, Schultheis JM, Bey MJ, Hawkins RJ. Electromyographic activity and applied load during shoulder rehabilitation exercises using elastic resistance. Am J Sports Med. 1998;26(2):210-20.

74. Moseley JB, Jobe FW, Pink M, Perry J, Tibone J. EMG analysis of the scapular muscles during a shoulder rehabilitation program. Am J Sports Med. 1992;20(2):128-34.

75. Myers JB, Pasquale MR, Laudner KG, Sell TC, Bradley JP, Lephart SM. On-the-field resistance-tubing exercises for throwers: an electromyographic analysis. J Athl Train. 2005;40(1):15-22.

76. Lear L, Gross M. An electromyographical analysis of the scapular stabilizing synergists during a push-up progression. J Orthop Sports Phys Ther. 1998;28(3):146-57.

77. Cronin JB, Owen GJ. Upper-body strength and power assessment in women using a chest pass. J Strength Cond Res. 2004;18(3):401-4.

78. Meyhew J, Bemben M, Piper F, Ware J, Rohrs D, Bemben D. Assessing bench press power in college football players: the seated shot put. J Strength Cond Res. 1993;7:95-100.

79. Negrete RJ, Hanney WJ, Kolber MJ, Davies GJ, Ansley MK, McBride AB, et al. Reliability, minimal detectable change, and normative values for tests of upper extremity function and power. J Strength Cond Res. 2010;24(12):3318-25.

80. Negrete RJ, Hanney WJ, Kolber MJ, Davies GJ, Riemann B. Can upper extremity functional tests predict the softball throw for distance: a predictive validity investigation. Int J Sports Phys Ther. 2011;6(2):104-11.

81. Chmielewski TL, Martin C, Lentz TA, Tillman SM, Moser MW, Farmer KW, et al. Normalization considerations for using the unilateral seated shot put test in rehabilitation. J Orthop Sports Phys Ther. 2014;44(7):518-24.

82. Reiman MP, Manske RC. Functional testing in human performance. London: Champaign Illinois. Human Kinetics; 2009.

83. Sawa TM. An alternate conservative management of shoulder dislocations and subluxations. J Athl Train. 1992;27(4):366-9.

84. DeCarlo M, Malone K, Hawkins RJ, Misamore G. Protective devices for the shoulder complex. Shoulder injuries in the athlete: surgical repair and rehabilitation. New York, NY: Churchill Livingstone; 1996. pp. 365-73.

85. Weise K, Sitler MR, Tierney R, Swanik KA. Effectiveness of glenohumeral-joint stability braces in limiting active and passive shoulder range of motion in collegiate football players. J Athl Train. 2004;39(2):151-5.

CHAPTER 5

Carpal Tunnel Syndrome

Judy L Matsuoka-Sarina

ABSTRACT

Carpal tunnel syndrome (CTS) is the most common upper extremity compressive neuropathy of adults in 2012. In 2000, almost 6% of this population opted for carpal tunnel release surgery. Symptoms may include one or both wrists and/or hands with intermittent to persistent numbness, tingling, burning, aching, shooting pain, edema, and/or radiating symptoms up the arms to the neck. The effectiveness of conservative treatment is limited in evidence to obtain long-term relief.

The assessment and conservative treatment of CTS is complex. Mild to moderate CTS may benefit from an orthosis at night, exercise, manual edema mobilization (MEM), deep tissue mobilization, physical agent modalities, nerve mobilization, and adjunctive therapies. To promote self-management, the certified hand therapist of occupational or physical therapy utilize and educate the basic science, brain perception, nervous system anatomy, correlating the patient's behaviors, habits, lack of awareness of the hand and body to activity and/or positioning to improve lifestyle changes.

■ INTRODUCTION

Carpal tunnel syndrome (CTS) is the most common upper extremity compressive neuropathy affecting between 3% and 6% of adults in the general population in 2012.[1] In 2000, it was reported up to 5.8% of the population opted for carpal tunnel release surgery.[2]

Symptoms are characterized in one or both wrists and/or hands with intermittent to persistent numbness, tingling, burning, aching, shooting pain, stiffness, swelling, edema, and/or radiating symptoms up the arms to their neck. Patients who repetitively use their fingers or wrists often report severe symptoms at night, and some during the day as well. Many patients frequently report dropping objects, including plates, cups, or coins

and papers, and are unable to sustain pinch or grasp for spontaneous reach, pickup and carry. Women may have an inability to manage or manipulate small jewelry fasteners.

Evidence regarding effectiveness of conservative intervention for CTS—outside of steroid injections—to obtain long-term relief, is frequently limited or conflicting.[1-15]

Epidemiology

There is conflicting data regarding causation of CTS related to work-related demands such as repetitive hand movements, use of vibratory tools, and extensive pinching or gripping. In one 2012 study, two-thirds of persons who were presumed to have occupational CTS were found to have other medical conditions and comorbidities capable of causing and/or contributing to carpal tunnel symptoms.[10]

Other anatomical problems that may contribute to the incidence of CTS are idiopathic in origin and include: aberrant muscles, rare soft tissue tumors, ganglion cysts, and a dislocated lunate.[8] Comorbidities may include diabetes, hypothyroidism, endocrine system pathology, rheumatoid arthritis, obesity, hypertension, depression, alcoholism, inactivity, age, work activities, hobbies,[4,16] repetitive maneuvers, pregnancy, trauma, amyloidosis, sarcoidosis, multiple myeloma, and leukemia.[2]

Anatomy

The carpal tunnel consists of the carpal bones arranged from scaphoid and trapezium to pisiform bones—considered the floor of the tunnel, with the transverse carpal ligament bridging across the carpus—considered the roof of the carpal tunnel, over its contents. The median nerve injured in this syndrome, lies just under the transverse carpal ligament (Fig. 1).

The flexor tendons of the hand slide inside the carpal tunnel (Figs 2 to 5) during dynamic hand function. The wrist bones are held together by a complex network of ligaments: the intercarpal, carpal-metacarpal, carpal-radio and carpal-ulnar ligaments maintain the respective

articulations. There are additional, longer, dynamic, diagonal, and strategically located ligaments across both the volar and dorsal surfaces of the carpus. The volar ligaments, including the transverse carpal ligament, which holds the carpal bones together, allow wrist and digit tendon movement and nerve excursion.

The arch of the hand, emanating from the carpal canal, allows the fingers and thumb to move freely. Insertion of the musculotendinous wrist extensors travel dorsally across the dorsal carpal tunnel, to provide lift of the carpus and hand allowing ease in movement when

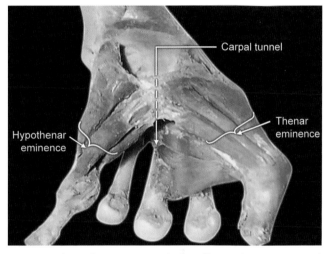

FIG. 2: Cadaver depicting muscular bundle attachments to carpal tunnel ligament. The dashed arrow indicates the location of the tunnel under the ligament
Source: Reproduced from Sydney Morning Herald via Wikipedia.

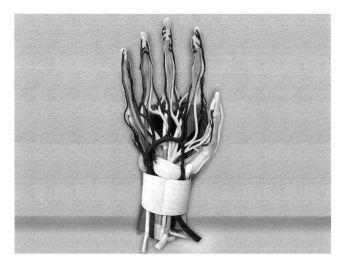

FIG. 1: The plastic anatomical model of the right hand depicts the carpal tunnel ligament and the more proximal flexor retinaculum as white bands (shown more distinctly than in cadaver photographs). The median nerve, (yellow) is located just under the carpal tunnel ligament. The nerve is more vulnerable to increased pressure and movement when flexor tendons are moving, or in combination of wrist positions and/or strong sustained fisting

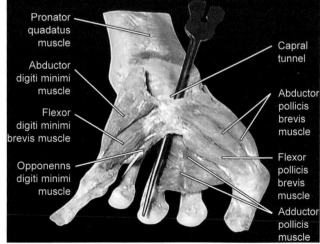

FIG. 3: Cadaver with embedded tool in computerized tomography. The surrounding musculature is identified
Source: Reproduced from Sydney Morning Herald via Wikipedia.

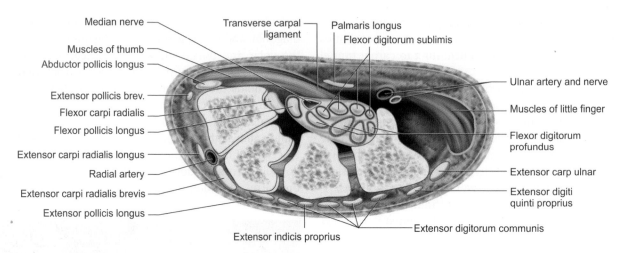

FIG. 4: Cross-section through distal carpal row. Greater multangular renamed trapezium. Lesser multangular renamed trapezoid
Source: Reproduced from Wikipedia via Gray's Anatomy.

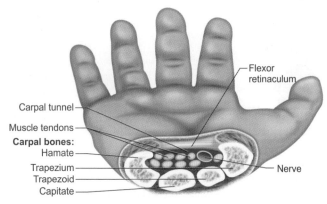

FIG. 5: Cross-section through distal carpal row facing distally
Source: Reproduced from Wikipedia from OpenStax College-Anatomy & Physiology, Connexions Website.

using the hand. These wrist and digit extensor tendons glide close to the bones and are contained by the extensor retinaculum. The extensors provide a balance of force against the stronger flexors, and lumbricals, which are attached to finger extensors through lateral bands (Fig. 6). Primary carpal and intercarpal ligaments, attaching from the radius to the base of the metacarpal bones, provide flexible stabilization allowing for the dynamic and smooth movements of coordination and dexterity. This flexible stability is combined with sensory perception to obtain final function.

The eight finger flexor tendons and one thumb flexor tendon glide through the carpal tunnel where the median nerve lies parallel and superficially to these flexor tendons. They are held inside the canal by the stabilizing

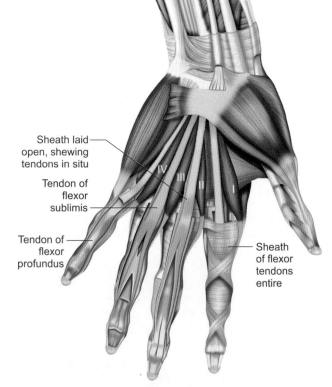

FIG. 6: Anatomical representation of the lumbrical muscles, attached to each finger flexor through lateral bands located laterally on the proximal phalanx. This delicate balance can be disrupted by overuse or shortening of these muscles, eliciting incomplete movement of the "hook fist" or the possibility of the lumbricals traveling into the carpal tunnel with full fisting. Lumbricals I, II, III, and IV inserted to lateral bands of extensor tendons
Source: Reproduced from Gray's Anatomy via Wikipedia.

carpal transverse ligament and, slightly more proximally, by the flexor retinaculum.

Anatomical variations of the median nerve in this area include: a course of the thenar motor nerve branch within the tunnel, an accessory variation of the thenar nerve branch, a high division of the median nerve with accessory branches proximal to the carpal tunnel, or a recurrent branch distal to carpal tunnel ligament which courses backward to the thenar eminance.[17]

Cadaver research has revealed aberrant muscle anatomy as a contributing factor to CTS: muscles arising from the floor tendons, a persistent median artery (the central median artery usually dies off), and a reverse palmaris longus arising off the tendon (causing the nerve to collapse under the extra structural pressure) are all potential contributing anomalies.[18]

The median nerve is one of three peripheral nerves providing sensory and motor components of hand function (Fig. 7). The sensory portion of the median nerve can be demonstrated by mapping its innervation of the volar thumb, index, and middle fingers, the radial half of the ring finger and dorsally distal to the proximal interphalangeal joints of the index, middle, and radial half of the ring finger tissues.

The median nerve innervates the following muscles of the hand:
- Index and middle finger lumbricals
- Opponens pollicis, abductor pollicis brevis, flexor pollicis brevis (superficial head).

Etiology

Carpal tunnel syndrome etiology is currently idiopathic. However, pathogenesis appears to be related to increased pressure within the carpal tunnel.

The features of the outer connective tissues of the nerve include the perineurium and epineurium. The epineurium provides a diffusion barrier to keep toxins out of the nerve and offers biomechanical support to resist tension or compression of the nerve.[19,20] The Schwann cell is the primary mediator of the neural response to prolonged compression, resulting in morphologic changes to the cell and of myelin.[16]

The transition zones of central nervous system (CNS) to peripheral nervous system are connective tissues protecting the nerve root against traction injuries. Generally, the projections of central tissue are absent in small motor rootlets, and longer in sensory and lower nerve rootlets.[21]

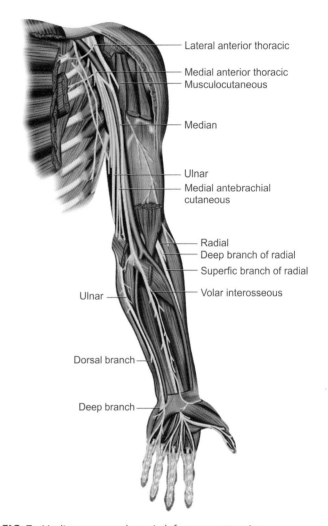

FIG. 7: Median nerve pathway in left upper extremity
Source: Reproduced from Gray's Anatomy via Wikipedia.

The classification of nerve compression includes varying states of pathophysiology. The primary factors are edema within the endoneurial compartment and decreased blood flow to the nerve. Most CTS are classified as type I neuropraxia injuries, with patients reporting mild to moderate sensory symptoms. Nerve compression at one segment along a nerve pathway may increase vulnerability to nerve compression injury at a site distal or proximal to the segment. This may indicate axoplasmic transport disruption. More severe injuries, which include motor impairment, are likely to be classified as type II axonotmesis.[16]

Carpal tunnel syndrome has been reported post-Colles' fracture, and coinciding with carpal arthritis, first carpometacarpal (CMC) joint inflammation, flexor tenosynovitis, and with lesser-known tumors. Non-inflammatory fibrosis of the subsynovial connective tissue is related to CTS and the subsynovial connective tissue volume or stiffness may be the source of median nerve compression. There is statistical association of diabetic conditions, obesity, hypothyroidism, pregnancy, renal disease, inflammatory arthritis, acromegaly, gender (women greater than men), genetic predisposition, age (>50 years of age), smoking, and work activities of forceful grip with wrist flexion, but not definitive as a cause-and-effect.

The controversial concept of double-crush phenomenon that was introduced 30 years ago, noted a high incidence of carpal and cubital tunnel syndrome with associated cervical nerve root abnormalities or irritations.[16]

Injuries to the median nerve can result from: lacerations, humeral fractures, elbow dislocations, distal radius fractures, and lunate dislocations into the carpal tunnel.[7]

■ CLINICAL PRESENTATION

Patients with CTS report swelling or edema, which is most visible in hands and wrist. Patients may also have difficulty wearing rings, bracelets or watches due to edema, skin irritation or hypersensitivity. Sustained compression of the nerve due to trauma or traction will induce the accumulation of edema into the endoneurial space of the trunk.[16] Wrist watches may also contribute to symptoms, via compression. The compression can elicit numbness either from a more proximal compression and/or edema combined with the more localized wrist compression.

The sympathetic nerve fibers may express changes in vasomotor function, e.g. skin color, skin temperature and edema, pseudomotor or sweat function, pilomotor function (goose flesh), and trophic changes.[17] The patient's skin sensitivity or detection of light touch pressure may be altered and symptoms can vary from no pain to hypersensitivity, or tingling to severe pain. The patient may report that they have always had cold hands, or acquired it thinking it was age-related. The pink (normal) color may decrease to darker pink, or reddish and blotchy, to bluish color. Digits may change in appearance from normal finger pulp shape with a quick rebound to shape after firm pressure is applied to the pad, to a slow response to capillary refill or remaining flat or atrophied after release of the firm pressure. The shape of the fingertip may change from round to pointed, observably blanched or white in appearance

and/or exhibit smooth friction ridges, tactile dryness, or wrinkling. It has been the author's experience that patients are usually unaware of any of these changes in their tissues.

■ CLINICAL EXAMINATION

History and Functional Questionnaires

The clinician performs an extensive review of the patient's medical history including: dates of occurrence of systemic disease, heart disease, cancers and their treatment, skin and joint disorders, CNS diagnoses, congenital diagnoses and any falls, trauma, automobile accidents or surgeries.

Michigan Hand Outcomes Questionnaire

The Michigan Hand Outcomes Questionnaire can be completed and scored online.[22] All questions must be answered to obtain an accurate score. A paper form can be printed from the website for clinic use. For patients who are not employed or who are retired, it is recommended that the word "work" may be substituted by "activities".

Work History

It is helpful for the clinician to review work history, activities or duties, length of sustained duties, active hours worked daily, total amount of time or percentage of day and/or of highly repetitive or sustained activities typical of a patient's routine day. The clinician can make inquiries into details such as what positions occur, how often, and/or of what duration, and whether activity breaks or lunch breaks are taken.

Computer Usage

Additional inquiries can be made about the workstation and the setup of the tasks performed by the patient.

- The clinician should determine if the workstation ergonomically assembled by the patient, or the company's designated ergonomic consultant.
- If work is being done in the home, the clinician should glean how, where, what type of setup is utilized in the home.
- The length of time the position for the work is sustained is also valuable data to gather.
- The clinician should also identify the frequency of interruptions.

Leisure Activities

Additional inquiries about the leisure activities performed by the patient can be significant.
- The clinician needs to determine how often, and for how long is the leisure activity performed.
- If the activities are performed in a seated position, the clinician will inquire about the following:
  - What these activities are, and for how long are these activities performed?
  - If television viewing is a regular activity, the position at which it is performed, and the shape and size of furniture can be relevant.
  - When electronics or computers are used frequently, the ergonomics of the setup are important. The clinician identifies where the device (electronic book, laptop, or smartphone) is placed, and whether seating adjustable.
  - With patients who read routinely, the clinician will want to know for how long, and in what positions, including if there is use of foot furniture.
  - If the patient sits on the floor or on the couch, the clinician will identify for how long, and how often.

Social and Recreational Activities

The clinician should inquire about the social and recreational activities of the patient.
- The length and frequency of relevant activities should be documented.
- The type of activity and location can be important (e.g. sitting, standing, walking, and jogging), and should be noted.

Driving

For patients who spend significant periods of time driving, the clinician will want to document the following details:
- The typical length and frequency of driving excursions should be determined.
- The type of transmission, manual or automatic, may impact CTS.
- The ergonomics of the car are important, and considerations include the seat support and fit specific to the driver, as well as if the seat itself is adjustable. The patient may sit in a relaxed or an upright position. The seat may be reclined. The clinician will want to know if the patient's knees rest higher or lower than their hips, and how their stature compares to the size of the seat. The clinician will ask the patient if they are aware of their positioning while driving, and if they feel it may contribute to their symptoms.
- The clinician will ask the patient what strategies they use for drives longer than 2 hours.

Caring for Family and/or Pets

Care-giving activities can contribute to CTS symptoms therefore the clinician will want detailed information about these activities.
- The size, age, and weight of the family member or pet for whom the patient cares are significant.
- The amount of time engaged in care-giving activity.
- The clinician will determine if the care-giving may incur sustained positioning of the hand, wrist, arm or body, and/or if repetitive motions are performed.
- The type of motion of the hand, wrist, forearm, shoulder, and head for the activities should be identified.

Body Type

The clinician will determine the size or stature of the person, such as petite, small, medium, large or tall. This will help in providing information to the patient about why their body size may not fit their seating or other furniture at home.

Provocative Testing and Nerve Compression Testing

Physical examination findings in a systematic review of properties of clinical tests for CTS found Phalen's maneuver has 68% sensitivity and 73% specificity.[23] Phalen's maneuver is performed by instructing the patient to flex both wrists, placing the backs of their hands together, and to hold this position for 30–60 seconds. The test is considered positive when pain, tingling, or numbness is reported in the thumb, index, long, and half of the ring finger.

To perform the Tinel's Test, the clinician lightly taps or applies a percussive force over the median nerve, eliciting tingling in the median nerve distribution of the hand. This test was found to be 50% sensitive and 77% specific.[23] When dermatomal regions are exhibited, the proximal path of the nerve should be considered and incorporated into the assessment. The symptoms are noted and this author presents a diagram of the corresponding dermatome mapping of the body to the patient, to educate the patient as to how the nervous system is connected from spinal cord to the skin and finger tips.

Carpal compression elicited 64% and 83% sensitivity and specificity, respectively.[23]

When diagnosing CTS, manual resistive strength testing of abductor pollicis brevis exhibited 75% specificity and 27% sensitivity, while atrophy of the muscle exhibited 88% specificity and 11% sensitivity.[23]

Berger's test is performed while wrist is in neutral position and the patient is asked to make a fist for 30–40 seconds. The test is considered positive when complaints of pain and paresthesia are reported. When Berger's test is positive, it is suspected that the lumbricals traveled into the carpal tunnel space and elicited the symptoms.[23]

The "hand elevation" test has been found to be 88% sensitive and 98% specific. This test is performed by asking the patient to elevate their hands overhead for 2 minutes. The test is positive if the symptoms are reproduced. The "hand elevation" test is an adjunctive test when combined with the Goloborodko test. The Goloborodko test is performed by the examiner, using their fingers to exert dorsal pressure on the first metacarpal and pisotriquetral complex, and volar pressure on the lunate. The test is considered positive if pain or paresthesia is reported.[23]

Reports or complaints of swelling in the affected hand and the distal metacarpal compression maneuver are helpful in diagnosis and also in designing an orthotic.[23] Girth measurements or volumetric measurements are obtained and compared to the other hand to document edema or swelling. Carpal tunnel compression has a higher correlation for the diagnosis of tenosynovitis than for CTS.[23]

In one study, the provocative tests of Tinel's, Phalen's, reverse Phalen's, the clinician asks the patient to perform wrist and digit extension, held for 2–3 minutes. The test is positive if reports of tingling, pain or numbness occur in the median nerve distribution.[20]

Evans studied the presence of four conditions, in patients with CTS. The presence of the following four conditions, increased the probability of a CTS diagnosis to 0.86.[23]

1. A positive Durkin's test.[24] The clinician presses their thumbs over the carpal tunnel and holds it for 30 seconds. The test is considered positive when pain or paresthesia is reported within 30 seconds, in the median nerve distribution of the hand.
2. Abnormal sensibility with Semmes-Weinstein monofilament style (touch-pressure) testing.[19,25] A standardized graded monofilament test of light touch sensation mapping the detection of light touch pressure of the hand. The clinician always begins from distal fingertips, ending proximally, using the normal light touch monofilament (2.83) until sensation is reported. A positive test is an inability to detect 3.61 or 4.31 or larger monofilament on the volar thumb, index, long, and radial half of the ring finger tips or pads. Significant loss is revealed when the full length of these fingers are involved.
3. An abnormal hand diagram, where a patient's mapping of the discomfort and quality of their symptoms is drawn. Radiating symptoms in the median nerve distribution pattern may be drawn as well.
4. Presence of nocturnal pain or symptoms of the hand and/or wrist.

Active Range of Motion Assessment and Palpation

Active range of motion (AROM) assessment may elicit symptoms. The clinician should identify any substitution patterns and should ask the patient to describe their symptoms in detail.

The clinician asks the patient to move the neck and head (Figs 8 and 9), and the thoracic spine. The clinician assesses scapular positioning and stabilization (by palpation, if the patient is clothed); the position of the first and second rib compared to that of the clavicle; glenohumeral joint motion—especially of flexion, internal and external rotation at side of body (to identify pectoralis major and/or minor tightness, and scapular stabilizer weakness or impairment condition); glenohumeral abduction and adduction; elbow extension overhead; forearm rotation with elbow at side of body (not in front of the rib cage); wrist extension and flexion with the hand relaxed; and ask the patient to form a gentle fist with the forearm positioned in neutral, and positioned in supination; and finally, the clinician observes the patient while performing an open extended hand with wrist extension, then gentle fisting combined with wrist flexion.

When assessing AROM, additional information may be gathered, such as:
- The clinician will ask the patient to identify the location of the tightness and ask them to point to it.
- Identifying the nature of the tightness as deep or superficial can be useful.
- The clinician will ask the patient in which direction he or she experiences the tightness, and if the tightness reproducible.
- The quality of the restriction limiting the movement— hard, bony block, in contrast to a sensation of muscle tightness—can provide the clinician with insight.

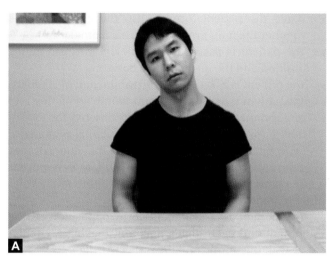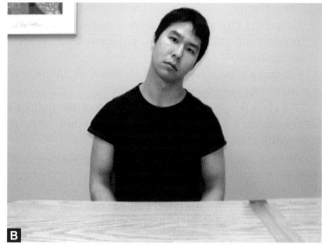

FIGS 8A AND B: Comparing—(A) Right; and (B) Left cervical long lateral flexion the clinician assesses loss and simultaneously inquires about the patient's symptoms

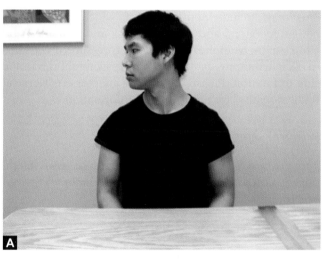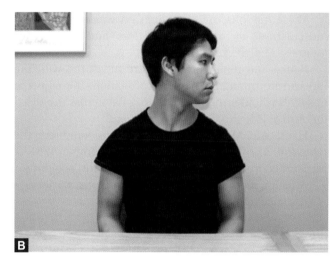

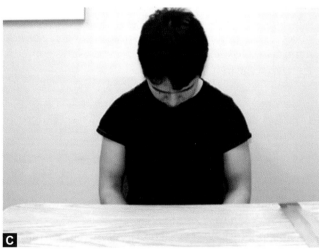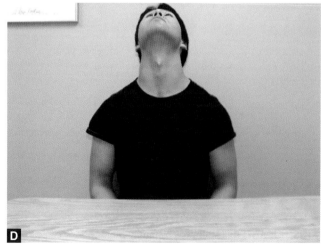

FIGS 9A TO D: (A and B) Comparisons between the two sides are made, visually by clinician, and by the patient; (C and D) The clinician and the patient work together to detect accommodations to neurodynamic tensions. Shortened and/or deconditioned musculature may elicit symptoms more proximally, asymmetrically, centrally or in a radiating symptom pattern down the arm

The clinician will want to know if the intensity of symptoms change with repeated motions, or if the location of the symptoms changes after several repetitions.

Providing a mirror for visual feedback at this time is meaningful to the patient's experience.

The clinician needs to consider whether the patient's ROM is normal for that person's background, and for their medical history.

When assessing wrist AROM, the elbow should be positioned at the side of body. The patient is asked to perform the following motions:

- Wrist extension and flexion in forearm neutral, supination, and pronation with gently relaxed fist.
- Composite digit extension combined with wrist motion.
- Composite digit flexion or fisting combined with wrist motion.

These motions can shed light on weakness of wrist musculature, or overuse of flexors and overuse or tightness of digit extensors.

Radial and ulnar deviations are measured with the forearm in pronation. While in pronation, the clinician observes whether the ulna is sitting flat across the distal forearm or is it visually more prominent.

Hand AROM is assessed with the hand on the table top, or off the table top with the elbow in flexion. Measurements should be taken in all forearm positions.

- A fisting motion or fingertips to touch palmar crease distance is measured for all the digits.

While the patient forms a fist, the clinician notes whether the nails are parallel to each other.
- The patient is asked to perform the intrinsic minus position and the intrinsic plus position.
- The patient is asked to perform abduction of all digits.
- The patient is asked to perform thumb abduction and opposition. The clinician should observe for loss of motion or a deformity in the metacarpal-phalangeal (MP) or basal joint of the thumb. The clinician also assesses for tightness in the palm and/or web space.

The patient is asked to oppose the thumb to the volar fifth MP joint.

The patient is asked to perform opposition of the thumbnail and each digit's nail, and making a circular shape with the thumb and the respective digit.

Cervical Spine Screening

This may include Spurling's test, which requires the patient to extend and rotate the neck and side bend, the clinician then applies manual overpressure downward to elicit symptoms radiating to the ipsilateral limb to the side of rotation. Please refer to the chapter on "Cervical Radiculopathy" for more detailed information.

Postural Screening

The posture screen should include front and lateral observation of patient's normal sitting position (Figs 10A and B).

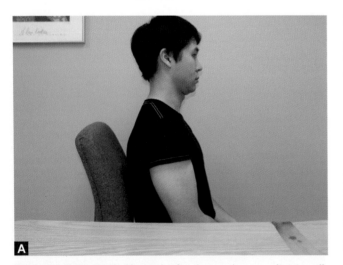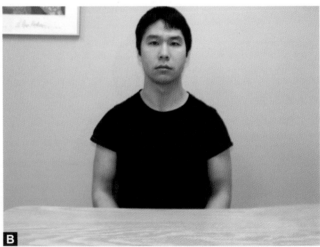

FIGS 10A AND B: (A) Photos by family members, or clinician allow the person to visually analyze their own relaxed posture. They can decide how they can use the photo to remind them, as they learn to improve their posture; (B) Notice the differences between the shoulder levels, and/or the angulation of the midline of neck and shoulder. A mirror can be used to point out the difference

The clinician can lightly slide the hand over the whole back and can detect atrophy, deconditioned scapular stabilization musculature or trunk musculature, and any acquired scoliosis. Identified abnormalities may require confirmation from the patient, for details of exact locations of abnormality based on previous testing, or further objective testing for musculature deficiency.

Grip Strength Testing

The clinician will note any symptoms that might be reproduced during grip strength testing. The author measures grip strength in the standardized position (Figs 11A and B). The patient is asked to alternate hands at each span level at all five spans of the dynamometer with maximal effort. The patient will report any symptoms and differences between the hands. This will increase their own awareness to detect differences in performance and strength of their hands. The patient's grip strength status for span two (female) and span three (male) should be measured. The patient is educated about what is expected over the five spans: a bell shaped curve of the five graduated spans/widths of grip strength performance.

Pinch Strength Testing

The patient will alternate between hands, while testing for lateral pinch, tripod or 3-jaw chuck pinch, pad to thumb pad of each digit in forearm and wrist neutral positions (Figs 12A and B). Standardized pinch of lateral, three-jaw chuck, and index tip to thumb tip pinch should be measured and a comparison between the affected and nonaffected hands should be performed. The author prefers additional finger opposition to demonstrate to the patient the differences in strength or weakness of each digit. Observation of each finger's ability to sustain midline demonstrates whether there is overcompensation to perform in this position.

Myofascial Pain Differentiation

Myofascial pain may elicit symptoms similar to CTS, hence requiring differentiation. Further discussion of myofascial pain is beyond the scope of this chapter. Travell describes pain mappings in detail in Myofascial Pain and Dysfunction: The Trigger Point Manual.

Differential Diagnosis

Other diagnoses that need to be ruled out when treating CTS include:
- Other peripheral neuropathies
- Pronator syndrome
- Anterior interosseous syndrome
- Cervical radiculopathy
- Cervical sprain and strain
- Thoracic outlet syndrome
- Hand-arm vibration syndrome
- Diabetic neuropathy
- CNS pathology.

It has been the author's experience that patients who do not tolerate their physician's prescribed and/or issued

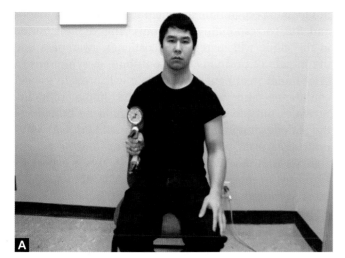 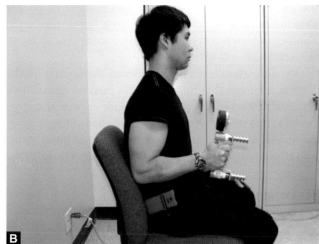

FIGS 11A AND B: (A) Front view; (B) Side view. Standardized positioning for maximal grip strength testing using the Jamar™ Dynamometer. The author prefers alternating hands for all five spans provide a bell shape curve of the muscular performance for each width. Neurodynamic accommodation can be observed

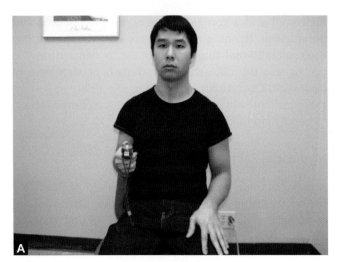 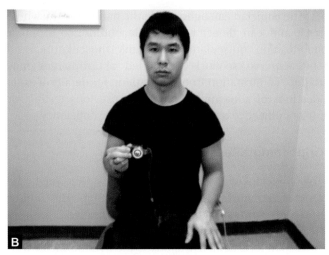

FIGS 12A AND B: Standardized—(A) Lateral pinch; and (B) Three-point pinch (thumb opposing index and middle finger pads) meter testing demonstrate strength of the upper quadrant nervous system distally. Neurodynamic accommodation and joint laxity can be observed

standard wrist brace may have a combination of local and more proximal involvement.

PHYSICAL THERAPY TREATMENT

Conservative management of CTS has been well documented. However, conservative approaches are not typically considered for the chronic moderate to severe CTS, when signs of muscle atrophy or significant sensory impairment (such as numbness or inability to detect a sharp pin prick) are present. Research has been inconclusive for or against using these measures to select the intervention strategy. Eighty-two percent of people respond to nonoperative management, but a substantial number experience symptom recurrence and progress to surgery.[1]

Rehabilitation techniques will vary depending on the findings of the evaluation. It is highly recommended that, on their first visit, the patient is made aware of factors contributing to progressive edema, pain, tingling, or numbness, (i.e. lack of movement, changes in positioning, and sustained positioning).

Treatment Planning

Initially, it is critical to explain, to illustrate and to demonstrate how the symptoms that the patient may be experiencing are related to the central and peripheral nervous system, and the corresponding dermatome mappings. Educating the patient on the impact of the entire nervous system and how it affects their whole body, not just an isolated part of the body, such as the hand, is an integral part of preliminary treatment. An illustration of the brachial plexus and its proximal and distal pathways will reinforce the importance of those body parts attached to it and how the pathways run in continuity between the neck and the hand. It has been the author's experience that many patients do not understand how the position of each proximal area, such as the spine and head, affects the distal parts, such as the wrist and hands. Instruction in resolving poor habits with the person by simulating the provocative positions should provide immediate recognition, and help to change these habits and the corresponding symptoms. This demonstration in the clinic will increase the patient's awareness and the impact of positions that contribute to symptoms. A brief initial treatment in the clinic will provide greater confidence and adherence to the home program. Activities outside of employment should be brought to the patient's attention with discussion of joint and nerve protection principles, problem solving and/or activity analysis with modifications as needed. This is especially a priority for those who are already involved in a regular exercise program. Many may benefit from additional emphasis on posterior upper quarter strengthening using free-weights, customized to the condition. Improving head, neck and trunk positioning prior to upper extremity movement and during cardiovascular workouts is a high priority to prevent reinjury and to sustain good general health.

Improving Activity Tolerance

Many patients report avoiding engaging in regular exercise, often due to another medical diagnosis, work, family, fatigue or because of personal preference. Positioning the patient in an improved posture, then asking if their symptoms change, is critical to the patient achieving independent management. The clinician should discuss how the rehabilitation techniques can be performed at work, and incorporated into commuting, and engaging in social activities. The author expects that the patient reports their effort and any changes in symptoms on their next follow-up visit.

Orthotic Considerations

- Wrist orthoses are customized to provide 2 degrees of wrist flexion and 3 degrees of ulnar deviation[23] and are used mostly for night-time wear.
- Lumbrical blocking orthoses: MP flexion is blocked between 20° and 40°. If Berger's test is positive and flexor synovitis is present, a combination of this position for all the digits and wrist orthoses positioned in neutral are recommended.[23]
- The thumb is positioned in CMC neutral position, when symptoms are associated with carpal-metacarpal joint osteoarthritis. This thumb position can be combined with a wrist orthotic for night-time wear.[23] A short opponens orthotic for day-wear will assist and prevent CMC dislocation, dissociation and limit adduction forces. This author has incorporated additional inserts by incorporating neoprene padding to prefabricated or off-the-shelf supports, when the manual support of specific areas provides a decrease in symptoms.
- Use of a full night resting hand pan orthotic or a wrist neutral, digits free brace for nocturnal pain[23] combined with instructions for improved sleep positioning can provide short-term relief as the patient improves.
- Strategies to maintain the wrist in neutral for keyboarding include light-weight biofeedback-type coated spring wire, splinting material or elastic taping. The flexible wire material, coated for comfort, is positioned on the dorsum of the wrist and hand extending over the third metacarpal, with a distal loop to fit around the proximal phalanx of the long finger, and the forearm portion is secured by strapping proximally.

Many patients will endure the use of braces, or soft neoprene thumb and/or wrist wraps during work.

These should be tapered quickly during day use, while progressing into independent management of posture correction, frequent stretches, upper quarter edema management, and interventions to address soft tissue dysfunction and/or weakness. It is not uncommon to hear patient complaints of bulkiness or interference with hand hygiene or cooking related to splints or orthoses. Clinically, the prolonged use of a splint or brace may often develop weakness of the extensors and small muscles of the hand. Weakness of these muscles may have been present prior to wrist support acquisition. Proximal edges of these supports can compress soft tissues, compromising the forearm structures and adding to the original symptoms.

Reports of intolerance of these orthoses may indicate a more proximal dysfunction to the clinician. An evaluation of the upper quadrant involvement of brachial plexus and cervical function needs to be performed in these cases. Reassessment of the functional, sustained positions in which the orthotic is worn may shed light on the involvement of the proximal tissues. Tolerance of the orthotic may improve as the proximal nerve dysfunction dissipates.

Nerve Mobilization and Gliding

Mobilization of the nervous system is a common hands-on treatment provided by a well-trained clinician.[26,27] The author has not formally used this technique, however, embraces the premise that the nervous system is designed for movement and entrapment can occur at any point along the nerve pathway.[16,19,23-25,28-33] A literature review comparing nerve mobilization and nerve gliding to nonmobilization yielded limited results. The review indicated that nerve mobilization and/or nerve gliding treatment could be utilized for a particular patient type preference. In this situation the patient would be informed of expectations to demonstrate its effectiveness.[12] The clinician should be aware that in addition to the direct and local tissues, other remote tissues innervated by the involved nerves may also be the source of the patient's symptoms.

Patient Education and Training

Stretching

This author prefers to emphasize repetitions or movement, which involves the whole body, rather than static isolated stretches. These stretches are to be performed every 20–30 minutes.[34-37] The purpose is to move large body parts for both sedentary patients and

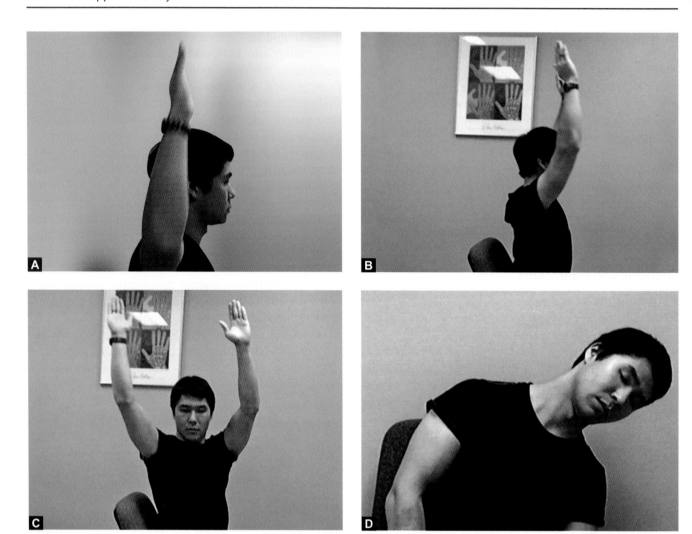

FIGS 13A TO D: (A) Active arm motions to assist in neurovascular movement and edema reduction; (B) Arm pumping overhead reach, and bringing the arm down to squeeze the armpit lymph nodes. The arm positioning is in tolerable external rotation and horizontal humeral abduction, then raised overhead. Each arm is to be moved separately for five repetitions, and then five times together; (C) Trunk rotation combined with both arms elevated; (D) Combining lateral flexion of the neck and torso

those who perform highly repetitive activities to increase circulation of the musculature and to increase lymph flow and decrease edema. To ensure regular interruption, of either static postures or repeated movements, the clinician may suggest the use of a timer or of a software program as a reminder. Prescribed stretches include reaching overhead, bringing hand down behind the back, and head and trunk rotations in isolation as well as in combination (Figs 13A to D).

Stretching hands and fingers into abduction (Figs 14A and B), wrist and digit extension, forearm supination, external rotation and overhead reaching every 15–30 minutes, while looking up or away will assist in preventing muscle shortening, edema and pain.

Hand and wrist stretches are recommended when performing long periods of keyboarding, 10-key numerical pad use, or mousing. Stretches may include forearm supination combined with digit flexor stretches against the table edge in front of body (Figs 14A and B) and to the side of the body on a wall or table. Figure 18A demonstrates the intrinsic minus stretch (MP hyperextension combined with full proximal and distal interphalangeal flexion of all and each individual finger).

These manual stretches may not be well-tolerated by the patient during the first visit. It might take a few sessions, depending on the adherence to the lifestyle modifications brought to their attention by the clinician, before they can be successfully implemented. The stretches are to be

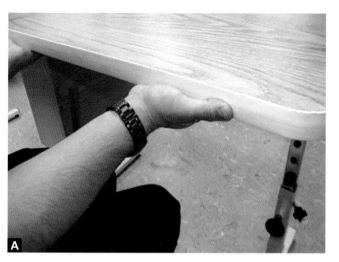 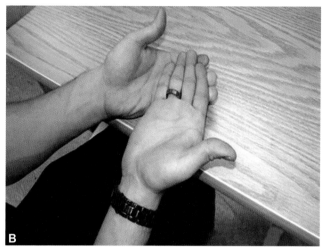

FIGS 14A AND B: (A) The thumb and palmar web and fascia stretches are depicted. Thumb abduction and digit-thumb abduction stretches are performed at edge of table. The thumb from carpometacarpal (CMC) to pad is placed on the table edge, with the rest of hand under table; (B) Fingers or contralateral hand pull digits and metacarpals as a group, and then each digit individually, toward the ulnar side of hand. The thumb remains stationary, the wrist and hand being stretched remain relaxed. The patient is told that the stretch sensation should be detected across the palm between the thumb and base of the finger being pulled

performed diligently by the patient, with the patient self-reporting the symptom intensity as a guide. Repetition will help detect the changes in symptoms. Overhead hand and arm pumping between hand stretches are helpful to improve neurovascular circulation.

Activity and Ergonomic Modifications

Activity and ergonomic modifications are important to decrease tendon and nerve loading, and to improve joint protection. It is the author's experience that all activities and positions of the patient, during their entire day should be explored and discussed. Ergonomic principles have been utilized successfully to address occupational injuries.[34-40] The biomechanical and human factors are emphasized in education of both, the patient and their employer. The job-site evaluation and/or treatment session should include the area where the job is performed, and the duties of the patient. Self-help checklists are personalized for the patient to use as a future reference. Ergonomic tools and furniture can be beneficial, however, in isolation, they do not always achieve complete resolution of symptoms.[41] This author has noted that some patients do not take the initiative to make their workstation or chair more comfortable, but would wait for permission to do so. It is the clinician's responsibility to educate the patient that an ergonomic furniture or adaptive aide may not completely resolve their symptoms.

It will be the patient's responsibility to monitor and modify how they use their bodies that will be most helpful while concurrently implementing rehabilitation techniques. The patient's awareness of symptoms can be demonstrated by asking the patient to verbalize symptom changes and report lifestyle changes. This will allow the patient to be independent with symptom management and with progressing toward recovery during each activity everyday.

Ergonomic Reaching and Fitting

The patient is advised to keep documents, keyboard, mouse, and supplies within easy horizontal reach, not more than 16–18 inches away. Ergonomists have designed strategies to improve the fit between workers and their jobs, including computer workstations.[10,38-41] The evidence is insufficient, but recommended based on consensus for ergonomic interventions in settings with combinations of risk factors, such as high force and high repetition.[7] Forearm support for frequent keyboard users is necessary for potential prevention of neck and/or shoulder symptoms.[7]

In the clinic, the patient may begin to detect changes in the symptoms. Becoming aware that changes in positions of the arms, especially, elevation on top of the table top, or "unloading" the weight of the arm from the upper torso during use, often decrease symptoms. This author has noted that armrests, in general, can pose problems for those unaware of how the armrest height and placement influences their posture. If the armrest is too low, the patient might lower him or herself, or shift his or her torso to lean on the armrests.

Recent manufacturing developments for products and workstation analysis have helped to minimize sustained seating, by incorporating an adjustable standing computer workstation, or counter. The long-term research to promote adaptive equipment is currently in progress.

Ergonomic Positioning and Adaptations for Interacting with Vision

The clinician educates the patient that monitors, tablets, smartphones, books and documents should be held or positioned upright, not flat on the table (Figs 15A to G).[38-41]

Poor eyesight can be a contributing factor to postural dysfunction, as the patient wants to move the head forward to adjust to changes in or loss of visual acuity. Consider reading and/or computer glasses for improved vision. Separate keyboards can be attached if the laptop monitor or tablet needs to be elevated and angled significantly. The patient should consider scanning the information, to be available for reading on the monitor.

For bed readers, the clinician should consider prism glasses. This will allow readers to lie flat on their back and to have the reading material propped up on their chest. The author prefers to limit reading to 20–30 minutes before falling asleep, or incorporating the 20-20-20 rule of eyesight (refer to vision care paragraph later).

Table-top readers may want to consider a cookbook holder, placed on a 4 inch box or stack of books. The recommended height of the box or stack of books will

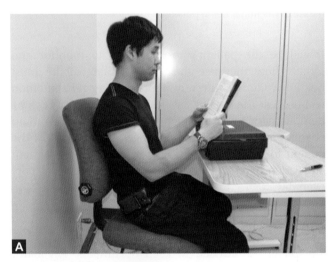

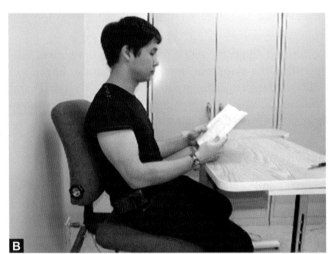

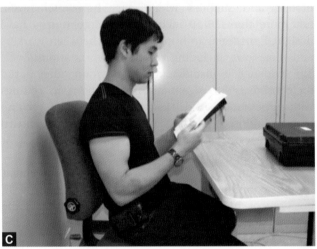

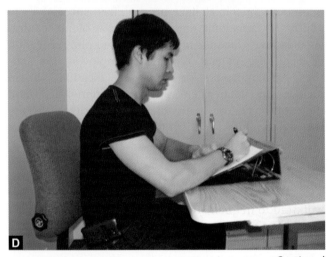

Continued

Continued

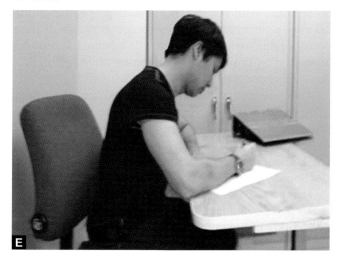

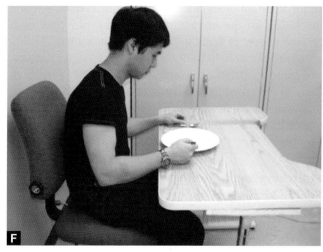

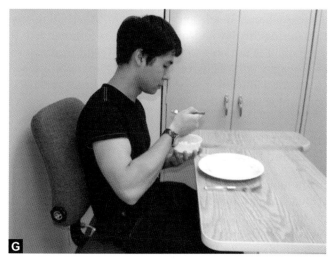

FIGS 15A TO G: (A to C) Exploring neurodynamic tension while performing functional activities such as reading a book with and without arm support increases awareness of cumulative symptoms or tightness; (D and E) Writing habits are persistent, however, people will adapt to their workstation, others will change their positioning to accommodate their changing visual acuity. The latter will need medical intervention to assist in lifestyle corrections in eye-hand positioning activities; (F and G) Eating positions with and without socialization can contribute to symptoms. Heightened awareness of this habitual sustained positioning is another demonstration to educate the patient in neurodynamics

depend on the torso height of the patient and on the type of glasses, if needed, for a proper ergonomic fit.

Standing to read instead of being seated provides a change in positioning. The same setup for the table top reader can be applied for the counter top. The clinician may advocate sitting on a stool, as doing so uses a different muscle set than sitting in a standard chair. Legs can be spread apart and dropped lower to provide greater variety of muscle engagement. The 20–30 minutes stretch rule applies here for both, the body and the eyes.

Reading or watching television on the couch and/or recliners can also pose problems over time. The patient will need to frequently move from a seated position to a standing position, and to stretch. Emphasis will be placed on standing, stretching and practicing proper posture. Educating the patient regarding the rules for vision care for sustained reading will decrease eye strain and incorporate an increased awareness of correcting head and neck positioning.

While reading, the vision care 20-20-20 rule must be followed. The rule states: after reading for 20 minutes, the eyes should look out at something 20 feet away for 20 seconds. This resets the balance of the eye focusing muscles. This would also be an opportunity for the patient to stand up and stretch.

Ergonomic Seating

To adequately address CTS, ergonomic seating modifications or variations might be required.[34-40] The patient will benefit from the clinician's exploration of proper seating guidelines. For a small person, a chair for their stature will provide more support and decrease strain of the spine and the neurodynamic system. Varying the height of the chair during the day can provide a greater variety of body and muscle engagement. Sitting on a wedge can help to obtain improved sitting posture. The clinician can trial the wedge with the patient provided there are no medical low back contraindications. When a patient experiences reduction in effort to maintain the desired posture, the adherence to the instruction and training for lifestyle modifications is improved.

Stretching and Restoration of Muscle Length for Seated Activities

Restoration of muscle length of tight hip flexors, and pectoralis major and/or minor can be combined with myofascial mobility to be performed while sitting and/or standing. While "unloading" or manually lifting and handling the relaxed proximal portions of the upper arm and shoulder, the clinician or patient can gently position the arm towards the chest. This may be performed in supine or sitting position. The pain or symptoms will reportedly decrease, and a notable ease in movement in the hand is discovered. To regain normal length of the pectoralis musculature either the clinician or patient can begin to actively assist to reestablish the normal flexibility easing compression over the proximal portions of the peripheral nerves.

Performing arm and hand movements while resting the arm on an elevated table top can be incorporated, to ease pain and symptoms. It is extremely important for the clinician to demonstrate this unloading for immediate decrease in symptom intensity and to heighten the patient's awareness. An example of unloading the proximal upper quadrant in a seated position can be demonstrated using 3–4 inches firm foam, pillows or books under the forearm, optimally at the patient's side. Positioning the elevated arm in front of the patient can help to decrease the neurovascular tension and to allow wrist and/or hand movement with reduced symptoms. Lowering the chair or elevating the table, combined with sitting upright can additionally help reduce symptoms. The goal should be to help the patient to detect the differences in symptoms in different positions.

Workload Reduction

It is critical to decrease the workload of the affected hand.[40] The clinician should recommend use of the other hand for gross hand activities, if possible, while the involved hand is rehabilitating. Examples should be explored with the patient, including opening doors, drawers, or windows, using the computer mouse, wiping down a table, or carrying plates. The patient should be instructed on proper trunk positioning while performing these activities.

The clinician may recommend that the patient consider using a voice-activated computer, tablet or cell phone program. However, the patient should be cautioned about the time involved in training the computer to the patient's voice, about change of voice when the patient has a cold, and about the greater demand on the vocal cords.

Use of a speaker-phone can help to decrease strain of the neck, shoulder, arm and hand from the sustained positioning of holding a handset or a cell phone. If this is not possible, a Bluetooth, ear cradled wireless or wired speaker to the ear, or an over-the-head headset can help decrease hand, head, and arm strain. Alternating the ears during the day and/or the week is recommended. If the patient is not able to tolerate the weight or pressure or unbalanced weight of the headset or over-the-ear piece, the clinician may want to assess head and neck positioning with its use.

Frequent Body Movements during Sustained Positions

Instructing the patient to utilize the trunk muscles, while seated, instead of relaxing them will assist in frequent posture corrections during the day. Activating the trunk muscles can help to provide strength and support throughout the day. The patient can be challenged to try sitting up taller for longer periods of time, or standing taller while walking.

Anecdotally, chair abdominal strengthening is often challenging for these patients. These can easily be completed in the workstation intermittently throughout the day (Fig. 16). Instruction can be given on how to correctly perform this exercise, incorporating proper posture and core strength, while performing a bicycling motion, to decrease the elevating ribs into the brachial plexus.

Modifications for Leisure Activities

The same principles of posture, hand and body mechanics, ergonomics and joint, tendon, and nerve protection can be applied to assist the patient to safely perform their leisure activities. Exploration of how to modify each leisure activity or skills with and without adaptations is strongly encouraged, unless it is contraindicated, for maximum relaxation and entertainment.

Increasing Upper Extremity Activity

Edema can increase throughout the upper extremity when workloads are sustained for long periods of time, such as in keyboarding. In order to decrease edema overflow in the entire limb, the patient is instructed to incorporate frequent overhead reaching, reaching backward—with

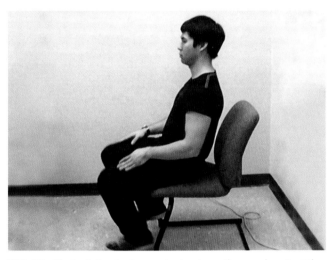

FIG. 16: Chair abdominals exercise to strengthen and protect the low back. Performing bicycling in an upright seated position away from the back of the chair. The clinician should reinforce correct head and spine alignment. This exercise should be performed for 30 seconds, at regular intervals throughout the day

and without trunk rotation—and turning the head in all directions. The author recommends that the patient should be taught how to palpate for edema buildup, comparing involved and non-involved arms and learn to address it with proper techniques.

Edema can increase during the night, as the activity level is significantly less. Patient education can explain increased intensity of symptoms at night. Instruction to perform general body stretches prior to bedtime, taking a shower at night and/or moving about more often during sleep can be beneficial. Increasing cardiac output by engaging in regular exercise may additionally assist to mobilize the edema.

A combination of MEM with intermittent head, neck, shoulder, arm, forearm, wrist, and digit movement will intensify efforts to decrease symptoms. These exercises include stretches of thumb, finger flexors and intrinsic minus positioning in supination, glenohumeral joint external rotation with scapular adduction and elevation and/or depression, performed every 30 minutes. This exercise is performed in the initial phase for 1–3 weeks, depending on severity of symptoms. Overhead reaching sequence can be combined with lateral torso stretches as well.

Movement of the upper torso will increase circulation. Exercises that can be performed include: sitting up as tall as possible, looking up to the ceiling while gently arching the upper back, tall sitting with lateral side movements of head (Figs 17A and B). The clinician should include lateral and rotational torso movements into the patient's regimen.

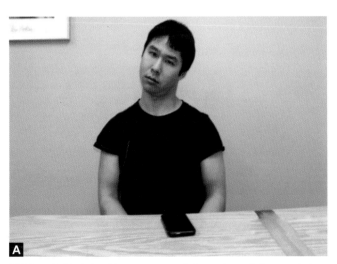
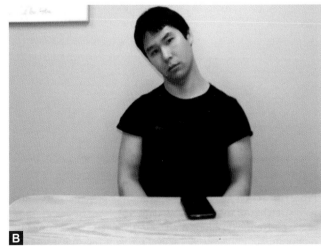

FIGS 17A AND B: Observation and discussion of detected shortened musculature or tight positioning. This is an example of shorter lateral cervical flexion. Note the coordination to move to the—(A) Left; compared to the (B) Right, he is not able to perform it in the exact same position due to possible tightness of right side limiting motion and weakness of the left

Awareness of tightness initially is optimal to detect changes in softness of tissues after each stretch and/or the same repetitive movement event. As the symptoms decrease, movement and activity can be increased.

Full Upper Quadrant Arm Stretch

The patient is asked to extend the elbow, to supinate the forearm, and to extend the hand and fingers, with thumbs pointing behind them. The hand is then placed flat on their seat pan behind the hips. The patient will need either verbal or tactile cues to bring the superior scapula, upward and backwards and into adduction towards the spine.

The activation of extensor digitorum communis (EDC) with finger hook presentation (intrinsic minus position) when forearm is supinated, elbow flexed at 90° and shoulder externally rotated with elbow pinned to their side can be challenging (Figs 18A to D). To ease this effort, elevation of the scapula will often support and relax the tension on the peripheral nervous system, unless there is glenohumeral joint limitation or scapulothoracic strain or weakness.

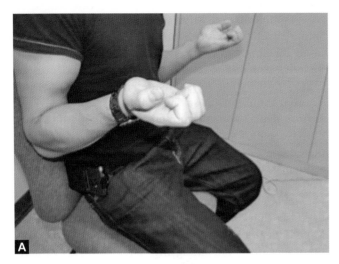
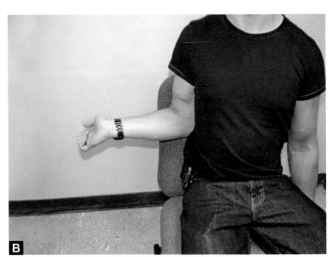
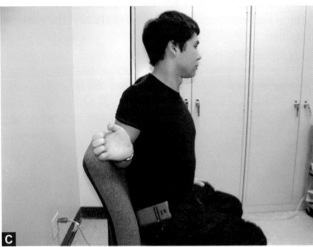
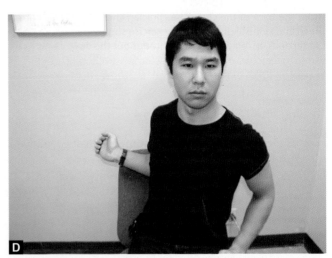

FIGS 18A TO D: Active range of motion of proximal upper quadrant with sustained distal wrist and digit extensor strength combined with stretches of the lumbricals, digit flexors, wrist flexors, pronator, and pectoralis major, and musculature for internal rotation. None of the end range positions should be sustained. Repetition of the movements with awareness of end tightness is preferred. (A) Extensor digitorum communis (EDC) activation with full metacarpal-phalangeal (MP) extension; (B) Adding gentle wrist extension with full external rotation; (C) Adding elbow behind rib cage with wrist extension; (D) Full scapular adduction with glenohumeral extension combined with external rotation positioning to detect tightness of superior upper quadrant

Manual Therapy

Manual Edema Mobilization

Manual edema mobilization techniques can be utilized to decrease ischemic fluid build-up of the entire upper extremity.[42] Periodic use of MEM can be combined with stretches throughout the day. Neck and trunk stretches can be performed to coordinate with diaphragmatic breathing. When edema does not resolve readily, especially of subacute and chronic phases, the upper quarter can be treated in individual segments. The sequence of moving edema should be from proximal area, including the trunk, followed by the shoulder/armpit area, then to the upper arm, and by sections, distally to the digits. Combinations of joint motions of the upper extremity are performed between each section of MEM completed. Many patients and clinicians are unaware of the accumulation of edema or protein fluid in their upper extremity.[43] Persistent edema throughout the upper torso would benefit from performing aquatic exercises, however, when not available, a shower before bedtime and again in the morning will assist in reducing superficial buildup. The patient is encouraged to increase water intake while trying to move the edema using MEM as maintaining hydration levels is beneficial. The author has recommended a long and thin nylon flexible towel or mild skin exfoliator-type towel (4 feet long by 5 inches wide) to assist in stimulating the superficial tissues along the back and torso with the larger movements of the extremities and torso. Instruction in self-soft tissue mobilization at this time can be very beneficial. Demonstration of changes in the swollen and painful tissues will be very motivating.

Taping

The clinician can apply elastic tape to swollen areas of the hand, wrist, or forearm. Taping can assist with joint stability to hypermobile or lax ulnar-carpal joint during hand function. Carpometacarpal radial taping support to the carpal tunnel has recently been demonstrated to decrease pain, edema, and provide light support. Taping can be used as a biofeedback aide to remind the patient to sustain wrist neutral or slight wrist extension position while keyboarding. The tape can assist in eccentric contractions of weakened musculature.[44,45]

Both static and dynamic taping can provide support and/or decrease pain, depending on the application and goals. When using tape, precautions against skin irritation are needed. Kinesio Tape®, one of the first elastic tapes,

provides a 2-way stretch. Dynamic Tape™ provides more comfort with 4-way stretch.[45] Wearing time may vary from a few hours to days.

Soft Tissue Mobilization

Soft tissue mobilization techniques, either manually or using a rigid tool (e.g. ASTYM™) have been incorporated targeting specific muscle structures and/or myofascial regions. The techniques may be applied under stretch or in the resting position, depending on the structures involved. Gently pulling tissues up away from the bone to decrease adhesive characteristics is beneficial. The patient may report an immediate change and decrease in hypersensitivity. If symptoms do not decrease immediately following the treatment session, it may suggest that there is more proximal issue and/or joint dysfunction. The author has incorporated these techniques combined in a particular sequence with traditional physical agent modalities to obtain reduction in pain and edema. The patient progresses more readily by incorporating the soft tissue mobilization techniques frequently throughout the day.

Physical Agents

Physical agents have been studied in isolation and in combination with other therapeutic interventions when treating the upper extremity; however, there is a need for more research to establish their efficacy.[46]

Ultrasound

Ultrasound has not been supported in current research for effectiveness in the treatment of CTS, neither for short- nor long-term relief.[13] However, other reviews have indicated that short-term relief is unknown.[10] Ultrasound has been used for acute, subacute and chronic CTS patients who have not responded to use of a splint, or have rejected an injection as a treatment modality.[7] Anecdotally, this modality has been helpful in reducing edema of the forearm and distal wrist, as in tenosynovitis, when combined with soft tissue mobilization, edema mobilization and repetitive overhead reaching and pumping of all upper extremity musculature. The settings will depend on the amount of edema, and the acuteness of the nerve irritability. Manual edema mobilization combined with large upper quarter movements immediately following ultrasound has been very beneficial.

Electrical Nerve Stimulation

Noxious-level stimulation, known as electro-acupuncture is used when other methods of pain modulation have failed. Research has indicated that applying a noxious-level stimulation, releases endogenous opiates.[43] Transcutaneous electrical nerve stimulation (TENS) and interferential current for pain modulation or electro-analgesia have been used. This author applies TENS simultaneously with active and passive stretches to achieve more movement with less pain.

Sensory re-education using transcutaneous electrical nerve stimulation[43-45,47]

For patients who report difficulty in detecting the location of their symptoms, the author has incorporated the use of TENS. It provides a stimulus at the wrist or hand to explore the location of tight musculature or weakened proximal area eliciting decreased sensation or pain. Some will need the arm to be unloaded, or supported by a 3–4 inch cushion while engaging in the gentle, slow and active movement. The patient is asked to detect the stimulus on their wrist/hand while performing head, neck, glenohumeral, and scapular motions, in combinations with the elbow and forearm movements.

Some patients who experience dysfunctional sensibility may benefit from traditional sensory re-education training combined with TENS. The use of TENS is perceived to enhance the detection of the stimulus distal to the electrode, or as a mode to discriminate between the monofilament and the simultaneous stimulus of the TENS to the same dysfunctional area. Pacini corpuscles, quickly-adapting nerve fiber, perceiving moving-touch, vibration, and tactile-gnosis, detect 256 Hz.[42,43] Most portable home TENS units offer 250 Hz. A home digital readout TENS unit that provides a customized setting can provide additional light touch stimulus with parameters of 200 Hz and below and 300 milliseconds pulse width and below. The progression of nerve repair has been described from moving-touch to moving two-point discrimination, constant-touch to classic two-point discrimination.[42,43] 30 Hz and 256 Hz vibratory stimuli were recommended to be present prior to moving two-point discrimination.[42] The combination of TENS and classic sensory re-education may enhance compliance.

Neuromuscular electrical stimulation

Neuromuscular electrical stimulation (NMES) is used to achieve a muscle contraction, increasing muscle strength, decrease disuse atrophy or deconditioned muscle, and decrease edema. Clinically, the author has found this beneficial application to shortened, trigger points and/ or deconditioned musculature. A typical example is applying the NMES to the flexor carpi radialis longus and brevis or to the pronator teres while combining wrist extension or grasping during a functional task. Sample tasks include the transfer of a small box to another height or location while rotating it in the air, or the grasping and lifting a glass or tumbler. The latter would be a goal in the strengthening stage.

Phonophoresis and Iontophoresis

Phonophoresis and iontophoresis, for the treatment of CTS, were not recommended by the American College of Occupational and Environmental Medicine (ACOEM). The intervention is recommended when other conservative treatment measures have been tried unsuccessfully.[7]

Contrast Bath

Contrast baths are widely recommended in the literature to treat CTS, however the quality of research supporting this intervention for management of CTS is lacking and it is not a recommended treatment under ACOEM, 2011. Currently, costs exceed benefits, based on limited evidence.[7]

Low-Level Laser Therapy

Low-level laser therapy received US Food and Drug Administration (FDA) approval in the United States for treatment of pain associated with CTS in 2002. It is a relatively new physical agent in the United States. The application and treatment parameters are not well-standardized.[42] Low-level laser therapy is not recommended on a routine basis.[7]

Exercises and Therapeutic Activities

Hand web exerciser and abduction manual stretches are taught and performed by slowly moving between each digit, and returning back to the first set to detect any change in palmar or web tightness. The author recommends this motion to be repeated three times, if tolerated. Pumping the hand overhead may allow additional repetitions. Although the self-stretching can be performed (Fig. 14), most report that they need another person to provide adequate relief of tightness. Intrinsic

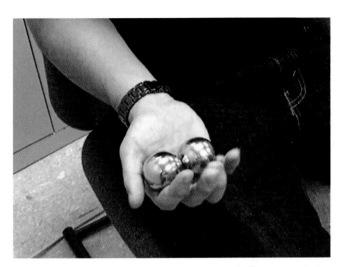

FIG. 19: Metal or ceramic Chinese exercise balls can easily be used for increasing circulation and coordination of the lumbricals and interosseous muscles. The weight adds extra sensory input (and often, the balls come with a chime that sounds each time the balls contact). The balls are sold in various sizes

minus stretches (hook fist) provide relief from tightness of the lumbricals.

Increasing circulation or movement of the intrinsic muscles of the hand is most easily performed by manipulating Chinese exercise balls, or golf balls (Fig. 19), moving them from the radial side of hand to the ulnar side in free-flowing coordination while watching a movie or television is usually acceptable as an exercise. When patients are not able to do this coordination activity, the progressive sponges can be used between the extended fingers in varying degrees of metacarpal phalangeal arcs of motion.

Use of three-block rectangular firm foam sponges increase intrinsic length and activation in longer grip spans. Functional use can be simulated using large 6-inch mouth jars or other containers to be opened.

Theraputty™ exercises (Figs 20A to D) are incorporated for both the hand intrinsic exercises, and for glenohumeral depression combined with the points of external rotation. The latter is performed by placing the putty under the ulnar side of the patient's hand, and instructing the patient to push and drag it on the table top, bringing the outstretched arm towards their body, allowing the elbow to flex and move toward the posterior rib cage. Patients can be given five points to work through from a start position with the arm in front of their body, to full external rotation with the shoulder abducted, as tolerated. Repetitions are performed in series, five times or 25 downward straight fist into the Theraputty™.

Isolated motions of digits, thumb and combined motions of fingers and wrist can be performed. Intrinsic and extrinsic muscles of hand and wrist are addressed.

Theraband® exercises for the upper quadrant posterior region are taught. These activities can be performed one- or two-handed. Overhead band resistive movements can also be implemented. The patient is advised to perform 5–7 movements every 1–2 hours, or more, assist to provide stretching and strengthening of posterior quadrant for the subacute phase.

An upper quadrant posterior strengthening series (Figs 21A to I) has proven helpful in the author's clinic. The patient often will be able to increase their grip strength of span two or three, assuming their symptoms have decreased enough to tolerate the exercises. Reaching or pushing a free-weight overhead can be taught for weakened upper trapezius and levator scapulae musculature. Adding abdominal toning simultaneously for sedentary workers is useful to assist in core strengthening and postural awareness.

Alternative and Complementary Medicine

Yoga exercise is a popular activity for increasing flexibility, relaxation and strength. Yoga exercises for acute, subacute, or chronic CTS have been documented to be beneficial, however, there is insufficient evidence for long-term use.[7] Some people enjoy this activity, self-directed, on a regular basis and do not understand why they may continue to have symptoms of CTS. It is the responsibility of the clinician to educate them regarding other factors, which may be contributing to their symptoms.

Yoga therapy,[48] is a form of movement therapy. It is considered a complementary and alternative medicine, as defined by the National Center for Complementary and Alternative Medicine (NCCAM). 40% of NCCAM members are occupational and physical therapy and speech and language pathologist. Many medical professionals are incorporating Yoga therapy for their patients. There are 84,000 positions documented.

Acupuncture and acupressure has been documented as an effective intervention for pain[1] and edema management. Both can be used in conjunction with the occupational or physical therapy treatments, however, it is preferred the treatments be provided on separate days, with 12–24 hours in between, especially when electrical stimulation is utilized. Medicinal herbs may be prescribed by an acupuncturist, to help to balance the body, and to provide a more effective acupuncture.

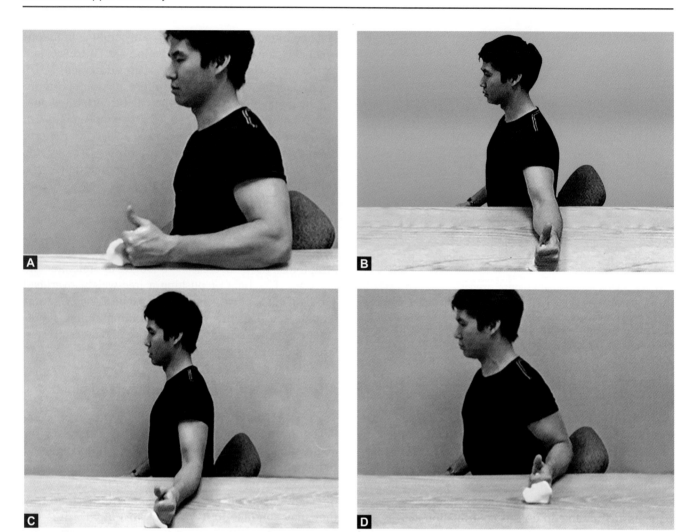

FIGS 20A TO D: Theraputy™ exercises. (A to D) The patient is positioned sideways to tabletop. Sustained proper upright posture is emphasized during the activity. The seat height is elevated to allow the forearm to slide posterior to the rib cage, just above the waistline. An ample amount of putty is trapped under the ulnar side of hand. The forearm is positioned in neutral throughout the drag-and-pull motion backward. The starting hand position is always away from the body and must be comfortable. Each time the goal is for the patient to move the elbow behind their back. The other arm also completes the same sequence for comparison. The clinician should assess and train patient about the contributing factors, explaining why symptoms may be experienced and how to alleviate them. No pain should occur

Additional adjunct medicine techniques include: active release therapy, craniosacral techniques, Reiki, Tai Chi, relaxation training and movement therapies (e.g. Feldenkrais). These and the those mentioned previously were not considered for a core component of hand therapy intervention, and recommended to be incorporated into treatment by an experienced hand therapist (minimum of 2 years of specialty practice).[49] The Hand Therapy Certification Commission will be publishing an updated list of techniques and tools used by current practicing certified hand therapist by early 2015.

The use of nutritional supplements, such as Vitamin B6, has been documented in the literature, but is not clearly more effective than other conservative treatments.[50]

Medical and Surgical Considerations

Medical treatment performed by the surgeon is a steroid injection with 40–80% relief of pain from tenosynovitis, however, within 18 months these numbers decreased to 22%.[50]

The most effective treatment for long-term relief of CTS is surgical decompression.[50] Decompression is

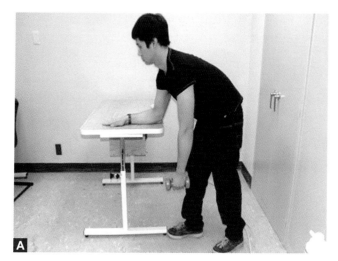

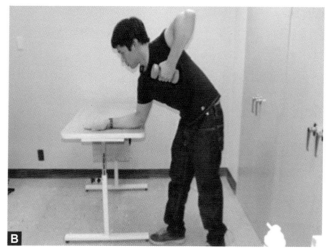

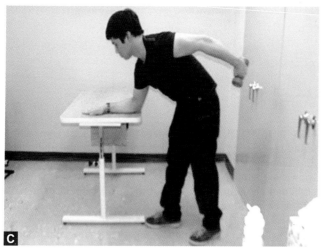

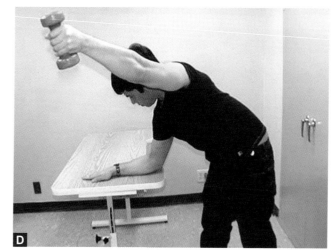

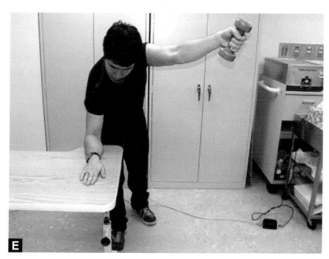

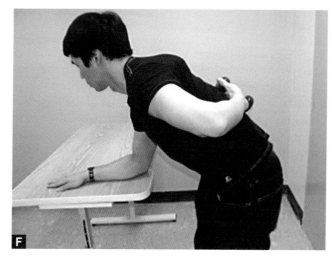

Continued

Continued

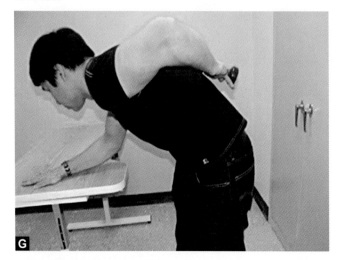

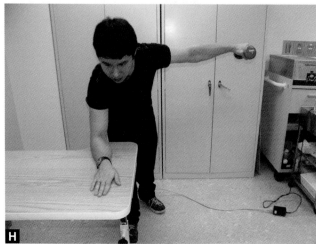

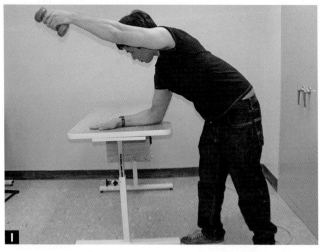

FIGS 21A TO I: Upper quadrant posterior strengthening series. (A) Starting position; (B) Humeral horizontal abduction; (C) Humeral extension with elbow extended; (D) Side view; (E) Top view of elbow extended with scaption and humeral flexion at 45 degrees abduction; (F) Starting position to lift entire arm off the back without extending elbow and sustaining scapular adduction; (G) Ending position of lifting arm off back; (H) Elbow extended with sustained 90 degrees humeral horizontal abduction; (I) Elbow extended sustained in full glenohumeral flexion to activate lower trapezius

achieved by sectioning the flexor retinaculum (transverse carpal ligament). The type of surgical release, open versus endoscopic, has been researched, and the functional outcome at 1 year is comparable for both types. Recurrent and unrelieved CTS needing repeat surgery in the studies ranges from 1.7% to 3.1% of cases.[50]

Postsurgical management may begin within hours, under the direction of the surgeon or therapist. It includes frequent digit and wrist movement without overuse or wound drainage. The wrist is either supported in neutral position during day and night between active motions, in forearm supinated position.[50] Some surgeons prefer an ace wrap over the gauze to secure the wound without the stabilization of a wrist orthotic, or volar wrist cast.

Many postoperative patients are able to recover without therapeutic intervention, however for those who

are referred to the hand therapy clinic, the emphasis on the first visit is the precautions and contraindications for the wound. Instruction and training in edema management then begin with whole arm upper extremity pumping, moving from arm resting at the side of the body to overhead reaching and then to return to waist. The patient is instructed to perform this activity several times, 5–10 repetitions every 30–45 minutes to increase lymph drainage until sutures are removed and/or edema is no longer visible or palpable. The patient is taught to manually detect pockets of edema, or thickened tissue, and to demonstrate management of localized edema of the forearm, wrist and hand without disturbing wound healing.

Direction is provided regarding sleep postures to protect the wound and healing nerve and the entire peripheral pathway. Optimal positioning goals are having the patient lying supine with the recovering arm in elevation (the height higher than the patient's abdomen) with the elbow slightly flexed, and the forearm in neutral. The side-lying position on the opposite side of the postoperative arm is also an option, provided the arm does not drop in front of the body and the elbow remains slightly flexed. Two or three pillows may be required to support the whole arm.

Activity level guidelines, including walking as tolerated to increase circulation and enhance wound healing, are provided. Sitting or lounging for hours does not allow the edema or lymph to move away, and therefore is discouraged. Drinking extra clear fluids may assist the patient in edema reduction. Emphasis on arm pumping and edema management is critical for pain reduction.

Typically, by the third postoperative day, AROM of wrist, forearm, and digits can be refined for all functional positions, and gentle tolerable stretches of the intrinsic musculature can be introduced. These include: AROM of proximal joints first—the neck and shoulders, then the elbow, progressing to forearm rotation and wrist motions. Finger motions are grouped for flexion or fisting, lumbrical positioning, intrinsic minus or hooked fist, abduction and adduction of all digits in forearm supination. The patient is instructed in moving fingers individually and in mobilizing every joint of each finger. Oppositional thumb exercises—touching the thumb to every fingertip, and ultimately, approximating the thumb to the palmar crease below the fifth digit—are then introduced. Emphasis on intrinsic minus positioning requires strength of the EDC to perform lengthening of all intrinsic musculature to regain a tight fist, with flexion of both proximal interphalangeal and distal interphalangeal joints.

Sutures are typically removed between 10 days and 14 days, though a sterile dressing often remains to hold the wound together for a longer period, if needed to prevent gapping.

Elastic taping such as Dynamic Tape™ may be used to assist in edema and pain reduction, however, hypersensitivity to the tape may occur with excessive swelling. Taping tolerance will depend on the soft tissue response to the surgery, incorporation of MEM to reduce edema, and the status of the wound. Pain reduction is usually reported immediately. As a precaution, the patient is educated to remove the tape if skin irritation or hypersensitivity occurs. The tape can be worn for several days to assist in increasing movement with less pain.

Physical agent modalities, such as ultrasound and TENS, can address troublesome edema or scar tissue formation, if followed by soft tissue mobilization. The objective remains to continue to progress to full motion and light activities. Continued elastic taping to assist with edema, pain, and offer light carpal stability may prove useful.

Posterior upper quadrant strengthening with wrist weights can be incorporated to assist with scapular and glenohumeral stabilization (Figure 21).

Progressive functional activities of gross and fine motor coordination can be incorporated as tolerated, and as needed, with light support, at 4-5 weeks. Full strengthening can be initiated by 5-6 weeks, with or without support.

Return to work will depend on the demands of work or functional activities required by the individual. This may be earlier than the 6 weeks, if the patient does not return to manual labor.

CONCLUSION

The conservative treatment of CTS is complex. Evidence-based practice is limited by the existing research and confounding variables. Mild to moderate CTS may benefit from resting orthoses and/or taping for the first week or longer, especially at night. Regular exercise is beneficial. Manual edema mobilization for extremity edema added to physical agent modalities and treatment methods including nerve mobilization and neurogliding, adjunctive therapies, steroid injections are all treatment considerations, and most complement one another. However, these are reportedly temporary, failing to provide complete resolution of symptoms in the long term, especially for the moderate to severe and chronic stages. It is this author's experience that these interventions alone may not be enough. Many factors contribute to the perpetuation of symptoms, including the patient's behaviors at work, habits outside of work, seated versus standing postures, walking mechanics or lack of proper positioning, lack of full body and/or upper torso movement, and lack of awareness of the positions or habits that elicit symptoms. The timing of implementation of newly learned rehabilitation techniques—the patient's understanding of when and how to intervene—may contribute to a slow recovery. Instruction, training and orientation of how the peripheral nervous system can respond during a clinical demonstration will emphasize changes in positioning and exercises that will continue to decrease symptoms and their intensity. When the clinician and patient work together and the patient's adherence to lifestyle changes improve, the patient will incorporate the rehabilitation techniques more often throughout the day. Techniques include strengthening the trunk muscles and upper quadrant help to sustain tabletop or sedentary activities that develop with the aging process.[51] The goal is to increase the patient's alternatives and choices for problem-solving and to assist with self-management throughout the entire day. A skilled clinician can provide the anatomy and physiology education to support lifestyle changes to remediate or delay the progression of severe symptoms. Traditional physical and occupational therapy and the intervention of physical agent modalities appear to provide initial benefit, however, the lifestyle changes are the variable most likely to sustain this initial benefit, or to delay the onset of more progressive CTS. Additional research for occupational and physical therapists to establish a gold standard is in progress. Research is beginning to demonstrate the interactive nature of individual patient behavior and neuroanatomical changes. As our understanding of the neuroanatomy and physiology at the cellular level develops, its influence on the surrounding tissues becomes more evident. Neuroplasticity of the brain is a growing field of research in the field of rehabilitation, giving insight to the importance of the brain and body connections. Use of computers and hands-held technology has accelerated in the recent years, and it has led to different hand and upper quadrant health conditions. On the other hand, this technology has a potential to aide in management of these conditions, e.g. use of self-monitoring and sensory feedback aides. Occupational and physical therapists are in a unique position to provide the needed guidance to improve the quality of life of a patient with CTS.

REFERENCES

1. LeBlanc KE, Cestia W. Carpal tunnel syndrome. Am Fam Physician. 2011;83(8):952-8.
2. Boyd, KU, Gan BS, Ross DC, Richards RS, Roth JH, MacDermid JC. Outcomes in carpal tunnel syndrome; symptom severity conservative management and progression to surgery. Clin Invest Med. 2005;28(5):254-60.
3. Peters SE, Johnston V, Coppieters MV. Interpreting systematic reviews: looking beyond the all too familiar conclusion. J Hand Ther. 2014;27:1-3.
4. National Guideline Clearinghouse. (2013). Carpal tunnel syndrome (acute & chronic). [online] Available from http://www.guideline.gov/content.aspx?id=47574. [Accessed October, 2014].
5. Hagman KT. Occupational Medicine practice guidelines. Evaluation and management of common health problems and functional recovery in workers. 3rd edition. Elk Grove Village (IL): National Guideline Clearinghouse. American College of Occupational and Environmental Medicine(ACOEM); 2011.p.1-73.
6. NIH-National Institute of Neurological Disorders and Stroke: reducing the burden of neurological disease. (2012). Carpal tunnel syndrome fact sheet. [online] Available from http://www.ninds.nih.gov/disorders/carpal_tunnel/detail_carpal_tunnel.htm. [Accessed October, 2014].
7. American Academy of Orthopedic Surgeons. Clinical practice guidelines on the treatment of carpal tunnel syndrome. National Guideline Clearinghouse; 2008.
8. Ott F, Mattiassich G, Kaulfersch C, Ortmaier R. Initially unrecognised lunate dislocation as a cause of carpal tunnel syndrome. BMJ Case Reports. 2013;3(18)pii:bcr2013009062.
9. Piazzini D, Aprile I, Ferrara P, Bertolini C, Tonali P, Maggi L, et al. A systematic review of conservative treatment of carpal tunnel syndrome. Clin Rehabil. 2007;21(4):299-314.
10. Harvard Health Publications. (2012). Hands: strategies for strong, pain-free hands. [online] Available from http://www.health.harvard.edu/special-health-reports/hands-strategies-for-strong-pain-free-hands. [Accessed October, 2014].
11. Gerritsen AA, de Krom MC, Struijs MA, Scholten RJ, de Vet HC, Bouter LM. Conservative treatment options for carpal tunnel syndrome: a systematic review of randomised controlled trials. J Neurol. 2002;249(3):272-80.
12. O'Connor D, Marshall S, Massy-Westropp N. Non-surgical treatment (other than steroid injection) for carpal tunnel syndrome. Cochrane Database Syst Rev. 2003;(1):CD003219.
13. Page MJ, Massy-Westropp N, O'Connor D, Pitt V. Splinting for carpal tunnel syndrome. In: The Cochrane Collaboration. Cochrane Database of Systematic Reviews. Chichester, UK: John Wiley & Sons Ltd; 2012. [online] Available from http://doi.wiley.com/10.1002/14651858.CD010003. [Accessed October, 2014].
14. Page MJ, O'Connor D, Pitt V, Massy-Westropp N. Exercise and mobilisation interventions for carpal tunnel syndrome. In: Cochrane Database of Systematic Reviews. Chichester, UK: John Wiley & Sons Ltd; 2012. [online] Available from http://doi.wiley.com/10.1002/14651858.CD009899. [Accessed October, 2014].
15. Page MJ, O'Connor D, Pitt V, Massy-Westropp N. Therapeutic ultrasound for carpal tunnel syndrome. In: Cochrane Database of Systematic Reviews. Chichester, UK: John Wiley & Sons Ltd; 2013. [online] Available from http://doi.wiley.com/10.1002/14651858.CD009601.pub2. [Accessed October, 2014].
16. Jacoby SM, Eichenbaum MD, Osterman AL. Basic Science of Nerve Compression. In: Skirvin T, Osterman AL, Fedorczyk JM (Eds). Rehabilitation of the Hand and Upper Extremity, 6th edition. Philadelphia, Penn: Elsevier Mosby; 2011. pp. 649-65.
17. Hentz V. The anatomy of upper extremity compression neuropathies. Lecture from All About Nerves, 4th Annual ASHT CA State Chapter Conference, March, 2014.
18. Duff SV, Estilow T. Therapist's management of peripheral nerve injury. In: Skirvin T, Osterman, AL, Fedorczyk, JM (Eds). Rehabilitation of Hand and Upper Extremity, 6th edition. Philadelphia, Penn: Elsevier Mosby; 2011. pp. 619-33.
19. Dellon AL. Evaluation of Sensibility and Re-education of Sensation in the Hand. Baltimore, MD: The Williams and Wilkins Company; 1981.
20. van der Heide B, Allison GT, Zusman M. Pain and muscular responses to a neural tissue provocation test in the upper limb. Manual Ther. 2001;6(3):154-62.
21. Hall T, Zusman M, Elvey RL. Adverse mechanical tension in the nervous system? Analysis of straight leg raise. Manual Ther. 1998;3(3):140-6.
22. Michigan Hand Outcomes Questionnaire. [online] Available from www.orthopedicscores.com. [Accessed October, 2014].

23. Evans R. Therapist's management of carpal tunnel syndrome: a practical approach. In: Skirvin T, Osterman AL, Fedorczyk JM (Eds). Rehabilitation of hand and upper extremity, 6th edition. Philadelphia, Penn: Elsevier Mosby; 2011. pp. 666-777.

24. Durkan JA. A new diagnostic test for carpal tunnel syndrome. J Bone Joint Surg Am. 1991;73(4):535-8.

25. Rosen B, Lundborg G. Sensory Re-education. In: Skirvin T, Osterman AL, Fedorczyk JM (Eds). Rehabilitation of hand and upper extremity, 6th edition. Philadelphia, Penn: Elsevier Mosby; 2011. pp. 634-45.

26. Topp KS, Boyd BS. Peripheral nerve: from the microscopic functional unit of the axon to the biomechanically loaded macroscopic structure. J Hand Ther. 2012;25(2):142-52.

27. Coppieters MW, Stappaerts KH, Wouters LL, Janssens K. Aberrant protective force generation during neural provocation testing and the effect of treatment in patients with neurogenic cervicobrachial pain. J Manipulative Physiol Ther. 2003;26(2):99-106.

28. Hall TM, Elvey RL. Nerve trunk pain: physical diagnosis and treatment. Manual Ther. 1999;4(2):63-73.

29. Greening J, Lynn B. Minor peripheral nerve injuries: an underestimated source of pain. Manual Ther. 1998;3(4);187-94.

30. Walsh MT. Nerve mobilization and nerve gliding. In: SkirvinT, Osterman AL, Fedorczyk JM (Eds). Rehabilitation of the hand and upper extremity, 6th edition. Philadelphia, Penn: Elsevier Mosby; 2011. pp. 1512-28.

31. Walsh MT. Interventions in the disturbances in the motor and sensory environment. J Hand Ther. 2012;25(2):202-19.

32. Kostopoulos D. Treatment of carpal tunnel syndrome: a review of the non-surgical approaches with emphasis in neural mobilization. J Bodywork and Movement Ther. 2004;8:2-8.

33. Miller TT, Reinus WR. Nerve entrapment syndromes of the elbow, forearm, and wrist. Am J Roentgenol. 2010;195(3):585-94.

34. Peddie S, Rosenberg CH. The repetitive strain injury sourcebook. Lincolnwood, Ill: Lowell House, a division of NTC/Contemporary Publishing Group, Inc.; 1998.

35. Mayfield M, Voge L. Computer comfort: a guide to working at your computer with less strain on your neck, back, hands, and eyes. Glenwood Springs, CO: UE Tech Upper Extremity Technology; 1993.

36. Stigliani J. The computer user's survival guide. Sabastopol, CA; O'Reilly & Associates Inc.; 1995.

37. Lacey JS, Dickson T, Levenson H. How to survive your computer workstation, 15 easy steps to workstation comfort, 2nd edition. Loredo, Texas: A CRT Serices, Inc. Publication; 1990.

38. Chaffin DB, Andersson GBJ. Occupational biomehanics. New York/Chichester/Brisbane/Toronto/Singapore: A Wiley-Interscience Publication, John Wiley & Sons; 1984.

39. Grandjean E. Fitting the task to the man: a textbook of occupational ergonomics, 4th edition. London/New York/Philadelphia: Taylor and Francis, Inc.; 1988.

40. Kasdan ML. Occupational hand and upper extremity injuries and diseases. Philadelphia, Penn: Handley & Belfus, Inc.; 1991.

41. Baker N. The effect of an alternative keyboard on musculoskeletal discomfort; A randomized cross-over trial. Work: A Journal of Prevention, Assessment & Rehabilitation. 2015;50(4):677-86.

42. Artzberger SM, Priganc VW. Manual edema mobilization: an edema reduction technique for the orthopedic patient. In: Skirvin T, Osterman, AL, Fedorczyk, JM (Eds). Rehabilitation of hand and upper extremity, 6th edition. Philadelphia, Penn: Elsevier Mosby; 2011. pp. 868-81.

43. Villeco JP. Edema: a silent but important factor. J Hand Ther. 2012;25(2): 153-62.

44. Coopee R. Elastic Taping (Kinesio Taping Method). In: Skirvin T, Osterman AL, Fedorczyk JM (Eds). Rehabilitation of hand and upper extremity, 6th edition. Philadelphia, Penn: Elsevier Mosby; 2011. pp. 1529-38.

45. Kendrick, R. Advanced dynamic taping guide for professional use only. Norfolk Island, Australia: Posture Pals Pty Ltd.; 2013.

46. Fedorczyk J. The use of physical agents in hand rehabilitation. In: SkirvinT, Osterman AL, Fedorczyk JM (Eds). Rehabilitation of hand and upper extremity, 6th edition. Philadelphia, Penn: Elsevier Mosby; 2011. pp. 1495-511.

47. Mannheimer JS, Lampe GN. Clinical transcutaneous electrical nerve stimulation. Philadelphia, Penn: F.A. Davis Company; 1984.

48. Taylor MJ, Galantino ML, Walkowich H. The use of yoga therapy in hand and upper quarter rehabilitation. In: Skirvin T, Osterman AL, Fedorczyk JM (Eds). Rehabilitation of hand and upper extremity, 6th edition. Philadelphia, Penn: Elsevier Mosby; 2011. pp. 1548-62.

49. Dimick MP, Caro CM, Kasch MC, Muenzen PM, Fullenwider L, Taylor PA, et al. 2008 Practice analysis study of hand therapy. J Hand Ther. 2009;22(4):361-76.

50. Amadio PC. Carpal tunnel syndrome: surgeon's management. In: Skirvin T, Osterman AL, Fedorczyk JM (Eds). Rehabilitation of hand and upper extremity, 6th edition. Philadelphia, Penn: Elsevier Mosby; 2011. pp. 657-65.

51. Day JM, Willoughby J, Pitts DG, McCallum M, Foister R, Uhl TL. Outcomes following the conservative management of patients with non-radicular peripheral neuropathic pain. J Hand Ther. 2014;27(3):192-200.

Section 2

Spine

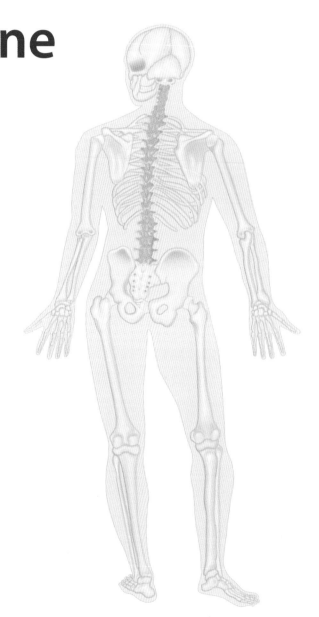

CHAPTERS

CHAPTER 6

Cervical Sprain and Strain

Rachel S Worman

ABSTRACT

Cervical pain arising from muscular or ligamentous soft tissue sources contributes to loss of function. Nearly one million cases of cervical spine sprain or strain as a result of whiplash injury occurred in North America in 2000, leading to significant economic costs, decreased work productivity and increased use of legal and medical services. Cumulative trauma disorders due to repeated tasks, sustained or constrained postures or forceful motions can also lead to cervical sprain and strain. Emerging evidence supports new tests and tools for diagnosis and treatment of cervical sprain and strain. Conservative management through physical therapy soft tissue mobilization and exercise, among other treatments, is an effective approach to manage pain and loss of function as a result of cervical sprain and strain.

■ INTRODUCTION

Cervical pain often presents clinically as arising from multiple soft tissue sources contributing to pain and loss of function. Ligaments, muscles, tendons, blood vessels, skin and articular cartilage are all considered soft tissues of the body.[1] The binding supportive structure to soft tissue is soft connective tissue made up of collagen and elastin fibers.[1] These are the primary fibers disrupted during cervical sprain and strain.

Sprain is defined as injury to the ligamentous structures supporting a joint. Strain is defined as injury to the musculotendinous unit.[2] Therefore, this chapter will focus on injury to ligamentous and musculotendinous soft tissues.

Sprains and strains can be classified as Grade I, II or III. Grade I is overstretched or minor tearing of the connective tissue fibers. Grade II is partial tearing of the

fibers. Grade III is a full tear that may require surgical intervention.[3]

Although sprain and strain are specific to muscular or ligamentous soft tissue, with either a sprain or strain, there is likely disruption to the related surrounding soft tissue, including the myofascial connective tissue, nerve, lymphatic, skin, cartilage and blood vessel tissue and these may need testing to rule in or rule out sprain or strain. In the case of injury to musculotendinous or ligamentous structures of the cervical spine, related surrounding soft tissue may also include injury to the bone and disk fibers. All of these structures together make up the motor unit.[4]

Epidemiology

Disruption of the soft tissue can occur in numerous ways, the most common being whiplash and cumulative trauma.

Whiplash Injury

Whiplash injury is a disruption of the bony and soft tissues of the cervical spine caused by rapid acceleration and deceleration of the neck.[5] It commonly occurs as the result of a sport injury or motor vehicle accident (MVA). Neck sprain and/or strain or whiplash injury is the most common injury in MVA. In 2000, there were an estimated 901,442 persons treated for whiplash in North American emergency rooms.[6] Following a whiplash injury, whiplash associated disorders (WADs) may result and occur at a rate of 600 per 100,000 people and 50% of these continue to chronicity.[7-10] WAD results in significant economic cost, decreased work productivity, increased medical care and legal services.[5] WADs are classified on a scale of 0–4 based on clinical presentations—0 is no complaint about the neck and no physical sign(s); 1 is complaint of neck pain, stiffness, or tenderness only but no physical sign(s); 2 is neck complaint and musculoskeletal sign(s); 3 is neck complaint and neurological signs(s); 4 is neck complaint and fracture or dislocation.[11] For the purposes of this chapter, we will focus on WAD grades 1–2.

Cumulative Trauma Disorders

Cumulative trauma disorders (CTDs) describe symptoms that may include discomfort, impairment, disability or persistent pain in joints, muscles, tendons and other soft tissues and occurs in connective soft tissues, primarily tendons and their sheaths. The local tissue damage will irritate proximal nervous tissue, and slow microcirculation. It is the result of repetitive motions such as vibration, sustained or constrained posture or forceful motions. Other risk factors are age, gender, acute trauma, chronic disease, use of birth control pills, circumstances of pregnancy and menopause.[12] CTDs may also be the result of cumulative vertical loading forces to the cervical joints and disks as a result of maintaining vertical posture against gravity.

Repetitive strain syndrome (RSS) or repetitive strain injury, are other terms to describe the same syndromes as CTD and refers to injury to the musculoskeletal soft tissue, as well as the nervous soft tissue.[13]

Precision work such as using a computer mouse requires static activation of multiple muscles including levator scapula and upper trapezius, which have attachments into the cervical spine and can result in strain.[14] Prolonged low force muscular contraction impairs perfusion and causes local tissue ischemia that may lead to muscle disorders such as myofascial dysfunction, trigger points and muscular weakness.[15]

Anatomy

Many anatomical structures of the cervical spine may be affected by WAD or RSS. Based on the definition of sprain and strain previously stated, this chapter will categorize primary anatomical structures as those specific to ligaments and muscles. Secondary anatomical structures involved will refer to other anatomical structures commonly involved in sprain and strain.

Primary Anatomical Structures

Tendons and ligaments

Tendons and ligaments are made up of dense fibrous connective tissue (Type I) fibers that are laid in parallel for optimal tensile strength.[16] Tendons and ligaments have firm fibrous attachments to periosteum and to bone via Sharpey's fibers.[16,17] Sharpey's fibers, also known as bone fibers or perforating fibers, are particularly dense at bone segments that receive the most motion force, such as intervertebral disks to vertebral bodies.[17] Each bone fiber travels with an arteriole and nerve fiber.[17] These fibers adhere so strongly to bone that during an injury, force, following the path of least resistance, will effectively disrupt the tendon or ligament before it will pull from the bone, as in an avulsion fracture.

Ligaments

Specific ligamentous structures relevant to MVA are the anterior and posterior longitudinal ligament, capsular ligament, interspinous, supraspinous ligaments and ligamentum flavum.

Made up of 80% elastin, the ligamentum flavum has the highest elastic qualities of all tissue in the human body.[18]

Relevant to MVA, frontal vehicle impact will affect the supraspinous ligament, interspinous ligament, and ligamentum flavum at C2–C3 through C7–T1.[18] During rear impacts the anterior longitudinal ligament and annular fibers will be strained.[18] Individuals who have their heads rotated during an impact, will have a higher incidence of alar and transverse ligament injury.[18]

Posterior cervical spine muscles

Three layers of muscles make up the posterior cervical spine: (1) the superficial, (2) intermediate, and (3) deep. Each layer may be involved in cervical muscle strain. The superficial posterior cervical muscles are splenius muscles, splenius cervicis, and splenius capitis. The intermediate posterior muscles are the spinalis cervicis and capitis, longissimus cervicis and capitis and iliocostalis cervicis. While, the deep posterior cervical muscles form the suboccipital triangle, which is made of four muscles, the rectus capitis posterior minor and major on the medial side and the inferior and superior oblique on the other two sides. The suboccipital triangle is deeper to the upper trapezius and semispinalis capitis muscle, and attaches to the skull just below the upper trapezius attachment point at the inferior nuchal line. The transversospinalis group, from superficial to deep, are the semispinalis, multifidus and rotatores.

Lateral cervical spine muscles

The superficial lateral cervical muscles are platysma, sternocleidomastoid and trapezius. The deep lateral muscles are the splenius capitis, levator scapula, posterior scalene, middle scalene and anterior scalene.

Anterior cervical spine muscles

Two layers of muscles make up the anterior cervical spine, the superficial and deep. The superficial layer consists of the platysma, sternocleidomastoid and trapezius muscles. The deep layer consists of cervical prevertebral muscles such as longus colli, longus capitis, rectus capitis anterior, and rectus capitis lateralis.

Longus capitis is noted for its action of cranio-cervical flexion and this action is what differentiates movement patterns from those of the deep anterior muscles compared to the superficial. This is important for differentially testing and treating. They are frequently found to be weak following whiplash injury and with repetitive strain. From computer models, the sternocleidomastoid and anterior scalene muscles comprise 83% of the cervical flexion action, suggesting longus capitis and colli assist with 17% of the movement.[19] Rectus capitis anterior also flexes the head. Rectus capitis lateralis flexes and stabilizes the head.

Secondary Anatomical Structures

While cervical sprain and strain refer directly to musculo-tendinous or ligamentous injury, many surrounding anatomical structures will also be affected as a result of cervical sprain and strain.

Joints and capsules

Facet or zygapophyseal joints are frequently disrupted during whiplash injury. Studies using medial branch nerve blocks have demonstrated that 60% of whiplash cases had pain stemming from one or more facet joints, 54% in patients with chronic neck pain after whiplash and 27% of

the cases with neck pain and/or headache were positive at the C2-3. These findings were also demonstrated in biomechanical studies where C5-6, C6-7 and C2-3 were most often affected.[8]

Fascia

Using ultrasonography, loss of fascial layers between semispinalis cervicis and cervical multifidus can be visualized in persons with chronic WADs.[20]

Nerves

Dorsal root ganglion may be disrupted by alterations in mechanical load following a whiplash injury.[18]

Arteries

The vertebral artery is a deep artery of the neck stemming from the first portion of the subclavian artery. It ascends in the pyramidal space formed by the scalenus anterior muscle and longus colli muscle and continues its course into the transverse process of the C6 to C1 vertebra. The suboccipital branch then courses along the posterior arch of the atlas before entering the foramen magnum to supply the brainstem, and joins the basilar artery to form a portion of the cerebral blood supply, the Circle of Willis.[21]

Injury to the vertebral artery during MVA whiplash may explain signs and symptoms of headache, dizziness, tinnitus, blurred vision and vertigo. Intimal tears of the vertebral artery are common at the atlantoaxial joint where axial rotation is occurring.[18]

CLINICAL PRESENTATION

Cervical sprain and strain may affect the neck or extend to the upper back, head, shoulders and upper extremities and may commonly present as pain in the neck, shoulder or as a headache.[22] Decreased cervical range of motion (ROM) is a common finding in persons with chronic neck pain.[23] Active ROM may be limited due to pain and/or swelling in localized soft tissue which may subsequently cause a secondary nerve root irritation and related radicular symptoms into the upper extremities. Particularly in the case of whiplash injury pain, altered movement patterns will be common for flexion and extension.[24] Common postural changes due to local muscle guarding may be one or two elevated shoulders. Supported extremities such as flexed elbow held to trunk or hand on head may indicate nerve root involvement. Prolonged static positions leading to repetitive strain will commonly present with kyphosis, excess upper cervical spine extension, forward shoulder posture, shoulder internal rotation, and forearm pronation. Ultimately these lead to repeated strain to the trapezius, levator scapulae muscles and are related to upper thoracic joint hypomobility.[12] This is often accompanied by visible creasing at the C5–6 and C6–7, where increased anterior translation has occurred repetitively and predictable segmental hypermobility is present, and thus ligamentous sprain and muscular strain are present.

■ CLINICAL EXAMINATION

Postural Observation

Anterior View

In the anterior view, the therapist will look for lateral flexion of the face. Forward shoulder posture will indicate excess internal rotation of the glenohumeral joint. This is also demonstrated with the forearms in excess pronation. The sternum will be a good reference for postural balance.

Posterior View

In examining cervical posture in the posterior view, the therapist should be sure to view the head as well as the thoracic spine. The posterior view may reveal asymmetries of edema present, muscular atrophy or hypertrophy and bony asymmetries. The posture of the thoracic spine will likely reveal information regarding the cervical spine.

Lateral View

From the side, the therapist should determine where the head is positioned in relationship to the shoulders and view shoulder position. This view will reveal kyphosis and lordosis of the thoracic and cervical spine. It will be easy to predict segments that will fold under load, at points of creasing.

Range of Motion Testing

Cervical ROM may be tested for cervical flexion, extension, lateral flexion and rotation using a number of validated tools. A systematic review of reliability and validity studies for measuring active and passive cervical ROM found that of 12 methods evaluated, the cervical ROM tools with good reliability and validity were the Cervical Range of Motion Instrument©, the Spin-T goniometer and the single inclinometer.[25]

Benefits of the Cervical Range of Motion Instrument© are that it is hands-free for the therapist which allows for fast readings, and that it eliminates shoulder and torso movement via a magnetic reference. However, it may be cost-prohibitive due to decreasing visit reimbursement rates, and it requires significant set-up time.

Smartphones are becoming more sophisticated, and several goniometer apps are available, which may offer more 3D graphs of ROM. This may allow the clinician to measure natural fluid ROM versus linear movements. These will require reliability and validity studies, but are worth mentioning as a future method of measurement that is easily accessible.

Testing to Determine Cervical versus Thoracic Range of Motion Mediated Symptoms

Flexion

When pain or restrictions in active ROM are present into cervical flexion or extension, it may be difficult to discern whether the pain or restricted ROM is a result of cervical spine dysfunction versus thoracic spine dysfunction. If a patient has restrictions in flexion, the therapist should ask the patient to return to their starting position. The therapist passively pre-positions the scapula into firm retraction, effectively stabilizing the thoracic vertebral segments into extension. The patient is then asked to flex the cervical spine again. If pain or restriction still exists while the thoracic spine was held steady, the cervical spine and/or its soft tissue can be ruled in as a strong mediator. If the cervical spine symptoms do not persist, a thoracic spine dysfunction could be suspected.

Extension

When pain or restriction in active ROM exists with cervical spine extension, the therapist should ask the patient to return to their starting position. The therapist positions the scapula into end range protraction while stabilizing the thoracic spine into flexion. The patient then repeats their attempt at cervical spine extension ROM. If the restriction persists, the cervical spine or soft tissue can be pursued for further specific testing. If the restrictions are not as severe or disappear, the thoracic spine warrants further investigation.

Special Tests

Ligament Sprain

Due to the nature of the mechanism of injury for many cervical sprains and strains, for instance a MVA or sports injury, special tests must be conducted in order to rule out grade III ligament lesions that can have more serious repercussions if not detected early.

The *transverse ligament stress test* is a stability test for the transverse ligament and assesses if the atlantoaxial articulation is hypermobile.[26]

The *Sharp-Purser test* is also a transverse ligament test to determine if subluxation of the C1 on C2 is present.[26]

Another test for atlantoaxial joint instability is the *lateral shear test.* [26] It is specific for testing odontoid dysplasia as in the case of the rare genetic Morquio's syndrome, however, it will also test for a fracture of the odontoid process. [27]

The *lateral flexion alar ligament stress test* identifies lateral flexion stability of the alar ligament, while the *rotational alar ligament stress test* assesses the rotational stability of the alar ligament.[26]

Vertebral Artery

Establishing the integrity of the vertebral artery vascularity is an important safety consideration before proceeding to manual interventions for the cervical spine. However, there is controversy surrounding vertebral artery testing. Understanding the purpose of the test and methods of performing the test must be established and utilized as needed.

Muscle Strain

A PubMed search for cervical muscle strain tests reveals no reliable testing methods to determine if a muscle strain is present. Testing that is beyond the scope of physical therapy practice, such as magnetic resonance imaging (MRI) or blood serum testing, may help to determine if strain or inflammation are present but is still being researched for reliability.

Evidence indicates that increased intramuscular pressures are associated with decreased muscular tissue oxygenation in prolonged static flexed postures, which may also contribute to muscular strain.[28] Physical therapy may be able to detect if strain is present during muscular strength testing.

Cervical Muscle Strength and Endurance Testing
Deep cervical neck flexor testing

Studies of persons with neck pain document diminished activity of deep cervical stabilizing muscles, while superficial musculature becomes increasingly active, leading to decreased endurance for activities of daily living.[29] A significant relationship exists between increased activity of superficial cervical muscles, anterior scalene and sternocleidomastoid, and neck pain intensity during the last stage of the craniocervical flexion test in persons with chronic pain.[30] Peolsson et al. determined age- and sex-specific reference values of neck muscle endurance for the first time and reported findings in 2007. They studied dorsal and ventral muscles. The average ventral endurance for men was 2.5 minutes and for women was 0.5 minutes. In 2011, Domenech et al. conducted a similar study to establish normative data using a similar method, the deep neck flexor (DNF) test, to determine DNF endurance and found that on average healthy men held for 38.9 seconds while women held for 29.4 seconds.[31] Reduced head steadiness is found during 40 seconds isometric cervical flexion testing in subjects with whiplash injury compared to non-traumatic neck pain and healthy controls.[32]

The craniocervical flexion test is a validated isometric endurance test for the DNF and deemed the most effective for testing DNF muscles but may also be categorized as a neuromotor control test, as it tests how the deep flexors are interacting with the superficial cervical flexors in a research setting.[33] It is performed using a pressure biofeedback device that is initially inflated to 20 mm Hg. The patient nods their head biasing toward flexion at 2 mm Hg increments, if they can sustain each level for 10 seconds for 10 repetitions, to a maximum of 30 mm Hg.[19,34] In persons with chronic tension-type headaches, isometric neck flexor training results in a quarter of the physiologic effect of manual therapy, therefore, testing for endurance is important.[35]

Deep cervical testing may also be performed using "the cup exercise" (described later in the chapter), which acts as a test and an exercise.

Posterior segmental testing

The therapist places fingers along the vertebral lamina bilaterally and asks the patient to contract the posterior cervical muscles at that level as if they were not going to let the therapist lift the vertebra. Muscular deficits, such as diminished contraction force may be palpated by the therapist. Often deficits are consistent with the level of injury to soft tissue or joint pathology, and can be felt unilaterally or bilaterally at that level. It is compared to the opposite side or another level to determine if the muscular deficit is present.

Respiratory Strength

Maximal inspiratory pressures and maximal expiratory pressures have been found to be diminished in persons with chronic neck pain, likely as a result of associated local and global muscular changes, and clinicians are advised to consider this in testing and in treatment.[36]

Neurologic

Doorbell sign test

The *doorbell sign test* (Fig. 1) is performed with the patient in supine and the knees slackened into flexion with a bolster under them to ensure the cervical spine tissue is slackened. Starting at C7, the practitioner gently places index fingers at the medial border of the sternocleidomastoid muscle and palpates anterior side of the transverse process at the groove of the spinal nerve in order to palpate the cervical nerve root. The practitioner asks the patient if the nerve root at that level feels equal from side to side. The practitioner then slides up to the next vertebral level, C6. A positive test is when the nerve root palpated is locally tender and/or refers pain and/or is different than the contralateral side. A painful nerve root will often correspond to disk lesion or neuroforaminal stenosis.

Peripheral Nerve

In order to rule out nerve root irritation from local swelling related to cervical spine ligamentous overstretch, the peripheral nerves can be palpated as in the doorbell sign test. Certain points of the upper extremity peripheral

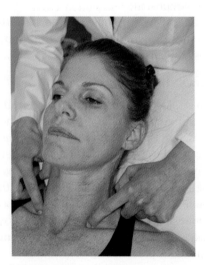

FIG. 1: Doorbell sign test

nerves are more superficial and will be the points to access for palpation.

The proximal peripheral radial nerve can be palpated approximately 1–2 finger widths inferior to the deltoid tuberosity, where the radial nerve is circumflexing anteriorly from its path in the radial groove on the posterior humerus and diving into the lateral intermuscular septum. It can be palpated again in the forearm just inferior to the lateral epicondyle, between the brachialis and brachioradialis muscles, and again in the anatomical snuff box.[37]

The ulnar nerve can be palpated just posterolateral to the medial epicondyle in the ulnar groove, and more distally, medial to the hook of the hamate bone.[37]

The median nerve is easily accessed just medial to the bicep tendon at the elbow.[37]

Soft Tissues

Soft tissue swelling is easily palpated following acute whiplash injury or in cases of repetitive strain or loading sprain or strain. Each tissue type in the body has a unique yield point along its unique stress or strain curve. It would follow then that each layer of tissue should be felt as an individual layer with its own grade of movement as the clinician gradually palpates the soft tissue.

Prior to touching any soft tissue, the practitioner can use the dorsal surface of the hand and hover just above the skin to sense any temperature changes that may be present. Following this, each layer of tissue should be individually and systematically assessed.

The skin can be palpated until its interface with the fascial layer below. The skin alone can be mobilized inferior, superior, and lateral to assess skin play, skin turgor. Regions where the fascia is restricted will develop erythema and be quite painful. This fascial dysfunction is then called subcutaneous panniculosis. It may be best to return and test for subcutaneous panniculosis once the deeper layers have been systematically tested. Subcutaneous panniculosis is painful, restricted fascia. Testing is best performed on patients who have moved into chronicity and with whom the clinician did not detect swelling, where they present as an "acute on chronic case". Once the therapist returns to test for subcutaneous panniculosis, the skin layer can be rolled. Points where there is not ease of movement between the fascial and muscle layers will often directly correlate to muscular trigger points below and are points of fascial "hang-ups".[38-40] Trigger points are identified in many cervical sprain and strain diagnoses: radiculopathy, joint dysfunction, disk pathology, tendonitis, tension headaches, carpal tunnel syndrome, computer-related disorders and whiplash associated disorders.[41]

Ligamentous

Coin test

The coin test (Fig. 2) is a palpation test where a coin is placed over the supraspinous ligament and gently pressed into the tissue. A positive test will result in patient complaint of local pain or tenderness and is often indicative of hypermobility and/or disk pathology at that segment.

Diagnostic Imaging

Frequent findings associated with WAD are diffuse hyperalgesia, fatty infiltrate into cervical muscles, and altered cervical spine postural lordosis as seen on X-ray studies.[7] Specific injury with WAD is often undetectable on imaging studies and thus, to date, treatment has reflected the concept that physical injury is not present. However, current MRI research demonstrating fatty infiltrate in cervical spine extensors and flexors following whiplash is underway and appears promising to identify changes associated with more subtle injury.[42,43]

Diagnostic Testing

Newer research demonstrates soft tissue damage may occur following a whiplash injury based on increased serum inflammatory biomarkers. Elevated serum pro-inflammatory markers tumor necrosis factor (TNF)-alpha

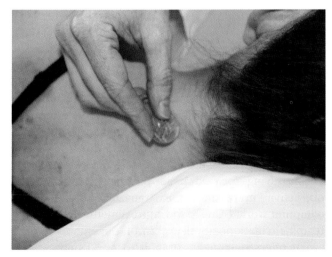

FIG. 2: Coin test

and interleukin-6 (IL-6) as well as anti-inflammatory markers IL-10 were present within 3 days following whiplash injury, similar to levels following an ankle sprain.[44] Further research testing acute (<3 weeks) and chronic (>3 months) serum inflammatory biomarkers indicate that these may play a role in whiplash injury outcomes and are associated with hyperalgesia and cervical extensor fatty muscle infiltrate.[45] Progressing research can aide practitioners in understanding the common complaints associated with WAD.[45]

Differential Diagnosis

Differential diagnosis should always start with a thorough patient history to determine if onset of symptoms are idiopathic versus traumatic.[46] Determining the date of onset and stage of healing will guide the therapist to rule in or out pathology. In the case of acute whiplash type injury pathologies such as ligamentous tears, zygapophyseal joint capsular strain, muscular strain, vertebral artery injury, thoracic outlet syndrome, nerve root injury and specifically dorsal root ganglion injury, disk pathology, facet joint injury, cervicogenic headache, tension headache, swelling related pain and fractures ought to be considered prior to testing, as information from the history may guide the types of testing considered.[8] In chronic whiplash type injury, the therapist may consider related injury such as postural changes leading to other pathology, carpal tunnel syndrome, tendonitis, arthritis and psychogenic sources of pain. With RSS, it is important to rule out the earlier listed pathologies, particularly those similar to chronic whiplash injury. These pathologies may coexist as a result of trauma or the chronic soft tissue changes that occur over time, often creating challenges for differential diagnosis and necessitating the therapist's attention to detail and diligence in locating the source for symptoms. The reader is directed to texts specific for differential diagnosis.[46]

■ PHYSICAL THERAPY TREATMENT

Physical therapy treatment consists of management of soft tissue disruption as well as targeted exercise. Evidence supports the use of manual therapy combined with exercise for the treatment of chronic neck pain and is found to offer improvement in pain, function and perceived effect.[47] It is important then that the subjective and objective portions of the examination are thoughtful and accurate to guide the therapist to the best treatment option. Categorizing exercise treatment options into stages of healing, in order to guide the therapist in safe procedures, will optimize outcomes for the patient.

Stages of Soft Tissue Healing

Ligament and tendon soft tissue undergoes stages of healing similar to other soft tissues. As there is not trauma to the skin, epithelialization will not occur.[48] During the proliferation phase, an injured region has the most type III collagen, which is laid down in a nonuniform pattern, and has about 15% of the normal tensile strength present, when compared to collagen fibers that are aligned in parallel, as they are prior to disruption from injury.[48] Physical therapy exercise treatment must be appropriately chosen to correspond to the stages of healing so as not to disturb the healing process.

Bracing

Studies comparing the use of a cervical spine soft collar, immediately following whiplash injury, to 10 treatments of physical therapy consisting of heat, lymphatic draining, massage and exercise, plus a Thera-Band® home exercise program for 14 days, show no difference in symptoms between groups after 1 week, but a significant improvement in pain and function in the group receiving physical therapy.[22]

Some controversy surrounds the use of a collar. Early return to movement has been largely promoted over stabilization in a soft collar. Contrary arguments suggest that stabilization is important while soft tissue heals, similar to stabilizing a healing ankle sprain. Studies have primarily centered around soft collar use versus other treatments, but not around collar and specific exercise.[49] Emerging research using imaging studies and serum markers may ultimately prove soft tissue damage does in fact occur, and stabilization or a combination of stabilization and exercise will have best outcomes. Reduction in pain and a reduction in the use of pain medication and nonsteroidal anti-inflammatory medications would be another positive outcome to using a collar versus early mobilization. At this time, it is best to defer to the patient and practitioner interaction to weigh the best option.[50]

Immediately following a cervical spine sprain and/or strain, the therapist may consider fitting the patient with a Philadelphia hard collar (Fig. 3) to aide in approximation of ligamentous soft tissue and to optimize healing length and reduce scarring. The patient is adamantly instructed that the collar is not to be used for resting, but rather as a

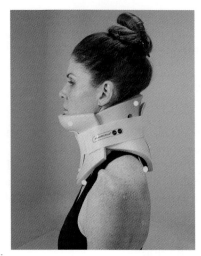

FIG. 3: Philadelphia collar worn as a guide to protect against excess cervical motion during healing. The collar should not have excess gapping or compression at each of the four points pictured

guide for movement. The patient is alerted to four points, one at the chin, sternum, occiput, and upper thoracic spine (Fig. 3). If the patient feels excess pressure at any one of the points, they must adjust their cervical spine position so there remains equal distance between the collar and each point. This will allow the cervical musculature to continue functioning, minimizing atrophy and aiding in vertebral positioning while the disrupted ligaments and facet capsules are allowed to heal in a shortened position. Patients are also instructed in a series of exercises that they can perform while wearing the collar. These exercises are discussed later in this chapter. The exercises will ensure that the patient is mindful, but not idle.

Taping

An alternative to bracing may be Kinesio Tape (KT), although KT has not been studied for whiplash injuries, only postural strain injuries. While KT is not well-researched to date, studies that are available indicate some benefit in enhancing proprioceptive and postural awareness and increasing local blood and lymphatic circulation. KT applied for neck retraction on subjects while in standing, at tape stretch of 15–25% to bilateral C4–T7 levels, has been found statistically significant in improving forward head posture and decreasing overactivation of the upper trapezius muscle during computer work.[51] Due to the improvements in blood and lymph circulation, as well as the proprioceptive guidance taping offers, one might extrapolate that KT may assist in post-whiplash recovery as well (Fig. 4).

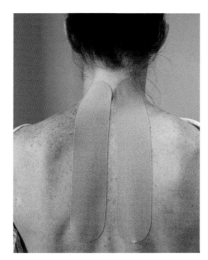

FIG. 4: Kinesio Tape applied from C4–T7 vertebral segments

Modalities

Ultrasound has been found to be efficacious in the early treatment of soft tissue disruption, has uses for pain control and to assist in lengthening shortened soft tissue.[48] Ice will be beneficial as an analgesic as well as to improve inflammation. Heat is a pain-reducer and can aide in soft tissue pliability. Electrical stimulation can assist in pain reduction as well as microcirculation.[48]

Manual Lymphatic Draining

Manual lymph draining (MLD) is a manual physical therapy technique that is founded on the theoretical basis that therapists will facilitate lymphatic circulation, hasten the removal of biochemical waste, reduce edema and decrease sympathetic nervous system response.[52] A search of current literature yields no results for high-level studies specific to validity of performing MLD for cervical sprain or strain. The Vodder method of MLD for acute ankle sprain yielded statistically significant changes in pain and edema after one session and improved ROM upon re-test at 1 week.[52] Due to known increases in swelling following cervical sprain and strain, MLD does warrant further specific study.

Intramuscular Manual Therapy

Dry needling (DN), also known as intramuscular manual therapy (IMT) or trigger point dry needling (TrP-DN) is a technique utilizing thin filiform needles to treat deep and superficial trigger points and connective tissue with the goal of minimizing neuromusculoskeletal pain and

restoring biomechanical function. The myofascial trigger point (MTrP) complex is made of taut tissue band and nodular tissue that often refer pain, creating hyperalgesic zones. MTrPs may develop from sudden injury, muscular overload, repetitive microtrauma, computer-related disorders and whiplash associated disorders, thus, DN may be a good treatment option for cervical spine sprain and strain.[41,53,54] In a randomized controlled clinical trial, TrP-DN of active trigger points in the upper trapezius was shown to be effective in the treatment of acute mechanical neck pain intensity, pressure sensitivity and in improving active cervical ROM.[55] DN must be performed by a specifically trained and skilled physical therapist, provided their jurisdiction allows it.[56]

Soft Tissue Mobilization

Manual soft tissue mobilization is an integral part of treatment for cervical spine sprain and strain. If the appropriate soft tissue mobilization technique is chosen and applied in accordance with the patient's stage of healing, it can facilitate a quicker return to normal movement patterns, ROM, strength and endurance. This in turn may enhance cervical stability and motion in persons with neck pain, allowing a safe progression to exercise.[57,58]

Physiologic soft tissue movement refers to movement that a soft tissue structure, such as muscle, tendon, ligament, fascia, would naturally move.[59] In the case of the cervical suboccipital muscles, for instance, physiologic soft tissue mobilization would lengthen the tissue in a caudal to cranial direction, the way it would move if the occipital-atlantal (OA) joint were flexed.[4,60]

Accessory soft tissue mobilization refers to movement that would not naturally occur with movement, such as if the muscle were manually bent laterally at the muscle belly.[59]

It is best to place the soft tissue in a slackened position prior to performing any soft tissue mobilization techniques. In the case of the cervical spine, in supine, placing a bolster under the knees will slacken the cervical soft tissue. The clinician's hands are placed gently on the posterior aspect of the patient's neck, and the soft tissue pliability is assessed. The therapist should feel that the posterior cervical spine fascia slackens inviting the therapist in for treatment. A pillow may be placed under the patient's head and the head-piece of the therapy table adjusted to accommodate various thoracic and cervical spine structures. In prone, a pillow is placed under the pelvis, bolster under the ankles and the headpiece adjusted to accommodate various thoracic and cervical spine structures.

Acute State Soft Tissue Mobilization

In the acute stage of healing, soft tissue treatment should be directed toward protection of soft tissue and managing pain and swelling. Soft tissue techniques appropriate for this stage are muscle broadening or muscle bending toward the spine or gentle nonischemic compression.

Muscle broadening—physiologic

During muscle broadening, the muscle to be addressed must be placed in a slackened position. The therapist uses a broad and gentle contact of two hands to sink into the layer of muscle to be addressed and then approximates the tissue. The muscle must be held in this position until the therapist has perceived that the intended change has occurred.

Muscle bending—accessory

Muscle bending will often be beneficial during acute muscle spasm. The therapist broadly contacts the lateral portion of the cervical paraspinals, for instance, and applies gentle compression force of the tissue toward the spine, placing slack into the nervous system, to decrease heightened neural sensitivity.

Nonischemic compression—accessory

Using a very broad flat surface contact, the therapist contacts the target treatment area engaging the tissue to the level of the muscle and holding this contact until the tissue softens or yields. If this does not occur, the therapist may change regions or attempt another approach. Muscles will often disengage.

Chronic State Soft Tissue Mobilization

In the chronic stages of healing, soft tissue treatment techniques may be directed toward manipulating stiff soft tissue to improve movement and function. These techniques may include cross-fiber massage (CFM), muscle lengthening, muscle pumping, muscle bending (J-stroke) (Fig. 5) and myofascial decompression (MFD).[60]

Cross-fiber massage—accessory

CFM, or deep transverse friction massage is meant to break-up chronic scar tissue with friction at the perpendicular plane of the muscle fiber.[61] In the cervical spine, the primary point of utilizing CFM is over the

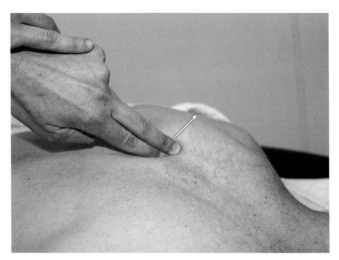

FIG. 5: J-Stroke. The therapist bends the paraspinal muscles from medial to lateral

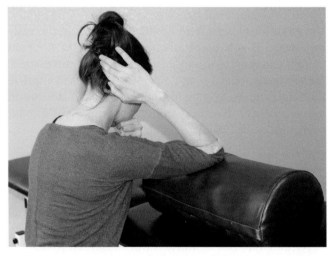

FIG. 6: Self-cross fiber massage (CFM) to suboccipital muscles

suboccipital muscle insertion into the base of the skull. This tissue is frequently found to be chronically shortened in persons who sit for prolonged periods in front of a computer monitor. The patient can also perform self-CFM at home by resting the chin in the left hand, and resting the right elbow on an elevated surface to minimize upper trapezius activation (Fig. 6).

Muscle lengthening—physiologic

Muscle lengthening can be performed by contacting a muscle with one hand (often close to the muscle origin or insertion) and "tacking" the tissue in place, while the therapist's other hand is contacting the muscle layer and gliding the opposite direction, stroking the muscle along the line of the muscle fibers. Alternately, this can be completed by "tacking" a muscle, and then moving the muscle across a joint, as in the case of suboccipital release, where the therapist's fingers contact the occipital insertion bilaterally, then move the head into OA flexion, causing the muscle to lengthen.

Muscle pumping—physiologic

Muscle pumping is soft tissue elongation that allows the patient to actively participate, facilitating antagonistic muscle contraction to assist. In the cervical spine, the suboccipital muscles can be "tacked", as mentioned in the muscle lengthening section. Once the therapist perceives the muscle is on stretch, the patient is asked to look toward the sternal notch in order to activate the deep cervical neck flexors, thus further elongating the suboccipital muscles. In the case of pumping the levator scapula, the therapist can contact the levator scapula at the scapular insertion site, biasing muscle contact in the cranial direction while the patient is asked to depress the scapula. This pattern is repeated as follows:

- Therapist tacks
- Patient depresses scapula
- Therapist removes hand
- Therapist manually replaces scapula in slightly elevated position.

Muscle bending—accessory

Whereas muscle bending can be used in acute soft tissue treatment by biasing the muscle bending toward the spine, muscle bending can also be biased away from the spine, as in the technique referred to by the Kaltenborn-Evjenth system as the "J-stroke" (Fig. 5). In treating the cervical spine, this technique would be best applied in the thoracic region to improve deep thoracic paraspinal mobility in order to decrease excessive mobility demands in the cervical spine. In another muscle bending technique for superficial thoracic paraspinal muscles, the therapist lines the thumb alongside the spinous processes and sinks down to come alongside the paraspinal. The therapist's force is directed away from the spine.

Myofascial decompression—accessory

MFD is a technique using dry suction cups to decompress the fascial system. 2 weeks of cupping coupled with exercise has been found more effective than heat in decreasing pain, and improving neck function in treating video display terminal users.[62] When using dry suction cups, do not allow the cups to remain in any one position for greater than 5 minutes. These techniques are best in the chronic stages of healing, as they will disrupt acutely healing tissue. Caution should be used when using these techniques in patients, such as the elderly, where skin integrity may be a concern.

MFD slide technique is used to decompress a large region of fascial stiffness. Preactive and postactive ROM testing is recommended prior to initiating treatment to determine improvement in myofascial restriction. The skin is prepped with a small amount of massage oil over the entire treatment area. The cup size is chosen based on the region to be treated.

Functional MFD uses a dry suction cup to decompress the fascia over a target muscle while the patient is instructed to functionally lengthen and broaden the muscle while decompressed. For instance, a small dry suction cup may be placed at the distal insertion of the right levator scapula muscle while the patient is instructed to move the cervical spine into left rotation and flexion, lengthening the levator scapula muscle while the dry suction cup frees the muscle from restricted fascia. The patient returns to the starting position and then repeats the procedure up to 5 minutes before the cup must be removed.

Gua Sha tools are made of jade or bone and come in many different shapes (Fig. 7). The tools are used in chronic stages of healing in order to initiate movement of stiff fascia, and are known to increase local microcirculation, which in turn may play a role is distal microcirculation and pain relief, although the mechanism is not well understood.[63,64] Further research is needed to determine pain-relieving effects.[65] A myofascial release cream is applied to the skin. The tool is held at a 20–30° angle to the skin and is applied to the layer of fascia just above the muscles in a dragging motion attempting to mobilize the

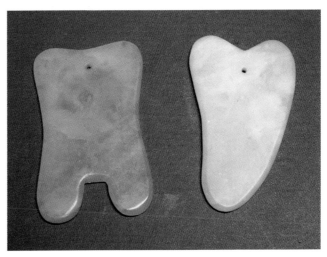

FIG. 7: Jade Gua Sha tools

fascia. It may have a similar effect to that of subcutaneous skin rolling. High level of disinfection for multiple patient use for Gua Sha and cupping tools is recommended.[66]

Subcutaneous skin rolling is a technique where the therapist drives the treatment point of their finger between the fascia and the muscle layer, freeing the fascia from restrictions hindering normal movement (Fig. 8).

Exercise Treatment

Tendons and ligaments undergo similar healing timeframes, which must be respected when prescribing exercise.[48] Early, safe, low-level activation of cervical muscles will minimize muscular atrophy, protect tendons

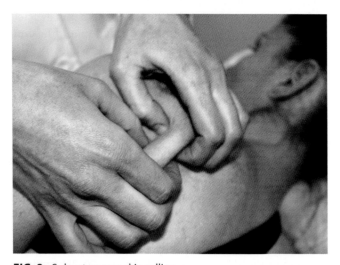

FIG. 8: Subcutaneous skin rolling.

and ligaments at their stage of healing, as well as aide in pumping inflammatory proteins. Exercise progression must be in accordance with the stage of healing, the patient's abilities, symptoms response and emotional or psychosocial state or status. Tissue will heal and may cease to be a pain source, however, pain associated with the nervous system may persist. While soft tissue strength may be altered following an injury, lowering its tolerance to force, the perception of threat following injury is signaled well before the actual ability of the tissue to accept force. Therefore, patients with chronic pain who are moving through a graded exercise program can be assured of their safety as they begin to initiate exercise.[67] Table 1 is a therapist guide for exercise prescription based on what is likely appropriate for tissue healing timeframes, however, the therapist must be a good judge of individual tissue tolerance, patient character and body awareness. Exercise challenge can be slowly increased by altering frequency, duration and intensity.[68] In trunk stability exercises, intensity can be altered by changing lever forces of the body and limbs. Altering the base of support of the body using balance devices and patient contact with floor can also change the intensity of the exercise.

Balance training ought to be incorporated into exercise routines to rehabilitate disrupted cervical spine tissue. Research has demonstrated that following whiplash injury, balance deficits are present in gaze stability and head-eye coordination.[69] Sway energy, especially with eyes closed in tandem stance, is altered in persons with idiopathic compared to whiplash-induced neck pain, however there is some difference in balance

TABLE 1: Sample cervical spine treatment and exercise options based on tendon and ligament tissue healing time frames[48]

Stage of healing	Time	Treatment	Exercise
Inflammation	(Days 1–6)	• Collar • Kinesio tape • Modalities • Manual lymphatic drainage • Soft tissue: muscle broadening, muscle bending, nonischemic compression	• Level 1 Cup exercise • Cardiovascular • Level 1 Foam exercises • Squats
Proliferation	(Days 3–20)		
Maturation	(Day 9 on, may persist over 1 year)		Level 2 exercises
Chronic inflammation	(May last for months or years)	• Muscle bending/J-stroke • Cross fiber massage • Manual muscle stretching • Psychosocial management • Patient education for lifestyle changes such as removal of repetitive tissue trauma	• Level 2–3 exercises • Therapist discretion based on the acuity of the chronicity

strategies between these groups.[70,71] Studies have also demonstrated improved cervical sensorimotor function in persons with neck pain, following balance training.[72]

During postural re-education training for repetitive strain, treatment should be centered around exercises that place the individual in mechanical positions that move away from the repetitive strain position. Also, a program for frequent movement should be established, such as hourly exercises to interrupt prolonged static postures. Utilizing a pen-grip mouse shows decreased electromyographic activity of the pronator teres by 46%, extensor digitorum by 46%, trapezius by 69%, levator scapulae by 82%, as compared to a normal computer mouse, minimizing strain.[14] A saddle chair helps to maintain a 120° thigh-torso angle, optimal for decreased low back pain, higher trunk activation, decreased upper trapezius and levator scapula activity.[73] The saddle chair has also been reported to provide optimal cervical and lumbar spine position, reducing muscular strain.[74]

Cup Exercise

The goal of this exercise is to initiate deep, primarily anterior, muscle function while protecting the joint position (Fig. 9). A partially supported, or unsupported, cervical spine during abdominal strengthening may cause neck pain, therefore, another goal of this exercise may be to strengthen the muscles so a patient can tolerate abdominal training for low back pain, as an example. The patient is placed supine with the knees supported. A cup, one-third full of water, is placed on the forehead and the

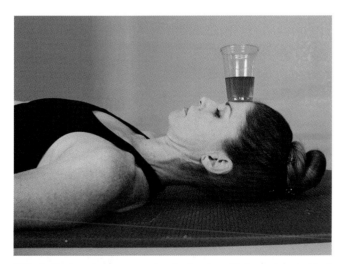

FIG. 9: During the cup exercise the forehead is brought to a level position. The head and neck are supported by towels, as necessary, for functional positioning

patient is asked to bring the water in the cup level, as if nodding the cervical spine "yes".

Level 1

The patient initiates cervical muscle flexion by looking down with their eyes only, aiming to the sternal notch. The therapist can gentle palpate at the anterior side of the transverse process to feel that the muscles are indeed activating. The patient is then instructed to look up under the brow line to deactivate or rest the cervical flexors, engaging the suboccipital muscles. The sequential contraction and relaxation of the extensor and flexor muscle groups acts like fluid pump to manipulate deep swelling.

Level 2

The patient is in the same starting position and holds their gaze on the sternal notch, then, while maintaining the water level, they are asked to nod the chin like they are saying "yes". The hold time start at 10 seconds and the duration progresses as tolerated.[19] If the patient only tolerates 5 seconds, the clinician may start with a shorter hold time but instruct the patient to more frequently through the day.[75] The patient should feel a "deep cramping in their throat", or deep cervical muscles. If the patient reports pain and points to the upper trapezius region or posterior cervical spine their positioning needs to be re-evaluated or they are not strong enough to maintain the position. Anecdotally, 10 repetitions at a 10 second hold time is often a good initial goal.

Supine Balance Training

The cervical spine is a relay center for neurologic balance information. The goal of this exercise is to facilitate deep spine muscles and to restore balance function while maintaining spinal alignment. The patient positions their spine lengthwise on a foam roller and attempts to find a functional cervical spine position. The functional cervical spine position is defined as the position where the joints are positioned to be the least symptomatic. The scapula are depressed and retracted in an attempt to stabilize the foam roller.

Level 1

Feet are positioned slightly apart (or together, if the patient is able) to maintain balance. The arms are positioned on abdomen, above shoulders or with little finger lightly resting on the floor to maintain balance (Fig. 10). The goal is to maintain balance.

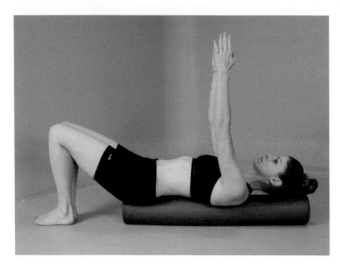

FIG. 10: Supine foam roller starting position

Level 2

Feet are placed together and one upper extremity is placed midline over sternum, then slowly stretched upward. The arm moves into horizontal abduction to a point when the knees begin to counter-balance and the contralateral trunk muscles have engaged. The arm is returned slowly to maintain balance. This motion is repeated for 1 minute and then the opposite upper extremity is challenged (Fig. 11).

Level 3

The patient maintains balance on the roller while she attempts to lift 1 foot off the ground 1 inch and then repeats with the opposite side, alternating for 1 minute (Fig. 12).

Prone Balance Training

Deep cervical extensor muscles have neural impairment with neck pain.[76] Therefore, specific training of the cervical extensor muscles should be considered when treating cervical sprain and strain.

The patient lies prone on a foam roller with the anterior surface of their chin resting on the edge of the foam roller. Shoulders are depressed and retracted while maintaining contact between the xiphoid process and the foam. The feet are together and the knees are extended, the gluteal muscles are maximally contracted and the abdominals are engaged from below. The thumbs are initially resting on the floor (Fig. 13). Patients often complain about bony pain over the chin, sternum or pubic bone with this exercise. It is important to explain that their tissue will remodel and adapt, similar to the bone and periosteal soreness experienced over the ischial tuberosities while riding a bike. The body will adjust with time.

Level 1

The hands are lifted, bringing the palms to rest on the lateral aspect of the thighs (Fig. 14). The arm is slowly moved away from the body to a point where the foam begins to move (Fig. 15). The arm is then slowly returned to the body.

Level 2

The upper extremities are level with the body in the "W" position (Fig. 16). The arms alternate, reaching overhead while maintaining the same distance from the floor (Fig. 17).

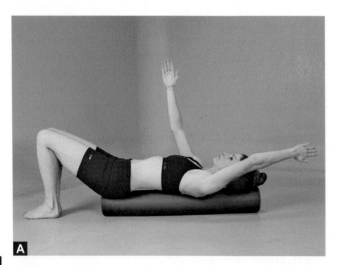

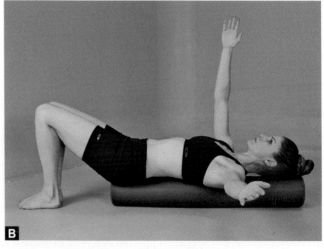

FIGS 11A AND B: Supine foam roller with upper extremity alternating—(A) Shoulder flexion; or (B) Abduction

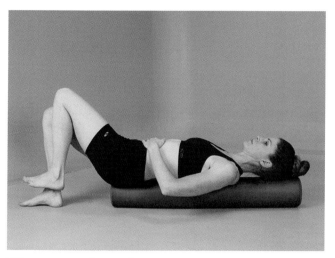

FIG. 12: Supine foam roller with lower extremity alternating hip flexion or marching

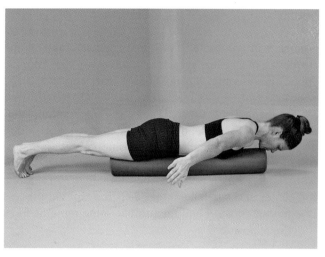

FIG. 15: Prone foam roller with alternating shoulder abduction

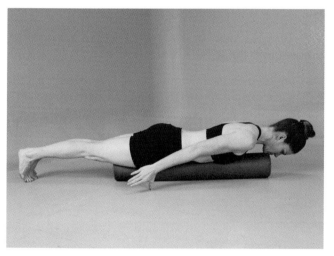

FIG. 13: Prone foam roller starting position

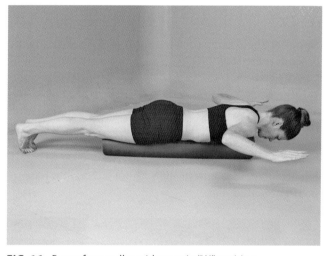

FIG. 16: Prone foam roller with arms in "W" position

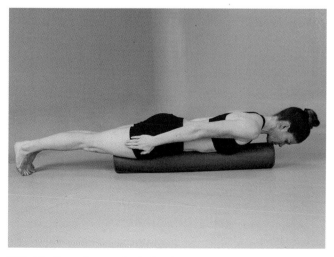

FIG. 14: Prone foam roller balancing

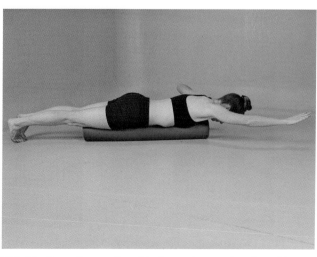

FIG. 17: Prone foam roller with alternating overhead reaching

Squats

Squats will promote continued activity and some cardiovascular exercise while protecting the cervical spine. Frequently, during squats the cervical spine will move into excessive extension, which may further irritate healing soft tissue. Using the Philadelphia collar four points as a guide, the patient can actively maintain a functional cervical spine position and enhance proprioceptive awareness. Heels are placed shoulder width apart with the toes externally rotated to 30°, aligning the center of the patella to toes 2–3. The xiphoid process is extended forward and the lumbar spine remains in its functional position.

Level 1

Squats are performed with the collar (Fig. 19A), or with the shoulders in flexion (Fig. 19B).

Level 2

Squats are held isometrically, on a balance board (Fig. 18) or foam roller (Fig. 19C).

Level 3

Squats are performed without a collar and while maintaining cervical spine position.

Level 4

Squats are held isometrically without a collar on balance board or foam roller.

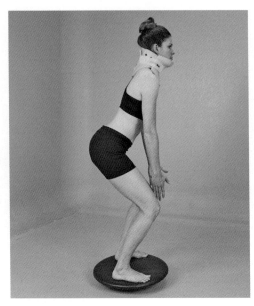

FIG. 18: Squat holds with collar on balance board

Single Limb Balance

This progression is similar to the squat progression. The balance starts out on a stable surface where the pelvis is level, sternum lifted and gluteal of the balancing leg is contracted.

Level 1

Single limb balance (SLB) is performed in a collar.

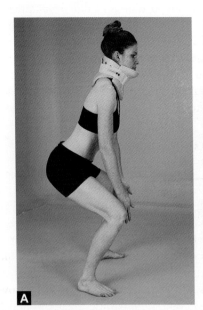
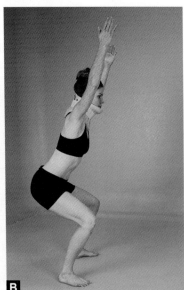
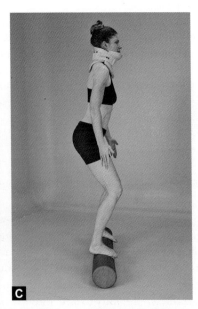

FIGS 19A TO C: The collar acts as a guide to maintain cervical alignment during—(A) Squat; (B) Squat with shoulder flexion; and (C) Partial squat on a foam roller

Level 2

SLB is performed while in a collar on balance board.

Level 3

SLB is performed without a collar.

Level 4

SLB is performed on balance board without a collar.

Rows

Pulley rows can be performed to reinitiate periscapular muscle function. In the wake of periscapular weakness, the upper trapezius muscles will often overactivate. The collar will serve as a reminder to activate the lower trapezius, inhibiting the upper trapezius, and allowing the exercise to target the periscapular weakness.

Triceps Press

It is not uncommon for the cervical spine to fall into subtle or excess extension at the terminal point of elbow extension. Provided that the patient is lifting an appropriate weight (no increased upper trapezius tone is visible), the triceps press is an unloading exercise for the spine and a therapeutic way to practice maintaining optimal posture.

Prone Ball or Balance Board

This is an exercise to transition a patient to unsupported cervical spine work. In the wake of disrupted proprioception, using the collar as a guide in the initial stages is appropriate, to guide the patient, especially while they work independently. The exercise aides in strengthening the spinal extensor and scapular retracting muscles that are often disrupted during cervical sprain and strain.

Level 1

The patient is positioned with the anterior superior iliac spine at the back edge of a gym ball so the body is at an angle as in the terminal point of a push-up (Fig. 20). The spine is aligned as if in a relative standing position. The hands are positioned next to the hips. The gluteals are maximally contracted and the abdominal muscles "hug" the ball. Without raising or lowering the chest, but allowing the whole body to sink into the ball, the arms are slowly raised to the lateral thigh.

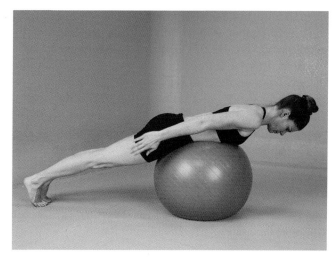

FIG. 20: Prone ball position

Level 2

The exercise is performed without a collar, with a therapist for cuing, and then progressed to the patient performing this exercise independently.

Level 3

The arm position is varied for increased balance challenge.

Supine Ball or Balance Board

Following the advanced level of the cup exercise, the patient has improved deep neck flexor strength and can be trialed in a supine position on a ball or balance board, maintaining alignment as if the cup were still in place, forehead level. The cervical collar can also act as a guide for cervical positioning. The patient is positioned initially so that the ball or board is just above the iliac crests. The position can be altered to increase or decrease the challenge, based on their ability.

Segmental Strengthening

Segmental strengthening targets muscles at each vertebral level. This is initially performed in a quiet treatment room as it requires significant concentration from the patient. The therapist places the lateral border of bilateral index fingers over the C2 lamina so that the fingers meet at the C2 spinous process. The therapist informs the patient that the clinician will make an attempt to lift the vertebra (in reality, it is soft tissue compression only, however, this cue will serve as a visual guide for the patient). The patient is told not to allow this to happen. Muscles that have become quite uncoordinated due to sprain or strain may need further facilitation, and this can be done by gently scratching the skin to bring tactile awareness to the segment. This can initially be used as a test to determine deficits from segment to segment, starting from C2 and moving toward C7, and from the left to the right sides. Often the segments with muscular deficit will also be the segments that have the most significant pathology (i.e. degenerative disk, degenerative joint, ligament sprain, muscle strain).

Level 1

The patient works with therapist as described earlier. The therapist facilitates where deficits are found.

Level 2

The patient is taught how to perform this at home. A narrow rope (such as a jump rope, old phone or Ethernet cord) looped around the posterior spine, just as the therapist's index finger was placed on the lamina. The patient's elbows are at rest on towels alongside the torso. The patient is instructed to hold the rope between the thumb and index finger, then to take up the rope slack using ulnar deviation alone so as to avoid any upper trapezius activation. The patient holds for 5 seconds. If one side needs more attention, the contralateral hand can tug the rope further, to cue the problem side (Figs 21 and 22).

Level 3

The exercise described in level 2 is performed on a foam roll.

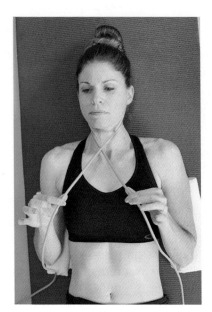

FIG. 22: Aerial view showing rope cross-over for cervical spine segmental strengthening

Segmental Extension over Ball

This exercise is designed to restore normal segmental motion of the cervical spine extensor muscles. With segmental strengthening, each vertebral segment is cued and thus encouraged to move in sequence, thus retraining the neuromotor system and restoring normal physiologic, and also accessory, movement patterns.

Hourly Exercises

Hourly exercises described by Dennis Morgan (DM), are designed to actively mobilize thoracic vertebra into extension or extension and side flexion to alleviate excess sprain and strain into the cervical spine region. It is recommended that they can be performed every hour in order to positively alter static posture, and thus blood, lymphatic and nerve flow, in addition to affecting joint position and muscle length. For patients who sit at a computer for prolonged periods, a reminder to perform these exercises can be set on the computer.

DM level 1

The patient is seated or standing in their functional position and instructed to sense functional head alignment. The arms start at the patient's side with the elbows flexed to 90°. The elbows maintain a fixed 90° as the shoulders begin to rise. At 90° of shoulder flexion, the elbows are flexed, and the arms are horizontally abducted

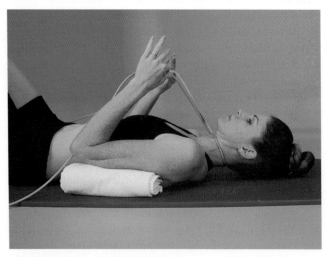

FIG. 21: Segmental strengthening set-up, with upper extremities positioned on a towel to avoid excess upper trapezius involvement

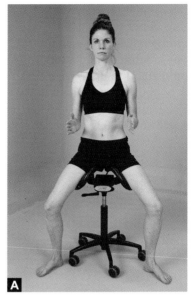 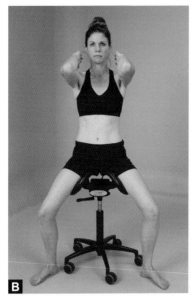 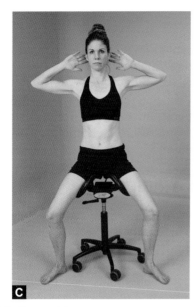

FIGS 23: Hourly exercises for thoracic extension—(A) Starting; (B) Mid; and (C) Ending position

so that the left and right finger-tips are approximated posterior to the cervical spine. It is important that the functional cervical position is maintained, not translated into excessive extension in order to target the thoracic spine for active extension mobilization. The exercise should be performed 10 times every hour (Figs 23A to C).

DM level 2

The patient is seated or standing in their functional position and instructed to sense functional head alignment. The left arm reaches to the ceiling into shoulder flexion, while the right arm reaches to the floor in shoulder extension, all while maintaining cervical functional position. The thoracic spine will actively be mobilized into extension and lateral flexion. The arms are alternated every 5 seconds and the exercise should be performed 10 times every hour.

Frog on Ball

This exercise will (maximally) contract thoracic and cervical spinal extensors, while attempting to protect the lumbar spine with hip flexion around the ball. The patient places the trunk prone on the ball and the knees are placed on each lateral side of the ball, relatively above the level of the pelvis. The xiphoid process maintains contact with the ball. The cervical spine maintains its functional position.

Level 1

The hands are placed folded over the sacrum, minimizing the lever force.

Level 2

The arms are lifted off the floor to the "W" position (Fig. 24). The patient holds this as long as they can while the therapist is timing. Based on the initial time to fatigue, the therapist will use this as the baseline time to instruct patient on holding goals and repetitions for home.

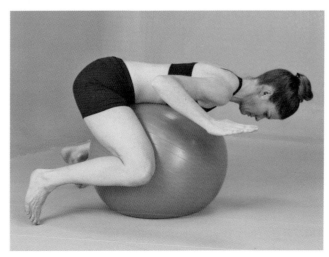

FIG. 24: Frog on ball exercise, Level 1

Level 3

The patient's arms can move out of the "W" position into alternating shoulder flexion.

Level 4

The patient's arms can go into a shoulder flexion hold position, increasing the spinal extensor muscle activity and endurance.

Cardiovascular Exercise

Perfusion of soft tissue via cardiovascular exercise is a key element in returning patients to function. Cardiovascular exercise not only facilitates circulation and perfusion of soft tissue, but reduces inflammation and releases natural pain-killers, endorphins, enkephalins and dynorphins, commonly referred to as "endorphins".[75,77] Education regarding cardiovascular exercise and initiation of exercise must occur early in treatment.

For patients in the acute or acute-on-chronic stages of cervical sprain or strain healing, the therapist can initiate cardiovascular exercise on a supine bike (Fig. 25). A cervical collar may assist in cervical alignment and can be worn on the stationary bike (Fig. 26), treadmill (Fig. 27), or Versa climber˚ (Fig. 28). While riding the stationary bike, the patient may be advised to sit upright and press into a front-wheel walker positioned on the backside of the bike in order to decompress the lower spine or activate the lower trapezius, thus inhibiting the upper trapezius

(Fig. 26). Careful attention by the therapist to ensure that overactivation of the upper trapezius does not occur, is imperative in treating cervical sprain.

Table 1 outlines treatment and exercise according to stages of healing. Table 1 is to be used as a guide. As always, judgment of the therapist and the therapist's understanding of the individual patient and available current research will ultimately determine the best treatment.

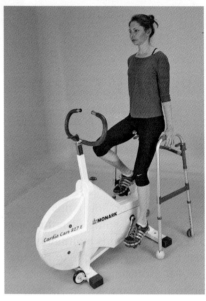

FIG. 26: Stationary bike with a front-wheel walker used as a decompression accessory

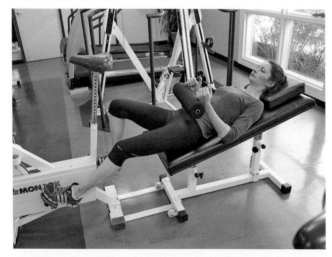

FIG. 25: Supine bike with decompression bar

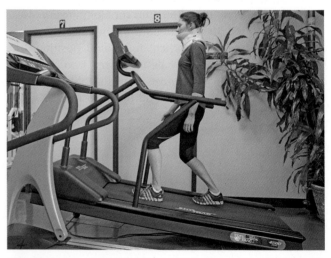

FIG. 27: Treadmill squat walk at 15% incline, with collar to guide cervical spine positioning

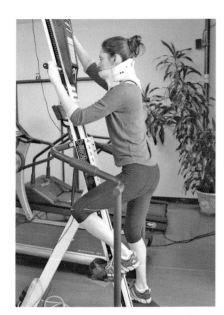

FIG. 28: Versa climber® with collar to guide cervical spine positioning

Surgical and Medical Considerations

Persistent symptoms that are not responding to conservative physical therapy management may require medical intervention.

Injections

In cases of myofascial pain, trigger point injections with lidocaine or B12 are a common medical intervention. In cases of persistent nerve disruption epidural may help to bathe the nerve often with cortisone medication. When performed using fluoroscopy, a facet block is a more accurate injection to tiny nerves surrounding the facet joint and is directed toward the medial nerve branch. If pain persists beyond potentially short-lasting injections, radiofrequency ablation is an option that uses radiofrequency to heat the offending nerve, effectively killing it and can have a more lasting effect, although the nerves will grow back overtime. Cryoanalgesia is a similar technique that uses liquid nitrogen to freeze the nerve.

Surgeries

When conservative management has been exhausted, severe cases of neck pain due to various structural pathologies may require surgical intervention such as cervical fusion, discectomy, or disk replacement.[75] While this chapter is not focused on rehabilitation following a cervical spine fusion, it should be noted that following a fusion, the adjacent cervical segment ligaments can become repetitively sprained and strained, although they were not initially the primary source of pain or lesion, and must be considered.[24]

◼ CONCLUSION

The process of evaluating and treating the human body and the human being is complex. In the study of cervical spine sprain and strain it becomes apparent that pain is multifactorial. New technologies in medical science are allowing us to understand how the biopsychosocial components of pain are working together. New research is guiding practitioners toward understanding how and why exercise that has been clinically observed to be beneficial for some time actually works. Initial manual treatment may be necessary to facilitate improved movement function, however, moving toward high-level exercise and prescribing a proper exercise program is what will empower patients to continue to maintain healthy movement function. High activity levels in a controlled environment such as a physical therapist supervised gym program or group exercise class that promotes a positive atmosphere that is sustained over time is the key to success in preventing acute cervical sprain or strain pain from becoming chronic and in changing the nervous system to move someone out of chronic states of pain. Support from and communication with other local health practitioners in promoting this type of treatment and intense exercise amongst patients will drive their success. Collaboration amongst the clinical and research communities is imperative to move research knowledge into a clinical setting and to allow the clinical setting to influence specific research concepts to enhance quality patient outcomes.

◼ REFERENCES

1. Holzapfel GA. Biomechanics of soft tissue. In: Lemaitre J (Ed). Handbook of material behavior: nonlinear models and properties. LMT-Cachan, France: Academic Press; 2000.
2. National Institutes of Health. (year). Sprains and Strains. [online] Available from http://www.nlm.nih.gov/medlineplus/sprainsandstrains.html. [Accessed January, 2015].
3. Goodman CC, Fuller KS, Boissonnault WG. Pathology: implications for the physical therapist, 2nd Edition. Philadelphia: Saunders; 2003.
4. Kaltenborn F, Evjength O. Manual mobilization of the joints: joint examination and basic treatment, 6th edition. Oslo, Norway: Norli; 2012.
5. Teasell RW, McClure JA, Walton D, Pretty J, Salter K, Meyer M, et al. A research synthesis of therapeutic interventions for whiplash-associated disorder (WAD): part 2-interventions for acute WAD. Pain Res Manag. 2010;15(5):295-304.

6. Quinlan KP, Annest JL, Myers B, Ryan G, Hill H. Neck strains and sprains among motor vehicle occupants—United States, 2000. Accid Anal Prev. 2004;36(1):21-7.

7. Kristjansson E, Jónsson H. Is the sagittal configuration of the cervical spine changed in women with chronic whiplash syndrome? A comparative computer-assisted radiographic assessment. J Manipulative Physiol Ther. 2002;25(9):550-5.

8. Curatolo M, Bogduk N, Ivancic PC, McLean SA, Siegmund GP, Winkelstein BA. The role of tissue damage in whiplash-associated disorders: discussion paper 1. Spine. 2011;36(25):S309-15.

9. Peolsson A, Ludvigsson ML, Overmeer T, Dedering Å, Bernfort L, Johansson G, et al. Effects of neck-specific exercise with or without a behavioural approach in addition to prescribed physical activity for individuals with chronic whiplash-associated disorders: a prospective randomised study. BMC Musculoskelet Disord. 2013;14(1):311.

10. Walton DM, Macdermid JC, Giorgianni AA, Mascarenhas JC, West SC, Zammit CA. Risk factors for persistent problems following acute whiplash injury: update of a systematic review and meta-analysis. J Orthop Sports Phys Ther. 2013;43(2):31-43.

11. Spitzer WO, Skovron ML, Salmi LR, Cassidy JD, Duranceau J, Suissa S, et al. Scientific monograph of the Quebec Task Force on Whiplash-Associated Disorders: redefining "whiplash" and its management. Spine. 1995;20(8):1S-73S.

12. Kroemer KH. Cumulative trauma disorders: Their recognition and ergonomics measures to avoid them. Appl Ergon. 1989;20(4):274-280.

13. Van Tulder M, Malmivaara A, Koes B. Repetitive strain injury. Lancet. 2007;369(9575):1815-22.

14. Ullman J, Kangas N, Ullman P, Wartenberg F, Ericson M. A new approach to the mouse arm syndrome. Int J Occup Saf Ergon. 2003;9(4):463-77.

15. Perrey S, Thedon T, Bringard A. Application of near-infrared spectroscopy in preventing work-related musculoskeletal disorders: brief review. Int J Ind Ergon. 2010;40(2):180-4.

16. Salter RB. Textbook of Disorders and Injuries of the Musculoskeletal System, 3rd edition. Baltimore: Lippincott Williams & Wilkins; 1999.

17. Wikipedia Free Encyclopedia. (2013). Sharpey's fibres. [online] Available from http://en.wikipedia.org/w/index.php?title=Sharpey%27s_fibres&oldid=563676933. [Accessed January, 2015].

18. Siegmund GP, Winkelstein BA, Ivancic PC, Svensson MY, Vasavada A. The anatomy and biomechanics of acute and chronic whiplash injury. Traffic Inj Prev. 2009;10(2):101-12.

19. Jull GA, O'Leary SP, Falla DL. Clinical assessment of the deep cervical flexor muscles: the craniocervical flexion test. J Manipulative Physiol Ther. 2008;31(7):525-33.

20. Kristjansson E. Reliability of ultrasonography for the cervical multifidus muscle in asymptomatic and symptomatic subjects. Man Ther. 2004;9(2):83-8.

21. Moore KL, Dalley AF. Clinically oriented anatomy, 4th edition. Philadelphia, PA: Lippincott Williams & Wilkins; 1999.

22. Vassiliou T, Kaluza G, Putzke C, Wulf H, Schnabel M. Physical therapy and active exercises—an adequate treatment for prevention of late whiplash syndrome? Randomized controlled trial in 200 patients. Pain. 2006;124(1-2):69-76.

23. Rudolfsson T, Björklund M, Djupsjöbacka M. Range of motion in the upper and lower cervical spine in people with chronic neck pain. Man Ther. 2012;17(1):53-9.

24. Sahrmann S. Movement system impairment syndromes of the extremities, cervical and thoracic spines. St. Louis, Missouri: Elsevier Mosby; 2011.

25. Williams MA, McCarthy CJ, Chorti A, Cooke MW, Gates S. A systematic review of reliability and validity studies of methods for measuring active and passive cervical range of motion. J Manipulative Physiol Ther. 2010; 33(2):138-55.

26. Magee DJ. Orthopedic physical assessment, 4th edition. St. Louis, Missouri: Saunders Elsevier; 2006.

27. Lipson SJ. Dysplasia of the odontoid process in Morquio's syndrome causing quadriparesis. J Bone Joint Surg Am. 1977;59(3):340-4.

28. Dupeyron A, Lecocq J, Vautravers P, Pélissier J, Perrey S. Muscle oxygenation and intramuscular pressure related to posture and load in back muscles. Spine J Off J North Am Spine Soc. 2009;9(9):754-9.

29. Peolsson A, Almkvist C, Dahlberg C, Lindqvist S, Pettersson S. Age- and sex-specific reference values of a test of neck muscle endurance. J Manipulative Physiol Ther. 2007;30(3):171-177. doi:10.1016/j. jmpt.2007.01.008.

30. O'Leary S, Falla D, Jull G. The relationship between superficial muscle activity during the craniocervical flexion test and clinical features in patients with chronic neck pain. Man Ther. 2011;16(5):452-5.

31. Domenech MA, Sizer PS, Dedrick GS, McGalliard MK, Brismee JM. The deep neck flexor endurance test: normative data scores in healthy adults. PM R. 2011;3(2):105-10.

32. Woodhouse A, Liljebäck P, Vasseljen O. Reduced head steadiness in whiplash compared with non-traumatic neck pain. J Rehabil Med. 2010;42(1):35-41.

33. Kelly M, Cardy N, Melvin E, Reddin C, Ward C, Wilson F. The craniocervical flexion test: an investigation of performance in young asymptomatic subjects. Man Ther. 2013;18(1):83-6.

34. Falla DL, Jull GA, Hodges PW. Patients with neck pain demonstrate reduced electromyographic activity of the deep cervical flexor muscles during performance of the craniocervical flexion test. Spine. 2004;29(19):2108-14.

35. Castien R, Blankenstein A, van der Windt D, Heymans MW, Dekker J. The working mechanism of manual therapy in participants with chronic tension-type headache. J Orthop Sports Phys Ther. 2013;43(10):693-9.

36. Dimitriadis Z, Kapreli E, Strimpakos N, Oldham J. Respiratory weakness in patients with chronic neck pain. Man Ther. 2013;18(3):248-53.

37. Butler DS. Mobilisation of the nervous system. London: Churchill Livingstone; 1991.

38. Herrera I. Ending female pain: a woman's manual. New York: Duplex Publishing; 2009.

39. Wise D, Anderson R. A headache in the pelvis: a new understanding and treatment for chronic pelvic pain syndromes, 6th edition. Occidental, California: National Center for Pelvic Pain; 2011.

40. Amy Stein. Heal pelvic pain. New York: McGraw-Hill; 2009.

41. APTA public policy, practice, and professional affairs unit. Description of dry needling in clinical practice: an educational resource paper. Alexandria, VA; 2013.

42. Elliott JM, O'Leary S, Sterling M, Hendrikz J, Pedler A, Jull G. Magnetic resonance imaging findings of fatty infiltrate in the cervical flexors in chronic whiplash. Spine. 2010;35(9):948-54.

43. Elliott J, Sterling M, Noteboom JT, Darnell R, Galloway G, Jull G. Fatty infiltrate in the cervical extensor muscles is not a feature of chronic, insidious-onset neck pain. Clin Radiol. 2008;63(6):681-7.

44. Kivioja J, Ozenci V, Rinaldi L, Kouwenhoven M, Lindgren U, Link H. Systemic immune response in whiplash injury and ankle sprain: elevated IL-6 and IL-10. Clin Immunol Orlando Fla. 2001;101(1):106-12.

45. Sterling M, Elliott JM, Cabot PJ. The course of serum inflammatory biomarkers following whiplash injury and their relationship to sensory and muscle measures: a longitudinal cohort study. PloS One. 2013;8(10):e77903.

46. Goodman C, Snyder T. Differential diagnosis for physical therapists: screening for referral, 4th edition. St. Louis, Missouri: Saunders Elsevier; 2007.

47. Miller J, Gross A, D'Sylva J, Burnie SJ, Goldsmith CH, Graham N, et al. Manual therapy and exercise for neck pain: a systematic review. Man Ther. 2010;15(4):334-54.

48. Cameron MH. Physical agents in rehabilitation: from research to practice, 2nd edition. St. Louis, Missouri: Saunders; 2003.

49. Schnabel M, Ferrari R, Vassiliou T, Kaluza G. Randomised, controlled outcome study of active mobilisation compared with collar therapy for whiplash injury. Emerg Med J EMJ. 2004;21(3):306-10.

50. Sackett DL, Straus S, Richardson WS, Rosenberg W, Haynes RB. Evidence-based medicine: how to practice and teach EBM, 2nd edition. Edinburgh: Churchill Livingstone; 2000.

51. Yoo WG. Effect of the neck retraction taping (NRT) on forward head posture and the upper trapezius muscle during computer work. J Phys Ther Sci. 2013;25(5):581-2.

52. Vairo GL, Miller SJ, McBrier NM, Buckley WE. Systematic review of efficacy for manual lymphatic drainage techniques in sports medicine and rehabilitation: an evidence-based practice approach. J Man Manip Ther. 2009;17(3):e80-89.

53. Kietrys DM, Palombaro KM, Azzaretto E, Hubler R, Schaller B, Schlussel JM, et al. Effectiveness of dry needling for upper-quarter myofascial pain: a systematic review and meta-analysis. J Orthop Sports Phys Ther. 2013;43(9):620-34.

54. Painful and tender muscles: dry needling can reduce myofascial pain related to trigger points muscles. J Orthop Sports Phys Ther. 2013; 43(9):635.

55. Mejuto-Vázquez MJ, Salom-Moreno J, Ortega-Santiago R, Truyols-Domínguez S, Fernández-de-las-Peñas C. Short-term changes in neck pain, widespread pressure pain sensitivity, and cervical range of motion after the application of trigger point dry needling in patients with acute mechanical neck pain: a randomized clinical trial. J Orthop Sports Phys Ther. 2014;44(4):252-60..

56. APTA Department of Practice and APTA State Government Affairs. Physical therapists & the performance of dry needling: an educational resource paper. Alexandria, VA; 2012.

57. Gong W. Impact of longus colli muscle massage on the strength and endurance of the deep neck flexor muscle of adults. J Phys Ther Sci. 2013;25(5):591-3.

58. Topolska M, Chrzan S, Sapuła R, Kowerski M, Sobo M, Marczewski K. Evaluation of the effectiveness of therapeutic massage in patients with neck pain. Ortop Traumatol Rehabil. 2012;14(2):115-24.

59. Morgan D. A Primer of Orthopedic Manual Therapy. 1993.

60. Kaltenborn F. Manuell Mobilisering Av Ryggraden. 2nd edition. Norway: Olaf Norlis Bokhandel; 1989.

61. Joseph MF, Taft K, Moskwa M, Denegar CR. Deep friction massage to treat tendinopathy: a systematic review of a classic treatment in the face of a new paradigm of understanding. J Sport Rehabil. 2012;21(4):343-53.

62. Kim TH, Kang JW, Kim KH, Lee MH, Kim JE, Kim JH, et al. Cupping for treating neck pain in video display terminal (VDT) users: a randomized controlled pilot trial. J Occup Heal. 2012;54(6):416-26.

63. Nielsen A, Knoblauch NT, Dobos GJ, Michalsen A, Kaptchuk TJ. The effect of Gua Sha treatment on the microcirculation of surface tissue: a pilot study in healthy subjects. Explore New York N. 2007;3(5):456-66.

64. Xu QY, Yang JS, Zhu B, Yang L, Wang YY, Gao XY. The effects of scraping therapy on local temperature and blood perfusion volume in healthy subjects. Evid-Based Complement Altern Med ECAM. 2012;2012:490292.

65. Lee MS, Choi TY, Kim JI, Choi SM. Using Gua Sha to treat musculoskeletal pain: a systematic review of controlled clinical trials. Chin Med. 2010;5:5.

66. Nielsen A, Kligler B, Koll BS. Addendum: Safety Standards for Gua sha (press-stroking) and Ba guan (cupping). Complement Ther Med. 2014;22(3):446-8.

67. Butler DS, Moseley L. Explain pain. NOI Australasia: NOI Group Publications; 2003.

68. Morgan D. Functional training and postural stabilization. Top Acute Care Trauma Rehabil. 1988;2(4):8-17.

69. Treleaven J, Jull G, Grip H. Head eye co-ordination and gaze stability in subjects with persistent whiplash associated disorders. Man Ther. 2011;16(3):252-7.

70. Field S, Treleaven J, Jull G. Standing balance: a comparison between idiopathic and whiplash-induced neck pain. Man Ther. 2008;13(3):183-91.

71. Silva AG, Cruz AL. Standing balance in patients with whiplash-associated neck pain and idiopathic neck pain when compared with asymptomatic participants: a systematic review. Physiother Theory Pract. 2013; 29(1):1-18.

72. Beinert K, Taube W. The effect of balance training on cervical sensorimotor function and neck pain. J Mot Behav. 2013;45(3):271-8.

73. Gadge K, Innes E. An investigation into the immediate effects on comfort, productivity and posture of the Bambach saddle seat and a standard office chair. Work Read Mass. 2007;29(3):189-203.

74. Annetts S, Coales P, Colville R, Mistry D, Moles K, Thomas B, et al. A pilot investigation into the effects of different office chairs on spinal angles. Eur Spine J. 2012;21(2):S165-70.

75. Fishman S. The war on pain. New York: Quill; 2001.

76. Schomacher J, Farina D, Lindstroem R, Falla D. Chronic trauma-induced neck pain impairs the neural control of the deep semispinalis cervicis muscle. Clin Neurophysiol. 2012;123(7):1403-8.

77. Wikipedia Free Encyclopedia. (2014). Endorphins. [online] Available at: http://en.wikipedia.org/w/index.php?title=Endorphins&oldid=603555163. [Accessed January, 2015].

CHAPTER 7

Cervical Radiculopathy

Powell J Bernhardt

ABSTRACT

The correct diagnosis and appropriate treatment is of extreme importance to people suffering with neck pain. With only 33–65% of people recovering from neck pain 1 year after onset, proper identification of the pathology and musculoskeletal impairments has a significant impact on the long-term prognosis. One cause of neck pain is cervical radiculopathy.

Cervical radiculopathy is a disorder that occurs secondary to nerve root compression, most commonly associated with a herniated disk or osteophyte formation. Subjective and objective findings include paresthesias, numbness, and other altered sensory changes in the neck and upper extremity. Although cervical radiculopathy might be the primary pathology, often the underlying cause is a myriad of musculoskeletal impairments—including postural dysfunction, restricted mobility, and cervical instability—that create various functional limitations and disability.

This chapter explores the anatomy, biomechanics, etiology, differential diagnosis, diagnostic imaging, and medical treatment, with an emphasis on the efficacy of physical therapy examination and treatment of cervical radiculopathy.

◼ INTRODUCTION

The correct diagnosis and appropriate treatment of neck pain is of extreme importance to those suffering from it. With only 33–65% of people recovering from neck pain 1 year after onset.[1] The proper identification of the pathology and associated musculoskeletal impairments has a significant impact on the long-term prognosis. One cause of neck pain is cervical radiculopathy.

The North American Spine Society (NASS) defines cervical radiculopathy as "pain in a radicular pattern in one or both upper extremities related to compression and/or irritation of one or more cervical nerve roots. Frequent signs and symptoms include varying degrees of sensory, motor and reflex changes, as well as dysesthesias and paresthesia related to nerve root(s), without evidence of spinal cord dysfunction (myelopathy)."[2]

Compression of the cervical nerve root(s) is often caused by cervical disk herniation, spondylosis, or stenosis, or some combination of these structural changes. Other common etiology includes trauma, cervical instability, and nonmusculoskeletal disorders.

Although cervical radiculopathy might be the underlying pathology, often, the underlying cause is a myriad of musculoskeletal impairments including postural dysfunction, restricted mobility, and cervical instability that create various functional limitations and disability.

Anatomy

Vertebrae

The cervical spine consists of seven vertebrae. Functionally, the atlas and axis move on the occiput and are commonly referred to as the craniovertebral region.

The third through the seventh cervical vertebrae will be described as the lower cervical vertebrae, for the purposes of this chapter. Figure 1 illustrates the basic anatomy of a typical cervical vertebra.

Intervertebral Disk

The intervertebral disk consists of the annulus fibrosus and the nucleus pulposus (Fig. 2). The outer annulus is composed of fibrocartilage and functions to create stiffness necessary to absorb compressive loads. The inner nucleus is a gelatinous material that functions to distribute compressive loads. While the morphology of the intervertebral disk is continuous in the thoracic and lumbar spine, it is unique in the cervical spine. The annulus fibrosus is a crescent-shaped structure that is thicker anteriorly as it extends toward the joints of Luschka. Posterolaterally, the annulus is deficient and does not provide any support.[3]

Flexion increases the intradiskal pressure, whereas extension reduces intradiskal pressure by transferring load to the neural arch and uncovertebral joints.[4] During flexion, if the integrity of the annulus fibrosus is compromised, the nucleus pulposus may extend posteriorly.

Nerve Roots

The cervical spine consists of seven cervical vertebrae and eight nerve roots (Fig. 3). 60% of cervical radiculopathy cases reportedly involve the C7 nerve root, while the C6 nerve root accounted for another 25%.[5-11] Although it is widely accepted that nerve root compression results in pain or paresthesias in a specific dermatomal distribution (Table 1), some evidence suggests that nerve root symptoms are not always specific to the dermatome of the affected root.[12]

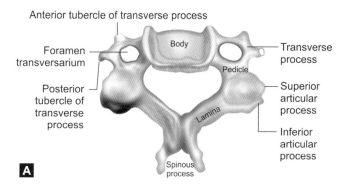

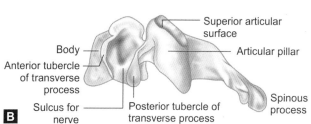

Figs 1A and B: (A) Superior view of cervical vertebra; and (B) Lateral view of cervical vertebra
Source: Gray's Anatomy via Wikimedia Commons.

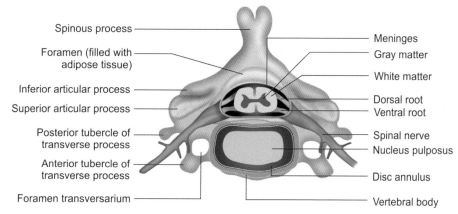

FIG. 2: Superior view of cervical vertebra and intervertebral disk
Source: From the Wikimedia Commons via Creative Commons Attribution-Share Alike 3.0 Unported.

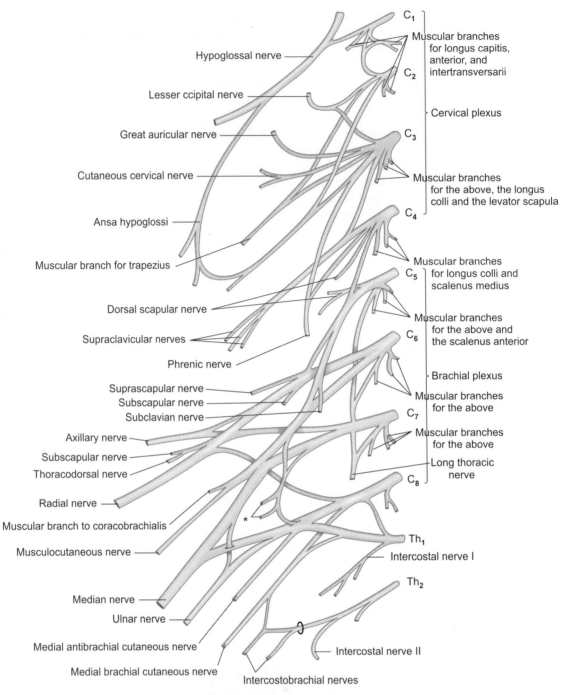

FIG. 3: Cervical nerve roots (· = anterior thoracic nerves)
Source: Gray's Anatomy via Wikimedia Commons.

Musculature

Cervical musculature consists of multiple layers that function to provide stability while facilitating neck motion.

Table 2 references the various layers and their respective muscles. Figures 4 to 6 illustrate the orientation of the respective muscles.

TABLE 1: Pain pattern, myotome, and reflexes associated with cervical nerve root

Nerve root	Pain pattern due to compression	Myotome	Reflexes
C2	The atlantoaxial and C2–3 zygapophyseal joints. May radiate from the occipital region to the parietal, temporal, frontal, and/or periorbital regions. May also present with ipsilateral eye lacrimation and conjunctival injection[13]	Scapular elevation	N/A
C3	The C2–3 zygapophyseal joint. May radiate to the occipital, temporal, frontal, and/or periorbital regions. This nerve root is most vulnerable in acceleration-deceleration injuries[13]	Scapular elevation	N/A
C4	Neck, trapezius[14]	Scapular elevation	N/A
C5	C5 dorsal ramus becomes cutaneous at the C6-7 spinous processes and descends into the suprascapular region. Symptoms may include superficial and deep pain at the suprascapula[13]	Weakness of the delotid[14]	Biceps brachii and brachioradialis
C6	Symptoms may include deep pain at the suprascapula and/or posterior deltoid.[13] Pain or paresthesia may also radiate into the superolateral upper extremity into the first and second digits[14]	Weakness of the biceps brachii,[14] elbow flexors, and wrist extensors	Biceps brachii and brachioradialis
C7	Symptoms may include deep pain at the interscapula.[13] Pain or paresthesia may also radiate into the dorsal upper extremity through the elbow into the third digit.[14]	Weakness of the triceps brachii,[14] elbow extensors, and wrist flexors	Triceps brachii
C8	C8 dorsal ramus becomes cutaneous at the T1–2 spinous processes and descends from the interscapula into the middle of the scapula. Symptoms may include superficial and deep pain at the interscapula and scapula.[13] Pain or paresthesia may also radiate from the inferomedial upper extremity into the 4th and 5th digit[14]	Weakness of the hand intrinsics, finger abduction, and grip[14]	Triceps brachii

TABLE 2: Musculature of the cervical spine[15]

Superficial	Deeper	Deepest	Deep neck flexors
• SCM • Scalenes • Trapezius • Levator scapulae	• Splenius capitis • Longissimus capitis • Semispinalis capitis	• Splenius cervicis • Longissimus cervicis • Semispinalis cervicis • Erector spinae • Iliocostalis • Longissimus • Semispinalis	• Longus colli • Longus capitis

SCM, sternocleidomastoid

Source: Adapted from Dutton with permission from McGraw Hill Medical.

Zygapophyseal Joints

The zygapophyseal, or facet, joint of the cervical spine is a diarthrodial synovial joint that enhances mobility, provides stability and absorbs compressive loads.

Although it has been widely accepted that cervical facet joints are oriented in the posterolateral direction, Pal G et al. identified that cervical facets more often face posteromedial at the third and fourth vertebrae, roughly in the frontal plane at C5, and posterolateral only at C6 and C7. They speculate that the posteromedial orientation of C3 facilitates craniovertebral rotation by stabilizing the C2 vertebra. When the facet orientation transitions at the fifth vertebra, movement occurs more easily due to the forward inclination. This degree of angulation also facilitates coupled motion.[16]

Intervertebral Foramen

The boundaries of the intervertebral (neural) foramen can be visualized in Figure 7. The respective nerve root occupies one-third of the intervertebral foramen in the normal cervical spine[17]

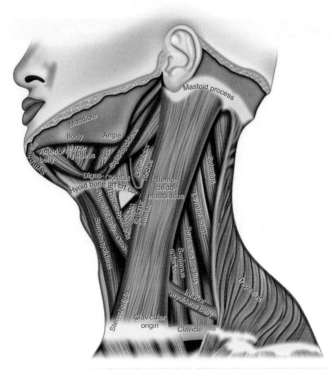

FIG. 4: Anterolateral musculature of the cervical spine
Source: Gray's Anatomy via Wikimedia Commons.

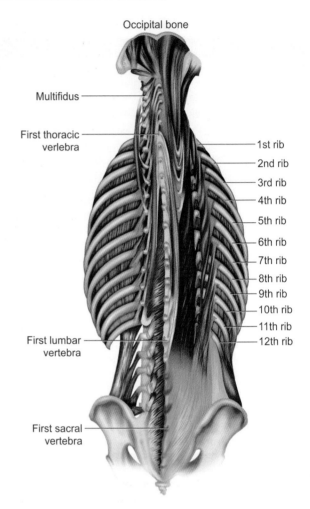

FIG. 5: Deep posterior musculature of the cervical spine
Source: Gray's Anatomy via Wikimedia Commons.

Uncovertebral Joint

The uncovertebral joints, or joints of Luschka, are formed between the uncinate processes of the cervical spine and the inferior portion of the superior vertebral body. Although these joints are well developed in the lower cervical spine, they can be found, but appear smaller, in the upper cervical spine.[18]

Biomechanics

The cervical spine has the greatest amount of mobility in comparison to other regions of the spine. The normative values for cervical mobility are 80°–90° of flexion, 70° of extension, 20°–45° of lateral flexion, and 90° of rotation.[19] A general understanding of the biomechanics of the cervical spine is necessary to properly evaluate and treat patients with cervical radiculopathy. Due to the higher frequency of cervical radiculopathy in the lower cervical spine, the biomechanics of the upper cervical spine will not be discussed in this chapter.

The cervical spine moves in the sagittal, coronal, and transverse planes to permit flexion, extension, lateral flexion, and rotation. During flexion of the lower cervical spine, the inferior facets of the superior segment glide superioanteriorly on the superior facets of the inferior segment. During extension, the inferior facets of the superior segment glide inferioposteriorly on the superior facets of the inferior segment. Furthermore, the boundaries of invertebral foramen widen during flexion and approximate one another during extension.[20-23] During side-bending, the ipsilateral superior facet glides inferioposteriorly on the superior facet of the inferior segment, while the contralateral inferior facet of the superior segment glides superioanteriorly. Cervical rotation occurs in a similar manner to lateral flexion.

Cervical radiculopathy is due to compression of the nerve root within the intervertebral foramen. The intervertebral foramen is maximally opened during cervical flexion coupled with contralateral rotation and

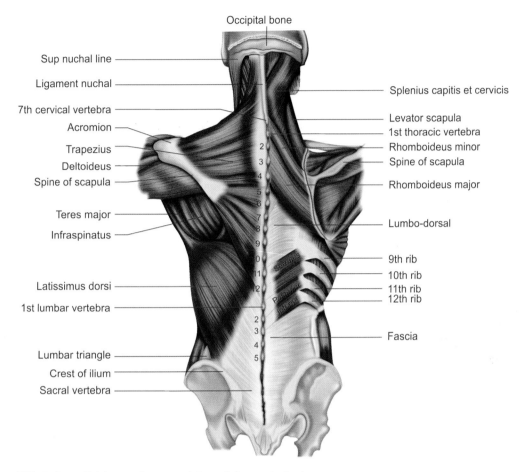

Occipital bone

Sup nuchal line

Ligament nuchal

7th cervical vertebra

Acromion

Trapezius

Deltoideus

Spine of scapula

Teres major

Infraspinatus

Latissimus dorsi

1st lumbar vertebra

Lumbar triangle

Crest of ilium

Sacral vertebra

Splenius capitis et cervicis

Levator scapula

1st thoracic vertebra

Rhomboideus minor

Spine of scapula

Rhomboideus major

Lumbo-dorsal

9th rib

10th rib

11th rib

12th rib

Fascia

FIG. 6: Superficial posterior musculature of the cervical spine
Source: Gray's Anatomy via Wikimedia Commons.

lateral flexion. Conversely, it is maximally compressed during cervical extension, ipsilateral rotation, and ipsilateral flexion.[23]

Due to the geometry of the facet joint and the axis of rotation, cervical rotation and lateral flexion occur together, which is an example of coupled motion.[24,25] Coupled motion, which requires greater amounts of motor control, allows for increased mobility while preserving stability in the cervical spine.[26] Coupled movement was shown to be the greatest during cervical rotation and the least during flexion and extension.[26] In addition to the orientation of the facet, coupled motion may also be facilitated by the crescent shape of the cervical intervertebral disk.[24] Coupled motion has been established in the lower cervical spine and should be considered in the application of manual therapy techniques.[27]

CLINICAL PRESENTATION

Signs and Symptoms

Subjective and objective findings of cervical radiculopathy include paresthesia, numbness, and other altered sensory changes in the neck and upper extremity. People with cervical radiculopathy typically identify the location of pain to include the neck and upper extremity, including the scapula and/or periscapular region, sometimes referred to as Cloward's areas.[28] These patients may also demonstrate decreased deep tendon reflexes of the upper extremity. In a retrospective review of 846 cases of people with cervical radiculopathy who received posterior-lateral foraminotomy, signs and symptoms of cervical radiculopathy were identified: arm pain (99.4%); sensory deficits (85.2%); neck pain (79.7%); reflex deficits (71.2%); motor deficits (68%); pain and/or paresthesias

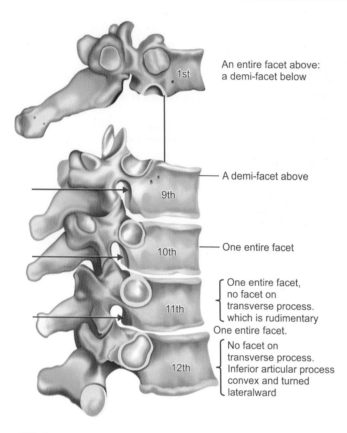

An entire facet above:
a demi-facet below

1st

A demi-facet above

9th

One entire facet

10th

One entire facet,
no facet on
transverse process.
which is rudimentary

11th

One entire facet.

No facet on
transverse process.
Inferior articular process
convex and turned
lateralward

12th

FIG. 7: Intervertebral foramen of the spine
Source: Gray's Anatomy via Wikimedia Commons.

in a dermatomal pattern (53.9%); scapular pain (52.5%), anterior chest pain (17.8%), headaches (9.7%), anterior chest and arm pain (5.9%); and left-sided chest and arm pain (1.3%).[29] It has also been suggested that lower cervical radiculopathy can be the source of some headaches.[30]

■ CLINICAL EXAMINATION

Prior to physical therapy intervention, it is imperative to perform a thorough examination. Nonmechanical sources of symptoms that mimic cervical radiculopathy include must be ruled out and include congenital abnormalities, metabolic, vascular, infectious, and oncologic diseases and disorders.[20] Patients suffering from myelopathy and/or pain of non-musculoskeletal origin should be referred to the appropriate practitioner(s).

Differential Diagnosis

During the examination of a patient with neck and upper extremity symptoms, the clinician should consider other possible neuromusculoskeletal disorders. The differential diagnoses that should be considered are described in Table 3. Other diagnoses not included in the table but discussed in detail in other chapters in this text include rotator cuff or impingement syndrome and thoracic outlet syndrome. Some of these diagnoses have signs and

TABLE 3: Musculoskeletal disorders included in differential diagnosis of cervical radiculopathy

Diagnoses	Brief description	Clinical presentation	Affected movements
Herniated nucleus pulposus	• Soft herniation—tears in the annulus fibrosis allow the nucleus pulposus to protrude or herniate upon various structures, including the nerve root or spinal cord. Typically result in motor loss (Fig. 8) • Hard herniation (see Cervical Spondylosis)	• Most often unilateral • Can be sudden when originates from the intervertebral disk • Often affects young and middle-aged people	• Although flexion or extension may increase pain, extension may result in centralization[31,32]
Cervical spondylosis	• Disk desiccation occurs. Osteophytic formation and sclerosis of vertebral body and facet joints result in thickening of ligaments and loss of cervical lordosis.[33] Increased joint motion, greatest between C5-C6 and C6-C7, exacerbates osteophytic formation[23] • Radiculopathy can occur due to formation of bone spurs in intervertebral foramen, also known as a hard herniation. Hard herniations often result in sensory loss[5,34]	• Often seen in the older population • Typically presents with restricted mobility. However, joint hypermobility coupled with cervical instability can also lead to cervical spondylosis • Demonstrates morning stiffness that improves with activity. As disease progresses, patient may experience a constant ache that increases with activity	• Pain typically occurs with extension or extension coupled with ipsilateral rotation.[17] Flexion may provide some relief as well[20-23]

Continued

Continued

Diagnoses	Brief description	Clinical presentation	Affected movements
Peripheral nerve entrapment	• Peripheral nerves are susceptible to injury secondary to their superficial location, narrowed pathway, or anatomical course through areas at higher risk of injury[35]	• May present with paresthesias or pain in distribution of affected peripheral nerve • Possible weakness of musculature innervated by affected peripheral nerve • See common sites of entrapment listed in Table 4	• Positive upper limb tension test(s) or special tests that compress or place tension on the affected peripheral nerve
Double crush syndrome	• Compression or traction of nerve centrally disturbs axonal transport, resulting in double-crush syndrome. Compression of the nerve root can result in remote effects of peripheral nerve originating from the injured root in one or more distal sites • Cervical radiculopathy may result in distal focal entrapment neuropathy, such as thoracic outlet syndrome, carpal tunnel syndrome, or ulnar neuritis at the cubital tunnel	• See Peripheral Nerve Entrapment and Table 4	• See Peripheral Nerve Entrapment and Table 4
Myofascial pain syndrome	• Characterized by pain secondary to myofascial trigger points[36] • A myofascial trigger point can facilitate central sensitization	• Muscle pain typically described as a tearing or cramping sensation difficult to localize[37] • Pain is reproduced by applying deep pressure to the trigger point • May restrict or impede muscle length, force production, and reflex inhibition. People suffering from myofascial pain syndrome may also exhibit autonomic symptoms[38]	
Cervical stenosis	• Narrowing of cervical spine vertebral canal due to degeneration • Although nerve root compression can occur, stenosis usually results in compression of the spinal cord, or cervical myelopathy	• Usually marked by periods of exacerbation followed long periods of intermission • Symptoms of cervical myelopathy include: gait and balance dysfunction, increased deep tendon and pathological reflexes, clonus, pain and paresthesia, leg and arm weakness with greater loss proximally in comparison to distally, bowel and bladder dysfunction, loss of dexterity, and hand intrinsic atrophy • Increased stiffness at the level affected may lead to a cycle of hypermobility, instability, and cord compression one or two levels above the stiff segment[33]	• Cervical stenosis often limits or causes painful cervical extension • Cervical flexion and distraction relieves symptoms
The fourth thoracic syndrome	• T4 syndrome is a condition characterized by paresthesia (unilateral or bilateral) in the upper extremity with or without neck or head pain.[39] Although the mechanism remains unclear, this disorder appears to affect the sympathetic nervous system[40]	• Paresthesia occurs in glove-like distribution, often accompanied by upper extremity weakness, clumsiness, coldness, and back stiffness.[41] Other symptoms include postural hypotension, peripheral edema, and/or diaphoresis[40] • During examination, chief pain complaint is reproduced or eliminated by mobilization of the affected thoracic segment.[40] Although "T4 syndrome" identifies the fourth thoracic vertebrae, it can be caused by any upper thoracic vertebra[40]	

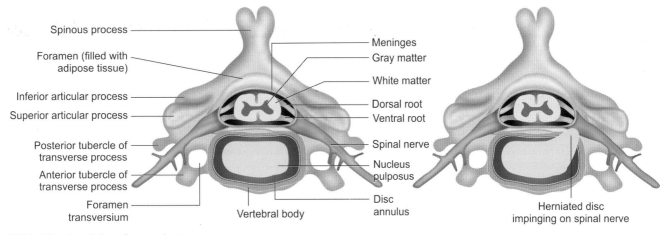

FIG 8: Herniated disc of cervical spine

Source: Wikimedia Commons via Creative Commons Attribution-Share Alike 3.0 Unported.

TABLE 4: Common sites of peripheral nerve entrapment[35,44]

Peripheral nerve	Areas of entrapment
Radial nerve (C5–C8, T1)	• Spiral groove • Radial tunnel • Brachioradialis • Supinator muscle • Arcade of Froshe* • Extensor carpi radialis brevis
Ulnar (C8, T1)	• Medial or accessory head of the triceps muscle • Arcade of Struthers • Cubital tunnel* • Flexor carpi ulnaris • Guyon's tunnel
Median (C6–8, T1)	• Bicipital aponeurosis • Pronator teres* • Flexor digitorum superficialis • Carpal tunnel

*Designates most common site of compression for each respective nerve.

symptoms that mimic cervical radiculopathy while others have been shown to lead to the disorder.

Jaw Pain and Headaches

Jaw pain and headaches often accompany neck pain due to compression of the upper cervical nerve roots as well as the dense neural connection via the trigeminal cervicocomplex. The grey matter of the trigeminal nerve is continuous the upper three cervical spinal nerves and is known as the trigeminocervical nucleus. This complex, which is housed in the C2–3 region, receives contributions from the seventh, ninth, and tenth cranial nerves. Nociceptive signals from cervical nerve roots as low as C7 can interact with the trigeminocervical complex, Because of this intricate plexus, upper cervical pain can refer into the head or jaw region and vice versa.[42,43]

As a result, it is important to query the cervical patient about the occurrence of jaw and/or head pain. However, it is beyond the scope of this chapter to discuss the treatment of these specific symptoms in detail.

The remaining portion of this chapter describes the examination and treatment of a patient presenting with cervical radiculopathy due to nerve root compression in the intervertebral foramen. Once sinister pathology has been eliminated as the source of the patient's symptoms, the purpose of the physical examination is to reproduce the patient's chief complaint pain, or comparable sign.[41] Because the severity of nerve compression can be time-dependent, a prompt and thorough examination is necessary to correctly diagnose the patient and to initiate appropriate intervention. The most common mechanical causes of cervical radiculopathy are soft or hard herniations in the intervertebral foramen.[14,34,45] While the biomechanical model of assessment can be useful, the patient response-based model is evidence-based.[46] Information presented in this chapter incorporates both ideologies but is predominantly grounded in the patient response-based model.

Postural Examination

The cervical spine demonstrates a modest amount of lordosis, which develops during infancy in response to

holding the head upright, prevents spinal cord injury and distributes loads.[23,47] Poor posture creates flattening of normal cervical lordosis and places increased stress on the intervertebral disks and facet joints.[48]

Postural control is a complex motor skill comprised of the integration of various sensorimotor systems.[49] Vladimir Janda, believed the musculoskeletal and central nervous system were interdependent and identified common muscular imbalances, or crossed syndromes.[44,50] Upper crossed syndrome is characterized increased postural changes, including forward head posture and winging of the scapulae. Janda found that tonic muscles, including the scalenes, sternocleidomastoid, levator scapulae, pectoralis major, and upper trapezius are prone to tightness; whereas phasic muscles, including the deep cervical neck flexors and lower scapular stabilizers, are prone to weakness.[50]

Postural examination involves the assessment of muscle length, flexibility, and muscle strength and stability of the entire vertebral column.[51] While symptoms of pathology may be localized to a particular segment, postural dysfunction typically affects multiple joints rather than a specific joint in isolation. The clinician should observe for asymmetry and identify postural faults from various angles.[52] The head should be in a neutral position while the neck should be in a mild lordosis with little muscular effort.[51] People with cervical radiculopathy may demonstrate a forward head posture.[47] This maladaptive posture places increased tension on the nerve roots,[53] and leads to tightness of the suboccipital muscles.[51]

Ergonomic Assessment

Part of the postural examination may also include an ergonomic assessment. The cervical spine and its musculature are often subjected to increased amounts of stress as a result of the postural demands of the workplace.

TABLE 5: Cervical myotomes[57]

Myotome	Muscle action
C1	Cervical rotation
C2–4	Scapular elevation
C5	Shoulder abduction
C5, C6	Elbow flexion
C6	Wrist extension
C7	Elbow extension, wrist flexion
C8	Thumb extension
T1	Finger abduction

Therefore, it is important to query patients about the demands of their occupation, and develop a plan of care that incorporates their specific ergonomic requirements.

Respiration Assessment

Improper breathing patterns may lead to increased use of secondary respiratory muscles, such as the sternocleidomastoid, and serratus anterior.[54] These muscles can also be taut in patients with deep cervical flexor weakness.[54] Therefore, assessment of respiration is relevant in patients with cervical radiculopathy. If the exam is abnormal, the patient should be educated on how to perform proper diaphragmatic breathing.

Neurological Examination

A neurological examination encompassing manual muscle testing, sensory testing, and deep tendon reflexes of the upper quadrant, as well as pathological reflexes, should be performed in the presence of suspected cervical radiculopathy.

Strength Testing for Neurologic Weakness

Since cervical radiculopathy involves compression of the nerve roots, weakness can occur specific to the musculature innervated by the compressed root. Motor loss in a myotomal pattern typically occurs with soft disk herniations,[34] therefore, strength testing is required. Although nerve root compression can lead to muscle weakness in a segmental distribution, this does not always happen because of the mixed innervation of terminal branches off the cervicobrachial plexus.[14]

Reflex Testing

Reflex testing (Fig. 9) should be performed with the patient in supine or sitting. Table 1 describes the spinal levels associated with each deep tendon reflex. If deep tendon reflexes are difficult to elicit, the patient can squeeze their knees together to facilitate a response.[55] People with cervical radiculopathy may demonstrate a hypoactive deep tendon reflex at the affected spinal level.

Sensory Testing

Sensory testing should be performed to identify if the patient exhibits afferent abnormalities. Testing should include exteroceptive (e.g. tactile, pain, temperature, and

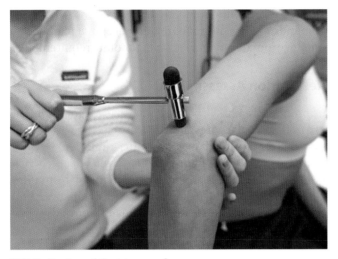

FIG. 9: Testing of the triceps reflex

sensory perversions), proprioceptive sensation (e.g. joint position sense, vibratory sense, kinesthesia), and cortical sensory functions (e.g. stereognosis, graphesthesia, two-point discrimination, touch localization, double simultaneous stimulation).[56] This is typically done in a randomized order from distal to proximal with the patient's eyes closed.[55] It is not necessary to test each dermatome (Fig. 10) unless sensory loss is noted. If that is the case, the specific boundaries and type of sensory loss should be identified.[55] Table 1 describes the dermatomal distribution of each respective spinal nerve.

Mobility Examination

James Cyriax was the first person to describe selective tissue tension testing as a means of determining the

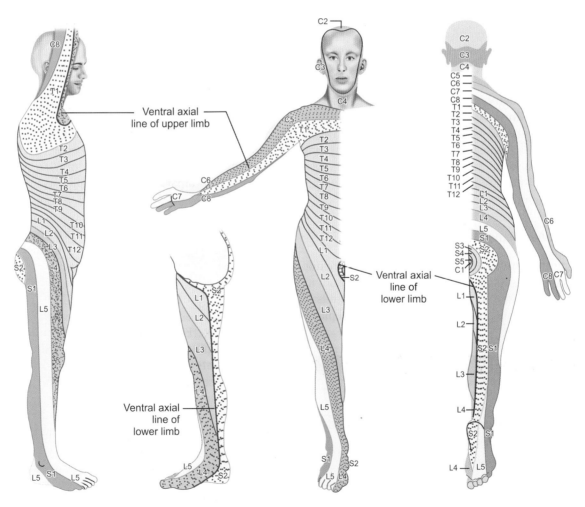

FIG. 10: Dermatome map
(Source: Reprinted from the Atlas of Anatomy by John Charles Boileau Grant via Wikimedia Commons.)

source of pain.[57] Physical therapists are uniquely qualified professionals to perform these manipulative techniques because of their training.[25] Based on information gathered from the movement examination and palpation, the practitioner can determine if the source of the pain is inert or contractile tissue. Inert tissues include the joint capsule, ligaments, and cartilage; while contractile tissues are comprised of musculature and its tendinous attachments. Typically, injured contractile tissue is painful during active contraction and passive elongation, whereas inert tissue usually is painful during passive elongation alone.[57] While often clinically useful, selective tissue testing was devised from clinical observations and not with supportive evidence.[58] As a result, these rules cannot be generally applied to all patients.

First, the physical therapist should have the patient move actively to measure the quantity and quality of motion. If the patient reports pain, the practitioner should determine the intensity of the pain, the amount of motion, as well as if it represents the patient's chief complaint. If the pain is acute, the practitioner may choose to defer further testing to prevent symptom exacerbation. If the motion is less reactive or painless, the practitioner should apply passive overpressure to determine if tissue elongation is provocative, as pictured in Figures 11 to 13. The practitioner should query the patient about the severity of their symptoms at the end range of the available passive range of motion (ROM). While applying overpressure, the practitioner should assess the quality and quantity of motion as well as end feel. If pain occurs during passive mobility testing only, the source of the pain is most likely noncontractile tissue. If pain occurs

with active contraction and passive elongation, it is more likely to be a contractile dysfunction.[56] Cervical motions to be tested include flexion, extension, rotation, and lateral flexion. Depending on the location of the patient's symptoms, the practitioner should also include upper cervical flexion and extension as well as thoracic flexion, extension, rotation, and lateral flexion.

Combined movements were first described by Brian Edwards.[59] The quadrant test, which consists of cervical extension, ipsilateral side-bending and ipsilateral rotation, is an example.[46] Movement in multiple planes may be necessary to reproduce the patient's symptoms when single-plane movements are not effective. Additionally, repeated movements at end-range may be necessary

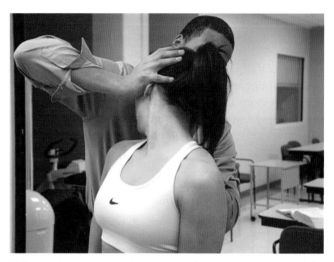

FIG. 12: Passive cervical rotation with overpressure applied by the clinician

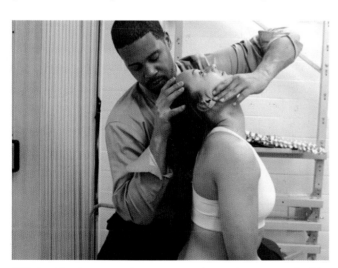

FIG. 11: Passive cervical extension with overpressure applied by the clinician

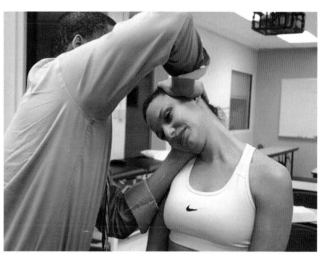

FIG. 13: Passive cervical lateral flexion with overpressure applied by the clinician

to reproduce the patient's symptoms, as described by Robin McKenzie. The patient should be queried to determine if their symptoms centralize, peripheralize, or are eliminated. The position that centralizes, reduces, or eliminates their chief complaint symptom is termed the direction of preference.[31,32] This concept will be further explored in the *treatment* section of this chapter.

Segmental Mobility

Prior to the testing joint accessory mobility, the vertebral artery test should be performed, as described in the *special tests* section. Following active and passive mobility testing, accessory mobility of each respective joint in the cervical spine should take place to localize the source of the pain. During a cervical spine evaluation, the practitioner should begin spring testing at the second cervical (C2) spinous process and proceed segmentally to the fourth thoracic spinous process (T4), secondary to the possibility of referral into the cervical spine.[40,41,46,60] Joint accessory mobility testing should be performed to determine the quantity and quality of mobility that occurs at each specific spinal segment. If pain is not reproduced, the level that is tested can be cleared as not being the cause of the comparable sign.[46,60] The clinician should note the stiffness of that particular level and then proceed to the inferior segment. Some studies have shown that for manual therapists, pain is a more reliable factor than stiffness to interpret during the assessment,[61-64] although intra-rater reliability was higher than inter-rater reliability for segmental mobility.[62] Once spring testing has been completed on the spinous process, the practitioner should perform unilateral posteroanterior (PA) along the zygapophyseal joint or articular pillar.[46] The clinician should assess for quality and quantity of movement as well as pain. This information should be synthesized with the result of pain-producing positions during gross mobility assessment to determine the source of the patient's chief complaint.

Jull et al. found that a highly trained manual therapist was able to accurately diagnose the level of the symptomatic cervical zygapophyseal joint utilizing spring testing with 100% specificity and sensitivity when compared to diagnostic blocks utilizing radiographs. However, the authors concluded more studies were needed to determine the inter-rater reliability, since the study only included one manual therapist.[65] King et al. performed a larger version of the previous study including 173 patients that found that the sensitivity was 89% and 47% specificity amongst practitioners identifying

the dysfunctional segment via manual examination.[65] Furthermore, Rey-Eiriz found a high sensitivity and low specificity for spring testing at the mid-cervical spine. They also concluded that PA glides of the cervical spine were as good as dynamic radiographic imaging for the assessment of hypomobility of the mid-cervical spine.[66]

Cervical Strength and Endurance Testing

Resisted isometric testing should be performed on the cervical flexors, extensors, rotators, and lateral flexors. In addition, it has been shown that poor cervical and scapular stabilization, including weakness of the middle and lower trapezius, can lead to a forward head and thoracic kyphosis.[50,51] Therefore the deep neck flexors, cervical extensors, and scapular stabilizers should be tested.

To test the deep cervical flexors, the examiner instructs the patient to perform a craniovertebral head nod, and to lift their head approximately an inch off the pillow, holding the position as pictured in Figure 14. Domenech et al. identified a mean hold time of 39 seconds for healthy men, and 29 seconds for healthy women.[67] The quality of muscle contraction is assessed to ensure that the patient is not compensating with other musculature.

To test the cervical extensors, the patient is pre-positioned in prone (Fig. 15). The patient is asked to retract their neck while maintaining neutral. The clinician assesses the quality of muscle contraction to ensure that the patient is not compensating with other musculature.

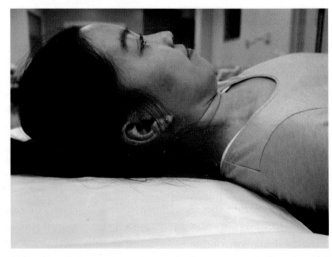

FIG. 14: Endurance testing of deep cervical flexors and strengthening position for the deep neck cervical flexors

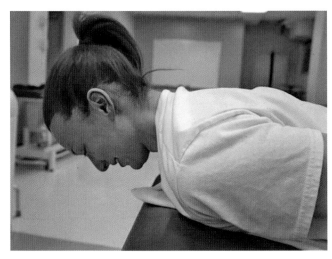

FIG. 15: Endurance testing of deep cervical extensors and strengthening position for the deep neck cervical extensors performed in prone

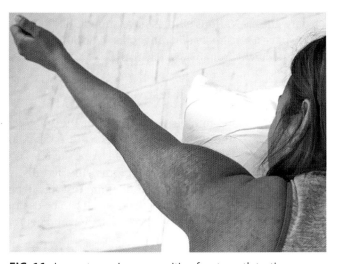

FIG. 16: Lower trapezius pre-position for strength testing

To perform testing of the lower trapezius, the patient should lie in prone with the arm placed diagonally overhead with the humerus parallel to the fibers of the tested muscle as described by Kendall (Fig. 16).[51] The clinician should apply a posterior to anterior force on the forearm.

To perform testing of the scapular retractors, the patient should lie in prone with the arm abducted to 90°. To bias the middle trapezius, the patient will externally rotate the shoulder to cause upward rotation of the scapula. To bias the rhomboid major and minor, the patient will medially rotate the shoulder to create downward rotation of the scapula. The clinician will apply a posterior to anterior force on the forearm.[51]

The ever-popular supine method of testing the scapular protractors, rarely identifies weakness. To perform testing of the serratus anterior, the preferred method by Kendall requires the patient to sit. While in sitting, the patient assumes a position of 120–130° of shoulder flexion in slight internal rotation. The clinician applies a downward force in the direction of extension as well as medial rotation of the scapula.[51]

If weakness is evident in any of the strength testing, the test position may be used to perform remedial strengthening exercises.

Special Tests

Provocative tests and orthopedic maneuvers increase the practitioner's ability to analyze information and make a proper diagnosis.

Sensitivity is the ability of a test to identify a true positive. When a test that is sensitive is negative, it allows the practitioner greater certainty that a disorder may be ruled out. In contrast, specificity is the ability of a test to identify a true negative. When a test that is specific is positive, the practitioner can rule in the specific disorder with greater confidence. Although some tests are more sensitive or specific than others, the ability to make a proper diagnosis is improved by clustering multiple tests as opposed to using the results of a single test. A study conducted to identify a clinical prediction rule for the diagnosis of cervical radiculopathy identified the following parameters: positive upper limb tension test, ipsilateral cervical rotation ROM less than 60°, a positive distraction test, and positive Spurling's test. When three and four of the four criteria were present, there was 94% and 99% specificity. There was low sensitivity, however.[68]

Orthopedic maneuvers used in the diagnosis of cervical radiculopathy validated by research include the following:

Vertebral Artery Testing[69]

Prior to the performance of manual therapy examination and treatment, the vertebrobasilar insufficiency (VBI) should be assessed for all patients who will be placed at end range cervical motion. If the patient reports symptoms (e.g. dizziness, diplopia, dysarthria, dysphagia, drop attacks and nystagmus) that clearly implicate VBI, special testing should not be performed, and the patient should be referred for further medical evaluation secondary to the stress placed upon the vertebral artery during testing.

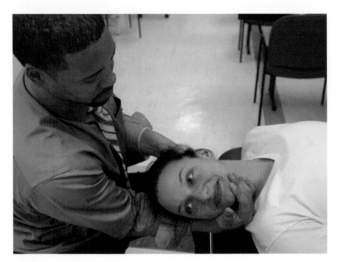

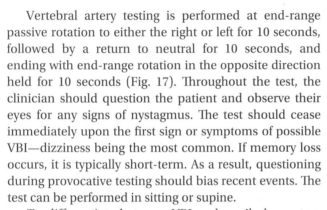

FIG. 17: Vertebral artery testing

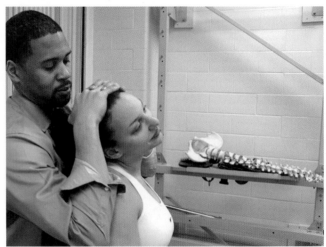

FIG. 18: The Spurling test

Vertebral artery testing is performed at end-range passive rotation to either the right or left for 10 seconds, followed by a return to neutral for 10 seconds, and ending with end-range rotation in the opposite direction held for 10 seconds (Fig. 17). Throughout the test, the clinician should question the patient and observe their eyes for any signs of nystagmus. The test should cease immediately upon the first sign or symptoms of possible VBI—dizziness being the most common. If memory loss occurs, it is typically short-term. As a result, questioning during provocative testing should bias recent events. The test can be performed in sitting or supine.

To differentiate between VBI and vestibular system dysfunction, the therapist can perform the neck torsion test. The test requires that the therapist stabilize the patient's head and have the patient rotate their body in both directions. As the test stabilizes the vestibular system, if there is dizziness with axial rotation, the patient would most likely have a cervicogenic dizziness.[70]

The Spurling Test (Fig. 18)

The Spurling test, which compresses the intervertebral foramen, has been described numerous ways in multiple sources.[71-75] The Spurling test is performed by placing the patient's neck in end-range extension, followed by performing lateral flexion to the involved side. If the patient does not have pain, the clinician should apply a downward compressive force to further sensitize the anatomical structures. This method of performing the Spurling test was suggested by Anekstein et al.[72] A positive test is the reproduction of the subject's chief complaint pain, which is typically neck and/or arm pain or paresthesia. Various studies have shown the Spurling test to have a sensitivity that ranges between 30% and 50% and a specificity from 85% to 93%.[72-74]

The Shoulder Abduction Test

The patient begins in a seated position in the *shoulder abduction test*. The examiner then asks the patient to place the involved hand on their head. A positive test is a reduction or elimination of symptoms. The sensitivity and specificity of the Shoulder Abduction Test has been reported as 17% and 92%, respectively.[76,77] It can be useful in diagnosing patients with cervical herniation and neural root tension.

Upper Limb Tension Tests (Figs 19 and 20)

Nerve function can be impaired by restrictions imposed by surrounding anatomical structures. Butler, Elvey and Maitland were pioneers of current understanding of the physiology and function of the nervous system. Butler identified "tension points", or anatomical landmarks that are more susceptible to neural tension to include tunnels (e.g. cubital tunnel), sites of nervous system branching (e.g. the brachial plexus), and sites where the nervous system is relatively fixed (e.g. C6, T6, and L4).[73,74,76]

During assessment of neurodynamic mobility, the practitioner should observe and palpate for atrophy and increased tone of the musculature innervated by the affected nerve root. As a result of restricted neural dynamics and/or compression, myotomal weakness and

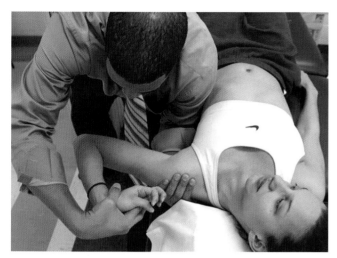

FIG. 19: Performance of upper limb tension test 3 (ulnar nerve)[71,78,79]

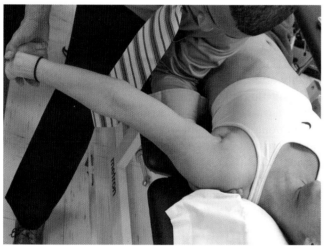

FIG. 20: Performance of upper limb tension test 1 (median nerve)[71,78,79]

TABLE 6: Upper limb tension tests[71,78,79]

Upper limb tension test 1 (median nerve bias)
- Scapular depression coupled with shoulder abduction to 110°, external rotation, and extension
- Elbow extension and supination
- Wrist extension
- Finger extension
- Contralateral cervical side-bending

Upper limb tension test 2a (median nerve bias)
- Scapular depression coupled with shoulder abduction to 10 degrees and external rotation
- Elbow extension and supination
- Wrist extension
- Finger extension
- Contralateral side-bending

Upper limb tension test 2b (radial nerve bias)
- Scapular depression coupled with shoulder abduction to 10° and internal rotation
- Elbow extension and pronation
- Wrist flexion and ulnar deviation
- Finger flexion
- Contralateral cervical side-bending

Upper limb tension test 3 (ulnar nerve bias)
- Scapular depression coupled with shoulder abduction to 90° and external rotation
- Elbow flexion and supination
- Wrist extension and radial deviation
- Finger extension
- Contralateral side-bending

restricted ROM can occur. It is important to note that Butler defined a positive finding as: demonstrating the patient's chief complaint pain; structural differentiation, or movement at a proximal location alters symptoms; and the patient's symptoms are different between the involved and uninvolved extremity.[78-80] However, it is common for healthy individuals to report symptoms, which include pain and paresthesias.[81]

The upper limb tension tests (ULTTs) described in Table 6 place additional tension on the median, radial, and ulnar nerves, respectively. ULTT1, which biases the median nerve, was found to have 97% sensitivity and 22% specificity.[68] Due to the sensitivity of the nervous system, the clinician must be extremely cautious when performing ULTTs. If the patient demonstrates chief complaint symptoms prior to performing movements at all joints, the clinician should instruct the patient to desensitize the movement proximally.

Cervical Distraction Test (Fig. 21)

The cervical distraction test can be performed in supine or sitting. When the patient is lying in supine, the practitioner should place one hand under the chin while the other hand is under the occiput. This movement is thought to decompress the cervical spine. Standing in a straddle position, the clinician should provide a gentle distraction force by leaning from their forward leg to the backward leg. A positive test is a decrease in or elimination of the patient's chief complaint symptoms. The cervical distraction test has a sensitivity of 44% sensitivity and specificity of 85–90%.[68,78]

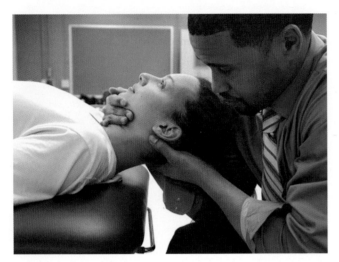

FIG. 21: Cervical distraction test

Tinel's Test

The sensitivity of peripheral nerves can be examined via tapping the nerve in areas where it is more superficial. Common sites of entrapment for the median, radial, and ulnar nerves can be found in Table 4.

Palpation

Palpation should be performed at the end of the examination.[57] The neck should be visualized for any skin abnormalities, such as surgical scars. Bony structures of importance that should be identified include the occiput, mastoid process, superior nuchal line, and spinous processes and articular pillars of each respective segment.[78] Soft tissue palpation should include the sternocleidomastoid, trapezius, suboccipital, scalenes, erector spinae, multifidus and any other structures the clinician feels may be involved in the disorder.[82] Musculature should be palpated in its entirety from the proximal to distal attachment.[51] Trigger points are found in the musculature of people with cervical radiculopathy.[83,84] The clinician should note areas of asymmetry, increased tone, or tenderness. Palpation has been found to demonstrate a low reliability in the spine.[62]

Following the examination, the physical therapist must analyze the information obtained and diagnose the patient. In addition to determining the pathological diagnosis, the physical therapist will employ the data garnered from the examination to develop short- and long-term goals that incorporate the patient's needs and are function-based.

Diagnostic Imaging and Electrodiagnostic Tests

Often, patients who are diagnosed with cervical radiculopathy are treated by a multidisciplinary team, not limited to family practice, internal medicine, orthopedic, rheumatologic, neurologic, pain management physicians, neurosurgeons and physical therapists. These other providers may use imaging studies and diagnostic tests that can enhance the clinician's understanding of the underlying pathology and help to guide intervention.

Imaging

A plain radiograph is usually one of the first imaging studies completed.[14] Anteroposterior and lateral views are useful to detect the presence of degenerative changes, such as disk desiccation, osteophytic formation within the intervertebral foramen and vertebral bodies, as well as the overall alignment.[14,85] Radiographs have low sensitivity for identifying disk herniation. Flexion and extension X-rays (Fig. 22) can provide the clinician with insight into quality and quantity of mobility in the cervical spine.[14] Utilizing this information, the health care practitioner can determine if instability exists at a particular segment. Limitations of X-ray include poor inter-rater reliability and increased rate of diagnostic errors.[14] Computerized tomography (CT) scans are useful in visualizing the relationship between bony structures and the spinal canal and intervertebral foramen. CT scans are the gold standard in evaluating foraminal compression.[86] X-ray and CT scans can be utilized with contrast, also known

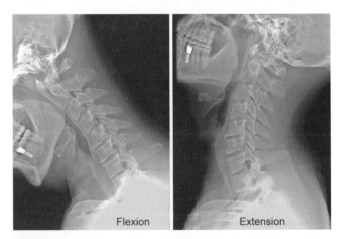

Flexion   Extension

FIG. 22: Flexion-extension cervical radiograph with degenerative changes at C5–6, but no evidence of instability

Source: Wikimedia Commons via Creative Commons Attribution-Share Alike 3.0 Unported.

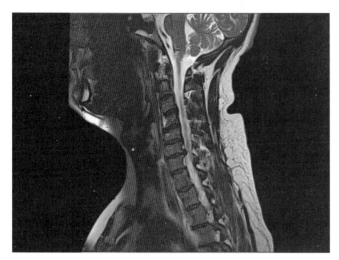

FIG. 23: Cervical magnetic resonance image with C6–7 herniated disk

Source: From Wikimedia Commons via Creative Commons Attribution-Share Alike 3.0 Unported.

as myelography, to improve visualization of the cervical spine (Fig. 23).[14]

Typically, a magnetic resonance imaging (MRI) is next diagnostic imaging ordered, after plain X-rays, due to its ability to identify soft tissue structures, including the spinal cord and intervertebral disks. MRI is the gold standard in the diagnosis of cervical radiculopathy.[86-88] However, Matsumoto et al. cautioned against using imaging alone for diagnosis, as their study found that 86–89% of asymptomatic subjects over 60 had cervical disk degenerative disease according to MRI findings.[88] In addition, Borenstein et al. found that the severity of a patient's condition could not be extracted from the stage and appearance of a lumbar disk herniation on the MRI.[89] While the latter study was not performed on the cervical spine, one can deduce the MRI results of the spine should never be used in isolation to diagnose the anatomical location and source of the patient's symptoms. To the contrary, this information should only provide additional information to be analyzed with other components of the physical examination. One study showed that although study participants had the presence of adolescent cervical disk degeneration on MRI, it could not be used to predict head and/or neck pain as adults.[90]

Electrodiagnostics

Electromyography (EMG) is a neurophysiologic test used to measure the electrical activity of skeletal muscle. This test can be performed intramuscularly via needle insertion or at the surface level through a superficial electrode. EMG is useful in detecting a myotomal pattern of weakness. However, it may not be as useful in early radiculopathies, because they usually present with greater sensory than motor dysfunction. The American Association for Neuromuscular and Electrodiagnostic Medicine found EMG to have only moderate diagnostic sensitivity in the diagnosis of cervical radiculopathy.[86]

Nerve conduction velocity (NCV) is an electro-diagnostic test used to measure the conduction of an electrical impulse through a specific nerve. Nerve damage can be detected based on abnormal findings with this test. Sensitivity and specificity are higher in the testing of proximal nerves compared to distal nerves. Sensory parameters are also less sensitive but more specific in comparison to motor parameters. NCV is also useful in ruling out peripheral nerve entrapment and other disorders.[91]

When CT is combined with myelography, it is 92% accurate in the diagnosis of the level and type of disease(s) involved in cervical radiculopathy.[82] However myelography alone was not as specific as MRI and CT. Although CT scans have been shown to be superior to MRI in assessment of the osteology, they too, have limitations, which include poor visualization of soft tissue structures and side-effects and risk due to its exposure to radiation.[14,85,87] In comparison, the sensitivity of MRI in preoperative patients with cervical radiculopathy is significantly higher than neurophysiologic tests (i.e. EMG and NCV tests); 93% compared to 42%. The authors concluded that neurophysiologic studies are not necessary to diagnose patients with cervical radiculopathy. They recommended that resources would be better allocated by performance of a sound clinical examination and correlating this with positive MRI findings.[92]

Often, health care practitioners will use radiographs, MRI, EMG, NCV and other studies to diagnosis patients but these tests should only be used to confirm or refute the clinician's hypothesis. The physical examination is the most important component needed to make the proper diagnosis.

■ PHYSICAL THERAPY TREATMENT

The physical therapy treatment of patients with cervical radiculopathy should be tailored to the individual needs of each patient. The plan of care can be developed based on the evaluation findings with the primary goal of improving the patient's chief complaint and overall function. For example, if the patient demonstrates chief complaint pain with closing of the right intervertebral foramen (i.e. extension, right rotation, and right lateral flexion) of the cervical spine, the plan of care should be tailored to increase those respective ranges. However, it may be necessary to avoid those positions early in the treatment secondary to the patient's irritability. In the acute stage of this case example, it may be beneficial to instruct the patient to perform movements that involve flexion, left rotation, and left lateral flexion to decompress the right cervical nerve root. As a result, prior to initiating treatment, the clinician must determine the patient's respective level of acuity. Treatment selection should be based on the patient's reproduction of pain during the examination.[39,46,61-64]

Patients with inflammatory conditions or central sensitization are often under medical management, taking medications such as nonsteroidal anti-inflammatory drugs (NSAIDs). From a physical therapy perspective, modalities can also be utilized to decrease pain and inflammation. These treatment interventions include, but should not be limited to: cold therapy, ultrasound, electrical stimulation, and laser therapy. Pain may also be decreased through the performance of desensitization techniques, such as the application of various textures along the affected dermatome. Patients with pain that is driven by inflammation or sensitization should also perform gentle pain-free ROM exercises to maintain range. Additionally, gentle joint mobilizations short of resistance, may help to decrease pain.

Patients with cervical radiculopathy who present with mechanical dysfunction often present with underlying impairments such as restricted mobility, weakness, sensory loss, and/or postural dysfunction, which result in functional limitations and disability.

There are a variety of well-established treatment techniques to improve the patient's impairments, which in turn impact the patient's function, including manual therapy, therapeutic exercise, and neuromuscular re-education.

Manual Therapy Treatment

Manual therapy techniques for patients with cervical radiculopathy can be utilized to decompress the nerve root, thereby improving their chief complaint symptoms, musculoskeletal impairments, functional limitations, and disability. The field of physical therapy has contributed to manual therapy via the tireless efforts of many clinicians, including Stanley Paris and Geoffrey Maitland.[25]

Often examination techniques, which reproduce or eliminate the patient's chief complaint, can be utilized as treatment interventions. After performing treatment interventions, including manual therapy techniques, the movement that recreated the patient's chief complaint should be reassessed for improvement. If the technique is not improving the patient's comparable sign, another intervention should be selected.[39,46] If the technique is effective, the manual therapy technique should be followed by a ROM or strengthening exercise to help maintain the recent gains. Various manual therapy techniques have been shown to be efficacious and are outlined in detail below.

Cervical Traction[39,46,52]

Manual distraction

Cervical distraction or traction is a generalized examination and intervention technique used to decompress the cervical spine. Often, manual cervical distraction will alleviate the patient's symptoms. Initially, cervical distraction can be employed in a neutral position, as pictured in Figure 21. Just enough force is applied to eliminate or reduce the patient's symptoms. This technique should be applied for approximately 1 minute.[46] As the patient's symptoms and mobility improve, the distractive force can be employed at end of the available ROM to decompress the nerve root in a provocative position. For example, if the patient has their chief complaint pain at 45° of right cervical rotation, the physical therapist may utilize traction at, or just short of, this barrier. Cervical distraction may also be employed using a towel to minimize the effect on the therapist's hands (Fig. 24). If the patient responds well to manual cervical distraction, mechanical cervical traction may be warranted.

Mechanical traction

Mechanical cervical traction is thought to improve neck pain and functional limitations by decompressing the cervical spine, affecting various structures including the vertebral body, facet joints, joint capsule, muscles, and ligaments.

Mechanical cervical traction is typically employed with the patient in supine. Various parameters, including angle of application, duration, frequency and the amount of the force, can be altered. One study that explored the amount of vertebral compression and separation created by mechanical traction suggests that 30 pounds of traction at 15° resulted in the greatest amount of

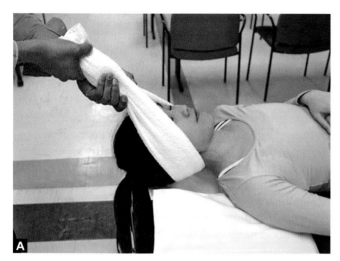 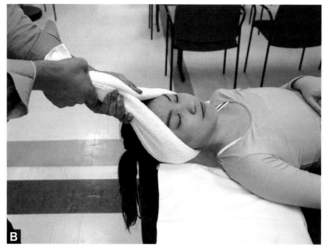

FIGS 24A AND B: Cervical traction provided with towel—(A) in Neutral; and (B) in Right rotation

anterior and posterior separation.[93] Although the force of pull during cervical traction can be continuous or intermittent, intermittent traction appears to be more effective in decreasing pain and improving disability.[94,95] Furthermore, the length of time and amount of force should be based on the patient's stage of irritability.[94] Typically, patients with acute conditions respond better to lesser duration and force while those with decreased reactivity tolerate greater force and treatment time. A force between 20 pounds and 45 pounds is necessary to distract the cervical spine.[7,93,94] Treatment time varies between 5 minutes and 10 minutes for patients with a herniated nucleus pulposus and 10–20 minutes for other treatment conditions.[52] Caution should be taken during initial trials and in patients with greater irritability.[7,93,94]

Although traction is widely used in clinical practice, its efficacy has been questioned.[96,97] Others have supported the benefits of cervical traction.[94,95,98,99] The effects of traction are greater when combined with other interventions.[94,98,99] A clinical prediction rule for intermittent cervical traction and exercise was initiated with factors that include—peripheralization with C4 through C7 mobility testing; positive shoulder abduction test; age more than or equal to 55 years; positive ULTT; and positive neck distraction test. Study results indicate a 79.2% and 94.8% post-test probability if patients had three and four of the five variables.[95]

Muscle Energy Technique

The muscle energy technique (MET) was developed as a safe and effective alternative to joint manipulation for the treatment of somatic dysfunction. By placing the joint at its restrictive barrier in three dimensions and eliciting an isometric or isotonic muscle contraction, MET can restore normal neurophysiological function at the respective joint. Through this technique, a number of dysfunctions—restricted ROM and muscle length, increased muscle tone, strength deficits, and improper lymphatic and venous pump activity to decrease fluid—can be restored.[100-102] Reciprocal and/or autogenic inhibition can be employed to restore normal joint mechanics (similar to proprioceptive neuromuscular facilitation techniques, described later). Assessment is typically performed by palpating the transverse processes in neutral, flexion, and extension to identify the restriction.[52,100-103] Muscle energy techniques can be classified as either direct or indirect. During the direct technique, the patient is placed at the restrictive barrier and the muscle contraction is elicited in the direction of the barrier. Direct MET utilizes reciprocal inhibition of the agonist muscle to promote relaxation of the antagonist. The theoretical mechanism of direct MET is through the muscle spindle. With indirect MET, the patient is placed at the restrictive barrier and the practitioner resists motion in the direction away from the barrier. Indirect MET employs autogenic inhibition is achieved through contraction of the antagonist muscle and leads to relaxation of that muscle group.[101] Indirect techniques are thought to influence the Golgi tendon organ or muscle spindles.[100-102] Other researchers think that MET influences the viscoelastic properties of musculature. Initially, MET techniques were utilized at the pelvis but over time have been applied to other joints, including the cervical spine.[102]

Following a comprehensive cervical evaluation, including palpation of the transverse processes of the cervical spine in neutral, flexion, and extension to determine the orientation of the dysfunctional vertebral segment, the practitioner should identify the restricted motions in the frontal, sagittal, and transverse plane.[52] For example, a patient who may be suffering from a left cervical facet lock (i.e. the left cervical facet will not open) may be restricted in cervical flexion, right rotation, and right side-bend. Once the restricted motions are identified, the patient should be positioned at those barriers, just shy of pain. The practitioner should then resist motion by creating a submaximal contraction in the specific direction (i.e. direct or indirect) for at least 6 seconds. The procedure should be repeated three times.[52]

The literature shows some variability in the success of MET in the treatment of neck pain. Burns et al. found that MET increased cervical ROM in asymptomatic subjects in comparison to the control group.[104] Additionally, Mahajan et al. found that MET was more effective than static stretching in increasing active ROM and decreasing pain in patients with subacute neck pain.[105] Still, only 46% of patients who received MET demonstrated improvement in a study performed by Cleland et al.[98] Although some results appear promising, further studies are needed to fully substantiate MET in the treatment of patients with cervical radiculopathy.

Neurodynamic Treatment

Neurodynamic treatment involves improving mobility and vascularization of the nerve root via myofascial release of the nerve at superficial tunnels.[78-80] Neural tissue management, joint mobilization of the affected joint segment, along with a host of other techniques can be utilized to improve neurodynamics.[46,60,78-80] For instance, the median nerve is composed of the nerve roots C5 through T1. The brachial plexus is susceptible to compression between the anterior and middle scalenes, as well as beneath the pectoralis minor musculature. Furthermore, the median nerve can be compressed along the medial epicondyle below the pronator teres and/or flexor carpi radialis musculature. In addition, the median nerve is often compressed as it passes through the carpal tunnel.[44] Possible treatment for median nerve tension might involve joint mobilization of the hypomobile cervical spine, myofascial release of the musculature involved, as well as neurodynamic techniques.[46,60,78-80]

When performing neurodynamic mobilizations, the practitioner should be cautious due the irritability of neural tissue. During testing, the clinician should place the minimal amount of tension on the nervous system to reproduce the patient's chief complaint. Table 6 lists the positions involved in ULTT1 that place maximal tension on the median nerve. During neurodynamic treatment, the physical therapist should take care not to simultaneously place tension on the peripheral nervous system proximally and distally. The patient may benefit from nerve gliding techniques where either contralateral flexion of the cervical spine or provocative upper extremity positions are performed in an alternating fashion.[78-80] If the clinician is not prudent, the patient could experience a significant increase in symptoms. In addition, the patient's symptoms should not be reproduced during intervention unless the clinician is cautiously performing a tensile loading technique.

A systemic review on the effectiveness of neurodynamic mobilization concluded that there is minimal evidence to support the use of specific techniques that included active nerve and flexor tendon gliding exercises for median nerve involvement, cervical contralateral glides (described later in this chapter), and ULTT 2b mobilization. Therefore, further studies are needed.[106]

Joint Mobilization

Joint mobilizations and manipulations involve performing passive movements to the joint capsule to achieve full, painless ROM. Joint mobilizations and manipulations are utilized to restore the arthrokinematics necessary to permit normal movement to occur. They also can be utilized to decrease pain via neurophysiological effects.[15,46,60,71,107-113] Spinal manipulation, involving high-velocity low amplitude thrusts and mobilizations, has been shown to be more effective than medications, including NSAID drugs, acetaminophen, or both, in the treatment of acute and subacute neck pain.[114,115] PA glides performed at C5 were shown to increase cervical lordosis and affect multiple segments, not just the targeted one. Most segments moved into extension while some moved into flexion.[116]

TABLE 7: Maitland joint mobilization grading scale[46,60]

Grades	Description
I	Small amplitude mobilization short of resistance
II	Large amplitude mobilization short of resistance
III	Large amplitude mobilization at 50% of R1-R2
IV	Small amplitude mobilization at 50% of R1-R2
V	High velocity thrust at end of resistance

Grading scales have been proposed and employed by various practitioners. The Maitland scale is defined in Table 7. Once the specific segment(s) and dysfunctional movement patterns have been identified during examination, the physical therapist must decide which techniques to employ to restore motion or decrease pain. PA mobilizations should not be prescribed to increase a specific anatomic motion, such as extension, rather they should be employed to increase generalized mobility of the spine. By utilizing these techniques in specific motions, or combined motions, the mobilizations are more specific to the targeted movements.[52] For example, performing a central PA on the C7 spinous process with the cervical spine in extension most likely increases that specific motion.

Numerous studies have found that joint mobilization and manipulation, including cervical lateral glides in upper limb neurodynamic position, cervical and thoracic spine manipulation, cervical and thoracic PA mobilizations, are effective.[98,106-123] Some suggest that manipulation is more effective than mobilization.[119] Other authors have concluded that cervical spine mobilization and manipulation had greater efficacy in comparison to thoracic spine mobilization and manipulation in the treatment of neck pain, although both were useful.[120,121] In conclusion, there is a large body of evidence to support the effectiveness of cervical and thoracic mobilization and manipulation in the treatment of mechanical neck pain.[98,106-123] A variety of joint mobilization and manipulation techniques described in detail follow. For each application, the practitioner should identify the resistance or pain barrier prior to initiating the maneuver. Based on the clinical findings, the physical therapist would then determine what grade is most appropriate. The practitioner should always err on the side of caution when performing joint mobilizations and manipulations.

Central posteroanterior glide[46,52,60]

The manual therapist positions the patient in prone, then places the thumb, or thumbs, on the spinous process as pictured in Figure 25.

Unilateral posteroanterior glides[46,52,60]

The therapist positions the patient in prone and using the thumb over thumb technique, places their digits on the articular pillar of the targeted segment (Fig. 26). To isolate the articular pillar, the thumb is placed approximately one thumb width laterally from the spinous process.

Unilateral anteroposterior glide[46]

Unilateral anteroposterior glides to the anterior aspect of the transverse process should be approached with care secondary to the vital structures in this region. The physical therapist should inform the patient about the placement of their hands near the throat. The therapist may have to move the sternocleidomastoid medially to palpate the transverse processes. The patient is positioned in supine. Using the thumb over thumb technique, the clinician places both thumbs on the anterior aspect of the transverse process of the targeted segment (Fig. 27).

Closing mobilization and manipulation with rotation bias:[46] The therapist places the metacarpophalangeal joint (MCP) of their second digit on the articular pillar of the inferior segment of the targeted facet joint. The clinician then induces contralateral lateral glide followed by ipsilateral lateral flexion until all the slack in

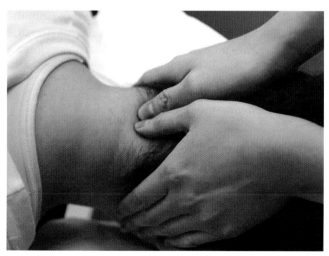

FIG. 25: Central posteroanterior glide performed in prone[46,60]

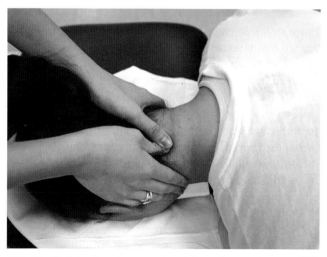

FIG. 26: Unilateral posteroanterior glide performed in prone[46,60]

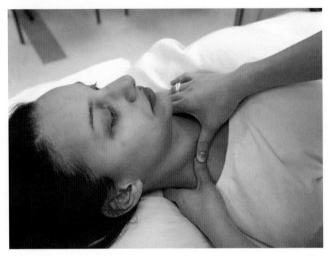

FIG. 27: Unilateral anteroposterior glide performed in supine[46]

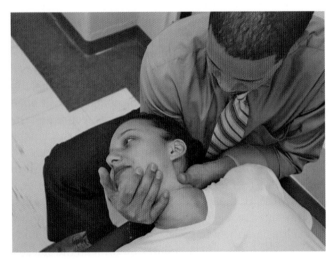

FIG. 28: Closing mobilization and manipulation with rotation bias[46]

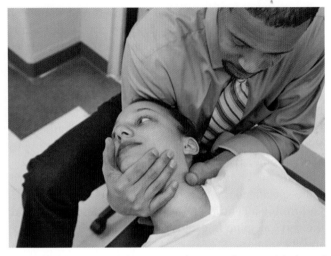

FIG. 29: Closing mobilization and manipulation with lateral flexion bias[46]

Closing mobilization and manipulation with lateral flexion bias[46]

The manual therapist places the MCP joint of the second digit on the articular pillar of the inferior segment of the targeted facet joint. A contralateral lateral glide is followed by ipsilateral lateral flexion until all the slack in the joint has been taken up in the joint capsule. In Figure 29, the clinician demonstrates a right translational force, accompanied by left lateral flexion. End-range range rotation is introduced next, followed by extension or flexion, depending on which portion of the capsule is restricted until the neck feels locked. In the lower cervical spine, typically extension is preferred, which biases the posterior capsule. The patient should be queried for any signs of VBI. If there are none, the mobilization force occurs from the MCP joint of the second digit or a combination of lateral flexion from the hand cradling the head and lateral flexion force from the MCP joint. This mobilization can be used to perform a grade V mobilization when applying a high velocity, low amplitude force.

Cervical retraction mobilization[96]

The therapist holds the head, with the stabilizing hand under the superior nuchal line and uses the first web space to apply a mobilizing force to the chin in a posterior direction. Before employing this technique, the clinician ensures that the patient does not have temporomandibular joint dysfunction or dental complications. If so, the mobilizing force may be applied to the maxilla instead.

the joint has been taken up in the joint capsule. In Figure 28, the clinician demonstrates a right translational force accompanied by left lateral flexion. Approximately 45° of contralateral rotation is then introduced, followed by extension or flexion, depending on which portion of the capsule is restricted, until the neck feels locked. The patient should be queried for any signs of VBI. If there are none, the mobilization force occurs from the MCP joint of the second digit, or a combination of lateral flexion from the hand cradling the head and lateral flexion force from the MCP joint. This mobilization can be used to perform a grade V mobilization when applying a high velocity, low amplitude force. Always obtain patient consent prior to performing Grade V mobilizations.

Cervical side-bending mobilization[52]

The therapist places the MCP joint of their second digit on the articular pillar of the inferior segment of the targeted facet joint. Ipsilateral lateral flexion is performed until all of the slack in the joint has been taken up in the joint capsule. The mobilization force occurs from the MCP joint of the second digit in an inferomedial direction to create lateral flexion. This mobilization can be used to perform a grade V mobilization when applying a high velocity, low amplitude force.

Lateral glide[52]

The clinician should place the MCP joint of second digit of their mobilizing hand on the articular pillar of the superior segment targeted joint. Performing a pure translatory movement, the practitioner glides the head and spine up to the location of the 2nd digits toward the asymptomatic side to decompress the affected nerve root. This is a good introductory technique to use with patients because it typically reduces or eliminates pain.[52] Cervical lateral glide mobilizations with the arm positioned to place tension on the median nerve were shown to effective in reducing subacute neural tension.[80,106,124]

Inferior glide of the first rib[46]

In supine, the therapist places the MCP joint of their mobilizing hand against the medial border of the first rib and applies an inferior directed glide towards the contralateral anterior superior iliac spine as pictured in Figure 30. The clinician must ensure that the force is being placed on the first rib and not the upper trapezius. If the scalenes are taut, the clinician may passively induce ipsilateral side-bend and contralateral rotation to reduce

muscular tension. This technique can also be performed in prone.

Thoracic spine manipulation

With the patient in side-lying and arms placed behind their head (or across their chest, in patients with glenohumeral laxity), the clinician makes a fist with the 3rd through 5th digits, placing the knuckles of the mobilizing hand in the area between spinous process and the transverse process (Fig. 31). The patient is turned onto their back, and their arms are leveraged to induce thoracic extension until the patient is over the mobilization hand (Fig. 32). Thoracic extension biases the upper thoracic spine. The patient is directed to inhale, and during the subsequent exhalation, a high velocity, low amplitude thrust is applied through the arms in a posterior direction.

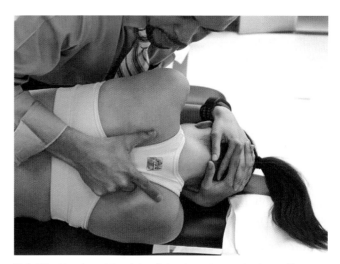

FIG. 31: Hand position (pistol) for thoracic manipulation[46]

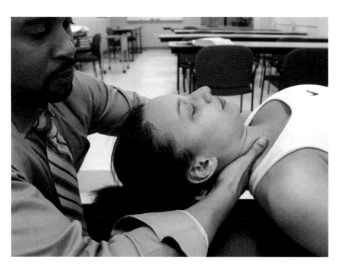

FIG. 30: Inferior glide of the first rib in supine[46]

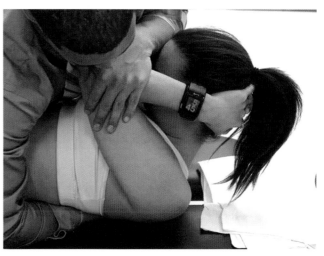

FIG. 32: Final position prior to thoracic manipulation[46]

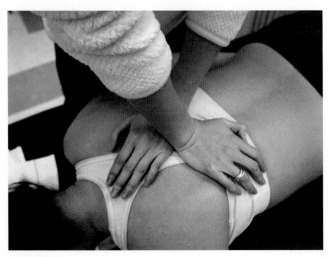

FIG. 33: Thoracic screw mobilization and manipulation in prone[46,52,60]

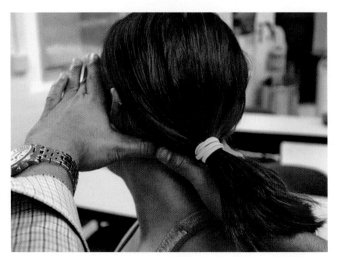

FIG. 34: Sustained natural apophyseal glide (SNAG) on left cervical facet to increase right rotation[125-127]

Thoracic screw mobilization

The therapist places the pisiform of one hand on the targeted aspect of the thoracic spine. Typically, this is performed on the transverse process. The pisiform of the other hand is then placed on the contralateral transverse process of the same segment, as pictured in Figure 33.[46,60] To induce rotation, the therapist places the other hand on the contralateral transverse process of the superior segment.[52] This mobilization can be used to perform a grade V mobilization when applying a high velocity, low amplitude force.

Natural apophyseal and sustained natural apophyseal glides (Fig. 34)

Brian Mulligan devised mobilizations in weight-bearing positions to restore the accessory component of normal joint movement. These pain-free mobilizations, called natural apophyseal glides (NAGs) and sustained natural apophyseal glides (SNAGs), are performed parallel to the plane of the facet joint with the goal of improving the painful movement during examination. The Mulligan techniques also include mobilizations with movement (MWMs), which involves a combination of a spinal accessory mobilization combined with peripheral joint movement. All mobilizations should be pain-free and are typically performed in sitting.[125]

NAGs are passive oscillatory techniques that are most useful in acute inflammatory conditions as well as when treating a stiff segment adjacent to a hypermobile segment.[125] Typically, these mobilizations work well in patients who do not tolerate PA glides performed in prone.[125] NAGs have been shown to be effective in the lower cervical spine.[126] Although SNAGs have been shown to be effective in the reduction of cervicogenic headache, the literature is scarce in their use for the lower cervical spine.[128]

To perform a NAG, the mobilizing thumb is placed on the articular pillar or spinous process of the affected segment. The opposite hand can be used to stabilize the upper segments in the anterior direction. The mobilizing force should be applied in the plane of the facet joint. NAGs are passive oscillatory techniques that are most useful in acute inflammatory conditions. NAGs are not as successful with patients demonstrating a forward head posture with secondary tightness of the suboccipital musculature.[125]

To perform a SNAG, the mobilizing thumb is placed on the articular pillar of the superior segment on the same side as the movement restriction. A sustained mobilizing force is applied along the plane of the dysfunctional facet joint as the patient actively moves in the desired direction, most often in the direction of movement loss. The SNAG should be maintained at end range for a few seconds and released as the patient returns to the initial position. If ROM does not improve, the clinician will apply a superoanterior glide to the superior segment on the opposite side of the movement restriction and repeat the active movement. If the mobility of the patient does not increase, the clinician will then apply superior glide to the spinous process of the superior segment.[129] For example, if a patient was limited with left rotation due to dysfunction of the C5–6 facet joint, the clinician will apply a superoanterior glide on the left articular pillar of C5 as the patient rotates their head to the left. If movement does not improve, the clinician will apply the same directed force to the right articular pillar of C6 as the patient moves to the left. Finally, if this does not improve mobility, the superior glide will be applied to the spinous process of C5.

SNAGs are recommended when symptoms are provoked with movement at a specific vertebral segment. Interventions at other levels besides the painful segment have also been effective.[125] For example, more than 40–45° of rotation occurs at the atlantoaxial joint.[19,85] In a patient with a restriction in rotation with C6 radiculopathy, greater gains may be achieved by treating C1–C2, than C5–C6. Although Mulligan techniques are typically described in a weight-bearing position, they can be performed in nonweight bearing as well.

Trigger Point Manipulation

Myofascial pain syndrome (MPS) is defined as pain that originates from a myofascial trigger point. A myofascial trigger point has two components: (1) a motor impairment, which results in a taut band of skeletal muscle; and (2) a sensory dysfunction, which most commonly creates pain. Trigger points can be local to the site or global. They can also be active, meaning they constantly generate pain, or latent, where they only elicit pain following compression.[130] Although the cause is unknown, it is theorized that a myofascial trigger point results from an increase in electrical activity at the neuromuscular junction, but this has not been confirmed via scientific evidence.[129] Myofascial trigger points are found in patients with cervical radiculopathy. In addition, MPS can mimic cervical radiculopathy.[83,84,130] Myofascial trigger points can be identified via flat or pincer palpation. It is important to reproduce the patient's pain during the examination through palpation. Treatment of a myofascial trigger point involves manipulation of the trigger point via soft tissue manipulation or by local anesthetic injection, or trigger point dry needling (see *Alternative Therapies*), to decrease or eliminate the motor and sensory dysfunction. When pain emanates from deeper structures, manual techniques may not be adequate.[130] Treatment of MPS should also involve postural re-education, ergonomics, manual therapy to increase joint accessory mobility and to alleviate tension due to trigger point. Modalities may also be employed in the presence of inflammation.

Trigger point dry needling

Trigger point dry needling, or intramuscular stimulation, involves inserting a monofilament needle into skeletal musculature until a local twitch response occurs to reduce or eliminate myofascial trigger points. It is theorized that by inserting the needle into the muscle, the trigger point improves via local stretch. This treatment should be performed to all myofascial trigger points of the functional muscle unit.[130] Some muscles that are more frequent in patients with cervical radiculopathy include the levator scapulae, splenius capitus, rhomboid minor and major, upper trapezius, and multifidus.[84] In addition, the teres minor is involved in C8 radiculopathy.[130] In this author's clinical experience, the scalenes, sternocleidomastoid, infraspinatus, supraspinatus, subscapularis, coraco-brachialis, pectoralis major and minor, common wrist flexors and extensors can also either mimic or occur in patients with cervical radiculopathy. A recent meta-analysis found trigger point dry needling superior to sham or placebo for decrease pain secondary to upper quarter myofascial pain syndrome immediately after and four weeks post-treatment.[131] Trigger point dry needling has also been shown to be effective in the treatment of a variety of musculoskeletal conditions.[35] Some contraindications to treatment via trigger point dry needling include vascular disease and local or systemic infections.[132]

Therapeutic Exercise

Therapeutic exercise is utilized to improve function, minimize complications, prevent future impairments, and minimize disability. Therapeutic exercise has been shown to increase ROM, muscular strength and endurance, improve posture, cardiovascular function, and neuromuscular control.[133] Exercises specific to the patient's impairments, functional limitations, and disability identified during the examination should be selected. Sequencing of exercises impacts the efficacy of treatment.[133] For instance, it may be more appropriate to perform stretching following a warm-up exercise on the upper body ergometer versus the start of the treatment session.

Research suggests that exercises performed with manual therapy are effective with patients with cervical radiculopathy.[53,96,98,117,121,122,134,135]

Range of Motion Exercises

Gentle ROM exercises are useful in maintaining or increasing mobility. Gentle mobility exercises without resistance, including neck retraction, extension, flexion, rotation, lateral flexion, and scapular retraction, performed 6–8 times a day as part of a home program was found to be similar to joint mobilization and manipulation in the treatment of acute and subacute neck pain.[115] ROM exercises are more useful during the initial stages of treatment and when patients demonstrate higher levels of irritability.[133] The clinician should instruct the patient to perform these exercises in a pain-free range. In addition, they can be used following other manual therapy techniques to maintain newly gained ROM.

Mechanical Diagnosis and Therapy

Mechanical diagnosis and therapy (MDT), formerly known as the McKenzie approach, utilizes repeated end range movements to determine a patient's direction of preference. The movement examination seeks to increase, reduce, centralize, peripheralize, or eliminate the patient's symptoms. Centralization is the reduction or alleviation of pain from the extremity toward the spine, whereas peripheralization is the movement of pain from the spine into the extremities. According to MDT, the treatment goal is to centralize or eliminate the patient's symptoms. Based on the patient's response to repeated end range movements, patients are classified into one of three categories: postural syndrome, derangement syndrome, or dysfunction syndrome. The ideal treatment involves exercises and mobilizations that bias the direction of preference identified during examination.[31,32]

A case study on the effect of MDT on a patient with left cervical radiculopathy (cervical spine derangement classification) adopted various treatment interventions, including repeated cervical retraction with rotation to the left, with the left arm horizontally adducted to decrease neural tension, resulted in centralization and pain-free function.[136] Other studies have shown the effectiveness of cervical retraction exercises on forward head posture and neck pain.[54,121] In addition, neck retraction decreases tension on cervical nerve roots.[53] Yet, a systematic literature review concluded that there was not enough research to determine the efficacy of MDT in neck pain.[137]

Stretching

Muscle spasm and myofascial trigger points often accompany cervical radiculopathy.[83,84,138] This may lead to restricted muscle length. Although the literature does not support stretching for neck pain, clinical observation by the authors of clinical practice guidelines from the American Physical Therapy Association's orthopedic section suggest that the scalenes, upper trapezius, levator scapulae, pectoralis minor, and pectoralis major often demonstrate decreased flexibility, and muscle length improves with stretching.[121] If decreased mobility is found during examination, flexibility exercises should be prescribed. Stretching can be effective at lengthening shorted tissue, decreasing stiffness, improving ROM, decreasing muscle spasm and decreasing pain.[133]

Cervical Strengthening

Isometric exercises

Isometric exercises can be utilized to maintain or increase strength as well as enhance stability via neuromuscular re-education.[133] They are most useful when movement is painful or weakness is present at a specified area in the patient's ROM.[133] Isometric exercises have been recommended in the treatment of people with cervical spondylosis.[17,139] Because cervical radiculopathy can result from spondylosis, these exercises may be useful in the initial stages of physical therapy treatment.

Isometric exercises can be performed with any movement of the cervical spine. To perform a cervical isometric exercise, the patient or clinician can place their hand on the patient's head and provide a counterforce to the desired direction that clinician wishes to strengthen. For example, to increase cervical lateral flexors isometric strength, the clinician may place their hand on the side of the patient's head. With the patient in a neutral position, the clinician will push the patient in the direction of contralateral lateral flexion while the patient contracts the cervical extensor. Care must be provided not to allow movement to occur. Isometric exercises can be executed at multiple angles as well, since strength gains are specific to the joint angle performed. Multiple-angle isometrics should be carried out every 15–20° throughout the ROM and held for 6 seconds.[133] The patient can provide their own isometric resistance as part of a home exercise program, as pictured in Figure 35. To perform cervical retraction exercises, the patient can hold the head in a neutral position. Exercises can be progressed by adding

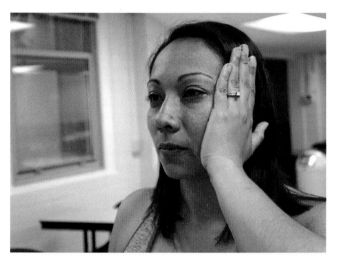

FIG. 35: Isometric cervical lateral flexion exercise

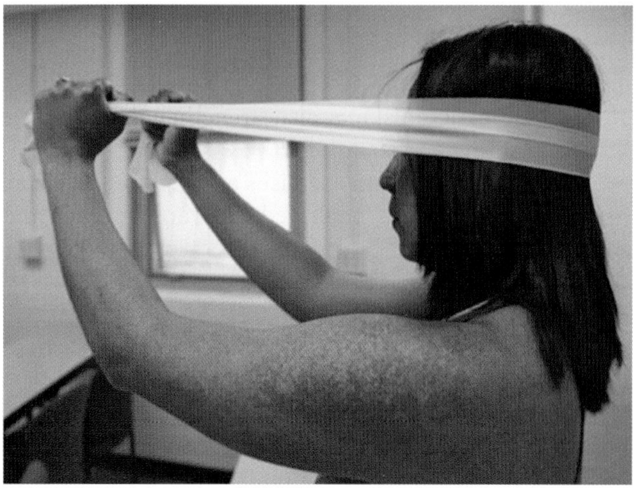

FIG. 36: Resisted neck retraction[54]

resistance, as pictured in Figure 36 or by altering positions (i.e. supine, sitting, and prone).

Stabilization of the Cervical Spine

Strengthening of the deep neck flexors

Numerous studies have found that the deep cervical flexors, which include the longus capitis, longus colli, rectus capitis anterior, and rectus capitus lateralis, play a significant role in the stability of the cervical spine. A study of manual therapy, cervical traction, and craniovertebral head nod in supine found that although the treatments were interdependent, 91% of the patients with cervical radiculopathy displayed reduced pain and improved function.[98] A similar study found there was a significant decrease in pain and increase in the peak-to-peak amplitude following the performance of a home exercise program including craniovertebral head nod in supine in patients with cervical radiculopathy who also exhibited forward head posture.[53] The craniovertebral head nod is an exercise that strengthens the deep cervical flexors, including the longus colli. A high density of muscle spindles have been found in the anterolateral region of the longus colli, and the information provided by these muscle spindles increases the quality of head control and proprioception for head-righting reactions.[140]

To perform the exercise, instruct the patient perform a craniovertebral head nod and hold for 5 seconds (Fig. 14). Observe for compensations, especially excessive firing of the sternocleidomastoid. To progress the exercise, instruct the patient to lift their head about an inch off of

the pillow after performing a craniovertebral head nod and to hold the position for 5 seconds.

Strengthening of the cervical extensors

In the prone position, the patient is instructed to retract their neck while maintaining neutral for 5 seconds (Fig. 15). Alter the sequence, frequency, intensity, and duration to bias increased muscular endurance.[133] This exercise can also be done in varied positions to be more functional or difficult. Stabilization exercises can be progressed by maintaining the cervical extension in other positions, such as side-lying, quadruped, sitting and standing.

Scapular Stabilization

Common exercises performed in studies espousing the benefits of manual therapy in conjunction with exercise were strengthening of the deep neck flexors and scapular musculature, including the scapular retractors, serratus anterior, and lower trapezius. Increasing scapular stability has also been found to improve forward head posture.[54,121] As a result, the testing positions listed in the *clinical examination* section can be utilized as strengthening exercises and progressed with resistance bands, physioballs, and weights. Exercises should be progressed according to the functional demands of the patient with cervical radiculopathy. Therefore, it may be more appropriate to strengthen the scapular retractors in sitting as opposed to prone or side-lying. To facilitate postural re-education, the therapist can increase the frequency, intensity, and duration for the previously mentioned exercises for cervical and scapular stability. Although these exercises have been demonstrated in an antigravity position, as described by Kendall, in Figures 15 and 16, the therapist may also strengthen these muscle groups in sitting and standing.[51]

Scapular stabilization exercises are explored in detail in the chapters of this book dedicated to shoulder and scapular dysfunction.

Proprioceptive Neuromuscular Facilitation

Proprioceptive neuromuscular facilitation (PNF) is a treatment technique that is utilized to increase ROM, flexibility, and strength. It has been theorized that PNF techniques improve joint mobility through the gate control theory or pain reduction, stress relaxation, autogenic inhibition, or reciprocal inhibition.[141] These techniques position the patient just short of the end-range restricted motion. There are a variety of PNF techniques, but contract-relax (CR) and contract-relax-agonist-contract (CRAC) appear in scientific literature more often.[141]

These generalized techniques are useful in multiple joints to increase motion and strength, including the cervical spine.[142] It is important to note that PNF techniques have been shown to decrease strength, power, and other variables when performed prior to high intensity exercise for up to 90 minutes.[141] As a result, it is important to properly institute PNF techniques at the correct time to achieve treatment goals. These techniques can also be incorporated into a home exercise program via use of a towel or a trained family member.[133]

Alternative Therapies

Roughly 38% of American adults utilized complementary alternative medicine (CAM) in 2007.[143] The use of various Chinese herbs, including compound Qishe tablet, Jingfukang, and compound Extractum Nucis Vomicae, lacks scientific evidence.[144]

A meta-analysis and systematic review on the safety, efficacy based on pain and disability, and cost-effectiveness of CAM in the management of low back and neck pain. The results established that manipulation was significantly better than placebo or no treatment in reducing pain and disability. Joint mobilization was found to be effective in reducing pain and disability with people with acute neck pain compared to placebo, but the results were equivocal in subjects with chronic neck pain. Massage was found to be no better than no

treatment, placebo, or exercise in terms of reducing pain or disability. The findings were inconclusive as to the effectiveness of acupuncture, with some studies showing decreased pain and others indicating no statistical difference.[145]

Although many studies appear to be of poor quality, adults in the United States spent $33.9 billion on CAM in 2007. These complementary treatments are likely to remain and to evolve. Therefore, it is important for health care practitioners to become familiar with interventions that their patients may be utilizing.[146]

Medical and Surgical Interventions

Patients often will be prescribed oral medication as an alternative or in addition to other conservative interventions. When conservative measures are not effective, patients may be referred for more invasive treatment procedures, such as steroid injections, epidural injections, and dorsal root rhizotomy.

Oral Medications

People with cervical radiculopathy who seek medical treatment often take NSAIDs to control inflammation and pain. In addition, they may also be prescribed muscle relaxants, narcotics, and other drugs (e.g. gabapentin, pregabalin) that help to control neuropathic pain. The literature is scarce and largely inconclusive regarding the efficacy of NSAIDs, opioid analgesics, muscle relaxants, antidepressants, anticonvulsants, and oral corticosteroids for the treatment of cervical radiculopathy and/or cervical spondylosis.[147]

Injections

Selective nerve root blocks (SNRB), which can also be diagnostic in nature, are used to decrease or eliminate pain associated with cervical radiculopathy. Predictors of good outcome from SNRB include the presence of radicular pain in the upper extremity, spondylosis, and a hard disk lesion. A retrospective study on the benefit of SNRBs on subjects with cervical disk herniation associated with radiating neck pain to the upper extremities was performed using the neck disability index and numerical pain rating scale. This research found an improvement in these measures over a 12 month period.[148] Another retrospective study found that the average symptom-free period following injection was 7.8 months, and that 50% of patients who received SNRBs were satisfied with the results of their SNRB at 12 months post-treatment.[149] In contrast, a prospective randomized study showed that there was no difference between subjects receiving transforaminal injections of saline and local anesthetic versus those receiving steroids and local anesthetic near the affected cervical spinal level in people diagnosed with cervical radiculopathy. Only 30% of subjects who received steroid and saline injections combined with a local anesthetic had continued relief 3 weeks post-injection.[150]

Surgeries

If conservative measures are unsuccessful in the treatment of cervical radiculopathy, surgery may be necessary. Dorsal root rhizotomy is a procedure in which the sensory nerves of the cervical spine that are involved in the transmission of pain are inactivated via radiofrequency. A dorsal root rhizotomy is typically performed when steroid injections are unsuccessful, or the benefits are short-lived. Dorsal root rhizotomy can provide months or years of relief to many patients, including those suffering from cervical radiculopathy. In one study, 68% of patients with degenerative disease of the cervical spine reported improvement following dorsal root rhizotomy, while 42% demonstrated complete relief.[151]

Other surgical procedures for patients suffering with cervical radiculopathy who have failed conservative measures include foraminotomy, anterior cervical discectomy (ACD), anterior cervical discectomy with fusion (ACDF), posterior cervical decompression, posterior cervical laminectomy, and total disk replacement. The NASS suggests that ACD and ACDF result in similar outcomes when performed at a single level. They also recommend both ACDF and posterior lamino-foraminotomy (PLF) for the treatment of soft disc herniations, while ACDF is preferred over PLF for cervical radiculopathy secondary to degenerative disorders. In addition, ACDF and total disk replacement have similar outcomes.[2]

Engquist et al. found that patients who received surgery combined with physical therapy secondary to cervical radiculopathy were significantly better 1 year post-surgery in comparison to the subject group that completed physical therapy alone. The subjects in this study in the surgical group had anterior cervical decompression and fusion procedures. However, there was no statistical difference between both groups after 2 years. As a result, the authors of this study suggest that physical therapy can be as effective as surgery in the treatment of cervical radiculopathy.[152]

CONCLUSION

Roughly, 25% of patients receiving outpatient physical therapy are being treated for neck pain.[134] Some of those patients have neck pain due to cervical radiculopathy. Patients with cervical radiculopathy often present with a host of signs and symptoms, including neck and upper extremity pain and paresthesia.

The physical examination is key in properly diagnosing this patient population.[46,60,92] To aid practitioners, a clinical prediction rule has been developed to assist clinicians with diagnosing patients with cervical radiculopathy.[68] The variables include a positive upper limb tension test, ipsilateral cervical rotation less than 60°, a positive distraction test, and a positive Spurling test. In conjunction with the subjective and objective information gathered during the evaluation, diagnostic imaging and electrodiagnostic tests can facilitate proper diagnosis.

Although determining the pathological diagnosis is important to the patient and clinician, there is no standard protocol for physical therapy treatment of this disorder. However, the patient response-based model appears to be more evidence-based in comparison to other treatment approaches.[46] A treatment-based classification has been studied to improve evidence-based practice as well.[122] Therefore, physical therapy treatment should be based on the causes of musculoskeletal impairments, functional limitations, and disability identified during the examination.

The literature suggests that physical therapy demonstrates efficacy in the treatment of patients with cervical radiculopathy. Physical therapy has been shown to have the same long-term benefits as surgery in the treatment of cervical radiculopathy.[152] Manual therapy has been shown to be more effective than medication alone in decreasing pain.[115] Combining manual therapy with therapeutic exercise is more effective than either intervention alone.[121,153] Manual therapy that targets not just the cervical but also the thoracic spine improves function and reduces patient pain.[121,134] Exercises that incorporate postural re-education and ergonomics are most relevant to a cervical radiculopathy diagnosis and should involve strengthening of the deep neck flexors and scapular stabilizers.[54,121] Other treatment interventions, such as trigger point dry needling, may help these patients, but lack sufficient scientific evidence. Overall, physical therapy has good efficacy in improving pain and function in patients with cervical radiculopathy and should be considered prior to pursuing more invasive measures.

REFERENCES

1. Hoy DG, Protani M, De R, Buchbinder R. The epidemiology of neck pain. Best Pract Res Clin Rheumatol. 2010;24(6):783-92.

2. Bono CM, Ghiselli G, Gilbert TJ, Kreiner DS, Reitman C, Summers JT, et al. An evidence-based clinical guideline for the diagnosis and treatment of cervical radiculopathy from degenerative disorders. Spine J. 2011;11(1):64-72.

3. Mercer S, Bogduk N. The ligaments and annulus fibrosus of human adult cervical intervertebral discs. Spine. 1999;24(7):619-26; discussion 627–8.

4. Fennell AJ, Jones AP, Hukins DW. Migration of the nucleus pulposus within the intervertebral disc during flexion and extension of the spine. Spine. 1996;21(23):2753-7.

5. Radhakrishnan K, Litchy WJ, O'Fallon WM, Kurland LT. Epidemiology of cervical radiculopathy. A population-based study from Rochester, Minnesota, 1976 through 1990. Brain. 1994;117 (2):325-35.

6. Abbed KM, Coumans JV. Cervical radiculopathy: pathophysiology, presentation, and clinical evaluation. Neurosurgery. 2007;60(1):S28-34.

7. Ellenberg MR, Honet JC, Treanor WJ. Cervical radiculopathy. Arch Phys Med Rehabil. 1994;75(3):342-52.

8. Malanga GA. The diagnosis and treatment of cervical radiculopathy. Med Sci Sports Exerc. 1997;29(7):S236-45.

9. Van Gijn J, Reiners K, Toyka KV, Braakman R. Management of cervical radiculopathy. Eur Neurol. 1995;35(6):309-20.

10. White AA, Panjabi M. Clinical Biomechanics of the Spine, 2nd edition. Philadelphia, PA: Lippincott Williams & Wilkins; 1990.

11. Parminder SP. Management of Cervical Pain. In: DeLisa JA, Gans BM (Eds). Rehabilitation Medicine: Principles and Practice, 3rd edition. Philadelphia, PA: Lippincott Williams & Wilkins; 1998.

12. Murphy DR, Hurwitz EL, Gerrard JK, Clary R. Pain patterns and descriptions in patients with radicular pain: does the pain necessarily follow a specific dermatome? Chiropr Osteopat. 2009;17(1):9.

13. Mizutamari M, Sei A, Tokiyoshi A, Fujimoto T, Taniwaki T, Togami W, et al. Corresponding scapular pain with the nerve root involved in cervical radiculopathy. J Orthop Surg Hong Kong. 2010;18(3):356-60.

14. Caridi JM, Pumberger M, Hughes AP. Cervical radiculopathy: a review. HSS J. 2011;7(3):265-72.

15. Dutton M. Orthopaedic examination, evaluation, and intervention, 3rd edition. New York: McGraw Hill Medical; 2012.

16. Pal GP, Routal RV, Saggu SK. The orientation of the articular facets of the zygapophyseal joints at the cervical and upper thoracic region. J Anat. 2001;198(4):431-41.

17. Levine MJ, Albert TJ, Smith MD. Cervical radiculopathy: diagnosis and nonoperative management. J Am Acad Orthop Surg. 1996;4(6):305-16.

18. Lyon E. Uncovertebral osteophytes and osteochondroses of the cervical spine. J Bone Joint Surg. 1945;XXVII(2):248-53.

19. Windle WF. The spinal cord and its reaction to traumatic injury. New York: Marcel Dekker; 1980. Also available online at: http://doi.wiley.com/10.1002/ana.410120233. [Accessed January, 2015].

20. Humphreys SC, Chase J, Patwardhan A, Shuster J, Lomasney L, Hodges SD. Flexion and traction effect on C5-C6 foraminal space. Arch Phys Med Rehabil. 1998;79(9):1105-9.

21. Yoo JU, Zou D, Edwards WT, Bayley J, Yuan HA. Effect of cervical spine motion on the neuroforaminal dimensions of human cervical spine. Spine. 1992;17(10):1131-6.

22. Farmer JC, Wisneski RJ. Cervical spine nerve root compression. An analysis of neuroforaminal pressures with varying head and arm positions. Spine. 1994;19(16):1850-5.

23. Langevin P, Roy JS, Desmeules F. Cervical radiculopathy: study protocol of a randomised clinical trial evaluating the effect of mobilisations and exercises targeting the opening of intervertebral foramen [NCT01500044]. BMC Musculoskelet Disord. 2012;13(1):10.

24. Bogduk N, Mercer S. Biomechanics of the cervical spine. I: normal kinematics. Clin Biomech. 2000;15(9):633-48.

25. Pettman E. A history of manipulative therapy. J Man Manip Ther. 2007;15(3):165-74.

26. Woodhouse A, Vasseljen O. Altered motor control patterns in whiplash and chronic neck pain. BMC Musculoskelet Disord. 2008;9:90.

27. Cook C, Hegedus E, Showalter C, Sizer PS. Coupling behavior of the cervical spine: a systematic review of the literature. J Manip Physiol Ther. 2006;29(7):570-5.

28. Cloward RB. Cervical diskography. A contribution to the etiology and mechanism of neck, shoulder and arm pain. Ann Surg. 1959;150:1052-64.

29. Henderson CM, Hennessy RG, Shuey HM, Shackelford EG. Posterior-lateral foraminotomy as an exclusive operative technique for cervical radiculopathy: a review of 846 consecutively operated cases. Neurosurgery. 1983;13(5):504-12.

30. Persson LC, Carlsson JY, Anderberg L. Headache in patients with cervical radiculopathy: a prospective study with selective nerve root blocks in 275 patients. Eur Spine J. 2007;16(7):953-9.

31. McKenzie R. The lumbar spine: mechanical diagnosis and therapy. Waikanae, NZ: Spinal Publications; 2003.

32. McKenzie R, May S. The cervical & thoracic spine: mechanical diagnosis & therapy. Raumati Beach, NZ: Spinal Publications; 2006.

33. McDonnell M, Lucas P. Cervical spondylosis, stenosis, and rheumatoid arthritis. Med Heal R. 2012;95(4):105-9.

34. Connell MD, Wiesel SW. Natural history and pathogenesis of cervical disk disease. Orthop Clin North Am. 1992;23(3):369-80.

35. Neal S, Fields KB. Peripheral nerve entrapment and injury in the upper extremity. Am Fam Physician. 2010;81(2):147-55.

36. Simons DG, Travel JG, Simons LS. Myofascial Pain and Dysfunction: the Trigger Point Manual; The Upper Half of Body, 2nd edition. Baltimore: LWW; 1998.

37. Mense S. Muscle pain: mechanisms and clinical significance. Dtsch Arztebl Int. 2008;105(12):214-9.

38. Dommerholt J, Bron C, Franssen J. Myofascial trigger points: an evidence-informed review. J Man Manip Ther. 2006;14(4):203-21.

39. Maitland GD. Vertebral Manipulation, 5th edition. Oxford England: Butterworth-Heinemann Medical; 1986.

40. Evans P. The T4 syndrome. Physiotherapy. 1997;83(4):186-9.

41. Mellick GA, Mellick LB. Clinical presentation, quantitative sensory testing, and therapy of 2 patients with fourth thoracic syndrome. J Manip Physiol Ther. 2006;29(5):403-8.

42. Bogduk N. Anatomy and physiology of headache. Biomed Pharmacother. 1995;49(10):435-45.

43. Biondi DM. Cervicogenic headache: mechanisms, evaluation, and treatment strategies. J Am Osteopath Assoc. 2000;100(9):S7-14.

44. Miller TT, Reinus WR. Nerve entrapment syndromes of the elbow, forearm, and wrist. Am J Roentgenol. 2010;195(3):585-94.

45. Benzel EC. Spine Surgery: Techniques, Complication Avoidance, and Management, 2nd edition. Philadelphia, PA: Churchill Livingstone; 2004.

46. Cook C. Orthopedic Manual Therapy: An Evidence Based Approach, 2nd edition. Upper Saddle River, NJ: Pearson Education; 2012.

47. Huelke DF. An overview of anatomical considerations of infants and children in the adult world of automobile safety design. Annu Proc Assoc Adv Automot Med. 1998;42:93-113.

48. Neumann DA. Kinesiology of the Musculoskeletal System: Foundations for Rehabilitation, 2nd edition. St. Louis, MO: Mosby/Elsevier; 2010.

49. Horak FB. Postural orientation and equilibrium: what do we need to know about neural control of balance to prevent falls? Age Ageing. 2006;35(2):ii7–ii11.

50. Janda J. Muscles and motor control in cervicogenic disorders. In: Grant R (Ed). Physical Therapy of the Cervical and Thoracic Spine, 2nd edition. Edinburgh; New York: Churchill Livingstone; 1994.

51. Kendall FP, Kendall FP. Muscles: Testing and Function with Posture and Pain, 5th edition. Baltimore, MD: Lippincott Williams & Wilkins; 2005.

52. Saunders D. Evaluation, Treatment, and Prevention of Musculoskeletal Disorders, 4th edition. Chaska, MN: Saunders Group; 2004.

53. Diab AA, Moustafa IM. The efficacy of forward head correction on nerve root function and pain in cervical spondylotic radiculopathy: a randomized trial. Clin Rehabil. 2012;26(4):351-61.

54. Page P. Cervicogenic headaches: an evidence-led approach to clinical management. Int J Sports Phys Ther. 2011;6(3):254-66.

55. O'Sullivan SB, Schmitz TJ. Physical rehabilitation, 5th edition. Philadelphia: F.A. Davis; 2007.

56. Walker HK, Hall WD, Hurst JW. Clinical methods: the history, physical, and laboratory examinations, 3rd edition. Boston: Butterworths; 1990. Also available online at: http://www.ncbi.nlm.nih.gov/books/NBK201/. [Accessed January, 2015].

57. Cyriax JH. Diagnosis of soft tissue lesions. London; Philadelphia: Baillière Tindall; 1982.

58. Fritz JM, Delitto A, Erhard RE, Roman M. An examination of the selective tissue tension scheme, with evidence for the concept of a capsular pattern of the knee. Phys Ther. 1998;78(10):1046-56; discussion 1057-61.

59. Edwards BC. Combined movements in the cervical spine (C2-7) their value in examination and technique choice. Aust J Physiother. 1980;26(5):165-71.

60. Maitland GD. Maitland's vertebral manipulation. Oxford; Boston: Butterworth-Heinemann; 2001.

61. Maher C, Latimer J. Pain or resistance—the manual therapists' dilemma. Aust J Physiother. 1992;38(4):257-60.

62. Seffinger MA, Najm WI, Mishra SI, Adams A, Dickerson VM, Murphy LS, et al. Reliability of spinal palpation for diagnosis of back and neck pain: a systematic review of the literature. Spine. 2004;29(19):E413-5.

63. Maher CG, Latimer J, Adams R. An investigation of the reliability and validity of posteroanterior spinal stiffness judgments made using a reference-based protocol. Phys Ther. 1998;78(8):829-37.

64. Maher C, Adams R. Reliability of pain and stiffness assessments in clinical manual lumbar spine examination. Phys Ther. 1994;74(9):801-9.

65. Jull G, Bogduk N, Marsland A. The accuracy of manual diagnosis for cervical zygapophysial joint pain syndromes. Med J Aust. 1988;148(5):233-6.

66. Rey-Eiriz G, Alburquerque-Sendín F, Barrera-Mellado I, Martín-Vallejo FJ, Fernández-de-las-Peñas C. Validity of the posterior-anterior middle cervical spine gliding test for the examination of intervertebral joint hypomobility in mechanical neck pain. J Manipulative Physiol Ther. 2010;33(4):279-85.

67. Domenech MA, Sizer PS, Dedrick GS, McGalliard MK, Brismee JM. The deep neck flexor endurance test: normative data scores in healthy adults. PM&R. 2011;3(2):105-10.

68. Wainner RS, Gill H. Diagnosis and nonoperative management of cervical radiculopathy. J Orthop Sports Phys Ther. 2000;30(12):728-44.

69. Magarey ME, Rebbeck T, Coughlan B, Grimmer K, Rivett DA, Refshauge K. Pre-manipulative testing of the cervical spine review, revision and new clinical guidelines. Man Ther. 2004;9(2):95-108.

70. Vidal P, Huijbregts P. Dizziness in orthopaedic physical therapy practice: history and physical examination. J Man Manip Ther. 2005;13(4):221-50.

71. Magee DJ. Orthopedic physical assessment, 5th edition. St. Louis, MO: Saunders Elsevier; 2008.

72. Anekstein Y, Blecher R, Smorgick Y, Mirovsky Y. What is the best way to apply the Spurling test for cervical radiculopathy? Clin Orthop Relat Res. 2012;470(9):2566-72.

73. Tong HC, Haig AJ, Yamakawa K. The Spurling test and cervical radiculopathy. Spine. 2002;27(2):156-9.

74. Ghasemi M, Golabchi K, Mousavi SA, Asadi B, Rezvani M, Shaygannejad V, et al. The value of provocative tests in diagnosis of cervical radiculopathy. J Res Med Sci. 2013;18(1):S35-8.

75. Scoville WB, Whitcomb BB. Lateral rupture of cervical intervertebral disks. Postgrad Med. 1966;39(2):174-80.

76. Beatty RM, Fowler FD, Hanson EJ. The abducted arm as a sign of ruptured cervical disc. Neurosurgery. 1987;21(5):731-2.

77. Viikari-Juntura E, Porras M, Laasonen EM. Validity of clinical tests in the diagnosis of root compression in cervical disc disease. Spine. 1989;14(3):253-7.

78. Butler D, Gifford L. The concept of adverse mechanical tension in the nervous system part 1: testing for "dural tension." Physiotherapy. 1989;75(11):622-9.

79. Butler D, Gifford L. The concept of adverse mechanical tension in the nervous system part 2: examination and treatment. Physiotherapy. 1989;75(11):629-36.

80. Nee RJ, Butler D. Management of peripheral neuropathic pain: integrating neurobiology, neurodynamics, and clinical evidence. Phys Ther Sport. 2006;7(1):36-49.

81. Davis DS, Anderson IB, Carson MG, Elkins CL, Stuckey LB. Upper limb neural tension and seated slump tests: the false positive rate among healthy young adults without cervical or lumbar symptoms. J Man Manip Ther. 2008;16(3):136-41.

82. Hoppenfeld S. Physical examination of the spine and extremities. New York: Appleton-Century-Crofts; 1976.

83. Gerwin RD. Classification, epidemiology, and natural history of myofascial pain syndrome. Curr Pain Headache Rep. 2001;5(5):412-20.

84. Sari H, Akarirmak U, Uludag M. Active myofascial trigger points might be more frequent in patients with cervical radiculopathy. Eur J Phys Rehabil Med. 2012;48(2):237-44.

85. Mullin J, Shedid D, Benzel E. Overview of cervical spondylosis pathophysiology and biomechanics. World Spinal Column J. 2011;2(3):89-97.

86. Hakimi K, Spanier D. Electrodiagnosis of cervical radiculopathy. Phys Med Rehabil Clin N Am. 2013;24(1):1-12.

87. Modic MT, Masaryk TJ, Mulopulos GP, Bundschuh C, Han JS, Bohlman H. Cervical radiculopathy: prospective evaluation with surface coil MR imaging, CT with metrizamide, and metrizamide myelography. Radiology. 1986;161(3):753-9.

88. Matsumoto M, Fujimura Y, Suzuki N, Nishi Y, Nakamura M, Yabe Y, et al. MRI of cervical intervertebral discs in asymptomatic subjects. J Bone Joint Surg Br. 1998;80(1):19-24.

89. Borenstein DG, O'Mara JW, Boden SD, Lauerman WC, Jacobson A, Platenberg C, et al. The value of magnetic resonance imaging of the lumbar spine to predict low-back pain in asymptomatic subjects : a seven-year follow-up study. J Bone Joint Surg Am. 2001;83-A(9):1306-11.

90. Laimi K, Pitkänen J, Metsähonkala L, Vahlberg T, Mikkelsson M, Erkintalo M, et al. Adolescent cervical disc degeneration in MRI does not predict adult headache or neck pain: a 5-year follow-up of adolescents with and without headache. Cephalalgia. 2014;34(9):679-685.

91. Pawar S, Kashikar A, Shende V, Waghmare S. The study of diagnostic efficacy of nerve conduction study parameters in cervical radiculopathy. J Clin Diagn Res. 2013;7(12):2680-2.

92. Ashkan K, Johnston P, Moore AJ. A comparison of magnetic resonance imaging and neurophysiological studies in the assessment of cervical radiculopathy. Br J Neurosurg. 2002;16(2):146-8.

93. Colachis S, Strohm M. A study of tractive forces and angle of pull on vertebral interspaces in cervical spine. Arch Phys Med. 1965;(46):820-30.

94. Moeti P, Marchetti G. Clinical outcome from mechanical intermittent cervical traction for the treatment of cervical radiculopathy: a case series. J Orthop Sports Phys Ther. 2001;31(4):207-13.

95. Graham N, Gross AR, Goldsmith C. Mechanical traction for mechanical neck disorders: a systematic review. Cervical Overview Group. J Rehabil Med. 2006;38(3):145-52.

96. Young IA, Michener LA, Cleland JA, Aguilera AJ, Snyder AR. Manual therapy, exercise, and traction for patients with cervical radiculopathy: a randomized clinical trial. Phys Ther. 2009;89(7):632-42.

97. Judovich B. Herniated cervical disc; a new form of traction therapy. Am J Surg. 1952;84(6):646-56.

98. Cleland JA, Whitman JM, Fritz JM, Palmer JA. Manual physical therapy, cervical traction, and strengthening exercises in patients with cervical radiculopathy: a case series. J Orthop Sports Phys Ther. 2005;35(12):802-11.

99. Raney NH, Petersen EJ, Smith TA, Cowan JE, Rendeiro DG, Deyle GD, et al. Development of a clinical prediction rule to identify patients with neck pain likely to benefit from cervical traction and exercise. Eur Spine J. 2009;18(3):382-91.

100. DeStefano LA. Greenman's Principles of Manual Medicine, 4th edition. Baltimore, MD: Lippincott Williams & Wilkins/Wollters Kluwer; 2011.

101. Chaitow L. Muscle energy techniques. Edinburgh; New York: Churchill Livingstone/Elsevier; 2006.

102. Fryer G. Muscle energy concepts: a need for change. J Osteopat Med. 2000;3(2):54-9.

103. Fryer G. Muscle energy technique: an evidence-informed approach. Int J Osteopat Med. 2011;14(1):3-9.

104. Burns DK, Wells MR. Gross range of motion in the cervical spine: the effects of osteopathic muscle energy technique in asymptomatic subjects. J Am Osteopath Assoc. 2006;106(3):137-42.

105. Mahajan R, Kataria C, Bansal K. Comparative effectiveness of muscle energy technique and static stretching for treatment of subacute mechanical neck pain. Int J Heal Rehabil Sci. 2012;1(1):16-24.

106. Ellis R, Hing W. Neural mobilization: a systematic review of randomized controlled trials with an analysis of therapeutic efficacy. J Man Manip Ther. 2008;16(1):8-22.

107. Bialosky JE, Bishop MD, Price DD, Robinson ME, George SZ. The mechanisms of manual therapy in the treatment of musculoskeletal pain: a comprehensive model. Man Ther. 2009;14(5):531-8.

108. Schmid A, Brunner F, Wright A, Bachmann LM. Paradigm shift in manual therapy? Evidence for a central nervous system component in the response to passive cervical joint mobilisation. Man Ther. 2008;13(5):387-96.

109. Perry J, Green A. An investigation into the effects of a unilaterally applied lumbar mobilisation technique on peripheral sympathetic nervous system activity in the lower limbs. Man Ther. 2008;13(6):492-9.

110. Moulson A, Watson T. A preliminary investigation into the relationship between cervical snags and sympathetic nervous system activity in the upper limbs of an asymptomatic population. Man Ther. 2006;11(3):214-24.

111. Coppieters MW, Stappaerts KH, Wouters LL, Janssens K. The immediate effects of a cervical lateral glide treatment technique in patients with neurogenic cervicobrachial pain. J Orthop Sports Phys Ther. 2003;33(7):369-78.

112. Sterling M, Jull G, Wright A. Cervical mobilisation: concurrent effects on pain, sympathetic nervous system activity and motor activity. Man Ther. 2001;6(2):72-81.

113. Vicenzino B, Collins D, Benson H, Wright A. An investigation of the interrelationship between manipulative therapy-induced hypoalgesia and sympathoexcitation. J Manip Physiol Ther. 1998;21(7):448-53.

114. Bronfort G, Haas M, Evans RL, Bouter LM. Efficacy of spinal manipulation and mobilization for low back pain and neck pain: a systematic review and best evidence synthesis. Spine J. 2004;4(3):335-56.

115. Bronfort G, Evans R, Anderson AV, Svendsen KH, Bracha Y, Grimm RH. Spinal manipulation, medication, or home exercise with advice for acute and subacute neck pain: a randomized trial. Ann Intern Med. 2012;156(1):1-10.

116. Lee RY, McGregor AH, Bull AM, Wragg P. Dynamic response of the cervical spine to posteroanterior mobilisation. Clin Biomech. 2005;20(2):228-31.

117. Costello M. Treatment of a patient with cervical radiculopathy using thoracic spine thrust manipulation, soft tissue mobilization, and exercise. J Man Manip Ther. 2008;16(3):129-35.

118. Suvarnnato T, Puntumetakul R, Kaber D, Boucaut R, Boonphakob Y, Arayawichanon P, et al. The effects of thoracic manipulation versus mobilization for chronic neck pain: a randomized controlled trial pilot study. J Phys Ther Sci. 2013;25(7):865-71.

119. Dunning JR, Cleland JA, Waldrop MA, Arnot CF, Young IA, Turner M, et al. Upper cervical and upper thoracic thrust manipulation versus nonthrust mobilization in patients with mechanical neck pain: a multicenter randomized clinical trial. J Orthop Sports Phys Ther. 2012;42(1):5-18.

120. Puentedura EJ, Landers MR, Cleland JA, Mintken P, Huijbregts P, Fernandez-De-Las-Peñas C. Thoracic spine thrust manipulation versus cervical spine thrust manipulation in patients with acute neck pain : a randomized clinical trial. J Orthop Sports Phys Ther. 2011;41(4):208-20.

121. Childs JD, Cleland JA, Elliott JM, Teyhen DS, Wainner RS, Whitman JM, et al. Neck pain: clinical practice guidelines linked to the international classification of functioning, disability, and health from the orthopaedic section of the american physical therapy association. J Orthop Sports Phys Ther. 2008;38(9):A1-A34.

122. Fritz JM, Brennan GP. Preliminary examination of a proposed treatment-based classification system for patients receiving physical therapy interventions for neck pain. Phys Ther. 2007;87(5):513-24.

123. Masaracchio M, Cleland J, Hellman M, Hagins M. Short-term combined effects of thoracic spine thrust manipulation and cervical spine nonthrust manipulation in individuals with mechanical neck pain: a randomized clinical trial. J Orthop Sports Phys Ther. 2013;43(3):118-27.

124. Allison GT, Nagy BM, Hall T. A randomized clinical trial of manual therapy for cervico-brachial pain syndrome—a pilot study. Man Ther. 2002;7(2):95-102.

125. Exelby L. The Mulligan concept: its application in the management of spinal conditions. Man Ther. 2002;7(2):64-70.

126. Miller J. The Mulligan concept–the next step in the evolution of manual therapy. Can Physiother Assoc Orthop Div Rev. 1999:9–13.

127. Hearn A, Rivett DA. Cervical SNAGs: a biomechanical analysis. Man Ther. 2002;7(2):71-9.

128. Hall T, Chan HT, Christensen L, Odenthal B, Wells C, Robinson K. Efficacy of a C1-C2 self-sustained natural apophyseal glide (SNAG) in the management of cervicogenic headache. J Orthop Sports Phys Ther. 2007;37(3):100-7.

129. Simons DG. Do endplate noise and spikes arise from normal motor endplates? Am J Phys Med Rehabil. 2001;80(2):134-40.

130. Dommerholt J. Dry needling—peripheral and central considerations. J Man Manip Ther. 2011;19(4):223-7.

131. Kietrys DM, Palombaro KM, Azzaretto E, Hubler R, Schaller B, Schlussel JM, et al. Effectiveness of dry needling for upper-quarter myofascial pain: a systematic review and meta-analysis. J Orthop Sports Phys Ther. 2013;43(9):620-34.

132. American Physical Therapy Association. Physical therapists & the performance of dry needling: an educational resource paper. Washington, DC: APTA; 2012.

133. Brody LT. Therapeutic exercise: moving toward function, 3rd edition. Philadelphia: Wolters Kluwer/Lippincott Williams & Wilkins Health; 2011.

134. Boyles R, Toy P, Mellon J, Hayes M, Hammer B. Effectiveness of manual physical therapy in the treatment of cervical radiculopathy: a systematic review. J Man Manip Ther. 2011;19(3):135-42.

135. Fritz JM, Thackeray A, Brennan GP, Childs JD. Exercise only, exercise with mechanical traction, or exercise with over-door traction for patients with cervical radiculopathy, with or without consideration of status on a previously described subgrouping rule: a randomized clinical trial. J Orthop Sports Phys Ther. 2014;44(2):45-57.

136. Schenk R, Bhaidani T, Melissa B, Kelley J, Kruchowsky T. Inclusion of mechanical diagnosis and therapy (MDT) in the management of cervical radiculopathy: a case report. J Man Manip Ther. 2008;16(1):e1–e8.

137. Clare HA, Adams R, Maher CG. A systematic review of efficacy of McKenzie therapy for spinal pain. Aust J Physiother. 2004;50(4):209-16.

138. Abdul-Latif AA. Dropped shoulder syndrome: a cause of lower cervical radiculopathy. J Clin Neurol. 2011;7(2):85.

139. McCormack BM, Weinstein PR. Cervical spondylosis. An update. West J Med. 1996;165(1-2):43-51.

140. Boyd-Clark LC, Briggs CA, Galea MP. Muscle spindle distribution, morphology, and density in longus colli and multifidus muscles of the cervical spine. Spine. 2002;27(7):694-701.

141. Hindle K, Whitcomb T, Briggs W, Hong J. Proprioceptive neuromuscular facilitation (PNF): its mechanisms and effects on range of motion and muscular function. J Hum Kinet. 2012;31:105-113.

142. Rezasoltani A, Khaleghifar M, Tavakoli A, Ahmadi A, Minoonejad H. The effect of a proprioceptive neuromuscular facilitation program to increase neck muscle strength in patients with chronic non-specific neck pain. World Journ Sport Sci. 2010;3(1):59-63.

143. Barnes PM, Bloom B, Nahin RL. Complementary and alternative medicine use among adults and children: United States, 2007. Natl Heal Stat Rep. 2008;(12):1-23.

144. Cui X, Trinh K, Wang YJ. Chinese herbal medicine for chronic neck pain due to cervical degenerative disc disease. Cochrane Database Syst Rev. 2010;(1):CD006556.

145. Furlan AD, Yazdi F, Tsertsvadze A, Gross A, Van Tulder M, Santaguida L, et al. A systematic review and meta-analysis of efficacy, cost-effectiveness, and safety of selected complementary and alternative medicine for neck and low-back pain. Evid Based Complement Altern Med. 2012;2012:953139.

146. Nahin RL, Barnes PM, Stussman BJ, Bloom B. Costs of complementary and alternative medicine (CAM) and frequency of visits to CAM practitioners: United States, 2007. Natl Heal Stat Rep. 2009;(18):1-14.

147. Hirpara KM, Butler JS, Dolan RT, O'Byrne JM, Poynton AR. Nonoperative modalities to treat symptomatic cervical spondylosis. Adv Orthop. 2012;2012:1-5.

148. Park EJ, Park SY, Lee SJ, Kim NS, Koh DY. Clinical outcomes of epidural neuroplasty for cervical disc herniation. J Korean Med Sci. 2013;28(3):461.

149. Chung JY, Yim JH, Seo HY, Kim SK, Cho KJ. The efficacy and persistence of selective nerve root block under fluoroscopic guidance for cervical radiculopathy. Asian Spine J. 2012;6(4):227.

150. Anderberg L, Annertz M, Persson L, Brandt L, Säveland H. Transforaminal steroid injections for the treatment of cervical radiculopathy: a prospective and randomised study. Eur Spine J. 2007;16(3):321-8.

151. Shin WR, Kim HI, Shin DG, Shin DA. Radiofrequency neurotomy of cervical medial branches for chronic cervicobrachialgia. J Korean Med Sci. 2006;21(1):119.

152. Engquist M, Löfgren H, Öberg B, Holtz A, Peolsson A, Söderlund A, et al. Surgery versus nonsurgical treatment of cervical radiculopathy: a prospective, randomized study comparing surgery plus physiotherapy with physiotherapy alone with a 2-year follow-up. Spine. 2013;38(20):1715-22.

153. Jette AM, Smith K, Haley SM, Davis KD. Physical therapy episodes of care for patients with low back pain. Phys Ther. 1994;74(2):101-10; discussion 110-5.

CHAPTER 8

Lumbar Strain and Sprain

Kristen M Branham

ABSTRACT

Spinal stability is achieved through three subsystems: the passive (viscoelastic structures: disks, facets, ligaments), the active (muscles), and the neural (central and peripheral nervous systems), each one separate yet directly related to the other. A thorough physical therapy examination classifies patients into subcategories, two of which are by the functional loss characteristics and the phase of healing, to help direct a treatment plan. This chapter discusses a physical therapy treatment progression of an acute lumbar strain or sprain through the phases of healing (inflammatory, fibroblastic, and remodeling). An array of treatment topics are discussed including appreciating risk factors, improving motor control deficits, incorporating balance and proprioception exercises, bracing options, patient education, manual techniques, managing peripheral nerve involvement, exercising intensely while limiting load to the disks, alternative treatments, and medical and surgical considerations.

■ INTRODUCTION

Most people will suffer low back pain (LBP) at some point in their lives and it is a main reason people miss work.[1,2] While acute episodes generally resolve on their own, it is very rare that people will describe a single episode of pain in their lifetime, as the rate of recurrence ranges between 24% and 80%.[1] The 2010 Global Burden of Disease has found LBP to be the number one leading cause of disability due to musculoskeletal conditions in all developed countries.[3] There is no doubt that treating LBP constitutes an enormous part of any orthopedic physical therapy practice.

A common classification system defines pain lasting less than 6 weeks as acute, 7–12 weeks as subacute, and greater than 3 months as chronic.[4] For the purposes of this chapter, the focus will be on the first 12 weeks of the acute and subacute phases of LBP, with an emphasis on treatment along the lines of healing phases.

Epidemiology

Though not necessarily predictors of pain, some common risk factors that have been identified with LBP include increased physical demands at work,[5] age,[6] psychosocial factors,[7] depression,[8] family history,[9] smoking,[10] and decreased educational status.[1,11,12] In addition, there is evidence linking decreased physical activity level,[13] high low-density lipoprotein (LDL) cholesterol,[14] high body mass index (BMI),[13,15] and atherosclerosis to the development of LBP as the arteries supplying to the lumbar spine become sclerosed.[16,17] These individual factors will influence treatment, but should not discourage the practitioner, as even in patients who possess a daunting list of comorbidities, their potential for a favorable clinical course of treatment can still be quite good.[18-20]

Anatomical Review

The anatomy of the lumbar spine is centered on the three joint motion segment—the two facet joints and the intervertebral disk in between. As Panjabi[21] described, spinal stability is achieved through three subsystems: the passive (viscoelastic structures: disks, facets, ligaments), the active (muscles), and the neural (central and peripheral nervous systems). While these sub-systems are separate entities, they are directly related to each other and when one is lacking there will be a concomitant effect on the other two. A review of some important points of the lumbar anatomy to consider is as follows:

Disk

The disk is an avascular structure consisting of an inner nucleus made up of a water and proteoglycan gel substance, an outer annulus made up of type 1 collagen fibers, and cartilaginous endplates. The sinuvertebral nerves supply the disk and are situated in the outer rings of the annulus fibrosus.

The disk goes through a natural degenerative process in all humans, beginning with tissue breakdown due to diminished blood supply in the first half of the second decade of life.[22-24] As the disk ages and loses height, pressure is distributed onto the posterior lateral annulus, which can create a weak area for bulging and mechanically compressing the sinuvertebral nerves.

Disk cell viability is related to nutrient supply through diffusion from the endplate, pores in the annulus fibrosus, and surrounding arteries through loaded and unloaded postures.[25-27] In a healthy disk, compressive load variations in a daily cycle are beneficial to disk maintenance.[28] Clinically, taking regular breaks to unload the spine can help transfer nutrients into the disk, as well as allow a person with weight-bearing sensitivity to be more functional.[29-31]

Facets

The lumbar facet joints are oriented more parallel to the sagittal plane in the upper lumbar region allowing for flexion and extension, and closer to the coronal plane in the lower lumbar spine providing rotation movement. The facet joint capsule helps to restrict motion into flexion and is lined with low-threshold afferent mechanoreceptors

involved in proprioception[32,33] and in sending reflexive activation signals to the muscles.[34]

The facets and the disks are directly related to each other and pathology in the disk frequently precedes that in the facets.[35] As the disk continues its natural degenerative process and becomes smaller in height, added load is placed onto the facet joints possibly giving rise to pain as a result of repetitive strain or low grade trauma accumulated over the course of a lifetime.[36] Along with mechanical changes at the joints, chemical inflammatory cytokines are released from the degenerative facet synovium, which can stimulate pain nociceptors and mimic radicular symptoms if it spreads to the adjacent nerve roots.[37,38] Inflamed facet joints can also refer symptoms to the lower extremities without nerve root involvement.[39]

Ligaments

Other than the facet joint capsule, the interspinous ligament, anterior longitudinal ligament, the posterior longitudinal ligament, the ligamentum flavum, the intertransverse ligament, and the supraspinous ligament also assist in the stability of the motion segment (Fig. 1). They are primarily made up of collagen fibers in a helical form and when stretched, the fibers begin to straighten providing stiffness.[40] Their primary role is in controlling flexion, rotation and posterior shear forces of the vertebrae.[33] Generally the supraspinous and interspinous ligaments are most susceptible to failure due to their inability to withstand the flexion forces on the spine.[33]

When the ligaments become taut, reflexive activation signals are sent via mechanoreceptors to the associated muscles to increase spine stability.[34] Research on the viscoelastic properties of the ligaments (creep, tension-relaxation, hysteresis, and length tension relation) has shown static and repetitive forward bending can disrupt these signals to the muscles. Jackson et al.[41] showed the stretch to the supraspinous ligament for 20 minutes resulted in a 50% decrease in multifidus activity, which took more than 7 hours of rest to regain prestretch conditions in both the ligament and muscle. Clinically, a therapist can have great impact on the health of the soft tissues by addressing postural issues at work and at home.

Muscles

Bergmark[43] described two muscle systems acting on the spine: the local muscles that directly attach to the lumbar spine and control segmental movement, and the global

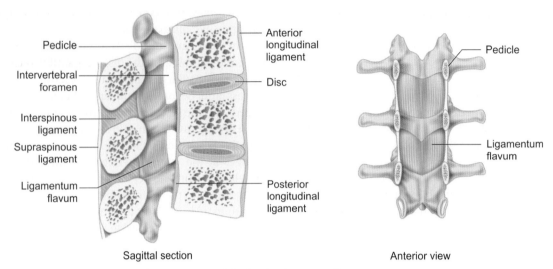

FIG. 1: Sagittal section and anterior view of the lumbar ligaments[42]
Source: Published with permission from Elsevier.

muscles which do not directly attach to but still have an effect on the lumbar spine. The local muscles include the lumbar multifidus, psoas major, quadratus lumborum, lumbar iliocostalis and longissimus, transversus abdominis, and the internal abdominal oblique. The global muscles are the rectus abdominis, external abdominal oblique, and the thoracic part of the lumbar iliocostalis. These local and global muscles, along with the diaphragm[44,45] and pelvic floor musculature,[46] work together to create active stability of the lumbar spine.

The spine muscles can show signs of atrophy, fatigue, spasm, active trigger points, and guarding and their changes can be precipitated by direct injury as well as indirectly due to pathological changes in neighboring joints.[47] Local concentration of inflammatory mediators, from other painful structures in the vicinity of muscle tissue, causes an increase in muscle nociceptor excitability and they easily become sensitized, hyperalgesic, and a pain-generating source themselves.[48]

The spine muscles can also demonstrate coordination insufficiency between the local and global systems. Particularly common are strength and motor control deficits of the transverse abdominis and lumbar multifidus.[49-51] As with the ligaments, if there is prolonged stretch on the muscle, usually involving flexion, then any of the involved mechanoreceptors become desensitized, and, hence, a decrease in muscle reflex activation is seen.[41,52] This can attribute to the local muscles exhibiting diminished postural control and in chronic cases proceeding to alteration of the organization in the primary motor cortex.[50] The global muscles then increase their activation in an attempt to compensate for the lack of stability.[53,54] This alteration in the motor cortex due to disrupted muscle activation patterns is one hypothesis for the high recurrence rate of LBP.

Nerves

The lumbar nerve roots arise from the spinal cord from the T10-L1 termination called the conus medullaris. These roots each comprise of a dorsal (efferent motor) aspect and a ventral (afferent sensory) aspect. The dorsal root ganglia location plays a significant role in its ability to become compressed. The more proximal to the spine the ganglia is located (intraspinal), the more vulnerable it is to compression, with the most common cause of compression being from the superior facet at the intervertebral foramen.[55] Although there is genetic variation in the position of the dorsal root ganglia, they are usually found more proximally placed as the spinal segments get more caudal, with S1 being mostly intraspinal.[55] The dorsal and ventral roots come together to exit as the spinal nerve at the corresponding level. The efferent sinuvertebral nerve then branches off the spinal nerve to supply the posterior longitudinal ligament, the outer disk annulus, and the periosteum.

It is important to remember that nerves can be involved anywhere along their pathways, not just the dorsal root ganglia, and signs of lumbar radiculopathy are produced with direct pressure, stretch, chemical inflammatory mediators, and can be mimicked by myofascial pain.[56]

CLINICAL PRESENTATION

Functional Loss Characteristics

When looking at mechanical causes of LBP, there have been many working models to help classify patients into subcategories based on acquired subjective and objective information.[57-60] Vollowitz[61] categorizes patients based on the clinical presentations of their functional loss characteristics. Vollowitz identified four key patterns of symptom behavior, one of which will fit every patient. These characteristics, described as follows, can overlap and change over time but they serve as a guide to what treatment strategies will be beneficial.

Position Sensitivity

These patients have a strong preference for flexion or extension postures. This finding is also supported by Long et al.,[62] who found exercising in the pain-free direction to be the most successful.

Weight Bearing Sensitivity

These individuals experience an aggravation of their LBP with compressive loading, regardless of their position.

Constrained Posture Sensitivity

These individuals report aggravated symptoms when in a static position, regardless of how supportive the position may be.

Pressure Sensitivity

These individuals have pain that is aggravated with direct pressure, especially on areas that have active inflammation.

Phases of Healing

In addition to functional characteristics, patients are also clinically classified based on what phase of healing they are in. Key points in each phase, ascertained from Hardy,[63] are as follows:

Inflammatory Phase

The first few days of an injury, including reinjury, involves bleeding of the injured vessels and vasodilation of the surrounding intact ones. If too much swelling occurs, there is potential for excessive scarring to ensue. Phagocytosis occurs to rid the wound of infection and macrophages stimulate the production of revascularization so that the wound is sealed off to signify the close of the inflammatory phase.

Repair Phase

This phase involves wound contraction and collagen production and lasts approximately from days 4 to 21.[64] At the end of this phase of healing there will be sufficient quantity of collagen to replace the damaged tissue, but the tensile strength is only at 15% and can be easily disrupted.

Remodeling Phase

In this phase, the scar changes to fit the tissue it is replacing. There is collagen turnover as the scar is rearranged due to internal and external forces acting on the tissue. Controlled mobilization of the scar during this time frame will allow for it to develop the qualities it will need for normal functioning. This final phase lasts approximately from day 21 up to 1 year.[64]

CLINICAL EXAMINATION

Evaluation

The subjective evaluation should thoroughly investigate the location (including the extremities), description, intensity, constancy, aggravating activities, easing activities, 24-hour behavior, medications, tests and procedures, occupation and activity level, past medical history, and description of previous episodes and the current complaint.[65] Additionally, it is necessary to rule out any red flag indicators for serious underlying pathology (tumors, severe neurologic symptoms, systemic disease, and fractures). This patient-therapist communication is the first step to developing a working hypothesis on what potential structures are involved, pathology, severity, irritability, nature, and the stage of healing.

The objective evaluation confirms the hypothesis from the subjective portion of the examination. A judgment needs to be made on how irritable the pain is, as someone in the inflammatory stage will likely flare up easily with simple, yet excessive, testing. In which case, prioritizing the exam should be done, saving further testing for a later time when the irritability is decreased. Examiners should be mindful that even less irritable patients may not be able to get into a specific "test position". Learning how to perform each test in an alternate position to accommodate for individual differences will help garner the sought after information. A basic objective guideline is as follows:

Observation

Performed from different angles with as much of the spine and legs visible to reveal postural deficits, scoliosis, shifting, amount and location of the spinal curves, where the spine hinges during movement and structural feedback in general.

Active Range of Motion

These measurements may be achieved via visual observation, video motion analysis, goniometry, linear measures, and inclinometry.[66] Recent advances in technology have even provided good intra-rater and inter-rater reliability data on the use of smartphone digital inclinometry applications for lumbar range of motion (ROM).[67,68] Range of motion findings will help to determine how they move and their direction of preference which will be important when developing a treatment program.[62,69]

Segmental Mobility

Segmental mobility testing measures the passive physiologic and accessory movements to determine the end feel, the quality, and the quantity of movement at the motion segment. The motion segments are determined to be either hypomobile, normal, or hypermobile.[70] Clinically, patients judged to have hypomobility at some level of the lumbar spine benefit from an intervention that involves mobilization plus stabilization, while those determined to have hypermobility benefit from treatment focused on stabilization exercises.[71-73] In the inflammatory stage, hypomobility may indicate local inflammation surrounding and within the facet joints not allowing for motion within the normal physiologic ranges, warranting treatment to decrease inflammation to restore mobility.

Palpation

Musculature and soft tissues of the spine, gluteal region, and along the path of the sciatic, tibial and peroneal nerves can be palpated to evaluate for pain, tension, and spasm. In an acute-type injury, signs of inflammation are assessed with light touch looking for any heat, swelling, and tautness in the local tissues.

Neurological Screening

Testing of sensation, reflexes, and muscle strength is necessary if you suspect radiculopathy or if the patient reports pain below the gluteal folds. Sensory integrity is assessed with light touch following the dermatome map of the body. Reflex testing of the patellar tendon, semitendinosus, and Achilles tendon is performed and assessed as hyperreflexive, hyporeflexive, or normal. Strength is tested following a myotomal chart, beginning in foot muscles furthest from the spine to minimize pain which may be provoked when testing the more proximal hip and thigh muscles that are directly attached to the spine and pelvis.[74]

Tension Signs

Tension signs are evaluated to determine the sensitivity and mobility of neurological structures. Disk pathology creating nerve root compression as well as inflammatory mediators in the area of the adjacent disk are causative for pain and decreased movement.[75] A positive test is determined when the symptoms are reproduced or there is an asymmetrical range of movement.

With the straight leg raise (SLR) test, ensure the patient is relaxed and lift the leg slowly, trying to determine the first sign of drag, or heaviness, of the leg as the nerve begins to get taut. It is recommended the end point of the SLR occur at the first sign of increased symptoms.[76] This test can be sensitized toward the tibial portion of the sciatic nerve with ankle dorsiflexion and toward the peroneal portion with ankle plantar flexion and inversion.[76]

On a cautionary note, Boyd et al.[77] studied individuals with type 2 diabetes mellitus and the distal symmetrical polyneuropathy associated with it and found that without the ability to discriminate the increases in neural loading with neurodynamic testing and sensitizing maneuvers, this population is at risk for injury from testing and the information gathered will be of limited use to the clinician anyway.

The presence of increased neural tissue mechano-sensitivity identified by nerve palpation is another key factor in identifying low back related leg pain.[78,79] The bowstring test (Fig. 2) is one means of testing the sciatic nerve through direct palpation in the popliteal space.[80] It is performed supine or side-lying by tensioning the sciatic nerve with hip flexion, dorsiflexion, and gradual

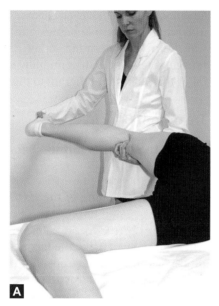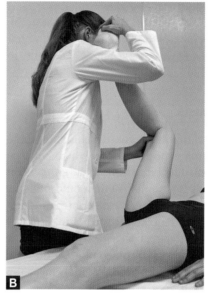

FIGS 2A AND B: Bowstring test. (A) Side-lying; (B) Supine

knee extension to bow the nerve in the popliteal space where the practitioner can apply compression. This test is positive when local or distal symptoms are reproduced with manual pressure on the tibial nerve in the central popliteal space and/or the common peroneal nerve in the posterior lateral popliteal space.

Special Tests

Special tests of the lumbar spine can provide further knowledge of the underlying structural integrity.

A Thomas test[81,82] can reveal muscular imbalances in the iliopsoas[83] and rectus femoris, and indirectly to the tensor fascia latae[84] if the hip presents abducted in the test position. Shortened iliopsoas muscles and can be problematic in individuals with increased sensitivity to the posterior joint structures, such as occurs with spinal or neuroforaminal stenosis for example.

The Coin test (Fig. 3) is a special test in which direct pressure with a coin or small finger is given to the interspinous spaces. While validity testing does not yet exist for this test, pain may be reproduced clinically as pressure is applied to the supraspinous and interspinous ligaments, indicating the possibility that they are directly sprained or there is underlying disk, ligamentous, or soft tissue inflammation at that level.

Provocation and/or alleviation testing determines the pain-producing structure by reproducing and alleviating the pain through specific movement, pressure, or load directly at that segment.[85,86] It is more reliable

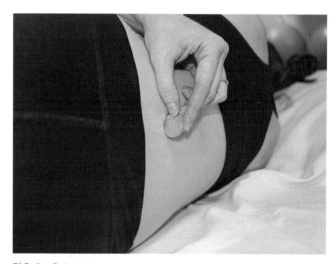

FIG. 3: Coin test

in individuals with mechanical (noninflammatory) symptoms when the inciting pain will increase and decrease with a specific change in direction of force.

Sacroiliac joint testing[87,88] is especially warranted if there is a history of pregnancy, fall or a sudden, unilateral force through a lower limb. The testing produces compression, distraction, and shear forces to the sacroiliac joints to determine their role in provoking pain.

Muscle endurance testing is more suited for patients who are pain-free or are in the chronic, non-inflammatory phase and may be suitable for an athlete ready to return to sport to determine global areas of weakness. There are many tests, but three are commonly used: the

Sorensen back extension test, the side bridge test, and the abdominal curl-up test.[89,90] A less rigorous test in the inflammatory phase is to have the patient perform a squat to reveal deficits in lower extremity strength and ability to use correct body mechanics.[91]

Differential Diagnosis

A typical doctor's referral to treat the lumbar spine can encompass a number of diagnoses, which may be overlapping and make it difficult to have a final conclusion for the exact source of the pain.[92] While some patients have a specific injury to recount, most report a sudden onset of pain due to an unknown reason.[93] This is likely due to low grade trauma that has occurred during regular activities over time, giving way to passive tissue damage that eventually results in pain. Imaging studies for acute and subacute pain are not performed unless indicated[94] and even in chronic stages, the diagnostic accuracy of magnetic resonance imaging (MRI) has the potential to lead to incorrect classification, as degeneration may be typical for a patient's age and not necessarily the pain producer.[95,96] Any innervated structure can be a source of pain and some investigation on the therapist's part will be necessary to determine potential stresses that are contributing to pain and disability.

The differential diagnosis for lumbar strain consists of a broad spectrum of pathologies including: disk bulge, herniated nucleus pulposis, facet and disk degeneration, spinal stenosis, instability, spondylolisthesis, muscle or ligamentous injuries, and sciatica/radiculitis. Examining every possible cause of LBP will not be explored in this chapter but can easily be found throughout literature. Using underlying knowledge of anatomy, patient presentations, and the soft tissue healing process, along with developing good manual therapy skills, will help to determine suitable treatment techniques for nonspecific LBP.

■ PHYSICAL THERAPY TREATMENT

Upon completing the examination, the clinician can formulate an assessment of the patient as they emerge primarily into one of three presentations: findings that indicate the inflammatory cycle, symptoms that are primarily arising from increased muscular tension or symptoms that are brought on by a mechanical hypomobility or hypermobility. Generally patients with a diagnosis of acute lumbar strain or sprain, as is the focus of this chapter, will initially present in the inflammatory cycle and treatment is chosen to allow the patient to safely

advance through that cycle. Reassessing the patient as the inflammatory episode settles and treatment progresses will help to determine other findings of increased muscular tension and/or mobility impairments to further tailor the treatment program to the individual needs.

Treatment Principles

Protect the Lumbar Motion Segments

Positions and activities that may generate repetitive shearing or stretching of the involved motion segments should be avoided in order to allow healing and to limit future flare ups.[97] Repetitive flexion, extension, or rotation will eventually damage the ligaments, muscles, annulus, disk, facet joints, joint capsules, or pars interarticularis as their respective structures are stressed to failure.[98] Even in the robust athletic population, if the athlete can learn to co-contract the abdominals and trunk stabilizers, repetitive spinal motions will be restricted, and disabling symptoms reduced.[99] For this reason, dynamic, rotatory exercises are not recommended in a treatment program as the goal is always to preserve the viscoelastic structures and avoid unnecessary low grade trauma.

Limit Spinal Loading

In the development of a physical therapy exercise program, care should be taken to provide a balance between achieving a strong muscle contraction while limiting the compressive loading on the spine. Recognizing that sitting, lumbar flexion, and flexion with rotation are going to load the intervertebral disks and viscoelastic structures, it is best to formulate an exercise program avoiding this undue stress.[97] Damage arising from repetitive loading is already a common phenomenon in everyday life, since compressive fractures and healing trabeculae are found in most cadaveric vertebral bodies.[98] Thus an exercise program and body mechanics training should strive to create a healthy environment, and not contribute to more everyday damage.

Instructing patients to limit spinal loading throughout the day is encouraged. Unloading has shown to promote disk cell proliferation and enhance nutrient supply by straightening the collagen fibers in the degraded annulus fibrosus and opening the annular pores.[25] This then aids in the drawing in of essential solutes across the endplates and into the disks, and unnecessary fluid out of the disks, in an ebb and flow fashion.[29] Unloading can be easily performed by using scapular depressors to deweight

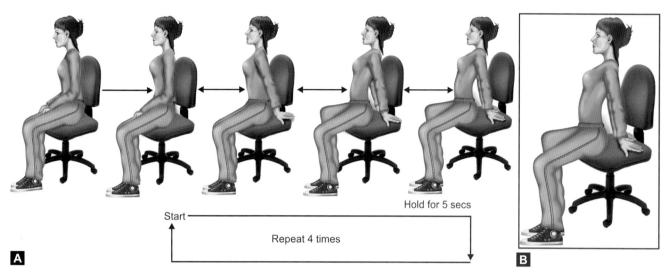

Start

Repeat 4 times

Hold for 5 secs

A

B

FIGS 4A AND B: (A) Chair-care exercise: Press into the seat cushions with your hands and relax the lower back while creating a distraction moment in the lumbar spine. The majority (60–80%) of your full weight should be supported by the shoulder girdles. Be sure to keep the chin retracted and arms externally rotated. Hold for 5 seconds. Gently return to neutral sitting posture for 1–3 seconds allowing the full weight to be resupported by the spine. Repeat 4 times; (B) Position of chair-care hold[29]

Source: Published with permission from Elsevier.

the lumbar spine by leaning or hanging from various apparatuses, such as leaning on the armrests of a chair or hanging from a towel over a door. These maneuvers are beneficial for everyone, but especially helpful for people whose occupations involve prolonged sitting.[100] Along with other occupational modifications that can be made, teaching regular unloading strategies on a regular basis (every 30–60 minutes), such as the Chair-care[29] (Fig. 4), can help promote the heath of the disks.

Limit Positions that Stretch the Neural Tissues

Limiting stretch on neural tissue is vital in individuals with nerve symptoms. Even in healthy subjects, neurological consequences can occur in positions and movements that tension the nervous system.[101] For example, many patients will describe stretching their hamstrings in a seated, straight-leg, forward flexed posture, not realizing they are also putting tension to the adjacent sciatic nerve and its branches. Awareness to avoid a full straight leg raise position, whether in supine, sitting, or standing, will allow the nerves to remain on slack and minimize their potential injury.

Attempt to Diminish Fear—Avoidance Behavior

Motor control (trunk stiffness, tissue flexibility, preferred movement strategies) and psychological factors (emotion,

cognition, behavior) both influence motor output and alter trunk mechanical behavior.[102] Some patients have strong underlying psychosocial issues driving their pain, eventually resulting in altered central processing and resultant motor dysfunction. Attempts to normalize their movement patterns alone will fail without the psychosocial issues being addressed.[103]

It is common that many patients have avoided activities due to the pain response they previously experienced with movement.[104] These individuals exhibiting protective postural strategies may have high levels of muscle guarding, creating muscular fatigue and pain due to these additional compressive loads to the spine. The goal of reducing fear of movement can be addressed by teaching safe, active movements as soon as possible with an emphasis on care provider reassurance of the condition.[105]

Begin with Local Muscles and then Move to Global Muscles

Begin with local muscle coordination and strength, and then move to global muscle contractions and movement patterns, addressing timing issues. The transverse abdominis and lumbar multifidus have received recognition for their dysfunctional role in LBP. Due to its horizontal fiber arrangement, the transverse abdominis contracts as a myofascial band that tightens upon contraction similar to a corset,[106] creating stability to the lumbar spine and sacroiliac joints.[107] Hodges[108] studied trunk muscle recruitment of the transverse abdominis and internal oblique and found that individuals without LBP initiated these muscles prior to limb movement, whereas the muscle contractions were delayed in individuals with LBP.

In addition, Hides[109,110] has shown the multifidus muscle to be diminished in size on the ipsilateral side of pain, even in first-time acute episodes of pain. This lack of localized muscle support and activation does not resolve on its own despite subjective reports of diminished symptoms and a return to prior activity levels.[111] Perhaps due to the weakness and poor motor control of these deeper muscles, there is compensatory overactivity shown in the larger global muscles of the spine.[112]

Treatment directed at addressing motor control deficits in the local muscles, to create dynamic segmental stability, has been shown to positively affect pain and function.[113-115] A stabilization training program specifically targeting the deeper muscles has been shown to decrease pain, increase cross-sectional area of the muscle, as well as return an individual to functional activities and sports.[110] Re-educating the transverse abdominis and multifidus to voluntarily contract with cognitive awareness prior to moving toward global muscle co-contractions will help to restore normal movement patterns, improve function, and decrease pain.[116,117] This can be accomplished through verbal and tactile feedback as well as with using neuromuscular biofeedback in the form of electromyography (EMG) and real time ultrasound.[118]

EMG involves the use of surface electrodes to detect skeletal muscle activity, which is then reported back to the user by a visual or auditory signal.[118] The signals are used to assist with increasing activity in weak muscles or to facilitate relaxation in spastic muscles.

Real time ultrasound also gives immediate feedback of muscle activity as well as the capability to see the muscle changes on a display.[118] It can effectively localize, give an assessment of their quality and activation pattern, and provide an opportunity for educational facilitation of the deeper multifidus and abdominals.[119]

Incorporate Proprioception and Balance Exercises

Proprioception is generally broken down to position sense and movement sense,[120] both of which are commonly coupled during daily activities. While joint position sense has not consistently proven to be related to LBP,[121] people with LBP have lower acuity for detecting changes in trunk position during motion perception (small changes in trunk position) testing.[120]

Impaired balance control, also known as postural control, has been found in LBP populations even including elite athletes.[104,122,123] The muscle spindles of the deep lumbar rotators are rich with mechanoreceptors[124] and their muscle contractions are executed when resisting rotation, as when having to maintain balance. Challenging patients by exercising on an unstable surface stimulates increased load to the spine through amplified trunk muscle activation striving for and creating stability.[125,126]

Patient Education

There is considerable variability in the nature and degree of motor control problems presenting in patients with LBP, highlighting the need for an individual problem-solving approach.[50] Patient education occurs at every visit and most individuals will benefit from information on pain expectations from exercises, the healing process,[63] and activity modification including controlling daily spinal loading,[29] limiting static end-range positions,[41,127] and instructing on the vast mechanical and ergonomic options at home/work/car to minimize load and repetitive strain.[128-133] In addition, every movement the patient makes in the clinic is a chance to instruct on body mechanics: how to put their bag down, how to get on/off the treatment table, floor, chair, and how to use exercise equipment.

Patients are educated to limit their bed rest in spite of their symptoms.[134-136] As reviewed by Waddell,[137] patients with LBP may have to modify their activities, and some may be confined to bed for a few days, but that should be an undesirable consequence of their pain and not a treatment. Wand et al.[138] found that individuals with LBP who participated in early, active physical therapy in the first 6 weeks of injury led to improved outcomes in disability, general health, social function, anxiety, depressive symptoms, mental health, and vitality compared with those who only received advice to stay active.

Treatment Outline through the Phases of Healing

Inflammatory Stage

For patients with active inflammation, the focus is on circulating fluid to control swelling as the injury prepares for healing. Limiting mobility is important in order to prevent disruption of the wound closure that is trying to occur. As in all phases of healing, individual modifications should be considered to keep pain from increasing. Some common treatments in this stage include:

Modalities directed at inflammation. If tolerated, the patient can ice multiple times a day on their own to encourage vasoconstriction and control excessive swelling.[139,140]

Manual therapy starting very superficially at the skin surface with effleurage to circulate the swelling back into the lymphatic system. The practitioner's pressure is gentle and force should go in a direction to shorten, or broaden, the tissue to prevent tension on the healing wound.

Bracing has been proven effective in the early stages of healing due to the analgesic effect of immobilizing the tissues leading to decreased medication consumption and earlier return to functional activity.[141] An elastic belt (Fig. 5) can provide vascular compression to limit excessive swelling of the tissues involved and can provide proprioceptive feedback,[142] while protecting the spine during the healing process. In the inflammatory stage, a brace can be worn 24 hours a day and is gradually weaned during the subacute phase. Bracing has not been proven as a preventative measure and patients should still have a home exercise program addressed at learning how to contract their deep spinal muscles as soon as they are able to without increased pain.

Postural taping during any stage can be a useful patient education tool, particularly if clients are having a difficult time relearning correct movement patterns,[143,144] considering the proprioceptive deficits found in this patient population.[120] Taping can also help decrease pain from muscle fatigue in the spinal extensors.[145] In the inflammatory stage, movement is controlled when the patient abides by the pull of the tape; their spine will maintain a neutral position as they learn to go about their daily activities without stressing the underlying inflamed structures.

Exercises are initially performed in the clinic with low velocity, low load, long rest, and few repetitions to remain safe without contributing to further repetitive lumbar injury.[97] Aleksiev[146] found that safely tolerated progressive isometric exercises performed by individuals at least four times a day, along with learning to brace their abdominal muscles during daily activities, demonstrated greater long term prevention of low back pain recurrences. The following exercises are highly modifiable by a skilled practitioner in order to suit the needs of each patient.

Diaphragmatic breathing

A first step to improving motor control is simply with proper breathing (Fig. 6).[45,147] Particularly in the early stages of healing this will control intra-abdominal pressure, assist with relaxation, and promote perfusion of oxygenated blood to healing structures.

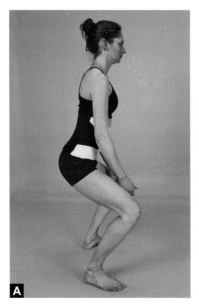 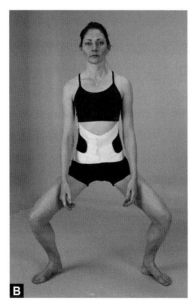

FIGS 5A AND B: Squat shown with lumbar corset in—(A) Frontal; and (B) Sagittal view. A wide base of support with the legs externally rotated (hip open pack position is 30) keeping feet and knees in line together. The lumbar spine is maintained in neutral as the knees are bent and the tailbone is directed posteriorly to get movement from the hips versus the lumbar spine. When pelvis begins to tilt posteriorly, that is the end of the safe motion

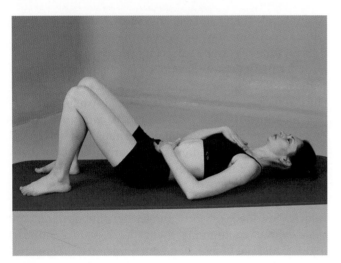

FIG. 6: Diaphragmatic breathing is shown with manual feedback on the chest and one at the level of the umbilicus. (1) The individual is instructed to take a relaxed breath creating excursion primarily through their belly. (2) Co-contraction training of the abdominals and pelvic floor occurs during expiration

Identify and teach lumbopelvic neutral range

The neutral zone of a spinal segment is the region of minimal stiffness in any direction (flexion-extension, torsion, lateral bending, shear, and compression).[148] Success has been demonstrated in individuals who have learned to control their neutral range in exercises and applied these skills to their daily lives.[149] Specifically, in the inflammatory stage, it is important for individuals to keep their spine in a mid-range position to decrease the irritation on healing structures and allow for inflammation to subside and a functional scar to form.

Clinically, it is helpful to experience the neutral range in different body positions, as it can change based on load, support, time of day, and stage of healing. The neutral range is found to vary among patients and, depending on the direction of preference found during ROM testing, patients may benefit from standing with slight knee flexion for a flexion bias, or sitting at the edge of a chair with the hips abducted for an extension bias, for example. Individuals should learn the muscular support necessary to maintain their lumbar neutral position as they transition from one movement to another, such as log rolling to get out of bed. From here, instruction on how to squat is also very useful on day one, as patients learn to function in their home and work environments while limiting repetitive flexion of the spine (Fig. 5).[97]

Active pumping of inflammatory fluid

Small bouts of unloading through the day by using the scapular depressors, as discussed earlier with the chair care exercise[29] (Fig. 4), will help to pump the inflammatory fluid out of the spine. Many positions can accomplish this, for example: hooklying gently pushing arms into an exercise ball (Fig. 7) or hooklying and pulling down from a Theraband® or towel; lying prone relaxed over an exercise ball; seated leaning on armrests or on elbows at a table; standing and leaning on a countertop, grocery cart, a walker, between two chairs, or hanging from a pull-up bar. The unloading should not be so strong to stretch underlying pathological structures at end range, but just enough so that the patient feels a release of pressure on the spine.

Muscle contraction

In the early phases of healing, gentle muscle contractions are beneficial to actively circulate inflammatory fluid that may have accumulated in the spine. Isometrically contracting the gluteals, abdominals, scapular depressors, and spinal extensors at a patient-chosen intensity for a short duration without increasing pain can assist in circulation of inflammatory exudates as the viscoelastic structures receive gentle compression and relaxation. Trunk muscle co-contraction increases the compression

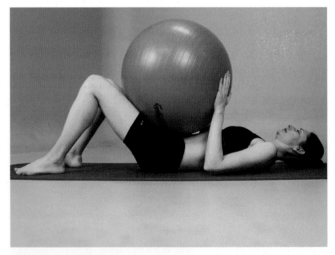

FIG. 7: (1) Unloading in hooklying: Both hands gently press the ball into the thighs, slowly building the distraction at the spine. The pressure is gentle and short of pain, abdominal muscle contraction, or lumbar movement. (2) Bracing: A contraction of the deep spinal muscles is maintained as both hands gradually press the ball with stronger force into the thighs

at the spine by 12–18%[150] and, while in the long run this will improve the stability of the spine, in the initial phases of healing a strong contraction will likely increase discomfort. For this reason, beginning in a low-load position such as hooklying will conservatively strive to limit any increase in pain from further compression (as with seated exercise) along with instructing the patient to contract their muscles at a lower intensity.

Contraction of the transverse abdominis without spinal movement serves to support the spine similar to a corset, as well as addresses the latency and motor control issues in this muscle.[151] Feedback to the patient can be given with tactile cues medial to the iliac crests. The exercises can be progressed in a variety of ways with co-contraction of the internal oblique, the pelvic floor, and multifidus muscles, in coordination with breathing (Fig. 6).

On a cautionary note, when the transverse abdominis contracts, there is an automatic firing of the pelvic floor muscles,[152] which help stabilize the spine.[46] In light of the common muscle imbalances that occur with LBP, the pelvic floor muscles may show signs of hypertonicity and continuing to contract them will only perpetuate the problem. Being attentive to the findings of elimination disorders, pelvic pain, cystitis, vulvodynia, or vaginismus can help to address their muscle imbalances and pain.[153]

Motor control training of the multifidus can begin initially in non-weight bearing positions with tactile cueing on the muscle as the patient imagines the tailbone moving posteriorly, the heels and back of skull coming closer together, or the spine moving toward the pubic bone. No actual spine movement occurs but a bulging of the muscle should be felt under the fingertips. This can be progressed to a co-contraction with the transverse abdominis, internal oblique, and pelvic floor muscles, in coordination with diaphragmatic breathing.

Because one muscle alone cannot provide stability to the spine,[154] movements that engage more global muscles can commence after the deeper muscle contractions have been established. Bracing involves the contraction of both deep and superficial muscles entirely,[155] with the extent of contraction related to the difficulty of the exercise. It should be instructed to begin with the deeper transverse abdominis and multifidus co-contraction and maintained as the muscle recruitment progresses to larger, more global muscles, depending on the exercise or activity. Individuals who learn to brace their abdominals with daily activities have been shown to have improved long-term decreases in LBP.[146]

Exercise progression

A variety of exercises can enhance the motor control and stability of the spine by co-contracting supporting muscles while maintaining the functional position. Contractions are all initiated with the deep transverse abdominis and multifidus first prior to bracing with other muscles. Care needs to be taken to choose an appropriate amount of muscle contraction as bracing the trunk muscles will also increase lumbar compression.[150] These can be started in the acute phase, though many will have better success in the subacute due to less pain with muscle contraction. Exercises such as pressing into the ball (Fig. 7) will contract a greater number of trunk muscles and allow the patient to feel their muscles having to stabilize against the natural tendency to move into lumbar extension. Other exercises are depicted in Figures 8 to 15, in order of increasing difficulty. While the load on the spine needs to be light in the inflammatory stage, the exercises can be modified for each individual by adjusting the number of exercises, strength of contraction, duration of holds, repetitions, and directional preference. All of these exercises can be done with a lumbar corset on, or with the spine taped for added stability, support, or proprioception as needed. Manual cueing by the practitioner is strongly encouraged to enhance the contraction of the desired muscles.

Cardiovascular

With fluid circulation and exchange of nutrients as the goal throughout treatment, gradual cardiovascular exercise will benefit the healing process. When patients are able to maintain a co-contraction of their trunk muscles and perform alternating lower extremity movements in a controlled and pain-free manner, they can progress to cardiovascular machines performed with controlling load in mind. In the inflammatory stage they may be unable to perform such exercise, but if so then 5–10 minutes of load-controlled motion is a good starting point and may include treadmill walking with body weight support,[156,157] a recline bike (Fig. 16), or an upright bike with walker support (Fig. 17).

Fibroblastic (Repair) Stage

This occurs from days 3 to 20, during the subacute phase. In this stage, patients are beginning to feel better but unfortunately this puts them at risk for reinjury as they

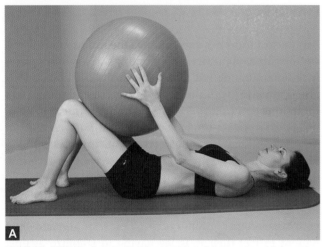
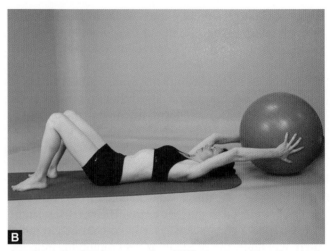

FIGS 8A AND B: Bracing with transitional movement of the arms overhead resisting lumbar extension. (A) The start position. Exercise is initiated with transverse abdominis and multifidus contraction; (B) The end position. Movement is slow and lumbar motion is controlled as the ball is raised overhead

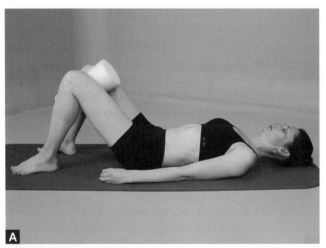
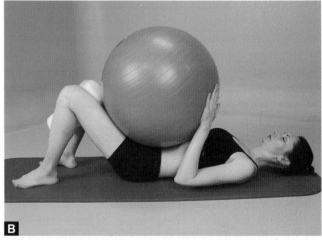

FIGS 9A AND B: (A) Transverse abdominis and multifidus activation initiates and contraction is maintained as the hips isometrically adduct; (B) Progress to adduction with a ball press into thighs

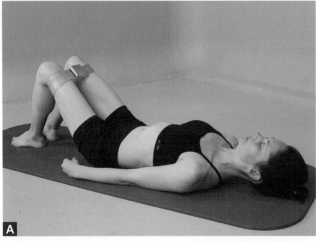
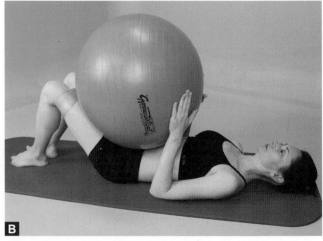

FIGS 10A AND B: (A) Transverse abdominis and multifidus activation initiates and contraction is maintained as the hips isometrically abduct against a belt; (B) Progress to abduction with a ball press into thighs

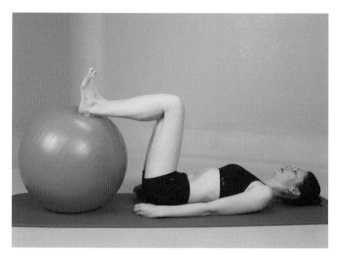

FIG. 11: Heel digs into ball. With the legs in 90° of hip and knee flexion it helps to pre-position the spine in slight flexion, however compensatory patterns, such as increased lumbar extension or increased lumbar flexion should be monitored

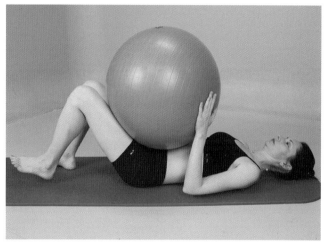

FIG. 13: Bracing with foot lifts. The deep spine muscles are activated prior to the arms pressing the ball into the thighs. The ball maintains equal pressure on each thigh as one foot is unloaded from the floor

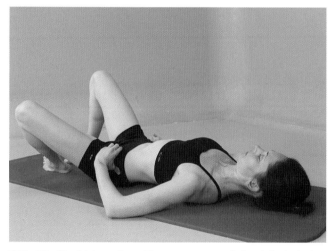

FIG. 12: Hooklying clam. The transverse abdominis is being monitored with self-palpation, to maintain the contraction while a single knee is abducted. Co-contraction with the multifidus and internal obliques is ideal

may resume previous poor habits. The collagen strength is only at 15% of normal at the end of the repair stage[63] and, thus, the scar may be easily stressed beyond capacity resulting in a setback.

Modalities and treatment directed at inflammation may still be necessary, though a gradual weaning from passive treatment to more active movement should occur through this stage.

Lumbar motion is still controlled, though not as strongly as in the inflammatory stage. Bracing with a corset is still a good option and will continue to provide proprioceptive feedback and external support to keep movement short of end ranges so patients are able to be more functional.[141,142]

Manual therapy may take a more prominent role depending on the findings. A common area of muscular issues (tension, pain, spasm, trigger points and guarding) is at the gluteus medius, maximus, minimus, and tensor fascia latae muscles on the same side as the LBP. There are many soft tissue techniques than can be employed, with the goal of limiting pull or stress at the healing lumbar joints. Functional massage is one technique in which the practitioner shortens the muscle, tacks the muscle with manual pressure, and then lengthens the muscle maintaining the tacked pressure (Fig. 18).

Exercises are gradually progressed in difficulty by increasing the subjective percent of maximum muscle contraction, increasing the speed, decreasing the support, and increasing the muscles necessary to maintain a position. See Figures 19 to 24 for examples.

Gradually incorporate balance exercises in the patient's controlled range. Balance can be challenged by decreasing the base of support, increasing the speed of movement, asymmetrical limb movements, and increasing the lever arm. See Figures 25 to 29 for examples.

Cardiovascular exercise can be increased per patient tolerance while still maintaining control of load on spine (Figs 16 and 17).

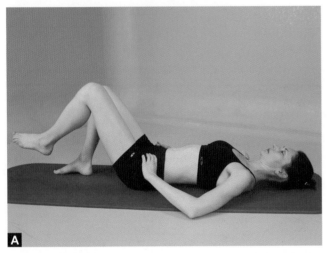 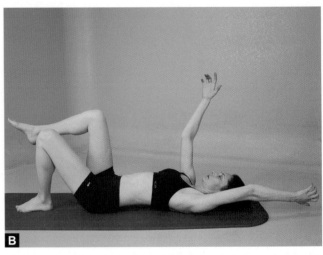

FIGS 14A AND B: Dead bug. (A) Marching by slowly lifting the foot in an attempt to minimize lumbar movement along with self-palpation of the transverse abdominis. (B) Progression of marching with alternating arm movement overhead. The practitioner can watch or feel to ensure neutral spine is maintained and give tactile cues at the transverse abdominis to encourage its firing

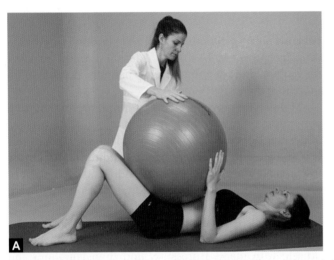 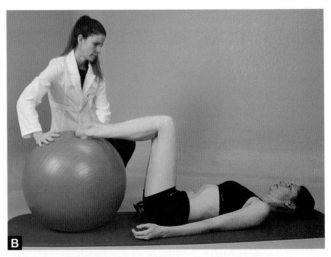

FIGS 15A AND B: Manual resisted exercises. (A) The individual initiates contraction of the deep spinal muscles and braces with the ball between hands and thighs; and (B) With a heel dig. The practitioner tells the patient what direction to expect as gradual resistance is applied to the ball and the patient resists the movement. An example of the verbal command would be "Don't let me move the ball toward your head." The force should start out very light—enough for the patient to feel slight added work. Initial movements should resist in caudal-cranial directions. As the patient is doing well, progression is then to resist medial-lateral directions, diagonals, and then finally resisting rotation, or twisting, of the ball. The practitioner will notice that slight changes in force, amplitude, and direction will create a challenging environment for the patient

Remodeling Stage

This occurs from weeks 6 to 12, at the latter end of the subacute phase. In this stage adequate tension needs to be placed on the healing tissue so as to allow for collagen remodeling to occur and provide a functional scar as the end product. Patients are still vulnerable to reinjury and increasing the resistance in this later stage should be done gradually to slowly toughen the tissues for normal forces in the daily routine of the individual.

Motion is controlled actively and no longer through external means of a brace.[158]

Advance the activation of local and global muscles at higher intensities. Many of the same exercises that have been shown in the earlier stages can be progressed to higher levels by increasing speed of movement, adding weights and resistance, adding asymmetrical movement, and decreasing the base of support. Figures 30 to 34 depict advanced exercises that a patient can be progressed to.

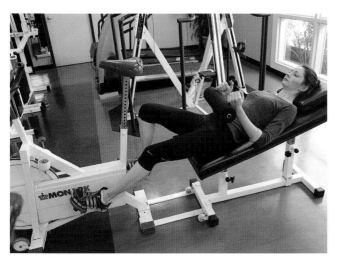

FIG. 16: Recline bike. A padded adjustable arm is attached to a bench to allow for self-unloading as the individual peddles. Training to get on and off safely, to find their functional range and to brace their deep and superficial spine muscles while peddling will limit unwanted movement at the lumbar spine. A lumbar corset may also be worn if there is poor endurance to maintain a safe position

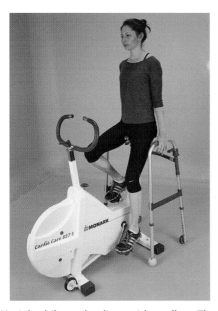

FIG. 17: Upright bike unloading with walker. The walker is adjusted to allow straight elbow unloading with the scapular depressors. Instruction is given to maintain co-contraction of trunk muscles when peddling. Initial training begins with light resistance and short duration, and progresses as symptoms and muscle control allow

Stretching exercises can be implemented at any time a tight muscle becomes a predominant aspect or is inhibiting correct form. It is important to stretch the adductors

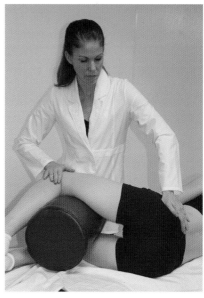

FIG. 18: Functional massage of the gluteus medius. The patient's leg is relaxed in an abducted position on the bolster, allowing it to be in a shortened position. The practitioner then manually tacks the muscle and holds this pressure while the patient adducts the knee into the bolster to create a lengthening effect and simultaneously inhibiting the gluteus medius from reflexively guarding

(Fig. 35), as tightness in these muscles can prevent full depth of squat, necessary for good body mechanics. A shortened iliopsoas is commonly found in individuals whose occupations involve sitting, and hence needs to be stretched (Fig. 36). Being able to stretch the hamstrings without increasing the flexion load on the lumbar spine is a common challenge and is addressed in Figure 37. Manually stretching these muscles may also be warranted, especially if the muscle tightness is preventing progression of treatment or is contributing to pain (Fig. 38).

Cardiovascular exercise in this phase can intensify, e.g., 30 minutes at a moderate intensity while still maintaining control of load on spine as in the earlier stages. The bicycles (Figs 16 and 17) can have increased tension. Aquatic exercises may be trialed in this phase if the patient has good trunk strength and coordination to brace against the resistance of the water. Treadmill walking on an incline (Fig. 39) and the Versa climber® (Fig. 40) are also good options.

Joint mobilization may also be warranted if hypomobility of the underlying segments is a predominant finding (versus inflammation or increased muscle tension).[71] There are many effective ways to mobilize a joint with the goals of reducing pain and lengthening

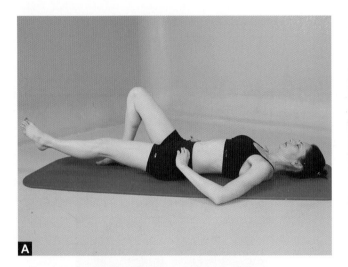

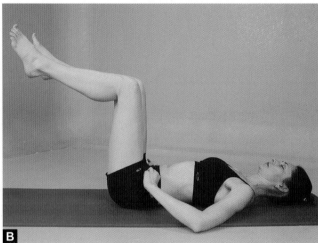

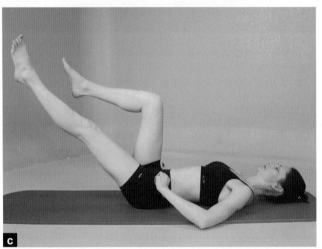

FIGS 19A TO C: Lower extremity dead bug progression. (A) The patient is monitoring a strong contraction of the transverse abdominis and limiting lumbar movement into extension and rotation, while keeping one foot on the floor and extending the other leg. Instructing the patient to keep both anterior superior iliac spines level can help minimize rotatory motion of the spine; (B) The patient has progressed to both legs raised to 90° hip and knee flexion as a starting point; (C) One leg moves out in front by straightening the knee, then returning to the start position, again monitoring for lumbar extension and rotation. As the patient becomes stronger, the extended leg can reach down closer to the ground

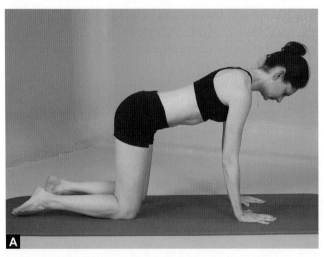

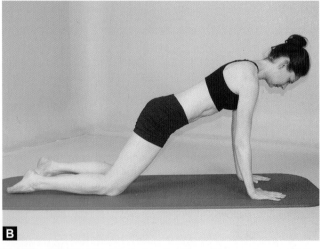

FIGS 20A AND B: Quadruped. (A) In the starting position the individual is advised to find their functional position and contract the deep muscles; (B) As the hips move forward in front of the knees, the gravitational force to fall into lumbar extension is great and the abdominal contraction becomes stronger to counteract the force

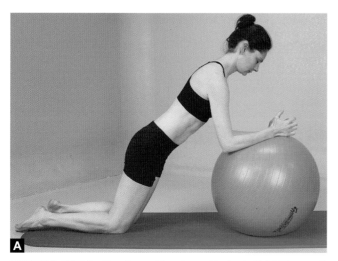 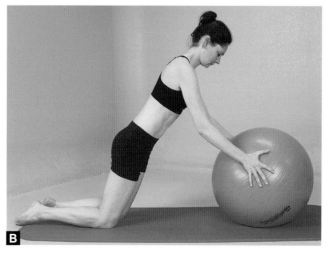

FIGS 21A AND B: Quadruped bracing with the ball. (A) The trunk muscles are braced as the individual moves the hips forward over the knees and onto the forearms on the ball. The further away the ball is from the individual, the more difficult the exercise with increased muscle activation; (B) The ball is squeezed laterally increasing difficultly as the base of support of the upper limbs is minimized

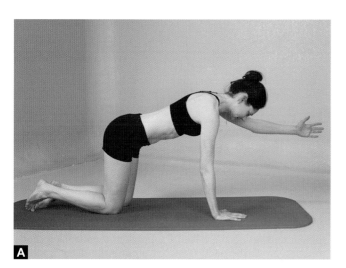 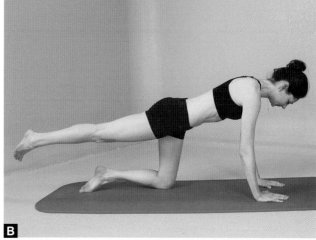

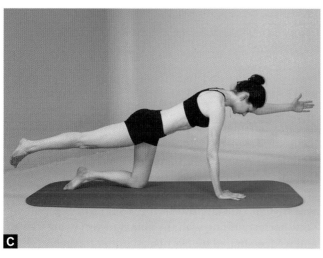

FIGS 22A TO C: Quadruped limb movement progression. The individual initiates deep spine muscle contraction of transverse abdominis and multifidus and then performs— (A) Arm movement alone; (B) Leg movement alone; and (C) Both opposing arm and leg

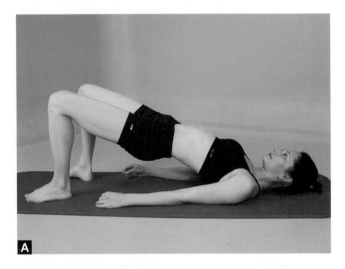
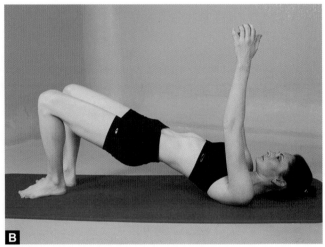
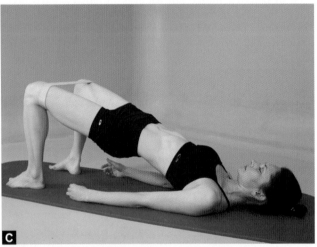
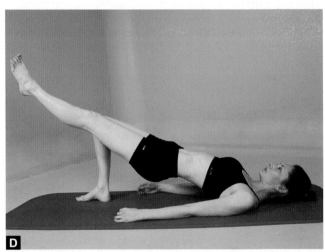

FIGS 23A TO D: Bridge progression. (A) With feet shoulder width apart, the deep spine muscles are contracted prior to the gluteals lifting the entire spine off the ground in one unit. The height achieved varies, with the patient maintaining their functional range short of pain; (B) The exercise is performed with bilateral arms in the air, decreasing the base of support and enhancing global muscle contraction for stability; (C) To further activate the gluteal muscles, an elastic band is placed around the distal thighs or the practitioner resisting abduction manually; (D) Resisting a rotatory component by lifting one leg prior to rising up, keeping the anterior superior iliac spines level

tightened connective tissue. One such way is with a treatment wedge to produce gapping at the facet joints (Fig. 41).

Alternative Treatments

Many patients often seek out complementary and alternative medicine in an adjunctive capacity with contemporary treatment.[159] Some common examples include chiropractic manipulation and acupuncture. These practitioners aim to achieve the same goals of long-term pain relief and functional improvement in people with LBP.

Chiropractors use a multimodal approach to therapy but many of the therapies they use have not been subjected to rigorous scientific scrutiny.[160] These include an Activator (a hand-held spring-loaded device that delivers an impulse to the spine), drop piece (a chiropractic treatment table with a segmented drop system that quickly lowers the section of the patient's body corresponding with the spinal region being treated) and wedge-shaped blocks placed under the pelvis.[160]

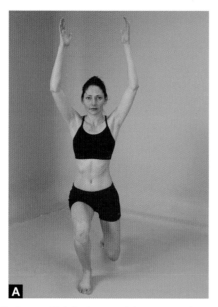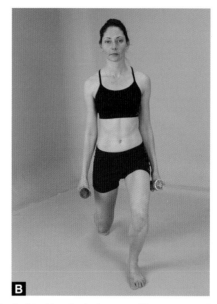

FIGS 24A AND B: Lunge. This is shown with a toe touch on the behind leg for balance and keeping nearly all of the weight on the front leg as the body is lowered toward the ground. The back leg returns to the forward position next to the front foot to complete the set. The practitioner watches that the knee does not fall into valgus, the chest does not fall into flexion, and that the anterior superior iliac spine remains nearly horizontal. (A) The beginning level with arms elevated to maintain upright thoracic posture; (B) In the remodeling stage, weights can be added

Acupuncture is based on the Chinese philosophy that energy flow, called Qi, courses in meridians (or channels) connecting the organs of the body.[161] This energy is a balance between dark (Yin) and light (Yang) and when the Qi is disrupted, disease is present.[161] Along the meridians are over 400 openings to the body and they are the acupuncture points.[161] Filiform needles are placed at the appropriate points based on evaluation and are manipulated to obtain the De Qi sensation from the patient, which is a feeling of heaviness, numbness, or tightness.[162] Evidence does show a positive effect on LBP in the chronic stages.[163]

In addition, dietary changes have also been encouraged. A high BMI has been shown to be associated with LBP,[13,164] and other symptoms of a poor diet are also related, such as atherosclerotic lesions in the abdominal aorta and the lumbar vessels themselves.[16] When this arterial supply becomes stenosed, diffusion of nutrients into the disk is impaired.[165] A whole foods plant-based diet (plant foods in their whole form, especially vegetables, fruits, legumes, and seeds and nuts) with vitamin B12 fortified foods/supplements[166] has shown to have many health benefits,[167,168] especially related to LBP is a decrease in the build-up of cholesterol in the bloodstream[169] and lower BMI.[170]

Medical and Surgical Considerations

Persistent, chronic LBP is frequently treated with minimally invasive procedures prior to surgical intervention. Injections are often initially diagnostic in nature to determine the pain producing structures and may take multiple trials to achieve the desired therapeutic effect. The lumbar disk and facet joint interventions described later are often performed in combination with a rehabilitation program in hopes that as the pain is lessened, the patient will become more functional as well as learn to modify activities that put undue stress on the healing structures.

Disk Interventions

Epidural steroid injections

Steroid medication has powerful anti-inflammatory effects and, unlike oral medication, it does not rely on blood flow to be delivered to a region where it may already be limited due to compression from a disk herniation[171] or atherosclerosis.[165] The epidural space is a continuous anatomic compartment extending from the base of the skull to the sacrum that can be entered at various levels and by various routes.[171] Injections of a corticosteroid and/or a local anesthetic are regularly performed with

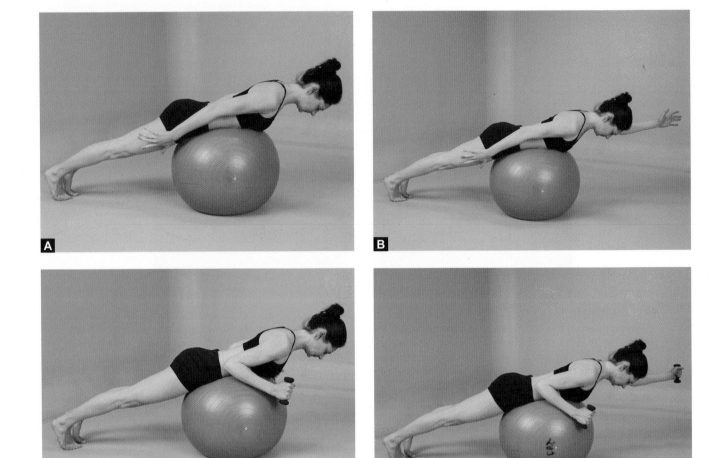

FIGS 25A TO D: Swim progression. The hands begin on the ground as the patient straightens the legs with feet together, contracts the quad and gluteal muscles, then pushes up onto their fingertips to align the body on an incline over the ball. (A) At this point, the arms are gradually raised while balance is maintained and manual cueing to the gluteals is done by the practitioner to keep their contraction strong. When the patient fatigues and is ready to rest, the arms are lowered to the ground first before gluteal contraction is relaxed to prevent excessive lumbar movement; (B) When demonstrating a strong gluteal contraction and steady with balance, the arms can alternate raising overhead in a swim fashion to progress the difficulty; (C) Progressing to weights and balancing; (D) Taking one weight at a time overhead

fluoroscopic visualization into the epidural space of the spine either by caudal, interlaminar, or transforaminal approaches.[172] Each of the three approaches show strong evidence for short-term pain relief (6 weeks or less)[171] with disk herniation or radiculitis, and show fair evidence for spinal stenosis, discogenic pain, and postsurgery pain syndrome.[173,174]

Selective nerve root blocks

This terminology commonly refers to a transforaminal epidural steroid injection, in which the anesthetic and corticosteroid are injected under fluoroscopy on a specific

nerve root, versus attempting to bathe the epidural space.[175]

Facet Joint Interventions

Intra-articular facet joint injections

Similar to an epidural injection, an intra-articular facet joint injection uses corticosteroids in combination with an anesthetic solution which is injected into the painful facet joint to block the nociceptors and produce an anti-inflammatory effect.[176] Immediately postinjection, the patient's LBP typically resolves completely mainly due to

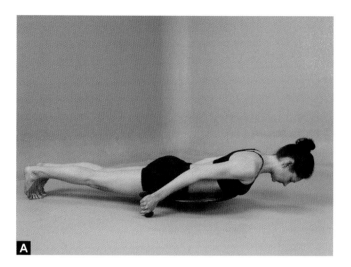

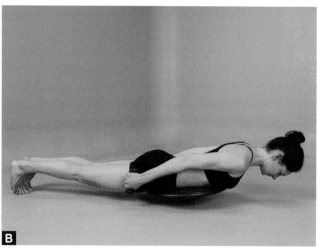

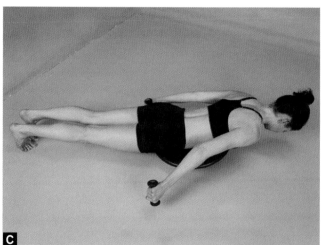

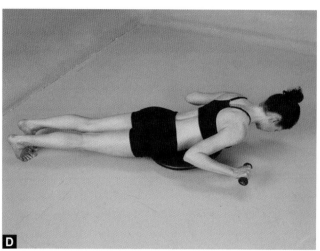

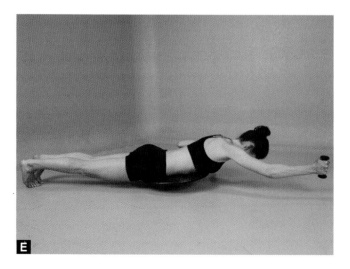

FIGS 26A TO E: Prone balance board progression. Prone position on the board with feet together, legs straight, and a neutral cervical posture. The gluteals and abdominals will work to counteract hyperextension. These pictures are depicted with weights but exercise should begin without weight and added to progress the difficulty as strength and balance improve. (A) Bilateral hands are contacting the ground as the patient gains control and balance; (B) Holding arms next to thighs; (C) Asymmetrical lateral arm movement only as far as they can maintain balance and control; (D) Bilateral arms near shoulders; (E) Asymmetrical arm movement overhead

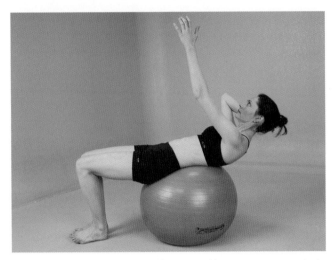 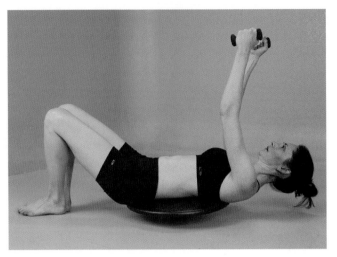

FIG. 27: Supine bracing on ball. Feet and knees are progressively brought close together as balance is achieved. A neutral lumbar spine is maintained with the deeper spinal muscles contracted and additional global, active bracing of the abdominal muscles to prevent lordosis. One arm supports the head, the other begins straight up, as shown, and the patient moves the arm laterally maintaining balance then returns to the starting position. The arm can also move overhead and back. The practitioner watches for signs of fatigue with the pubic bone or the shoulder blades dropping. Exercise progression may include: a hand-held weight, manual resistance applied to the arm, or an increase in arm movement speed

FIG. 28: Supine bracing on board. This picture shows the patient in a high level position with both arms raised and with weights. Beginners should start with feet and knees together, one hand behind the head, the other straight up and without weight. Balance is challenged with asymmetrical arm movements overhead and lateral with the distance the arm is moved depending on how well balance in maintained. The practitioner should watch for compensatory knee swaying to the opposite side of arm movement as well as increase in lumbar lordosis as the abdominals fatigue

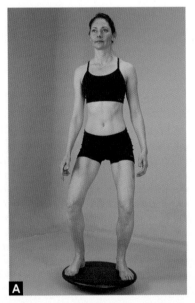 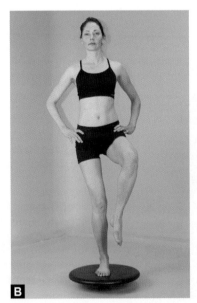 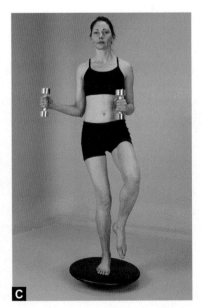

FIGS 29A TO C: Standing balance. (A) Beginning level with slight knee bend and abdominals engaged. Initially this is performed with fingertip support on a stationary object; (B) Single leg balance; (C) Remodeling stage progression with lateral arm movements followed by weights in both double limb and single limb balance exercises

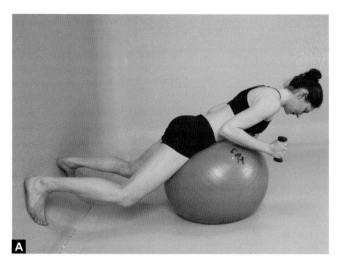
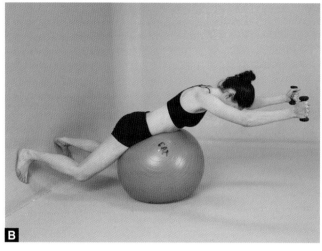

FIGS 30A AND B: Ball on wall. The ball is positioned under the abdominals. The knees are slightly bent, gluteals squeezed tight, and the thoracic spine is held to attain a neutral lumbar position. (A) Start position; (B) Progression with arms overhead

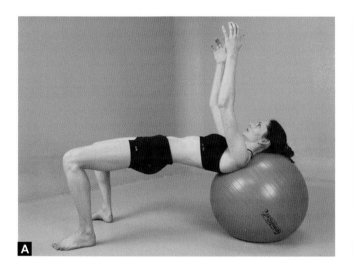
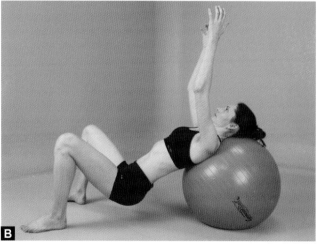

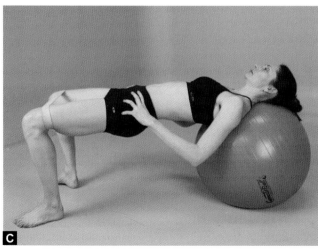
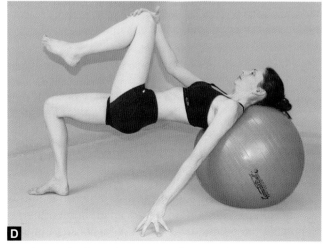

FIGS 31A TO D: Bridge on ball progression. (A) The starting position with muscles braced to support the neutral spine; (B) The end position with the patient hinging at the shoulder blades to keep the spine in neutral; (C) Progressed to resisting abduction with elastic band around thighs; (D) Single limb bridge is advanced with opposite hand and knee contact

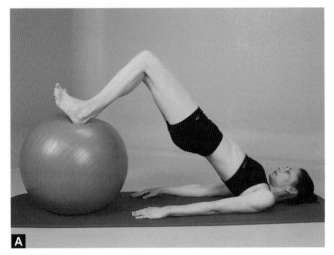 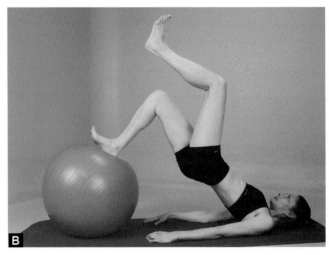

FIGS 32A AND B: Reverse bridge. (A) The patient begins with heels on the ball and lifts the entire spine up hinging at the shoulder blades. When the patient is able to, they can roll the ball away and return limiting movement in the lumbar spine; (B) Single limb reverse bridge is a higher level progression and the ball rolls in and out without lumbopelvic motion

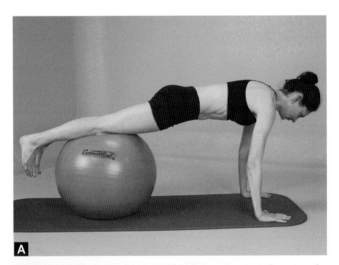 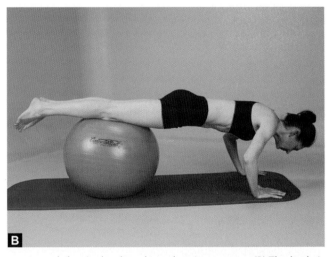

FIGS 33A AND B: Push up. (A) The deep spine muscles, scapular protractors, abdominals, gluteals are bracing to start; (B) The body is lowered and raised without lumbopelvic motion

the anesthetic effect, while the effect from the steroid may take 1–5 days to develop.[177] Pain relief can last as long as 1–2 years, though some never achieve relief despite positive effects with the anesthesia.[177] If steroid injections fail to control the pain, more advanced management may be needed with radiofrequency ablation.[177]

Facet joint nerve blocks/medial branch block

This diagnostic procedure involves the injection of an anesthetic solution to the medial branch nerves supplying the painful facet joints. A response of at least 80% improvement in pain indicates the procedure will be useful for further therapeutic injections with a

steroid,[178] as well as respond favorably to radiofrequency ablation.[179]

Radiofrequency ablation/neurotomy

This temporary denervation to the nerves supplying the facet joint involves using energy in the form of radio waves to perform necrosis of the medial branches of the dorsal rami.[180] A successful outcome is considered to be at least 50% reduction in pain which may last up to 1 year.[177] With the multifidus muscle also receiving innervations from the medial branches, atrophic changes are frequently found after this procedure and return as the axons regenerate.[181,182]

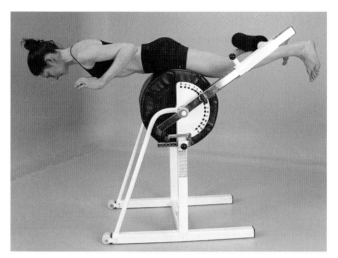

FIG. 34: Back trainer. This specialized equipment has a dial to change the amount of knee flexion and the leg pad at the calf can be adjusted to raise or lower to limit or enhance leg muscle involvement in the stabilization. The practitioner ensures strong gluteal activation with manual cues and that the spine maintains a neutral position. Patients do not move the spine but maintain the suspended position as shown in the picture. Handheld weights moved overhead and laterally can progress the exercise

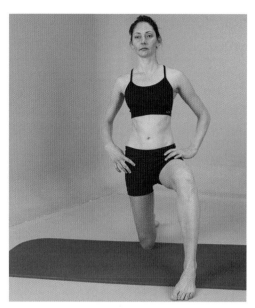

FIG. 36: Iliopsoas stretch shown on the individual's right leg. The back foot can be taken laterally to increase hip internal rotation. The right gluteal muscles are strongly contracted to promote a posterior pelvic tilt and that position is maintained as the individual lunges forward bringing the pelvis over the knee. A slight lateral bend away can intensify the stretch further

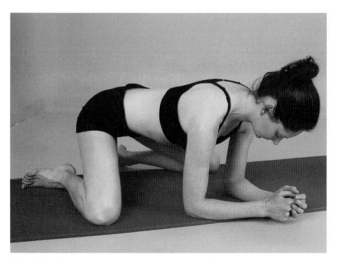

FIG. 35: Short adductor stretch. In kneeling and on elbows, the patient gently slides the knees apart until the onset of muscular tension. The tailbone is directed up toward the ceiling as the patient gently sits back posteriorly toward the heels to intensify the stretch

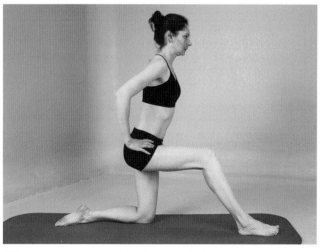

FIG. 37: Hamstring stretch. The individual strives to tilt the pelvis anteriorly to achieve a stretch while maintaining knee flexion to keep the sciatic nerve on slack. Holding a stationary object (chair) to maintain balance can be helpful

Ligament Intervention

Prolotherapy

This involves the injection of various types of solutions (irritant, chemotactic, osmotic) into the damaged ligaments and tendons to facilitate the body's healing process through inflammation of the connective tissue.[159] This is particularly useful in painful, hypermobile joints to toughen the tissues and promote joint stability.

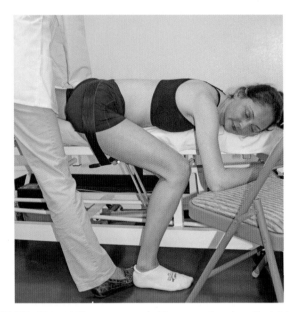

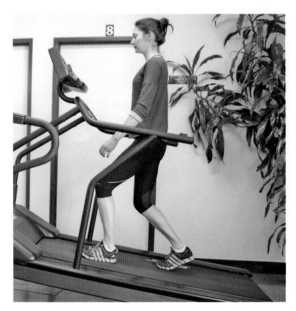

FIG. 38: Manual iliopsoas stretch. The set-up involves the table at a height to allow forward flexion of the uninvolved leg to prevent lumbar lordosis during the stretch. The patient has the upper body side-bent away and resting on a chair. A belt is wrapped under the table and on the patient below the posterior superior iliac spines and is tightened considerably to allow for relaxation as well as to keep the spine in neutral. The leg on the table is internally rotated and held in place with pressure on the greater trochanter. The leg-piece of the table is slowly lifted until a stretch is felt to the anterior hip and pelvis region. The patient can be asked to press the leg into the table to contract the muscle and then on relaxation the leg-piece may be moved higher or added pressure at the posterior hip joint may be applied

FIG. 39: Treadmill exercise is done on an incline (shown at 15% grade) to promote a squat walk for increased muscular shock absorption to minimize load on the spine. In addition the trunk muscles are braced and the individual is taught to limit the body from moving up and down with every step by stabilizing their gaze

Surgical Procedures

Discectomy

The primary goal of this type of surgery is to retrieve the herniated disk fragments and decompression of the nerve roots in patients with radicular pain from disk herniation, protrusion, or prolapse.[174] While the evidence is limited, exercise programs starting at 4–6 weeks postsurgery lead to faster decreases in pain and disability.[183]

Laminectomy

This surgery removes the lamina to widen the spinal canal and is considered the gold standard for patients with lumbar spinal stenosis.[184] The goal of surgery is to decrease radicular leg symptoms, but a decrease in LBP is also common.[184]

Foraminotomy

Those with radiculopathy due to lumbar foraminal stenosis may benefit from a foraminotomy, where the

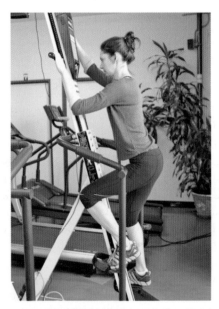

FIG. 40: The Versa climber® allows the individual to brace the trunk muscles while the legs and arms move in opposition to each other. The squat is maintained to prevent lateral bending and the arms are able to pull down providing some unloading to the spine during exercise

hypertrophied part of the facet and ligamentum flavum is removed to widen the foramen for the exiting nerve root.[185]

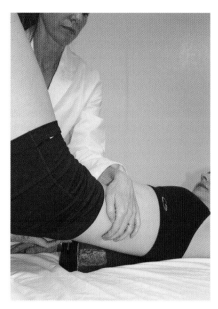

FIG. 41: Anterior-posterior vertebrae mobilization with treatment wedge. The leg-piece of the table is lifted to help the patient raise the spine up. The wedge is placed under the spine and contacts the transverse processes of the superior vertebrae at the desired hypomobile level. The practitioner palpates the interspinous space to feel for movement as pressure is directed posteriorly from the abdomen. The patient is instructed to maintain a posterior pelvic tilt to ensure the segments below (which may be hypermobile) do not fall into extension. Mobilization is coordinated with exhalation of a deep breath and the patient may need to do this multiple times a day to get the desired effect

Lumbar interbody fusion

In order to achieve stabilization of a degenerated motion segment, all disk material is removed and is replaced with an autogenic, allogenic, or synthetic bone graft.[186,187] There are many different approaches to achieve this, with most using rods, screws, plates, or cages to hold the graft material in place in order for it to fuse to the upper and lower vertebral bodies. With the elimination of painful motion at the fusion site, a complication is adjacent segment disease in which the increased stress is place on the nonoperated segments above and below.[188,189] Thus, a rehabilitation program focused on lumbar stabilization will continue to be the goal postsurgically.

Total disk arthroplasty

As an alternative to fusion, this surgery replaces the degenerated disk with an intervertebral prosthesis in an attempt to decrease pain while preserving ROM to reduce adjacent segment disease.[186]

CONCLUSION

Due to the complex nature of LBP, treating this population in physical therapy may present as a daunting task. There are many different risk factors that set up an individual for experiencing LBP, as well as occupational and psychosocial factors that may pose as difficult hurdles to overcome in therapy.

A thorough examination will help to understand the individual's functional loss characteristics and stage of healing as avenues to help categorize patients into treatment groups. In addition, patients are categorically determined based on their primary source of dysfunction as either due to inflammation, muscle guarding or tension, or a mobility issue, either hypermobility or hypomobility. This chapter discussed a treatment progression through an acute inflammatory presentation and there are far more treatment techniques that could have benefit if a patient's main finding was primarily muscle guarding or mobility dysfunction.

Regardless of the stage of healing, the goals of a treatment program are to protect the spinal segment, limit the spinal load, protect the neural structures, diminish fear avoidance behavior, motor control of the deep spine stabilizers prior to global muscle contractions, challenge proprioception and balance, and patient education.

Physical therapy treatment in the inflammatory acute and subacute stages is aimed at understanding the healing process and enabling the patient to remain active while allowing a functional scar to form. Early physical therapy intervention can help in many ways, but specifically to restore normal movement patterns that do not automatically return on their own and provide patient reassurance with education, both of which have been shown to decrease the acute LBP from turning into a chronic condition.

The treatment presented in this chapter is easily modified and can be an adjunct to other complementary and alternative treatments, as well as minimally invasive procedures and surgeries, to fit individual needs.

REFERENCES

1. Hoy D, Brooks P, Blyth F, Buchbinder R. The epidemiology of low back pain. Best Pract Res Clin Rheumatol. 2010;24(6):769-81.
2. Nachemson AL. The lumbar spine: an othopaedic challenge. Spine. 1976; 1(1):59-70.
3. US Burden of Disease Collaborators. The state of US health, 1990–2010: burden of diseases, injuries, and risk factors. J Am Med Assoc. 2013; 310(6):591-608.

4. Dionne CE, Dunn KM, Croft PR, Nachemson AL, Buchbinder R, Walker BF, et al. A consensus approach toward the standardization of back pain definitions for use in prevalence studies. Spine. 2008;33(1):95-103.

5. Guo HR. Working hours spent on repeated activities and prevalence of back pain. Occup Environ Med. 2002;59(10):680-8.

6. Waterman BR, Belmont PJ, Schoenfeld AJ. Low back pain in the United States: incidence and risk factors for presentation in the emergency setting. Spine J. 2012;12(1):63-70.

7. Gilkey DP, Keefe TJ, Peel JL, Kassab OM, Kennedy CA. Risk factors associated with back pain: a cross-sectional study of 963 college students. J Manipulative Physiol Ther. 2010;33(2):88-95.

8. Hirsch O, Strauch K, Held H, Redaelli M, Chenot JF, Leonhardt C, et al. Low back pain patient subgroups in primary care-pain characteristics, psychosocial determinants and health care utilization. Clin J Pain. 2014;30(12):1023-32.

9. Adams MA, Dolan P. Intervertebral disc degeneration: evidence for two distinct phenotypes. J Anat. 2012;221(6):497-506.

10. Abate M, Vanni D, Pantalone A, Salini V. Cigarette smoking and musculoskeletal disorders. Muscles Ligaments Tendons J. 2013;3(2):63-9.

11. Andersson GB. Epidemiological features of chronic low-back pain. The Lancet. 1999;354(9178):581-5.

12. Matsui H, Kanamori M, Ishihara H, Yudoh K, Naruse Y, Tsuji H. Familial predisposition for lumbar degenerative disc disease. A case-control study. Spine. 1998;23(9):1029-34.

13. Smuck M, Kao MC, Brar N, Martinez-Ith A, Choi J, Tomkins-Lane CC. Does physical activity influence the relationship between low back pain and obesity? Spine J. 2014;14(2):209-16.

14. Kauppila LI, Mikkonen R, Mankinen P, Pelto-Vasenius K, Mäenpää I. MR aortography and serum cholesterol levels in patients with long-term nonspecific lower back pain. Spine. 2004;29(19):2147-52.

15. Roffey DM, Ashdown LC, Dornan HD, Creech MJ, Dagenais S, Dent RM, et al. Pilot evaluation of a multidisciplinary, medically supervised, nonsurgical weight loss program on the severity of low back pain in obese adults. Spine J. 2011;11(3):197-204.

16. Kurunlahti M, Tervonen O, Vanharanta H, Ilkko E, Suramo I. Association of atherosclerosis with low back pain and the degree of disc degeneration. Spine. 1999;24(20):2080-4.

17. Kauppila LI. Atherosclerosis and disc degeneration/low-back pain--a systematic review. Eur J Vasc Endovasc Surg. 2009;37(6):661-70. doi:10.1016/j.ejvs.2009.02.006.

18. McIntosh G, Hall H, Boyle C. Contribution of nonspinal comorbidity to low back pain outcomes. Clin J Pain. 2006;22(9):765-9.

19. Kent PM, Keating JL. Can we predict poor recovery from recent-onset nonspecific low back pain? A systematic review. Man Ther. 2008;13(1):12-28.

20. Waris E, Eskelin M, Hermunen H, Kiviluoto O, Paajanen H. Disc degeneration in low back pain: a 17-year follow-up study using magnetic resonance imaging. Spine. 2007;32(6):681-4.

21. Panjabi MM. The stabilizing system of the spine. Part I. Function, dysfunction, adaptation, and enhancement. J Spinal Disord. 1992;5(4):383-9; discussion 397.

22. Boos N, Weissbach S, Rohrbach H, Weiler C, Spratt KF, Nerlich AG. Classification of age-related changes in lumbar intervertebral discs: 2002 Volvo Award in basic science. Spine. 2002;27(23):2631-44.

23. Twomey L, Taylor J. The lumbar spine: structure, function, age changes and physiotherapy. Aust J Physiother. 1994;40:19-30.

24. Vernon-Roberts B, Moore RJ, Fraser RD. The natural history of age-related disc degeneration: the influence of age and pathology on cell populations in the L4-L5 disc. Spine. 2008;33(25):2767-73.

25. Kuo YW, Hsu YC, Chuang IT, Chao PH, Wang JL. Spinal traction promotes molecular transportation in a simulated degenerative intervertebral disc model. Spine. 2014;39(9):E550-6.

26. Jackson AR, Yuan TY, Huang CY, Brown MD, Gu WY. Nutrient transport in human annulus fibrosus is affected by compressive strain and anisotropy. Ann Biomed Eng. 2012;40(12):2551-8.

27. Jackson AR, Huang CY, Brown MD, Yong Gu W. 3D finite element analysis of nutrient distributions and cell viability in the intervertebral disc: effects of deformation and degeneration. J Biomech Eng. 2011;133(9):91006.

28. Malandrino A, Noailly J, Lacroix D. The effect of sustained compression on oxygen metabolic transport in the intervertebral disc decreases with degenerative changes. PLoS Comput Biol. 2011;7(8):e1002112.

29. Fryer J, Zhang W. Preliminary investigation into a seated unloading movement strategy for the lumbar spine: a pilot study. J Bodyw Mov Ther. 2010;14(2):119-26.

30. Arun R, Freeman BJ, Scammell BE, McNally DS, Cox E, Gowland P. 2009 ISSLS prize winner: what influence does sustained mechanical load have on diffusion in the human intervertebral disc?: an in vivo study using serial postcontrast magnetic resonance imaging. Spine. 2009;34(21):2324-37.

31. Ferrara L, Triano JJ, Sohn MJ, Song E, Lee DD. A biomechanical assessment of disc pressures in the lumbosacral spine in response to external unloading forces. Spine J. 2005;5(5):548-53.

32. Ianuzzi A, Little JS, Chiu JB, Baitner A, Kawchuk G, Khalsa PS. Human lumbar facet joint capsule strains: I. During physiological motions. Spine J. 2004;4(2):141-52.

33. Sharma M, Langrana NA, Rodriguez J. Role of ligaments and facets in lumbar spinal stability. Spine. 1995;20(8):887-900.

34. Solomonow M. Time dependent spine stability: the wise old man and the six blind elephants. Clin Biomech Bristol Avon. 2011;26(3):219-28.

35. Butler D, Trafimow JH, Andersson GB, McNeill TW, Huckman MS. Discs degenerate before facets. Spine. 1990;15(2):111-3.

36. Cohen SP, Raja SN. Pathogenesis, diagnosis, and treatment of lumbar zygapophysial (facet) joint pain. Anesthesiology. 2007;106(3):591-614.

37. Igarashi A, Kikuchi S, Konno S, Olmarker K. Inflammatory cytokines released from the facet joint tissue in degenerative lumbar spinal disorders. Spine. 2004;29(19):2091-5.

38. Tachihara H, Kikuchi S, Konno S, Sekiguchi M. Does facet joint inflammation induce radiculopathy?: an investigation using a rat model of lumbar facet joint inflammation. Spine. 2007;32(4):406-12.

39. Schäfer A, Hall T, Briffa K. Classification of low back-related leg pain--a proposed patho-mechanism-based approach. Man Ther. 2009;14(2):222-30.

40. Solomonow M. Ligaments: a source of musculoskeletal disorders. J Bodyw Mov Ther. 2009;13(2):136-54.

41. Jackson M, Solomonow M, Zhou B, Baratta RV, Harris M. Multifidus EMG and tension-relaxation recovery after prolonged static lumbar flexion. Spine. 2001;26(7):715-23.

42. Ebraheim NA, Hassan A, Lee M, Xu R. Functional anatomy of the lumbar spine. Semin Pain Med. 2004;2(3):131-7.

43. Bergmark A. Stability of the lumbar spine. A study in mechanical engineering. Acta Orthop Scand Suppl. 1989;230:1-54.

44. Boyle KL, Olinick J, Lewis C. The value of blowing up a balloon. North Am J Sports Phys Ther. 2010;5(3):179-88.

45. Janssens L, Brumagne S, McConnell AK, Hermans G, Troosters T, Gayan-Ramirez G. Greater diaphragm fatigability in individuals with recurrent low back pain. Respir Physiol Neurobiol. 2013;188(2):119-23.

46. Bi X, Zhao J, Zhao L, Liu Z, Zhang J, Sun D, et al. Pelvic floor muscle exercise for chronic low back pain. J Int Med Res. 2013;41(1):146-52.

47. Mense S. Muscle Pain: mechanisms and clinical significance. Dtsch Ärztebl Int. 2008;105(12):214-9.

48. Mense S. Pathophysiology of low back pain and the transition to the chronic state-experimental data and new concepts. Schmerz Berl Ger. 2001;15(6):413-7.

49. Leinonen V, Kankaanpää M, Airaksinen O, Hänninen O. Back and hip extensor activities during trunk flexion/extension: effects of low back pain and rehabilitation. Arch Phys Med Rehabil. 2000;81(1):32-7.

50. Jull GA, Richardson CA. Motor control problems in patients with spinal pain: a new direction for therapeutic exercise. J Manipulative Physiol Ther. 2000;23(2):115-7.

51. Hides J, Gilmore C, Stanton W, Bohlscheid E. Multifidus size and symmetry among chronic LBP and healthy asymptomatic subjects. Man Ther. 2008;13(1):43-9.

52. Williams M, Solomonow M, Zhou BH, Baratta RV, Harris M. Multifidus spasms elicited by prolonged lumbar flexion. Spine. 2000;25(22):2916-24.

53. Park RJ, Tsao H, Cresswell AG, Hodges PW. Changes in direction-specific activity of psoas major and quadratus lumborum in people with recurring back pain differ between muscle regions and patient groups. J Electromyogr Kinesiol. 2013;23(3):734-40.

54. Richardson CA, Jull GA. Muscle control-pain control. What exercises would you prescribe? Man Ther. 1995;1(1):2-10.

55. Kikuchi S, Sato K, Konno S, Hasue M. Anatomic and radiographic study of dorsal root ganglia. Spine. 1994;19(1):6-11.

56. Lauder TD. Musculoskeletal disorders that frequently mimic radiculopathy. Phys Med Rehabil Clin N Am. 2002;13(3):469-85.

57. Spitzer W. Scientific approach to the assessment and management of activity-related spinal disorders. A monograph for clinicians. Report of the Quebec Task Force on Spinal Disorders. Spine. 1987;12(7):S1-59.

58. Waddell G. 1987 Volvo award in clinical sciences. A new clinical model for the treatment of low-back pain. Spine. 1987;12(7):632-44.

59. Koes BW, van Tulder M, Lin CW, Macedo LG, McAuley J, Maher C. An updated overview of clinical guidelines for the management of non-specific low back pain in primary care. Eur Spine J. 2010;19(12):2075-94.

60. Karayannis NV, Jull GA, Hodges PW. Physiotherapy movement based classification approaches to low back pain: comparison of subgroups through review and developer/expert survey. BMC Musculoskelet Disord. 2012;13:24.

61. Vollowitz E. Furniture prescription for the conservative management of low back pain. In: Topics in Acute Care and Trauma Rehabilitation. Netherlands: Aspen Publishers, Inc.; 1988. pp. 18-37.

62. Long A, Donelson R, Fung T. Does it matter which exercise? A randomized control trial of exercise for low back pain. Spine. 2004;29(23):2593-602.

63. Hardy MA. The biology of scar formation. Phys Ther. 1989;69(12):1014-24.

64. Reinke JM, Sorg H. Wound repair and regeneration. Eur Surg Res. 2012;49(1):35-43.

65. Maitland G, Hengeveld E, Banks K, English K. Maitland's Vertebral manipulation, 7th edition. Oxford: Butterworth-Heinemann; 2005.

66. Clarkshon H. Joint motion and function assessment: a research based practical guide. Philadelphia, PA: Lippincott Williams & Wilkins; 2005.

67. Bedekar N, Suryawanshi M, Rairikar S, Sancheti P, Shyam A. Inter and intra-rater reliability of mobile device goniometer in measuring lumbar flexion range of motion. J Back Musculoskelet Rehabil. 2014;27(2):161-6.

68. Kolber MJ, Pizzini M, Robinson A, Yanez D, Hanney WJ. The reliability and concurrent validity of measurements used to quantify lumbar spine mobility: an analysis of an iphone (R) application and gravity based inclinometry. Int J Sports Phys Ther. 2013;8(2):129-37.

69. Werneke MW, Hart DL, Cutrone G, Oliver D, McGill T, Weinberg J, et al. Association between directional preference and centralization in patients with low back pain. J Orthop Sports Phys Ther. 2011;41(1):22-31.

70. Haneline M, Cooperstein R, Young M, Birkeland K. An annotated bibliography of spinal motion palpation reliability studies. J Can Chiropr Assoc. 2009;53(1):40-58.

71. Fritz JM, Whitman JM, Childs JD. Lumbar spine segmental mobility assessment: an examination of validity for determining intervention

72. Childs JD, Fritz JM, Flynn TW, Irrgang JJ, Johnson KK, Majkowski GR, et al. A clinical prediction rule to identify patients with low back pain most likely to benefit from spinal manipulation: a validation study. Ann Intern Med. 2004;141(12):920-8.

73. Hicks GE, Fritz JM, Delitto A, McGill SM. Preliminary development of a clinical prediction rule for determining which patients with low back pain will respond to a stabilization exercise program. Arch Phys Med Rehabil. 2005;86(9):1753-62.

74. Frost DM, Beach T, Fenwick C, Callaghan J, McGill S. Is there a low-back cost to hip-centric exercise? Quantifying the lumbar spine joint compression and shear forces during movements used to overload the hips. J Sports Sci. 2012;30(9):859-70.

75. Walsh J, Hall T. Agreement and correlation between the straight-leg raise and slump tests in subjects with leg pain. J Manipulative Physiol Ther. 2009;32(3):184-92.

76. Boyd BS, Wanek L, Gray AT, Topp KS. Mechanosensitivity of the lower extremity nervous system during straight-leg raise neurodynamic testing in healthy individuals. J Orthop Sports Phys Ther. 2009;39(11):780-90.

77. Boyd BS, Wanek L, Gray AT, Topp KS. Mechanosensitivity during lower extremity neurodynamic testing is diminished in individuals with type 2 diabetes mellitus and peripheral neuropathy: a cross sectional study. BMC Neurol. 2010;10:75.

78. Hall T, Elvey R. Management of mechanosensitivity of the nervous system in spinal pain syndromes. In: Modern Manual Therapy of the Vertebral Column. Edinburgh: Churchill Livingstone; 2005. pp. 413-31.

79. Walsh J, Hall T. Reliability, validity and diagnostic accuracy of palpation of the sciatic, tibial and common peroneal nerves in the examination of low back related leg pain. Man Ther. 2009;14(6):623-9.

80. Supik LF, Broom MJ. Sciatic tension signs and lumbar disc herniation. Spine. 1994;19(9):1066-9.

81. Magee D. Orthopedic physical assessment, 5th edition. St. Louis, MO: Saunders Elsevier; 2008.

82. Ferber R, Kendall KD, McElroy L. Normative and critical criteria for iliotibial band and iliopsoas muscle flexibility. J Athl Train. 2010;45(4):344-8.

83. Jorgensson A. The iliopsoas muscle and the lumbar spine. Aust J Physiother. 1993;39(2):125-32.

84. Huang BK, Campos JC, Michael Peschka PG, Pretterklieber ML, Skaf AY, Chung CB, et al. Injury of the gluteal aponeurotic fascia and proximal iliotibial band: anatomy, pathologic conditions, and MR imaging. Radiographics. 2013;33(5):1437-52.

85. Evjenth O, Gloeck C. Symptom localization in the spine and in the extremity joints. First. Orthopedic Physical Therapy Products; 2006.

86. Schneider M, Erhard R, Brach J, Tellin W, Imbarlina F, Delitto A. Spinal palpation for lumbar segmental mobility and pain provocation: an interexaminer reliability study. J Manipulative Physiol Ther. 2008;31(6):465-73.

87. Laslett M, Williams M. The reliability of selected pain provocation tests for sacroiliac joint pathology. Spine. 1994;19(11):1243-9.

88. Cleland J. Orthopaedic clinical examination: an evidence-based approach for physical therapists. Philadelphia, PA: Saunders; 2007.

89. McGill S. Low back disorders: evidence-based prevention and rehabilitation. Illinois: Human Kinetics; 2002.

90. Evans K, Refshauge KM, Adams R. Trunk muscle endurance tests: reliability, and gender differences in athletes. J Sci Med Sport. 2007;10(6):447-55.

91. Straker LM. A review of research on techniques for lifting low-lying objects: 2. Evidence for a correct technique. Work Read Mass. 2003;20(2):83-96.

92. Binder DS, Nampiaparampil DE. The provocative lumbar facet joint. Curr Rev Musculoskelet Med. 2009;2(1):15-24.

93. Dunn KM, Hestbaek L, Cassidy JD. Low back pain across the life course. Best Pract Res Clin Rheumatol. 2013;27(5):591-600.

94. Chou R, Fu R, Carrino JA, Deyo RA. Imaging strategies for low-back pain: systematic review and meta-analysis. Lancet. 2009;373(9662):463-72.

95. Wassenaar M, van Rijn RM, van Tulder MW, Verhagen AP, van der Windt DA, Koes BW, et al. Magnetic resonance imaging for diagnosing lumbar spinal pathology in adult patients with low back pain or sciatica: a diagnostic systematic review. Eur Spine J. 2012;21(2):220-7.

96. Fu MC, Buerba RA, Long WD, Blizzard DJ, Lischuk AW, Haims AH, et al. Inter-rater and intra-rater agreement of magnetic resonance imaging findings in the lumbar spine: significant variability across degenerative conditions. Spine J. 2014;14(10):2442-8. doi:10.1016/j.spinee.2014.03.010.

97. Solomonow M, Zhou BH, Lu Y, King KB. Acute repetitive lumbar syndrome: a multi-component insight into the disorder. J Bodyw Mov Ther. 2012;16(2):134-47.

98. Adams MA. Biomechanics of back pain. Acupunct Med. 2004;22(4):178-88. doi:10.1136/aim.22.4.178.

99. McGill SM. Low back stability: from formal description to issues for performance and rehabilitation. Exerc Sport Sci Rev. 2001;29(1):26-31.

100. Ferrari S, Vanti C, O'Reilly C. Clinical presentation and physiotherapy treatment of 4 patients with low back pain and isthmic spondylolisthesis. J Chiropr Med. 2012;11(2):94-103.

101. Shacklock M. Improving application of neurodynamic (neural tension) testing and treatments: a message to researchers and clinicians. Man Ther. 2005;10(3):175-9.

102. Karayannis NV, Smeets RJ, van den Hoorn W, Hodges PW. Fear of movement is related to trunk stiffness in low back pain. PLoS ONE. 2013;8(6):e67779.

103. O'Sullivan P. Classification of lumbopelvic pain disorders--why is it essential for management? Man Ther. 2006;11(3):169-70.

104. Moseley GL, Hodges PW. Are the changes in postural control associated with low back pain caused by pain interference? Clin J Pain. 2005;21(4):323-9.

105. Guzman J, Hayden J, Furlan AD, Cassidy JD, Loisel P, Flannery J, et al. Key factors in back disability prevention: a consensus panel on their impact and modifiability. Spine. 2007;32(7):807-15.

106. Hides J, Wilson S, Stanton W, McMahon S, Keto H, McMahon K, et al. An MRI investigation into the function of the transversus abdominis muscle during "drawing-in" of the abdominal wall. Spine. 2006;31(6):E175-8.

107. Richardson CA, Snijders CJ, Hides JA, Damen L, Pas MS, Storm J. The relation between the transversus abdominis muscles, sacroiliac joint mechanics, and low back pain. Spine. 2002;27(4):399-405.

108. Hodges PW, Richardson CA. Altered trunk muscle recruitment in people with low back pain with upper limb movement at different speeds. Arch Phys Med Rehabil. 1999;80(9):1005-12.

109. Hides JA, Richardson CA, Jull GA. Multifidus muscle recovery is not automatic after resolution of acute, first-episode low back pain. Spine. 1996;21(23):2763-9.

110. Hides JA, Stanton WR, McMahon S, Sims K, Richardson CA. Effect of stabilization training on multifidus muscle cross-sectional area among young elite cricketers with low back pain. J Orthop Sports Phys Ther. 2008;38(3):101-8.

111. Moreside JM, Quirk DA, Hubley-Kozey CL. Temporal patterns of the trunk muscles remain altered in a low back-injured population despite subjective reports of recovery. Arch Phys Med Rehabil. 2014;95(4):686-98.

112. Silfies SP, Squillante D, Maurer P, Westcott S, Karduna AR. Trunk muscle recruitment patterns in specific chronic low back pain populations. Clin Biomech Bristol Avon. 2005;20(5):465-73.

113. Hides J, Stanton W, Mendis MD, Sexton M. The relationship of transversus abdominis and lumbar multifidus clinical muscle tests in patients with chronic low back pain. Man Ther. 2011;16(6):573-7.

114. Hides JA, Jull GA, Richardson CA. Long-term effects of specific stabilizing exercises for first-episode low back pain. Spine. 2001;26(11):E243-8.

115. Hides JA, Stanton WR, Wilson SJ, Freke M, McMahon S, Sims K. Retraining motor control of abdominal muscles among elite cricketers with low back pain. Scand J Med Sci Sports. 2010;20(6):834-42.

116. Hall L, Tsao H, MacDonald D, Coppieters M, Hodges PW. Immediate effects of co-contraction training on motor control of the trunk muscles in people with recurrent low back pain. J Electromyogr Kinesiol. 2009;19(5):763-73.

117. Ferreira P, Ferriera M, Maher C, Herbert R, Refshauge K. Specific stabilization exercise for spinal and pelvic pain: a systematic review. Aust J Physiother. 2006;(52):79-88.

118. Giggins OM, Persson UM, Caulfield B. Biofeedback in rehabilitation. J Neuro Engineering Rehabil. 2013;10:60.

119. Hides JA, Richardson CA, Jull GA. Use of real-time ultrasound imaging for feedback in rehabilitation. Man Ther. 1998;3(3):125-31.

120. Lee AS, Cholewicki J, Reeves NP, Zazulak BT, Mysliwiec LW. Comparison of trunk proprioception between patients with low back pain and healthy controls. Arch Phys Med Rehabil. 2010;91(9):1327-31.

121. Silfies SP, Cholewicki J, Reeves NP, Greene HS. Lumbar position sense and the risk of low back injuries in college athletes: a prospective cohort study. BMC Musculoskelet Disord. 2007;8:129.

122. Della Volpe R, Popa T, Ginanneschi F, Spidalieri R, Mazzocchio R, Rossi A. Changes in coordination of postural control during dynamic stance in chronic low back pain patients. Gait Posture. 2006;24(3):349-55.

123. Oyarzo CA, Villagrán CR, Silvestre RE, Carpintero P, Berral FJ. Postural control and low back pain in elite athletes comparison of static balance in elite athletes with and without low back pain. J Back Musculoskelet Rehabil. 2014;27(2):141-6.

124. Nitz AJ, Peck D. Comparison of muscle spindle concentrations in large and small human epaxial muscles acting in parallel combinations. Am Surg. 1986;52(5):273-7.

125. Cholewicki J, Simons AP, Radebold A. Effects of external trunk loads on lumbar spine stability. J Biomech. 2000;33(11):1377-85.

126. Cho M, Jeon H. The effects of bridge exercise on an unstable base of support on lumbar stability and the thickness of the transversus abdominis. J Phys Ther Sci. 2013;25(6):733-6.

127. Dunk NM, Kedgley AE, Jenkyn TR, Callaghan JP. Evidence of a pelvis-driven flexion pattern: are the joints of the lower lumbar spine fully flexed in seated postures? Clin Biomech Bristol Avon. 2009;24(2):164-8.

128. Cambron JA, Duarte M, Dexheimer J, Solecki T. Shoe orthotics for the treatment of chronic low back pain: a randomized controlled pilot study. J Manipulative Physiol Ther. 2011;34(4):254-60.

129. Lengsfeld M, Frank A, van Deursen DL, Griss P. Lumbar spine curvature during office chair sitting. Med Eng Phys. 2000;22(9):665-9.

130. Gadge K, Innes E. An investigation into the immediate effects on comfort, productivity and posture of the Bambach saddle seat and a standard office chair. Work Read Mass. 2007;29(3):189-203.

131. Annetts S, Coales P, Colville R, Mistry D, Moles K, Thomas B, et al. A pilot investigation into the effects of different office chairs on spinal angles. Eur Spine J. 2012;21(2):165-70.

132. O'Sullivan K, McCarthy R, White A, O'Sullivan L, Dankaerts W. Can we reduce the effort of maintaining a neutral sitting posture? A pilot study. Man Ther. 2012;17(6):566-71.

133. Castanharo R, Duarte M, McGill S. Corrective sitting strategies: an examination of muscle activity and spine loading. J Electromyogr Kinesiol. 2014;24(1):114-9.

134. Belavý DL, Bansmann PM, Böhme G, Frings-Meuthen P, Heer M, Rittweger J, et al. Changes in intervertebral disc morphology persist 5 mo after 21-day bed rest. J Appl Physiol (1985). 2011;111(5):1304-14.

135. Dahm KT, Brurberg KG, Jamtvedt G, Hagen KB. Advice to rest in bed versus advice to stay active for acute low-back pain and sciatica. Cochrane Database Syst Rev. 2010;(6):CD007612.

136. Hides JA, Lambrecht G, Richardson CA, Stanton WR, Armbrecht G, Pruett C, et al. The effects of rehabilitation on the muscles of the trunk following prolonged bed rest. Eur Spine J. 2011;20(5):808-18.

137. Waddell G, Feder G, Lewis M. Systematic reviews of bed rest and advice to stay active for acute low back pain. Br J Gen Pract. 1997;47(423):647-52.

138. Wand BM, Bird C, McAuley JH, Doré CJ, MacDowell M, De Souza LH. Early intervention for the management of acute low back pain: a single-blind randomized controlled trial of biopsychosocial education, manual therapy, and exercise. Spine. 2004;29(21):2350-6.

139. Bailey SR, Eid AH, Mitra S, Flavahan S, Flavahan NA. Rho kinase mediates cold-induced constriction of cutaneous arteries role of 2C-adrenoceptor translocation. Circ Res. 2004;94(10):1367-74.

140. Hodges GJ, Zhao K, Kosiba WA, Johnson JM. The involvement of nitric oxide in the cutaneous vasoconstrictor response to local cooling in humans. J Physiol. 2006;574(3):849-57.

141. Calmels P, Queneau P, Hamonet C, et al. Effectiveness of a lumbar belt in subacute low back pain: an open, multicentric, and randomized clinical study. Spine. 2009;34(3):215-20.

142. Newcomer K, Laskowski ER, Yu B, Johnson JC, An KN. The effects of a lumbar support on repositioning error in subjects with low back pain. Arch Phys Med Rehabil. 2001;82(7):906-10.

143. Kang MH, Choi SH, Oh JS. Postural taping applied to the low back influences kinematics and EMG activity during patient transfer in physical therapists with chronic low back pain. J Electromyogr Kinesiol. 2013;23(4):787-93.

144. Paoloni M, Bernetti A, Fratocchi G, Mangone M, Parrinello L, Del Pilar Cooper M, et al. Kinesio Taping applied to lumbar muscles influences clinical and electromyographic characteristics in chronic low back pain patients. Eur J Phys Rehabil Med. 2011;47(2):237-44.

145. Alvarez-Álvarez S, Jose FG, Rodríguez-Fernández AL, Güeita Rodríguez J, Benjamin JW. Effects of Kinesio® Tape in low back muscle fatigue: randomized, controlled, doubled-blinded clinical trial on healthy subjects. J Back Musculoskelet Rehabil. 2014;27(2):203-12.

146. Aleksiev AR. Ten-Year follow-up of strengthening versus flexibility exercises with or without abdominal bracing in recurrent low back pain. Spine. 2014;39(13):997-1003.

147. Mantilla CB, Sieck GC. Impact of diaphragm muscle fiber atrophy on neuromotor control. Respir Physiol Neurobiol. 2013;189(2):411-8.

148. Smit TH, van Tunen MS, van der Veen AJ, Kingma I, van Dieën JH. Quantifying intervertebral disc mechanics: a new definition of the neutral zone. BMC Musculoskelet Disord. 2011;12:38.

149. Suni J, Rinne M, Natri A, Statistisian MP, Parkkari J, Alaranta H. Control of the lumbar neutral zone decreases low back pain and improves self-evaluated work ability: a 12-month randomized controlled study. Spine. 2006;31(18):E611-20.

150. Granata KP, Marras WS. Cost-benefit of muscle cocontraction in protecting against spinal instability. Spine. 2000;25(11):1398-404.

151. Hides JA, Stanton WR, Mendis MD, Gildea J, Sexton MJ. Effect of motor control training on muscle size and football games missed from injury. Med Sci Sports Exerc. 2012;44(6):1141-9.

152. Sapsford RR, Hodges PW. Contraction of the pelvic floor muscles during abdominal maneuvers. Arch Phys Med Rehabil. 2001;82(8):1081-8.

153. Butrick CW. Pelvic floor hypertonic disorders: identification and management. Obstet Gynecol Clin North Am. 2009;36(3):707-22.

154. Kavcic N, Grenier S, McGill SM. Determining the stabilizing role of individual torso muscles during rehabilitation exercises. Spine. 2004;29(11):1254-65.

155. Koh HW, Cho SH, Kim CY. Comparison of the effects of hollowing and bracing exercises on cross-sectional areas of abdominal muscles in middle-aged women. J Phys Ther Sci. 2014;26(2):295-9.

156. Flynn TW, Canavan PK, Cavanagh PR, Chiang JH. Plantar pressure reduction in an incremental weight-bearing system. Phys Ther. 1997;77(4):410-6.

157. Ruckstuhl H, Kho J, Weed M, Wilkinson MW, Hargens AR. Comparing two devices of suspended treadmill walking by varying body unloading and Froude number. Gait Posture. 2009;30(4):446-51.

158. Mok NW, Hodges PW. Movement of the lumbar spine is critical for maintenance of postural recovery following support surface perturbation. Exp Brain Res. 2013;231(3):305-13.

159. Marlowe D. Complementary and alternative medicine treatments for low back pain. Prim Care. 2012;39(3):533-46.

160. French S, Werth P, Walker B. Approach to low back pain—chiropractic. Aust Fam Physician. 2014;43(1):43-44.

161. Wu JN. A short history of acupuncture. J Altern Complement Med. 1996;2(1):19-21.

162. Lao L. Acupuncture techniques and devices. J Altern Complement Med. 1996;2(1):23-5.

163. Carlsson CP, Sjölund BH. Acupuncture for chronic low back pain: a randomized placebo-controlled study with long-term follow-up. Clin J Pain. 2001;17(4):296-305.

164. Heuch I, Heuch I, Hagen K, Zwart JA. Body mass index as a risk factor for developing chronic low back pain: a follow-up in the Nord-Trøndelag Health Study. Spine. 2013;38(2):133-9.

165. Kurunlahti M, Karppinen J, Haapea M, Niinimäki J, Autio R, Vanharanta H, et al. Three-year follow-up of lumbar artery occlusion with magnetic resonance angiography in patients with sciatica: associations between occlusion and patient-reported symptoms. Spine. 2004;29(16):1804-8; discussion 1809.

166. M dry E, Lisowska A, Grebowiec P, Walkowiak J. The impact of vegan diet on B-12 status in healthy omnivores: five-year prospective study. Acta Sci Pol Technol Aliment. 2012;11(2):209-12.

167. Tuso PJ, Ismail MH, Ha BP, Bartolotto C. Nutritional update for physicians: plant-based diets. Perm J. 2013;17(2):61-6.

168. NutritionFacts.org. (year). The Latest in Nutrition Related Research. [online] Available from http://nutritionfacts.org/. [Accessed January, 2015].

169. Ornish D, Brown SE, Billings JH, Billings JH, Armstrong WT, Ports TA, et al. Can lifestyle changes reverse coronary heart disease?: the lifestyle heart trial. The Lancet. 1990;336(8708):129-33.

170. Sabaté J, Wien M. Vegetarian diets and childhood obesity prevention. Am J Clin Nutr. 2010;91(5):1525S-9S.

171. Abdi S, Datta S, Trescot AM, Schultz DM, Adlaka R, Atluri SL, et al. Epidural steroids in the management of chronic spinal pain: a systematic review. Pain Physician. 2007;10(1):185-212.

172. Rho ME, Tang CT. The efficacy of lumbar epidural steroid injections: transforaminal, interlaminar, and caudal approaches. Phys Med Rehabil Clin N Am. 2011;22(1):139-48.

173. Chou R, Atlas SJ, Stanos SP, Rosenquist RW. Nonsurgical interventional therapies for low back pain: a review of the evidence for an American Pain Society clinical practice guideline. Spine. 2009;34(10):1078-93.

174. Manchikanti L, Abdi S, Atluri S, Benyamin RM, Boswell MV, Buenaventura RM, et al. An update of comprehensive evidence-based guidelines for interventional techniques in chronic spinal pain. Part II: guidance and recommendations. Pain Physician. 2013;16(2):S49-283.

175. Datta S, Manchikanti L, Falco FJE, Calodney AK, Atluri S, Benyamin RM, et al. Diagnostic utility of selective nerve root blocks in the diagnosis

of lumbosacral radicular pain: systematic review and update of current evidence. Pain Physician. 2013;16(2):SE97-124.

176. Ribeiro LH, Furtado RN, Konai MS, Andreo AB, Rosenfeld A, Natour J. Effect of facet joint injection versus systemic steroids in low back pain: a randomized controlled trial. Spine. 2013;38(23):1995-2002.

177. Stone JA, Bartynski WS. Treatment of facet and sacroiliac joint arthropathy: steroid injections and radiofrequency ablation. Tech Vasc Interv Radiol. 2009;12(1):22-32.

178. Manchikanti L, Boswell MV, Singh V, Benyamin RM, Fellows B, Abdi S, et al. Comprehensive evidence-based guidelines for interventional techniques in the management of chronic spinal pain. Pain Physician. 2009;12(4):699-802.

179. Cohen SP, Huang JH, Brummett C. Facet joint pain--advances in patient selection and treatment. Nat Rev Rheumatol. 2013;9(2):101-16.

180. Poetscher AW, Gentil AF, Lenza M, Ferretti M. Radiofrequency denervation for facet joint low back pain: a systematic review. Spine. 2014;39(14):E842-9.

181. Gossner J. The lumbar multifidus muscles are affected by medial branch interventions for facet joint syndrome: potential problems and proposal of a pericapsular infiltration technique. Am J Neuroradiol. 2011;32(11):E213.

182. Dreyfuss P, Stout A, Aprill C, Pollei S, Johnson B, Bogduk N. The significance of multifidus atrophy after successful radiofrequency neurotomy for low back pain. PM R. 2009;1(8):719-22.

183. Oosterhuis T, Costa LO, Maher CG, de Vet HCW, van Tulder MW, Ostelo RW. Rehabilitation after lumbar disc surgery. Cochrane Database Syst Rev. 2014;3:CD003007.

184. Jones AD, Wafai AM, Easterbrook AL. Improvement in low back pain following spinal decompression: observational study of 119 patients. Eur Spine J. 2014;23(1):135-41.

185. Ahn Y, Oh HK, Kim H, Lee SH, Lee HN. Percutaneous endoscopic lumbar foraminotomy: an advanced surgical technique and clinical outcomes. Neurosurgery. 2014;75(2):124-33.

186. Lykissas MG, Aichmair A. Current concepts on spinal arthrodesis in degenerative disorders of the lumbar spine. World J Clin Cases. 2013;1(1):4-12.

187. Phillips FM, Slosar PJ, Youssef JA, Andersson G, Papatheofanis F. Lumbar spine fusion for chronic low back pain due to degenerative disc disease: a systematic review. Spine. 2013;38(7):E409-22.

188. Xia XP, Chen HL, Cheng HB. Prevalence of adjacent segment degeneration after spine surgery: a systematic review and meta-analysis. Spine. 2013;38(7):597-608.

189. Mannion AF, Leivseth G, Brox JI, Fritzell P, Hägg O, Fairbank JC. Long-term follow up suggests spinal fusion is associated with increased adjacent segment disc degeneration but without influence on clinical outcome: results of a combined follow-up from 4 RCTs. Spine. 2014;39(17): 1373-83.

Section 3

Lower Extremity

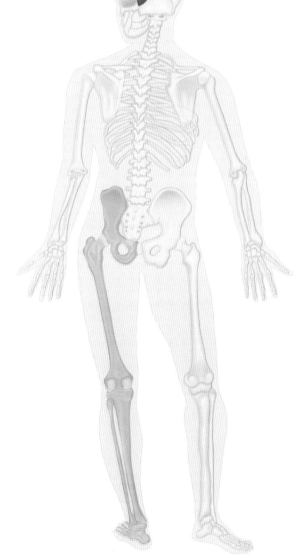

CHAPTERS

CHAPTER 9

Osteoarthritis of the Hip and Knee

JH Abbott

ABSTRACT

Osteoarthritis (OA) is among the most common presentations in musculoskeletal care, and is the single greatest cause of disability in older adults. This chapter begins with a brief summary of the epidemiology, etiology, prognosis and progression of OA. The clinical presentation and diagnosis of hip and knee OA is comprehensively described, accompanied by a guide to assessment. The clinical management of hip and knee OA is comprehensively covered, with an emphasis on physical therapy treatment. The author is a physical therapist active in producing, reviewing and summarizing clinical research evidence. The chapter is extensively referenced to recent peer-reviewed literature.

▓ INTRODUCTION

Osteoarthritis is a complex, active disease process involving the whole joint structure: bone, cartilage, synovium, ligaments, and muscles supporting and surrounding the affected joint.

Epidemiology

Osteoarthritis (OA) is among the most common presentations in musculoskeletal care,[1] with hip and knee OA the most common forms of OA. In any 1 year approximately 5% of the total adult population age 55 years or older will consult their family practice doctor or other primary health practitioner about knee OA.[2]

The prevalence of OA increases with age: it affects around 10% of adults aged 35–45 years, over 40% of adults 45–55 years, rising rapidly in older adulthood to over 80% in those older than 75 years.[3,4] As the population distribution of many countries is aging, by the middle of this century we will see the proportion of people age over 65 years increase to around a quarter of the overall population, while the number of people over 85 years will quadruple. This "gray tsunami" will have a dramatic effect on the prevalence of OA.

As a highly prevalent and painful condition, OA has a significant impact on the nation's health and disability burden.[3,5] Of all conditions presenting in primary care, it has one of the greatest effects on overall impaired physical health.[1] This combination of high prevalence and high disability burden makes OA the single greatest cause of disability in adults.[2] With an increasing number of working-age adults suffering OA, there is an increasing disability burden on society resulting from lost productivity, other indirect financial costs, and premature death.[4] Helping to manage the OA with effective nonsurgical care is therefore especially important for a "gray tsunami" future.

Etiology

Osteoarthritis is the most common form of arthritis. OA can be primary, or can be secondary to trauma or other joint disease. The disease process of OA is characterized by progressive structural joint changes, including degeneration and loss of articular cartilage. The limited early understanding of OA as a "wear and tear" disease of the cartilage, associated with aging has been overturned, and it is now accepted that OA is a disease of the whole joint, associated with adverse biomechanical forces.[6] It is now clear that OA is a complex, active disease process involving the bone, cartilage, synovium, ligaments and muscles supporting and surrounding the affected joint.

Osteoarthritis is primarily a disease of patho-mechanics.[7] It develops as a result of biomechanical insult to the cartilage and underlying bone, causing degeneration at a faster rate than the body is able to repair it. While heritable genetic and dietary factors play a role in susceptibility to OA, these are wholly overwhelmed by the dominant role of mechanical factors.[7] The abnormal stresses leading to joint degeneration can be either or both focal and general. Examples of focal stresses are those caused by congenital or acquired joint incongruity, such as meniscal defects or joint dysplasia. Examples of general adverse joint stresses are overweight and obesity, or excessive loading imparted by certain work- or sport-specific demands. These mechanical factors can act individually or in concert.

Focal and general pathomechanical stresses cause surface damage, matrix disruption, proteoglycan loss, and chondrocyte death.[6] Degeneration of the internal joint structure leads to altered joint kinematics and loss of function.[8,9] Kinematics of the joint are affected by joint capsule contracture, loss of periarticular flexibility, and increased intracapsular pressure.[9-13] Pain and disability have been shown to be associated with increased intracapsular pressure, altered joint kinematics and impaired muscle function.[13,14]

The body's response to this imbalance between the mechanical forces acting on the joint, and the ability of the cartilage to withstand them, is manifest not only in various microscopic and macroscopic features of the cartilage, but also in the subchondral bone, synovium, capsule, ligaments and the muscles acting across the joint. Age is certainly a risk factor associated with OA, but the exact mechanism is unknown. Studies point to a generally reduced healing capacity of the joint tissues and the accumulation of mechanical risk factors over years of life.[6]

Prognosis and Progression of Osteoarthritis

The course of OA is heterogeneous: it ranges from asymptomatic (as an incidental finding on medical imaging) to rapidly progressive disease resulting in structural joint failure.[6]

It is important to note that in its early, mild to moderate stages, the long-term outcome of the disease is not inevitable worsening. Research in population cohorts and in early hip or knee OA has shown that around one-fourth of people with symptoms of early OA will worsen, around ½ will remain unchanged, and around ¼ will improve or resolve.[15] In most cases the course of the disease is relatively slow, with very little change in the first 3 years, and worsening progression after more than 3 years follow-up.[16] At the individual level, however, there is considerable variation. Although there is no cure for OA, treatment can be targeted to alleviating symptoms and changing modifiable risk factors for progression.[6,17] There is considerable potential for reversing the cellular and structural damage of OA by decreasing adverse mechanical factors, optimizing supportive and advantageous mechanical factors, and ensuring the best conditions for the body's natural constructive metabolism to turn over and lay down new tissue.

Left unmanaged, or managed poorly, OA can become a chronically painful, disabling condition that can result in a cascade of effects, described by Gruber and Hunter as a comorbidity matrix (Fig. 1).[18]

Progression of knee OA has been shown to be associated with varus knee (mal)alignment and obesity.[20] Patients presenting at an older age, with worse radiographic features, and with OA at multiple joints are more likely to experience greater disease progression.[20] Muscle weakness, not only at the quadriceps but also of hip muscles, has been shown to be associated with knee OA.[6] On the positive side, there is strong evidence that exercise, physical activity and sports participation are not associated with disease progression, and some evidence that they are protective.[20]

In hip OA, patients presenting at an older age, with higher levels of pain and functional limitation, and with worse radiographic features are more likely to experience greater disease progression.[21] Femoroacetabular impingement is an example of congenital joint incongruity associated with focal cartilage damage. Overweight and obesity are not strongly associated with progression of hip OA, whereas they are in knee OA.[20,21] On the positive side, exercise therapy has been shown to delay or prevent the need for hip joint replacement surgery.[22,23]

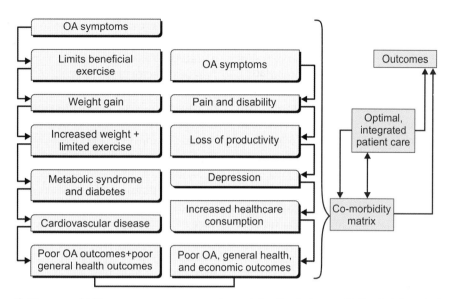

FIG. 1: Osteoarthritis comorbidity consequences cascade and feedback loops. Optimal, integrated care drives the comorbidity matrix down, and outcomes up
Source: Adapted from Gruber and Hunter[18] and reproduced with permission from The Clarity Group.[19]

Further to prediction of disease progression is prediction of outcome from intervention. There is only preliminary evidence that there may be patient-related factors that help predict outcome from physical therapy interventions in patients with knee OA, but these remain unconfirmed.[20,24,25]

The first such study, in patients with knee OA, indicated that favorable response to manual therapy treatment of the hip joint may be indicated by the presence of one or more of five variables: hip or groin pain or paresthesia, anterior thigh pain, passive knee flexion less than 122°, passive hip medial (internal) rotation less than 17°, and pain with hip distraction.[25] Based on the pretest probability of success (68%), the presence of one variable increased the probability of a successful response to 92% at 48-hours follow-up, while presence of two variables increased the probability of success to 97%.[25]

A later study of patients with knee OA receiving exercise therapy and/or manual therapy indicated that six criteria may be predictive of a successful outcome[26]: posterior knee pain; duration of symptoms (> 5 years); female sex; instability affecting activity; disturbed sleep; and absence of previous knee injury.[26] Presence of four predictor variables nearly doubled the post-test probability of success, from 35% to 58%. If less than three predictor variables were present, post-test probability of success decreased to 21.5%.[26]

A similar study of patients with hip OA receiving exercise therapy and/or manual therapy reported preliminary definition of a cluster of baseline variables that may identify patients with hip OA more likely to respond positively to physical therapy interventions.[24] That study found that combinations of unilateral hip pain, age less than or equal to 58 years, pain ≥ 6/10, a time of less than or equal to 25.9 seconds on a 40 m fast-paced walk test, and duration of symptoms less than or equal to 1 year were associated with a favorable response to physical therapy treatment in patients with hip OA [defined by the Outcome Measures for Arthritis Clinical Trials (OMERACT)-Osteoarthritis Research Society International (OARSI) criteria].[27,28] When at least two out of those five predictor variables were present, the probability of a successful response to physical therapy doubled from a pre-test probability of 32% to a post-test probability of 65%. Presence of more than or equal to 3 predictor variables increased the post-test probability to more than 99%.[24]

However, it must be emphasized that these are preliminary studies that must be successfully validated in future research before they can be confidently used in clinical practice. It should be noted that the variables identified differs among these studies, which may be a warning sign that some or even all may be chance findings that do not withstand the scrutiny of subsequent validation studies. Indeed, a recent study of patients with hip OA, receiving exercise therapy and/or manual therapy, found four baseline variables were predictive of a positive outcome at 9 weeks: male sex, pain with activity

(<6/10), Western Ontario and McMaster Universities Osteoarthritis Index physical function subscale score (<34/68), and psychological health (Hospital Anxiety and Depression Scale score <9/42), but no predictor variables were identified at the 18-weeks follow-up.[29] It is notable that the only comparable variable revealed in the two hip OA studies was the patient-reported pain level, with directly opposite findings: one found that pain ≥ 6/10 was associated with treatment success,[24] while the other found pain with activity <6/10 was associated with success.[29] These disparate findings highlight the danger of accepting any findings from the preliminary development of clinical prediction rules until they have been reproduced and independently verified.[30]

CLINICAL PRESENTATION

Osteoarthritis generally presents as pain at or about the joint, impacting quality of life, with reported and clinically evident functional limitation. Clinical features of the patient with OA include pain, stiffness and loss of motion of the affected joint, loss of muscle strength, decreased flexibility of muscles about the joint, loss of aerobic capacity, disability and weight gain.[8,9] The pain experienced is of two quite distinct types: intermittent, intense pain of relatively short duration; and chronic, persistent ache. Typically, the patient experiences three clinical stages[6,31]:

- Stage 1 characterizes early OA: Discrete episodes of predictable, sharp pain associated with biomechanical stresses, such as turning or bending movements during sport or work. Although acutely painful, these intermittent events have relatively little effect on function but eventually limit high impact activities.
- Stage 2 or mild OA: The joint pain becomes more constant and begins to affect daily activities. The joint is often reported to feel stiff after inactivity, e.g. upon waking and after periods of sitting. The joint pain may become more unpredictable and may be accompanied by locking or the sensation of "giving way".
- Stage 3 or advanced OA: The pain becomes more constant—dull, and aching in nature—punctuated by intermittent, unpredictable episodes of intense pain. The unpredictable exacerbation of pain is distressing and exhausting, and results in significant functional limitations.

Presentation is, however, widely variable with respect to the severity of pain, functional limitation, and radiographic evidence.

It is common for patients to present with OA already at Stage 2. In some cases, the patient has discussed dull or intermittent hip or knee pain with his or her family practice doctor, but referral to physical therapy rarely occurs.[32] Patients often do not seek care from private providers due to: (1) inadequate understanding of the disease and what can be done to alleviate and manage it, and (2) out-of-pocket costs often further limit uptake if access to insurance- or publicly-funded treatment is limited or unavailable.[33] For the small proportion accessing physical therapy, current physical therapist practice typically does not comply with that seen in the successful trials underpinning OA clinical guidelines.[34,35]

As the patient endures OA for longer, many patients become anxious, fearful of falling or of the leg giving way, and develop low mood.[31] Sleep is often negatively affected. Depression is a common consequence of both the unremitting nature of the joint achiness, sleep loss, fear of worsening, and the limitations to work and social participation. In the author's research, around 50% of patients revealed evidence of depression, and loss of confidence was a strong theme in qualitative interviews.[36]

It is important to recognize that the symptoms and limitations affecting patients are manifold, including a poor or inaccurate knowledge of the causes, effects, and course of the disease, pain of two distinct types, movement impairments, limitations of physical function, limitations to social and occupational participation, and significant psychological ramifications. Clearly, a holistic assessment and multimodal management plan are necessary, and this is largely within physical therapists' scope of expertise.

CLINICAL EXAMINATION

Diagnosis

The main clinical findings are reduced range of motion (ROM), tenderness, crepitus, bony swelling, and deformity. Diagnosis of OA can be made confidently on the basis of clinical signs and symptoms alone.[6]

Evidence-based diagnosis of knee OA has been defined in many national and international clinical practice guides.[37-39] The most established are the American College of Rheumatology (ACR) criteria.[37,38,40] The 1986 ACR clinical criteria for knee OA state that clinical diagnosis can be made with confidence on the basis of knee pain present on most days for greater than 1 month, plus three of the following six criteria: age more than 50 years, morning stiffness of less than 30 minutes, crepitus on active movement, tenderness of the bony margins of the joint, bony enlargement of the joint noted on examination, lack of palpable warmth of the synovium.[37] These criteria have a sensitivity of 95% and specificity of 69%. As an example, based on these criteria, a subject who is less than 50 years but has knee pain and three of the other five criteria would also be classified as having knee OA. The 1991 ACR clinical criteria for hip OA are either: hip pain present on most days for greater than 1 month, plus hip flexion limited to less than 115° and hip internal rotation limited to less than 15°; or hip pain with internal rotation, plus morning stiffness of less than or equal to 60 minutes duration, and age 50 years or older.[40] The use of these clinical criteria has the additional benefits of avoiding unnecessary costs and exposure to ionizing radiation that occur with radiographic assessment of knee OA.

In many cases, radiographs may be available. While these may be useful to gauge the extent of joint structural loss, and help estimate prognosis, radiographs are unnecessary for the physical therapist's diagnosis or treatment planning.[39] It is also worth noting that radiographs can be misleading, as some people with radiographic evidence of OA remain asymptomatic, and others can have significant symptoms but no radiographically evident disease.

A weakness of the 1986 ACR criteria[37,38] is that they were developed using hospital-referred patients, which may introduce bias in application to a primary care population. The more recent 2010 European League against Rheumatism (EULAR) guidelines for the diagnosis of knee OA used systematic review evidence, and ensured optimal generalizability to the primary care setting by emphasizing evidence from primary care and from population-based studies.[39 41,42] The research evidence supporting the accuracy of each individual clinical sign or symptom indicates that none are strong enough alone to support a diagnosis of OA. Diagnostic strength is expressed as the likelihood ratio (LR) for a positive test. A test with a LR of 1 makes no contribution at all—it is completely uninformative—while an LR from 2 to 5 is modestly strong, greater than 5 moderately strong, and greater than 10 very strong. The LR for each these findings are of modest strength (Table 1), but cumulatively they become powerful when 3 or more are present.[37-39] Joint-line tenderness and pain on patella-femoral compression were also considered informative signs, but no statistical LR was available. The EULAR guidelines conclude that the three most informative symptoms (persistent knee pain, limited morning stiffness and reduced function)

TABLE 1: Accuracy of clinical findings for the diagnosis of osteoarthritis (OA)

History

- Age 50 years or more has a likelihood ratio for a positive test (LR+) of 1.20
- Knee pain has been present for most days of the past month (defined as *persistent*) has a LR+ of 1.67
- Knee pain is "usage-related", i.e. it gets more painful following home-life, occupational or sporting usage, has a LR+ of 1.16
- Morning stiffness that lasts ≤30 minutes, has LR+ of 1.84
- Report of a feeling of the knee "giving way", has a LR+ of 1.25

Physical tests

- Palpation of crepitus with active range of motion (ROM) has a LR+ of 2.23
- Bony enlargement has a LR+ of 11.81

Measures of impairment, functional limitation

- Restricted ROM has a LR+ of 4.4
- Functional limitation, by patient history or as indicated by, for example, the Western Ontario and McMaster (WOMAC), has a LR+ 1.5

Source: Adapted from the EULAR recommendations, 2010.[39]

and three most informative signs (crepitus, restricted movement and bony enlargement) could diagnose knee OA with an estimated probability of 99%, when all six symptoms and signs were present (assuming a patient aged ≥45 years and the background prevalence of knee OA in adults is 12.5%).[39]

More succinctly, a clinician can confidently make a working diagnosis of hip or knee joint OA on the basis of three simple criteria[43]:

1. Persistent joint pain that is worse with use
2. Age 45 years and more
3. Morning stiffness lasting no more than half an hour.

These criteria do not provide a definitive diagnosis, but do provide an entirely adequate working diagnosis for the provision of primary care and other physical therapy outpatient care, in the absence of signs or suspicion of alternative diagnoses (Table 2). All diagnosis is subject to uncertainty: presence of other signs and symptoms mentioned in the ACR and EULAR criteria, earlier, increases the level of diagnostic certainty.

Assessment

Best-practice management of OA, as recommended in rigorous clinical practice guidelines,[44,45] should begin with a holistic, multifaceted assessment that identifies

TABLE 2: Differential diagnoses

Differential diagnoses
The following differential diagnoses should be considered:
• Acute injury: Meniscal tear, cruciate or collateral ligament tear   ○ Rule out if not acute, and if there is an insidious history of onset; no report of "locking"; or negative diagnostic tests
• Other common musculoskeletal conditions   ○ e.g. patellar tendonitis, patellofemoral pain syndrome, prepatellar bursitis, pes anserinus bursitis, semimembranosus bursitis, iliotibial band friction syndrome
• Inflammatory arthritis, primarily rheumatoid arthritis, pigmented villonodular synovitis   ○ Rule out if not hot or swollen (in osteoarthritis the joint may be slightly warmer than usual, but not hot)
• Gout   ○ Rule out if not hot or swollen (joint was warmer than usual, but not hot), not intensely painful
• Osteochondritis dissecans   ○ Risk factors: Most common in young men, adolescents and children; assess history of locking, movement block, swelling
• Avascular necrosis   ○ Risk factors: Long-term steroid use, excessive alcohol use, blood clotting disorders
• Infection   ○ Rule out if not hot or swollen (joint was warmer than usual, but not hot), long insidious onset
• Tuberculosis of the bone (femur)   ○ Rule out if no history of living in high risk geographic area
• Referred knee pain from hip osteoarthritis   ○ Cleared by clinical examination
• Referred hip or knee pain from the lumbar spine   ○ Cleared by clinical examination

the salient problems and modifiable risk factors present for each individual, and serves to direct targeted interventions. The assessment should include age, sex, sociodemographic, psychological and social factors (anxiety, depression, self-efficacy, fatigue and social support), cognitive and visual impairments, general health comorbidity and overweight, health behaviors, physical activity, injury history, physical impairments (pain, stiffness, reduced muscle strength, laxity of the knee joint, proprioceptive inaccuracy, history of locking or giving way of the limb, poor standing balance and impaired range of joint motion), and level of optimism/pessimism for improvement, as all of these are associated with outcome.[46]

Validated, self-reported questionnaire instruments represent the optimal method of assessing pain and physical function. The Western Ontario and McMaster (WOMAC) OA index is the most widely used and validated outcome measure for assessing pain and physical function in patients with osteoarthritis. It includes pain, stiffness, and physical function subscales; the greatest number of items is in the "function" subscale.[47,48] The minimum important change is considered around 15% change from baseline score for physical function and around 20% change for pain.[49] The lower extremity functional scale (LEFS) can also be used.[50,51] Recent reports also support use of the patient-specific functional scale (PSFS—Appendix B).[52-54] A pain rating index is also recommended,[55] if not explicitly covered already by, e.g., the WOMAC. Information on outcome measures for OA is available at: http://www.oarsi.org/research/outcome-measures. (See Appendices B and C for example of forms for the PSFS and numeric pain rating scale).

Because of the prevalence of depression in older adults presenting to physical therapy with musculoskeletal conditions,[56] and particularly high risk in OA,[31,36] screening for mood and psychological function is indicated. The two-question depression screen is a quick and sensitive way to screen patients for the presence of clinically relevant depression.[57,58] In the event of a positive result, a third question is recommended, regarding the patient's wishes to discuss the issues with another health professional.[59] The physical therapist must have a policy in place regarding how to deal with positive screening results. Communication with or referral to the patient's referring doctor should notify the doctor about the screening test result and its meaning.

Psychological function in the domains of self-efficacy, fear-avoidance, anxiety and catastrophizing have an effect on outcomes in hip and knee OA.[60] Many instruments can assess these. The pain beliefs screening instrument (PBSI), see Appendix D, is one tool that can efficiently be used to assess pain intensity, disability, self-efficacy, fear avoidance, and catastrophizing.[61,62] PBSI is a screening instrument that has been shown to be sensitive to elevated levels of pain intensity, disability, self-efficacy, fear avoidance, and catastrophizing that may require additional or modified intervention (such as a cognitive behavioral therapy approach to exercise therapy) or referral to another health professional for cotherapy.[61,62] Again, the physical therapist must have a policy in place regarding how positive screening results will be addressed—whether by adjusting the treatment plan and/or by referral.

The physical therapist should also take a medications history, as clinical practice guidelines have established that medications are an important second-line of intervention for OA, and patients are very often not utilizing these optimally, whether by not being on an optimum plan or not following the plan as prescribed. Again, the clinician needs to be prepared to intervene by counseling and educating the patient and/or referral. Although it is outside the scope of practice, in most jurisdictions, for physical therapists to prescribe or be perceived to be recommending medicines, it is reasonable to provide education to patients regarding the purpose of the medications they have already been prescribed by their physician, about the concepts of attaining and maintaining therapeutic levels of medication in the bloodstream, duration of effect, relative effectiveness of each medication prescribed, and to counsel patients on adherence.[63-65]

Physical performance tests are recommended in the assessment of all patients with hip or knee OA. A consensus study has established a core set of recommended physical performance tests endorsed by the OARSI and are intended to be complementary to self-report measures.[66] These are:
- 30-second chair stand test
- 40 m fast-paced walk test
- Stair climb test
- Timed up-and-go test and
- 6-minute walk test.

The first three tests are recommended as a minimal core set of tests that should be used as performance-based outcome measures in OA research and clinical practice. The latter two tests are commonly used in clinical practice and research in OA as well as other health conditions affecting older adults.[66] The timed up-and-go test encompasses more than one activity dimension, including transitions between sit-to-stand, walking short distances, balance and turning while walking, so can be considered a multi-dimensional ambulatory transitions test. This makes it very useful for assessing physical function in non-surgical patients with OA. The 6-minute walk test was considered the best available test of walking over long distances, but does require more time and physical space to perform. Instructions and instructional videos are available at: http://www.oarsi.org/research/physical-performance-measures.

The consensus study was unable to recommend a specific stair climb test due to lack of sufficient data in the literature. Assessment of stair climbing is an important safety consideration, and is often important to patients'

physical function, however a subsequent study suggests that timed stair climb tests may not be sufficiently responsive to change to be useful as an outcome measure.[67]

Key impairments of physical function that should be assessed include:
- Quadriceps and hamstrings muscle strength and length
- Hip abductor, extensor, flexor, and rotator muscle strength, adductor and flexor length
- Ankle plantarflexor muscle strength and length
- Hip, knee, and ankle ROM.

Quadriceps strength is crucial to muscular control and support of the knee, and has been shown to be associated with the development, progression and outcome of OA. Hip muscle strength has also been shown to be associated with knee OA outcomes. Muscle strength of the ankle plantarflexors and dorsiflexors are underappreciated in their influence on knee control, support, and shock absorption. A recommended test of ankle plantarflexion is to assess the patient's ability to perform 10 unilateral heel raise repetitions to full height with full heel inversion/adduction. Generally it is recommended to assess bilateral ability first, progressing to unilateral ability to complete the test, failing which exercises targeting tibialis posterior, gastrocnemius and soleus muscle strength are indicated.

Lumbosacral spine strength and ROM should also be assessed, with careful note of any referred pain present during loaded, end-of-range assessment, as referred back pain can easily be misdiagnosed as hip or knee OA, or may summate to exacerbate hip or knee OA symptoms.

PHYSICAL THERAPY TREATMENT

Best-practice management of OA, as recommended in contemporary clinical practice guidelines[44,45] (Fig. 2), should begin with:
- A holistic, multifaceted assessment that identifies the salient problems and modifiable risk factors present for each individual, and serves to direct targeted interventions, consisting principally of:
  - Patient education and advice—including about weight loss if indicated, *and*
  - Exercise therapy as the first line of management, followed by;
  - Medications as second-line interventions, with the addition of any adjunctive interventions that are: (a) indicated by the thorough assessment, and (b) supported by evidence of effectiveness; plus

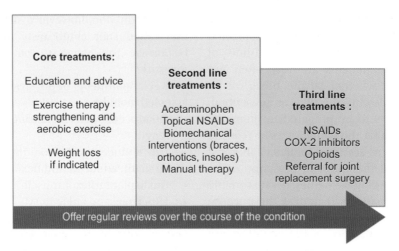

FIG 2: Summary of the UK National Institute for Health and Clinical Excellence (NICE) guidelines[44,68]
Source: Reproduced with permission from The Clarity Group.

○ A management plan and periodic review; and finally,

○ Joint replacement surgery is recommended before established disability and severe pain.[44]

Education

While patient education alone has been shown to have only very small, clinically insignificant effects, it is still widely accepted as a key component of OA management by all major clinical practice guidelines.[6,69] Clinical experience, conventional wisdom and qualitative research all maintain that both the disease and the interventions must be clearly explained to patients to enhance adherence and outcomes. The main objectives of patient education are to dispel misinformation and myths about the disease, its treatment, progression and outcomes, and to reinforce the importance of lifestyle changes around physical activity, exercise and weight loss.[6] It is important to distinguish a genuine therapeutic educational process from simply providing information such as basic trifold pamphlets.[6]

Weight Loss

Weight loss can have a strong influence on OA-related symptoms, and can influence the effectiveness of other cointerventions.[6] Weight loss is recommended for all overweight and obese individuals, particularly with knee OA. Diet modification and weight loss are difficult to achieve, however the combination of diet plus exercise results in better physiological and clinical outcomes compared with either intervention alone.[70]

Exercise Therapy

Exercise therapy, specifically strengthening and aerobic exercise, is the number one recommendation in practically all contemporary OA guidelines. An adequate dose and duration of a known effective exercise therapy protocol should be the first line of treatment for hip and knee OA.[17,44,71]

Exercise is known to be effective in reducing pain and increasing physical function in OA of the hip and/or knee,[72,73] through improvement of muscle strength, flexibility and endurance, joint ROM, aerobic fitness and neuromuscular coordination.[6,8,9] Most research has focused on land-based exercise programs, whether clinic-, class- or home-based, although water-based exercise programs can also be effective. Exercise therapy has an effect size equivalent to or greater than that of analgesic medications.[69]

A systematic review of nonsurgical, nonpharmacological interventions for OA[74] concluded that exercise therapy has the most evidence for cost-effectiveness, and is probably highly cost-effective and possibly a cost-saving intervention from the health system perspective,[75,76] with the cost of intervention being more than recouped by savings in other health services over 12 months.[75] Notably, long-term follow-up of exercise therapy interventions has shown it can delay or, in a small proportion, possibly prevent the need for joint replacement surgery.[22,23]

Although supervised, individualized, multimodal programs of exercise therapy are generally considered the "ideal standard of clinical practice"[11,77,78] the most effective content and method of delivery remains unclear.[8,9,72,73,78-84] Although the short-term effectiveness of exercise therapy has been established, few studies have followed participants up to 12 months, and very few to 2 years or longer.[82] Of studies with long-term follow-up, most have failed to show sustained benefit, however exercise programs that have maintained adherence through additional booster sessions show moderate evidence of sustained effects on pain and physical function.[82] There is evidence, from two studies following patients for 5 or more years, that exercise therapy may delay or prevent the need for joint replacement surgery.[22,23]

It is commonsense that a higher dose and duration of exercise is more likely to result in better outcomes, provided significant symptom exacerbation, overtraining and injury are avoided. Evidence of this is borne out among the many trials evaluated in systematic reviews of hip and knee OA. Significantly greater improvements in pain and physical function were found when patients received 12 or more therapist-supervised treatment sessions, compared with fewer sessions.[85] Additionally, there is some evidence of better outcomes with individual, supervised treatment, compared with a home program. Importantly, it has been shown that physical therapists' patterns of practice typically do not reflect well the interventions delivered in the evidence and guidelines,[34] and therefore may be far less effective than is possible, and may in many cases be ineffective due to inadequate content, dose and duration.

Clinical trials indicate that, in patients with hip or knee OA, a moderately strong dose of well-prescribed, well-monitored exercise therapy is well-tolerated and beneficial. The recently reported management of osteoarthritis (MOA) trial investigated the effectiveness of providing exercise therapy treatment (and/or manual therapy) in addition to usual care.[36] The exercise therapy provided in that trial (Table 3) was developed from the most effective protocols reported in earlier studies of exercise therapy,[85,86] and resulted in good effectiveness at short-term and 1 year follow-up,[36] which was still maintained at 2 year follow-up.[87] Each exercise had 3 or more levels of difficulty, so that patients could be progressed over time as they improved. Each level began with three sets of 10 repetitions, which is arbitrary but common practice used in place of more formal "repetition maximum" protocols, starting each patient on the level they could achieve with some effort, but without deviation from the correct plane and form for each exercise. Treatment sessions were 45–55 minutes. The standardized effect size produced by the exercise therapy protocol on the MOA trial was 0.31 at 1 year, which is equivalent to analgesic medications. This improved to 0.57 at 2 years, compared with usual care, in

part due to maintenance of positive effect in the treatment group and in part due to continued deterioration of the control group receiving no physical therapy care.[87] These data indicate a greater and longer lasting effect than most interventions trialed in most earlier studies.[45,80,88,89] An economic evaluation conducted alongside the MOA trial found that the exercise therapy and manual therapy protocols described earlier were highly cost-effective.[90] The content of the MOA trial hip and knee OA exercise therapy protocols are provided in Table 3.

Manual Therapy

The role of manual physical therapy in OA is to restore lost joint motion, optimize joint kinematics, reduce focal concentrations of compressive forces on articular cartilage, and reduce intracapsular pressure.[11,12] Manual therapies can also be targeted to increase the length and flexibility of the soft tissues surrounding the affected joint(s), including musculotendinous connective tissues and the joint capsule. Manual therapy is defined as skilled therapist-applied manual procedures intended to modify the quality and ROM of the target joint and associated soft tissue structures, provided by physical therapists trained in delivering manual therapy procedures. These interventions are therefore intended to reduce pain and disability by correcting impairments of the musculoskeletal system.

At the publication date of contemporary clinical practice guidelines, the effectiveness of manual physical therapy had not yet been well established.[72] Two seminal studies by the same group were the first randomized clinical trials (RCTs) to examine the combined effect of exercise plus manual therapy in knee OA.[91,92] The first study[91] compared exercise plus manual physical therapy to an inactive placebo control. It found manual therapy plus exercise to be superior to an inactive sham intervention, and reported the need for knee joint replacement surgery at 1year was reduced by 75% in the manual therapy plus exercise group, compared to the sham control group.[91] This represents a number needed to treat of seven patients [95% confidence interval (CI) 4–134] in order to prevent one knee replacement surgery at 1 year, but the second study,[92] which compared manual physical therapy plus exercise to an individually instructed home exercise program (including a detailed booklet, an exercise log and a follow-up consultation at 2 weeks) could not replicate the finding of any difference in knee replacement surgery rates between the groups. Although that second study found manual therapy plus exercise to be superior at

TABLE 3: Brief description of the management of osteoarthritis (MOA) trial exercise therapy interventions*

Supervised exercise therapy

Mandatory interventions

1. Aerobic exercise: Up to 10 minutes cycle or walk
2. Strengthening: 3 sets of 10 repetitions of
   - *Hip:* hip abduction (AI, AII); hip extension; hip lateral rotation; knee extension.

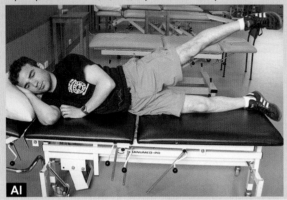
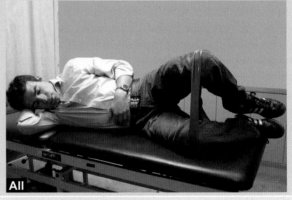

   - *Knee:* Knee extension (B); hip extension (C); knee flexion. Resistance adjusted as appropriate.

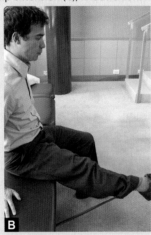
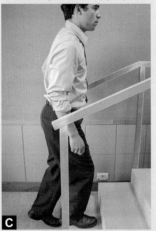

3. Stretching: 60 seconds passive stretch of
   - *Hip:* Hip flexors; knee extensors; hip extensors; hip adductors (D); knee flexors (E) and lateral rotators; ankle plantar flexors.

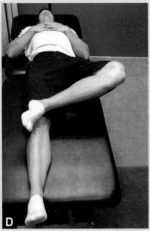
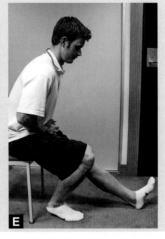

Continued

Continued

Supervised exercise therapy

Mandatory interventions

– *Knee:* Knee flexors; knee extensors (F); ankle plantarflexors (G);

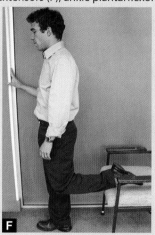
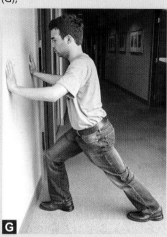

4. Neuromuscular coordination control exercises

Hip or knee: 3 sets of 2 minutes of (choose from): Standing weight-shifting exercises (H); standing balance on uneven surfaces; side-stepping (I), forward-backward and shuttle-walking drills; or stair walking

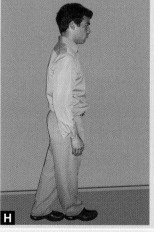
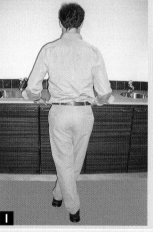

Secondary (non-mandatory) interventions, prescribed when indicated by assessment findings:

Hip: Trunk muscle strengthening (J); ankle plantarflexor muscle group strengthening; hip flexor strengthening.

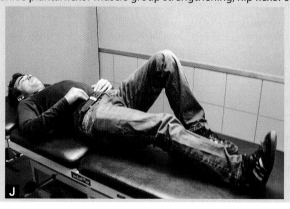

Continued

Continued

Supervised exercise therapy

Mandatory interventions

Knee: Ankle plantarflexor muscle group strengthening (K); hip abductor strengthening; hip lateral rotator strengthening; hip flexor and knee extensor stretching; trunk muscle strengthening.

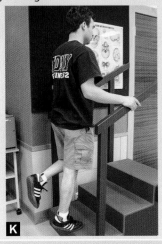

Home exercise program:

• Prescribed up to six of the above activities to reinforce clinic interventions.

*Treatment protocol used in the MOA trial.[36] Space does not permit full reproduction of the treatment protocols. A full description and illustrations of the intervention protocol and procedures is available at http://cmor.otago.ac.nz/moa.

Source: Reproduced with permission from the Clarity Group.

8 week follow-up there were no significant differences evident at 1 year follow-up.[92] A weakness in both of these studies is that it is not possible to differentiate the effect of manual therapy from that of exercise.

A 2004 study of hip OA did directly compare the effectiveness of manual therapy to exercise therapy and demonstrated superior effectiveness of manual therapy over exercise at 6 month follow-up.[11] The results of the MOA trial were consistent with the impression that manual therapy has a stronger treatment effect than exercise therapy at short-term and 1 year follow-up,[36] but with practically equivalent results at 2 year follow-up.[87] This was evident both for patients with hip OA or with knee OA.[36] In the MOA trial treatment protocols (Table 4), each manual therapy technique had 3 or more grades of force, plus alternative positions, and therapists ensured that patients were progressed over each treatment session. The protocol began with 3 sets of 30 repetitions, which is arbitrary but common practice. Treatment sessions were 40–50 minutes, which is a greater cumulative dose than is common practice in most countries. The standardized effect size produced by the manual therapy protocol on the MOA trial was 0.60 at 1 year, which is considerably greater than analgesic medications. This was maintained

to 0.55 at 2 years, compared with usual care.[87] A recent hip OA trial found similar effects for both exercise therapy alone and exercise therapy plus manual therapy, with both superior to no intervention at 9 weeks follow-up,[93] however the manual therapy component was limited to only 15 minutes in each of eight treatment sessions, considerably less than was delivered in the other trials.

While both manual therapy and exercise therapy (in addition to usual medical care) in the MOA trial were shown to be both effective and cost-effective individually, compared with usual care only, this was not the case for combined manual therapy plus exercise therapy.[36,90] Combined manual therapy plus exercise therapy generally resulted in weaker outcomes than either intervention delivered individually, and was neither clinically nor statistically better than usual care only at 1 year follow-up.[36] This surprise finding is most likely due to the reduced dose of both manual therapy and exercise therapy that was necessary in order to deliver both within the same treatment session. This was supported by the finding that a combined manual therapy plus exercise therapy intervention for hip OA, delivered in a reduced format of ten 30 minute sessions, produced outcomes no better than a sham intervention delivered by attentive

TABLE 4: Brief description of the management of osteoarthritis (MOA) trial manual therapy interventions*

Manual therapy**	
Hip:	

Mandatory interventions:
- Long-axis hip distraction with thrust (A)
- Lateral hip distraction, nonthrust
- Anteroposterior directed force to the proximal femur, nonthrust (C)
- Posteroanterior directed force to the proximal femur, nonthrust
- Medial hip rotation, nonthrust (B)
- Soft tissue manipulation to hip and thigh musculature and fascia (F)
- Manual stretches to connective tissue of hip and thigh (D)

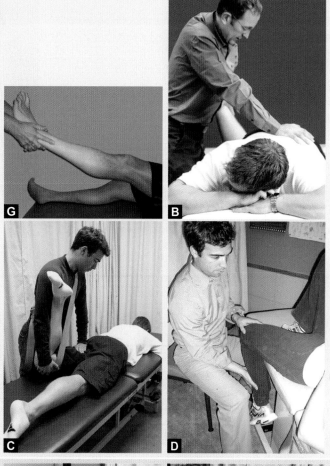

Secondary (non-mandatory) interventions prescribed when indicated by assessment findings:
- Knee flexion, nonthrust (E)
- Proximal tibiofibular joint manipulation, thrust or nonthrust
- Knee extension, nonthrust
- Patellar gliding force, nonthrust
- Ankle and talocalcaneal joint distraction, thrust or nonthrust
- Ankle talocrural anteroposterior directed force, nonthrust
- Anteroposterior directed force to distal fibula, tibiofibular joint, nonthrust
- Soft tissue manipulation, ankle plantarflexor muscle group
- Lumbopelvic rotation thrust manipulation

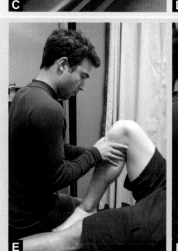

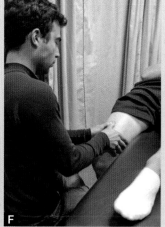

Home program of reinforcing activities:
- Prescribed up to six range-of-motion activities to reinforce clinic interventions.

Continued

Continued

Manual therapy**	
Knee:	

Mandatory interventions:
- Knee flexion, nonthrust (G)
- Anteroposterior directed force to the tibia, tibiofemoral joint, nonthrust
- Knee extension, nonthrust
- Posteroanterior directed force to the tibia, tibiofemoral joint, nonthrust
- Patellar gliding force, nonthrust
- Manual stretch to quadriceps, hamstring, triceps surae muscle groups
- Soft tissue manipulation, quadriceps (H) and peripatellar connective tissue, hamstring, hip adductor and triceps surae muscle groups

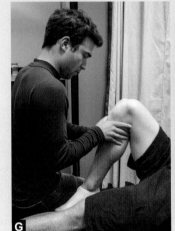 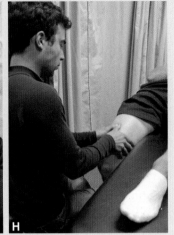

Secondary (non-mandatory) interventions prescribed when indicated by assessment findings:
- Long-axis hip distraction with thrust
- Lateral hip distraction, nonthrust
- Anteroposterior directed force to proximal femur, nonthrust
- Posteroanterior directed force to proximal femur, nonthrust (I)
- Medial hip rotation, nonthrust (J, K)
- Soft tissue manipulation to hip and thigh musculature and fascia
- Manual stretches to connective tissue of hip and thigh
- Ankle and talocalcaneal joint distraction, thrust or nonthrust
- Ankle talocrural anteroposterior directed force, nonthrust
- Anteroposterior directed force to distal fibula, tibiofibular joint, nonthrust
- Soft tissue manipulation, ankle plantarflexor muscle group
- Lumbopelvic rotation thrust manipulation

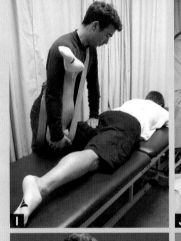 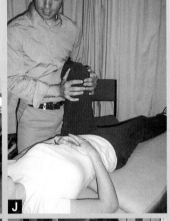

Home program of reinforcing activities:
- Prescribed up to six range-of-motion activities to reinforce clinic interventions (e.g. L)

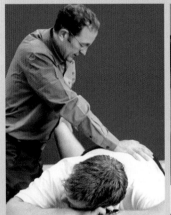 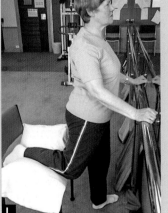

*Treatment protocol used in the MOA trial.[36] Space does not permit reproduction of the entire treatment protocol. A full description and illustrations of the intervention protocol and procedures is available at http://cmor.otago.ac.nz/moa

**The brief description and illustrations provided are no substitute for formal instruction in manual physical therapy, taught by qualified providers.

Source: Reproduced with permission from The Clarity Group.

physical therapists over an equivalent attention time.[94] The lesson therein is that it is very important to deliver a strong, progressive dose of exercise therapy in order to achieve good treatment effects—this may also be true for manual therapy—and it may not be possible to achieve this by attempting to deliver both forms of intervention at the same time. The results of these trials raise the question of what combination of interventions should be provided, and in what order. This has not yet been answered in the research.

Braces, Orthotics, and Insoles

Given the key role of mechanical forces to disease progression and symptoms of OA, particularly knee OA, biomechanical treatments targeting knee alignment and shock absorption may be very important. However, to date only modest progress has been made in this area.

In patients with medial tibiofemoral knee OA, lateral wedge insoles or orthoses may have a small benefit, but probably no greater benefit than simple nonwedged insoles.[95,96] Overall, however, the low quality of some studies and the heterogeneity among study findings suggest that any benefit of lateral wedge insoles may not be significant or clinically important.[95,96]

Shock absorbing insoles have been shown to decrease pain and disability, but medial arch supports do not appear to be useful for patients with medial tibiofemoral knee OA.[97]

There are a variety of knee braces available for people with knee OA. Not all have any published evidence of efficacy, but in general it appears that simple knee sleeves, for example neoprene supports, may decrease pain slightly but do not appear to offer any physical function benefits.[98] For patients with medial tibiofemoral knee OA, valgus knee braces are more effective than knee sleeves, with at least some medium-term benefits to pain and disability.[98,99] Valgus knee braces also provide mechanical benefits, improving gait symmetry, muscle strength and proprioception, and decreasing compressive loads to the medial joint space, although the data are quite inconsistent and low quality at this point in time.[98]

For patients with significant pain, the use of a walking cane has good face validity for decreasing mechanical forces through the hip or knee.[100,101] A recent RCT supports the clinical effectiveness of a walking cane for improving pain and physical function.[102] Although energy expenditure was substantially increased in the first month of use, patients soon became accustomed to its use, and energy expenditure returned to close to normal levels after around 2 months of use.[103]

Tape

Other interventions may be useful in addition to the core treatments and supplementary treatments described earlier. Taping has been shown to be effective for patellofemoral OA.[103-105] Methods vary, however, in general the tape is used to apply a medially-directed force to the patella, to alter contact forces between the patella and the patellar groove of the femur. A useful resource summarizing the evidence and describing the procedures can be found online in the Australian Family Physician website.[106]

Thermal Modalities

The effectiveness of therapeutic ultrasound (US) for knee OA has been studied in six small, generally low-quality trials. The data indicate that US provides a moderate benefit for reducing pain (around 1.2 points on a 0–10 pain scale), and perhaps a similar benefit for function, although the data on function have more variability and less precision.[107,108] Effects may persist beyond 10 months after the US treatment has concluded.[108]

Other thermal modalities are generally recommended in most clinical practice guidelines,[109,110] although these are based on only a small number of low quality studies. Short-wave diathermy has weak evidence of small effects on pain.[111]

Alternative and Medical Interventions

Acupuncture

Acupuncture has grown in acceptance for many musculoskeletal conditions, but there a great deal of skepticism remains among academics and clinicians. A meta-analysis of 16 RCTs of acupuncture indicate that acupuncture does show small to moderate treatment effects for relief of pain in knee OA. There is much less but generally consistent evidence for hip OA.[69,112] Most trials report only short-term outcomes.[69] Earlier studies had indicated the effect size to be similar to nonsteroidal anti-inflammatory drugs (NSAIDs), at around 0.35,[69] however, with more trials now completed, acupuncture appears less effective than first thought, at around 0.28. Although for most patients the percent change in pain and function is, on average, smaller than what can be considered clinically meaningful,[113] it may still be useful for a subset of patients who respond to acupuncture, at least in the short term. However, the most recent National

Institute for Health and Clinical Excellence (NICE) guideline recommends against offering acupuncture.[68] Acupuncture as an adjuvant to an exercise therapy program does not result in any additional benefits over exercise therapy alone.[112] Given the stronger evidence for, and effects of, exercise therapy, treatment time would be better spent doing a good job of providing exercise intervention.

Pharmacological Interventions

Acetaminophen (paracetamol) and NSAIDs are recommended,[113] although it is notable that the effect sizes for these medications in patients with OA has weakened as more studies are added to the literature.[69,113] New evidence shows the risks of harm with long-term use, particularly to the stomach and liver, have been underappreciated.[69,113] Topical capsaicin is effective for decreasing pain, but around half of users will experience skin reactions, with around 15% of users discontinuing because of these local adverse effects.[69,113] Glucosamine sulfate has been studied widely now, with many more recent negative trials balancing out earlier, poorer quality positive trials, with the result that glucosamine sulfate is not recommended.[69,113] The case is similar for chondroitin sulfate.[69,113]

Surgical Considerations

Joint replacement surgery is recommended before established disability and severe pain.[44] Joint replacement surgery for the hip and knee are both highly effective and cost-effective interventions, where indicated.[114] For many people with established pain and disability that cannot be managed by conservative therapies, it will be the best treatment. However, it is important to stress that not all cases of OA will progress to the point where joint replacement surgery is necessary or desired. Indeed, not all cases of OA will progress. Joint replacement surgery is more successful when provided neither too early nor too late in the progression of the disease; however the best timing has not been clearly established. What is clear is that revision surgeries are generally very much less effective and cost-effective in comparison to primary joint replacement surgery.[115]

Intra-articular corticosteroid injections are recommended by contemporary clinical practice guidelines,[113] however it is recommended these be provided no more than three times, and with a long period between injections, as effects generally to diminish with each subsequent use.

They appear to be most effective in people with a reasonable amount joint space remaining. There is still too little good evidence on intra-articular injection of hyaluronic acid to adequately inform recommendations.[69,113]

Similarly, as yet there is not enough high-quality evidence to support recommendations for other palliative surgeries such as microfracture, or alternatives to total joint arthroplasty such as resurfacing or unicompartmental procedures.

There is high quality evidence that arthroscopic lavage or debridement is ineffective, and, considering the risk of harm, these treatments are now consistently not recommended.[69,113]

■ CONCLUSION

For the vast majority of people with OA, medical management means long-term reliance on pain-relieving medications.[116] Family practice physicians rarely refer OA patients to physical therapy,[32] access to publicly funded treatment is limited by competing resource demands,[33] and out-of-pocket costs further limit access to private providers. For the small proportion accessing physical therapy, current physical therapist practice typically does not comply with that seen in the successful trials underpinning OA clinical guidelines.[34,35] It is not efficient to allocate the specialized resource of orthopedic surgeons' time to nonsurgical cases, yet generalist family practice doctors cannot reasonably be expected to attain expert depth of knowledge in OA management, or have the time or facilities to deliver the comprehensive level of care indicated.

There are numerous barriers to the delivery of the optimal care described in guidelines that may explain these shortcomings.[117,118] A significant barrier causing the gap between the recommendations in OA guidelines and actual health delivery is that guidelines encompass multiple forms of interventions, and implementation requires a holistic assessment and expert decision-making to target treatment effectively.[44] Both of these steps require expertise across multiple fields of knowledge that we cannot reasonably expect every primary care practitioner to possess, nor have the time and facilities to deliver. Indeed it is well recognized that medical education in musculoskeletal diseases is deficient,[119-122] and general physical therapists' knowledge, beliefs, and practice in OA are deficient.[34,35] OA care needs a paradigm shift.[123]

Although OA does not directly reduce length of life, it does impact strongly on quality of life in the years lived.

Where it persists to become a chronically painful, disabling condition, OA is implicated in a cascade of effects, described earlier (Fig. 1),[18] associated with comorbidities. Some comorbidities associated with OA, such as obesity, diabetes and depression, affect both length and quality of life. An intervention effective for treating all of those examples is exercise as a lifestyle change. Notably, it has been shown that a single weekly bout of specific exercise reduces the risk of cardiovascular death, both in men [relative risk (RR) 0.61, 95% CI 0.49–0.75], and women (RR 0.49, 95% CI 0.27–0.89), compared with those who reported no activity.[124] The form of exercise does not have to be especially frequent or intense, as research has shown that increasing the duration or the number of exercise sessions per week provides little added benefit in regards to cardiovascular risk[124]: compared with vigorous exercise, walking is associated with similar risk reductions.[125] The case for diabetes is similar.[126,127] The lifestyle change of maintaining regular exercise to manage OA will improve overall health and wellbeing and therefore will improve the cost-effectiveness of interventions over a longer term.

OA is a chronic condition requiring ongoing re-evaluation and review of treatment targeting.[44,128,129] International experts recommend that management of OA is best suited to a chronic care model (CCM) approach from early intervention to accessing secondary care.[123,128,129] There is sound basis to propose that the most efficient way of delivering this kind of multidisciplinary patient management model, with the focused expertise, time and facilities to deliver the core interventions, is within a clinic dedicated to OA, provided by physical therapy specialist practitioner.

Ideally, such a clinic would employ a CCM patient management approach explicitly guided by clinical practice guidelines.[129] Assessment and decision-making should be conducted by clinicians trained in deep and focused knowledge of OA clinical management and research.[44] The provision of the core education and exercise therapy, and adjunct manual therapy, bracing, canes and insoles, will be by physical therapists trained to faithfully deliver established effective treatment protocols. Attention must be paid to dose, progression, duration, and adherence. It is necessary to conduct a medications review and work in a collaborative multidisciplinary partnership with the referring medical doctor to ensure pharmaceutical management is optimal.[44]

The OA clinician must provide comprehensive education and advice, including around weight loss, and refer to dietitians where indicated to achieve this.[44,130,131] While challenging, there is good evidence that weight

management can be effective in people with OA,[132,133] although it is not often implemented.[134,135] Lifestyle change to include regular exercise is essential.

There is a wide range of known modifiable risk factors for functional decline in people with hip or knee OA that can be modified by core OA treatments.[21,46,136] These include physical impairments (e.g. reduced muscle strength, proprioceptive inaccuracy, and impaired range of joint motion), overweight and comorbidity, and psychological and social factors (e.g. depression, anxiety, poor self-efficacy and health behaviors).[46] These, alongside reduced pain and disability, should result in decreased consumption of other healthcare resources, increased social and occupational participation, and thereby increased health and well-being. Hence, such a holistic, integrated chronic care management approach to the management of OA, has clear potential to improve cost-effectiveness markedly over the lifetime of the patient population.[137-139]

This is an area well suited to physical therapists expertise. Research reports from the British, Australian, Canadian, and the US Military healthcare systems demonstrate the feasibility and advantages of an advanced physical therapy practitioner model. Examples have been developed to address a range of needs in orthopedic care,[140] including assessment and nonsurgical management of OA[141] and low back pain,[142] and have reported high levels of patient, general practitioner and consultant surgeon satisfaction.[142-144] Most research has been in secondary care, showing efficiency gains such as reductions in unnecessary referrals (i.e. those not requiring surgery or medical intervention) and decreased waiting times,[142,143,145] even in projects that resulted in referral volumes increasing.[143] Even in secondary care settings, the majority of patients were independently managed by physical therapists [146,147,142,143,145] and concerns with regard to X-ray investigation volume increases or excessive onward referral proved unfounded.[146] Reports have shown good agreement between advanced physical therapy practitioners and orthopedic surgeons regarding diagnostic and management decisions.[144-146,148]

More recently, a New Zealand example of a multi-disciplinary patient management clinic dedicated to OA within a secondary care hospital setting, has shown results consistent with those stated earlier.[149] In that model, a physical therapist with focused OA training and expertise assessed each patient, initiated and coordinated management and follow-up. Patients were referred to in-house facilities to deliver the core interventions. A formal program evaluation of this clinic, which serves a population of patients with moderate to severe hip or knee OA, has demonstrated very positive outcomes.[149]

In summary, osteoarthiritis is a very common, painful condition that increases in prevalence with advancing age. Osteoarthritis is a complex, active disease process involving the whole joint structure: bone, cartilage, synovium, ligaments, and muscles supporting and surrounding the affected joint. Progression can differ greatly between individuals. OA generally presents as pain at or about the joint, impacting quality of life, with reported and clinically evident functional limitation. After ruling out differential diagnoses, it can be confidently diagnosed on the basis of three simple criteria: persistent joint pain that is worse with use; age 45 years and more; and morning stiffness lasting no more than half an hour. Best-practice management of OA should begin with a holistic, multifaceted assessment that identifies the salient problems and modifiable risk factors present for each individual, and serves to direct targeted interventions. Given that:

- The strongest single feature of OA is an imbalance between adverse and advantageous biomechanical forces acting around joint;
- The body is responding with an ongoing, active repair process;
- The core recommended interventions are nonsurgical and mostly non-drug interventions, including exercise therapy; and
- There is strong evidence that the recommended interventions provided by physical therapists—most notably exercise therapy—are effective and cost-effective, clearly there is a strong role for physical therapy in the management of OA.

▨ REFERENCES

1. Grimaldi-Bensouda L, Begaud B, Lert F, Rouillon F, Massol J, Guillemot D, et al. Benchmarking the burden of 100 diseases: results of a nationwide representative survey within general practices. BMJ Open. 2011;1(2):e000215.
2. Peat G, McCarney R, Croft P. Knee pain and osteoarthritis in older adults: a review of community burden and current use of primary health care. Ann Rheum Dis. 2001;60(2):91-7.
3. Buckwalter JA, Saltzman C, Brown T. The impact of osteoarthritis: implications for research. Clin Orthop Relat Res. 2004;(427):S6-15.
4. Access Economics. The economic cost of arthritis in New Zealand in 2010. Arthritis New Zealand; 2010.
5. Access Economics. The economic cost of arthritis in New Zealand. Arthritis New Zealand; 2005.
6. Osteoarthritis Research Society International. OARSI Primer on Osteoarthritis. In: Henrotin Y, Hunter D, Kawaguchi H (Eds). Osteoarthritis Research Society International; 2010. Also available online at: http://primer.oarsi.org/content/oarsi-primer.
7. Felson DT. Osteoarthritis as a disease of mechanics. Osteoarthritis Cartilage. 2013;21(1):10-5.
8. Brosseau L, Pelland L, Wells G, Macleay L, Lamothe C, Michaud G, et al. Efficacy of aerobic exercises for osteoarthritis (part II): a meta-analysis. Physical Therapy Reviews. 2004;9:125-45.
9. Pelland L, Brosseau L, Wells G, Macleay L, Lambert J, Lamothe C, et al. Efficacy of strengthening exercises for osteoarthritis (part I): a meta-analysis. Physical Therapy Reviews. 2004;9:77-108.
10. Ralphs JR, Benjamin M. The joint capsule: structure, composition, ageing and disease. J Anat. 1994;184 (3):503-9.
11. Hoeksma HL, Dekker J, Ronday HK, Heering A, van der Lubbe N, Vel C, et al. Comparison of manual therapy and exercise therapy in osteoarthritis of the hip: a randomized clinical trial. Arthritis Rheum. 2004;51(5):722-9.
12. Hoeksma HL, Dekker J, Ronday HK, Breedveld FC, van den Ende CH. Manual therapy in osteoarthritis of the hip: outcome in subgroups of patients. Rheumatology (Oxford). 2005;44(4):461-4.
13. Robertsson O, Wingstrand H, Onnerfalt R. Intracapsular pressure and pain in coxarthrosis. J Arthroplasty. 1995;10(5):632-5.
14. Steultjens MP, Dekker J, van Baar ME, Oostendorp RA, Bijlsma JW. Range of joint motion and disability in patients with osteoarthritis of the knee or hip. Rheumatology (Oxford). 2000;39(9):955-61.
15. van Dijk GM, Veenhof C, Spreeuwenberg P, Coene N, Burger BJ, van Schaardenburg D, et al. Prognosis of limitations in activities in osteoarthritis of the hip or knee: a 3-year cohort study. Arch Phys Med Rehabil. 2010;91(1):58-66.
16. van Dijk GM, Dekker J, Veenhof C, van den Ende CH. Course of functional status and pain in osteoarthritis of the hip or knee: a systematic review of the literature. Arthritis and Rheumatism. 2006;55(5):779-85.
17. Hunter DJ, Felson DT. Osteoarthritis. BMJ. 2006;332(7542):639-42.
18. Gruber WH, Hunter DJ. Transforming osteoarthritis care in an era of health care reform. Clinics in Geriatric Medicine. 2010;26(3):433-44.
19. Abbott JH. Management of osteoarthritis: a guide to non-surgical intervention. Dunedin, New Zealand: The Clarity Group; 2014.
20. Chapple CM. Physiotherapy for osteoarthritis of the knee: predictors of outcome at one year. Dunedin: School of Physiotherapy, University of Otago; 2011.
21. Wright AA, Cook C, Abbott JH. Variables associated with the progression of hip osteoarthritis: a systematic review. Arthritis Rheum. 2009;61(7):925-36.
22. Pisters MF, Veenhof C, Schellevis FG, De Bakker DH, Dekker J. Long-term effectiveness of exercise therapy in patients with osteoarthritis of the hip or knee: a randomized controlled trial comparing two different physical therapy interventions. Osteoarthritis and Cartilage. 2010;18(8):1019-26.
23. Svege I, Nordsletten L, Fernandes L, Risberg MA. Exercise therapy may postpone total hip replacement surgery in patients with hip osteoarthritis: a long-term follow-up of a randomised trial. Ann Rheum Dis. 2013.
24. Wright AA, Cook CE, Flynn TW, Baxter GD, Abbott JH. Predictors of response to physical therapy intervention in patients with primary hip osteoarthritis. Phys Ther. 2011;91(4):510-24.
25. Currier LL, Froehlich PJ, Carow SD, McAndrew RK, Cliborne AV, Boyles RE, et al. Development of a clinical prediction rule to identify patients with knee pain and clinical evidence of knee osteoarthritis who demonstrate a favorable short-term response to hip mobilization. Phys Ther. 2007;87(9):1106-19.
26. Chapple CM, Baxter GD, Nicholson H, Abbott JH. Will this patient with knee osteoarthritis benefit from physiotherapy? Rotorua: New Zealand Manipulative Physiotherapists Association Conference; August 27-28, 2011.
27. Pham T, van der Heijde D, Altman RD, Anderson JJ, Bellamy N, Hochberg M, et al. OMERACT-OARSI initiative: Osteoarthritis Research Society International set of responder criteria for osteoarthritis clinical trials revisited. Osteoarthritis Cartilage. 2004;12(5):389-99.

28. Pham T, Van Der Heijde D, Lassere M, Altman RD, Anderson JJ, Bellamy N, et al. Outcome variables for osteoarthritis clinical trials: The OMERACT-OARSI set of responder criteria. J Rheumatol. 2003;30(7):1648-54.

29. French HP, Galvin R, Cusack T, McCarthy GM. Predictors of short-term outcome to exercise and manual therapy for people with hip osteoarthritis. Phys Ther. 2014;94(1):31-9.

30. Stanton TR, Hancock MJ, Maher CG, Koes BW. Critical appraisal of clinical prediction rules that aim to optimize treatment selection for musculoskeletal conditions. Phys Ther. 2010;90(6):843-54.

31. Hawker GA, Stewart L, French MR, Cibere J, Jordan JM, March L, et al. Understanding the pain experience in hip and knee osteoarthritis--an OARSI/OMERACT initiative. Osteoarthritis Cartilage. 2008;16(4):415-22.

32. Shrier I, Feldman DE, Gaudet MC, Rossignol M, Zukor D, Tanzer M, et al. Conservative non-pharmacological treatment options are not frequently used in the management of hip osteoarthritis. J Sci Med Sport. 2006; 9(1-2):81-6.

33. Brand C. Translating evidence into practice for people with osteoarthritis of the hip and knee. Clinical Rheumatology. 2007;26(9):1411-20.

34. Holden MA, Nicholls EE, Hay EM, Foster NE. Physical therapists' use of therapeutic exercise for patients with clinical knee osteoarthritis in the United kingdom: in line with current recommendations? Phys Ther. 2008;88(10):1109-21.

35. Walsh NE, Hurley MV. Evidence based guidelines and current practice for physiotherapy management of knee osteoarthritis. Musculoskeletal Care. 2009;7(1):45-56.

36. Abbott JH, Robertson MC, Chapple C, Pinto D, Wright AA, Leon de la Barra S, et al. Manual therapy, exercise therapy, or both, in addition to usual care, for osteoarthritis of the hip or knee: a randomized controlled trial. 1: clinical effectiveness. Osteoarthritis and Cartilage. 2013;21(4):525-34.

37. Altman R, Asch E, Bloch D, Bole G, Borenstein D, Brandt K, et al. Development of criteria for the classification and reporting of osteoarthritis. Classification of osteoarthritis of the knee. Diagnostic and Therapeutic Criteria Committee of the American Rheumatism Association. Arthritis Rheum. 1986;29(8):1039-49.

38. Altman RD. Criteria for classification of clinical osteoarthritis. J Rheumatol Suppl. 1991;27:10-2.

39. Zhang W, Doherty M, Peat G, Bierma-Zeinstra MA, Arden NK, Bresnihan B, et al. EULAR evidence-based recommendations for the diagnosis of knee osteoarthritis. Ann Rheum Dis. 2010;69(3):483-9.

40. Altman R, Alarcon G, Appelrouth D, Bloch D, Borenstein D, Brandt K, et al. The American College of Rheumatology criteria for the classification and reporting of osteoarthritis of the hip. Arthritis Rheum. 1991;34(5):505-14.

41. Peat G, Thomas E, Handy J, Wood L, Dziedzic K, Myers H, et al. The Knee Clinical Assessment Study--CAS(K). A prospective study of knee pain and knee osteoarthritis in the general population. BMC Musculoskeletal Disorders. 2004;5:4.

42. Peat G, Croft P, Hay E. Clinical assessment of the osteoarthritis patient. Best Pract Res Clin Rheumatol. 2001;15(4):527-44.

43. Royal College of Physicians. Osteoarthritis: National clinical guideline for care and management in adults. London: Royal College of Physicians of London; 2008.

44. National Institute for Health and Clinical Excellence. Osteoarthritis: the care and management of osteoarthritis in adults. NICE clinical guideline. 2008;59:1-22.

45. Zhang W, Moskowitz RW, Nuki G, Abramson S, Altman RD, Arden N, et al. OARSI recommendations for the management of hip and knee osteoarthritis, Part II: OARSI evidence-based, expert consensus guidelines. Osteoarthritis Cartilage. 2008;16(2):137-62.

46. Dekker J, van Dijk GM, Veenhof C. Risk factors for functional decline in osteoarthritis of the hip or knee. Curr Opin Rheumatol. 2009;21(5): 520-4.

47. Angst F, Aeschlimann A, Steiner W, Stucki G. Responsiveness of the WOMAC osteoarthritis index as compared with the SF-36 in patients with osteoarthritis of the legs undergoing a comprehensive rehabilitation intervention. Ann Rheum Dis. 2001;60(9):834-40.

48. Angst F, Ewert T, Lehmann S, Aeschlimann A, Stucki G. The factor subdimensions of the Western Ontario and McMaster Universities Osteoarthritis Index (WOMAC) help to specify hip and knee osteoarthritis. a prospective evaluation and validation study. J Rheumatol. 2005;32(7): 1324-30.

49. Tubach F, Ravaud P, Martin-Mola E, Awada H, Bellamy N, Bombardier C, et al. Minimum clinically important improvement and patient acceptable symptom state in pain and function in rheumatoid arthritis, ankylosing spondylitis, chronic back pain, hand osteoarthritis, and hip and knee osteoarthritis: results from a prospective multinational study. Arthritis Care Res (Hoboken). 2012;64(11):1699-707.

50. Binkley JM, Stratford PW, Lott SA, Riddle DL. The lower extremity functional scale (LEFS): scale development, measurement properties, and clinical application. Phys Ther. 1999;79(4):371-83.

51. Williams VJ, Piva SR, Irrgang JJ, Crossley C, Fitzgerald GK. Comparison of reliability and responsiveness of patient-reported clinical outcome measures in knee osteoarthritis rehabilitation. J Orthop Sports Phys Ther. 2012;42(8):716-23.

52. Abbott JH, Schmitt J. The patient-specific functional scale is valid for group-level change comparisons and between-group discrimination. J Clin Epidemiol. 2014;67(6):681-8.

53. Fairbairn K, May K, Yang Y, Balasundar S, Hefford C, Abbott JH. Mapping patient-specific functional scale (PSFS) items to the international classification of functioning, disability and health (ICF). Phys Ther. 2011;92(2):310-7.

54. Horn KK, Jennings S, Richardson G, Vliet DV, Hefford C, Abbott JH. The patient-specific functional scale: psychometrics, clinimetrics and application as a clinical outcome measure. J Orthop Sports Phys Ther. 2011;42(1):30-42.

55. Downie WW, Leatham PA, Rhind VM, Wright V, Branco JA, Anderson JA. Studies with pain rating scales. Ann Rheum Dis. 1978;37(4):378-81.

56. Walsh RM, Abbott JH. Screening for depression in a musculoskeletal outpatient physical therapy clinic: Point prevalence and comparison of two instruments. J Back Musculoskelet Rehabil. 2008;21(3):171-4.

57. Arroll B, Khin N, Kerse N. Screening for depression in primary care with two verbally asked questions: cross sectional study. BMJ. 2003;327(7424):1144-6.

58. Whooley MA, Avins AL, Miranda J, Browner WS. Case-finding instruments for depression. Two questions are as good as many. J Gen Intern Med. 1997;12(7):439-45.

59. Arroll B, Goodyear-Smith F, Kerse N, Fishman T, Gunn J. Effect of the addition of a "help" question to two screening questions on specificity for diagnosis of depression in general practice: diagnostic validity study. BMJ. 2005;331(7521):884.

60. Scopaz KA, Piva SR, Wisniewski S, Fitzgerald GK. Relationships of fear, anxiety, and depression with physical function in patients with knee osteoarthritis. Arch Phys Med Rehabil. 2009;90(11):1866-73.

61. Sandborgh M, Lindberg P, Denison E. The pain belief screening instrument (PBSI): predictive validity for disability status in persistent musculoskeletal pain. Disabil Rehabil. 2007:1-8.

62. Sandborgh M, Lindberg P, Denison E. Pain belief screening instrument: development and preliminary validation of a screening instrument for disabling persistent pain. J Rehabil Med. 2007;39(6):461-6.

63. Braund R, Abbott JH. Analgesic recommendations when treating musculo-skeletal strains and sprains. N Z J Physiother. 2007;35(2):54-60.

64. Braund R, Abbott JH. Recommending NSAIDs and paracetamol: a survey of New Zealand physiotherapists' knowledge and behaviours. Physiother Res Int. 2011;16(1):43-9.

65. Braund R, Abbott JH. Nonsteroidal anti-inflammatory drugs (NSAIDs) and paracetamol for acute musculoskeletal injuries: physiotherapists' understanding of which is safer, more effective, and when to initiate treatment. Physiother Theory Pract. 2011;27(7):482-91.

66. Dobson F, Hinman RS, Roos EM, Abbott JH, Stratford P, Davis AM, et al. OARSI recommended performance-based tests to assess physical function in people diagnosed with hip or knee osteoarthritis. Osteoarthritis Cartilage. 2013;21(8):1042-52.

67. Abbott JH, Van der Esch M, van der Leeden M, Knoop J, Lems WF, Roorde LD. Clinimetrics of the stair climb test in the Amsterdam Cohort. Osteoarthritis Cartilage. 2014;22:S186-7.

68. National Institute for Health and Care Excellence. Osteoarthritis: care and management in adults. NICE clinical guideline 177. London: National Institute for Health and Care Excellence; 2014.

69. Zhang W, Nuki G, Moskowitz RW, Abramson S, Altman RD, Arden NK, et al. OARSI recommendations for the management of hip and knee osteoarthritis: part III: Changes in evidence following systematic cumulative update of research published through January 2009. Osteoarthritis Cartilage. 2010;18(4):476-99.

70. Messier SP, Mihalko SL, Legault C, Miller GD, Nicklas BJ, DeVita P, et al. Effects of intensive diet and exercise on knee joint loads, inflammation, and clinical outcomes among overweight and obese adults with knee osteoarthritis: the IDEA randomized clinical trial. JAMA. 2013;310(12):1263-73.

71. Zhang W, Moskowitz RW, Nuki G, Abramson S, Altman RD, Arden N, et al. OARSI recommendations for the management of hip and knee osteoarthritis, part I: critical appraisal of existing treatment guidelines and systematic review of current research evidence. Osteoarthritis Cartilage. 2007;15(9):981-1000.

72. Ottawa Panel. Ottawa panel evidence-based clinical practice guidelines for therapeutic exercises and manual therapy in the management of osteoarthritis. Phys Ther. 2005;85(9):907-71.

73. Pencharz JN, Grigoriadis E, Jansz GF, Bombardier C. A critical appraisal of clinical practice guidelines for the treatment of lower-limb osteoarthritis. Arthritis Res. 2002;4(1):36-44.

74. Pinto D, Robertson MC, Hansen P, Abbott JH. Cost-effectiveness of nonpharmacologic, nonsurgical interventions for hip and/or knee osteoarthritis: systematic review. Value Health. 2012;15(1):1-12.

75. McCarthy CJ, Mills PM, Pullen R, Richardson G, Hawkins N, Roberts CR, et al. Supplementation of a home-based exercise programme with a class-based programme for people with osteoarthritis of the knees: a randomised controlled trial and health economic analysis. Health Technol Assess. 2004;8(46):iii-iv, 1-61.

76. Hurley MV, Walsh NE, Mitchell HL, Pimm TJ, Williamson E, Jones RH, et al. Economic evaluation of a rehabilitation program integrating exercise, self-management, and active coping strategies for chronic knee pain. Arthritis Rheum. 2007;57(7):1220-9.

77. Roddy E, Zhang W, Doherty M, Arden NK, Barlow J, Birrell F, et al. Evidence-based recommendations for the role of exercise in the management of osteoarthritis of the hip or knee--the MOVE consensus. Rheumatology (Oxford). 2005;44(1):67-73.

78. Tak E, Staats P, Van Hespen A, Hopman-Rock M. The effects of an exercise program for older adults with osteoarthritis of the hip. J Rheumatol. 2005;32(6):1106-13.

79. Jamtvedt G, Dahm KT, Christie A, Moe RH, Haavardsholm E, Holm I, et al. Physical therapy interventions for patients with osteoarthritis of the knee: an overview of systematic reviews. Phys Ther. 2008;88(1):123-36.

80. Fransen M, McConnell S, Bell M. Exercise for osteoarthritis of the hip or knee. Cochrane Database of Syst Rev. 2003(3):CD004286.

81. Vignon E, Valat JP, Rossignol M, Avouac B, Rozenberg S, Thoumie P, et al. Osteoarthritis of the knee and hip and activity: a systematic international review and synthesis (OASIS). Joint Bone Spine. 2006;73(4):442-55.

82. Pisters MF, Veenhof C, van Meeteren NL, Ostelo RW, de Bakker DH, Schellevis FG, et al. Long-term effectiveness of exercise therapy in patients with osteoarthritis of the hip or knee: a systematic review. Arthritis Rheum. 2007;57(7):1245-53.

83. van Baar ME, Assendelft WJ, Dekker J, Oostendorp RA, Bijlsma JW. Effectiveness of exercise therapy in patients with osteoarthritis of the hip or knee: a systematic review of randomized clinical trials. Arthritis Rheum. 1999;42(7):1361-9.

84. Zhang W, Doherty M, Arden N, Bannwarth B, Bijlsma J, Gunther KP, et al. EULAR evidence based recommendations for the management of hip osteoarthritis: report of a task force of the EULAR Standing Committee for International Clinical Studies Including Therapeutics (ESCISIT). Ann Rheum Dis. 2005;64(5):669-81.

85. Fransen M, McConnell S. Exercise for osteoarthritis of the knee. Cochrane Database Syst Rev. 2008(4):CD004376.

86. Fransen M, McConnell S, Hernandez-Molina G, Reichenbach S. Exercise for osteoarthritis of the hip. Cochrane Database Syst Rev. 2009(3):CD007912.

87. Pinto D, Robertson MC, Abbott JH, Hansen P, Campbell AJ, for the MOA Trial Team. Manual therapy, exercise therapy, or both, in addition to usual care, for osteoarthritis of the hip or knee. 2: Economic evaluation alongside a randomized controlled trial. Osteoarthritis & Cartilage. 2013;21(10):1504-13.

88. Abbott JH, Chapple C, Pinto D, Wright AA. The MOA Trial: management of osteoarthritis using exercise therapy, manual therapy, or both. New Orleans, Louisiana: The Combined Sections Meeting of the American Physical Therapy Association; 9-12 February 2011.

89. Abbott JH, Robertson MC, Chapple C, Pinto D, Wright AA, Leon de la Barra S, Baxter GD, Theis J-C, Campbell AJ, for the MOA Trial Team. Manual therapy, exercise therapy, or both, in addition to usual care, for osteoarthritis of the hip or knee: a randomized controlled trial. 1: clinical effectiveness. Osteoarthritis & Cartilage. 2013;21:525-34.

90. Pinto D, Robertson MC, Abbott JH, Hansen P, Campbell AJ, MOA Trial Team. Manual therapy, exercise therapy, or both, in addition to usual care, for osteoarthritis of the hip or knee. 2: economic evaluation alongside a randomised controlled trial. Osteoarthritis Cartilage. 2013;21(10):1504-13.

91. Deyle GD, Henderson NE, Matekel RL, Ryder MG, Garber MB, Allison SC. Effectiveness of manual physical therapy and exercise in osteoarthritis of the knee. A randomized, controlled trial. Ann Intern Med. 2000;132(3):173-81.

92. Deyle GD, Allison SC, Matekel RL, , Ryder MG, Stang JM, Gohdes DD, et al. Physical therapy treatment effectiveness for osteoarthritis of the knee: a randomized comparison of supervised clinical exercise and manual therapy procedures versus a home exercise program. Phys Ther. 2005;85(12):1301-17.

93. French HP, Cusack T, Brennan A, Caffrey A, Conroy R, Cuddy V, et al. Exercise and manual physiotherapy arthritis research trial (EMPART) for osteoarthritis of the hip: a multicenter randomized controlled trial. Arch Phys Med Rehabil. 2013;94(2):302-14.

94. Bennell KL, Egerton T, Martin J, Abbott JH, Metcalf B, McManus F, et al. Effect of physical therapy on pain and function in patients with hip osteoarthritis: a randomized clinical trial. JAMA. 2014;311(19):1987-97.

95. Penny P, Geere J, Smith TO. A systematic review investigating the efficacy of laterally wedged insoles for medial knee osteoarthritis. Rheumatol Int. 2013;33(10):2529-38.

96. Parkes MJ, Maricar N, Lunt M, LaValley MP, Jones RK, Segal NA, et al. Lateral wedge insoles as a conservative treatment for pain in patients with medial knee osteoarthritis: a meta-analysis. JAMA. 2013;310(7):722-30.

97. Hinman RS, Bardin L, Simic M, Bennell KL. Medial arch supports do not significantly alter the knee adduction moment in people with knee osteoarthritis. Osteoarthritis Cartilage. 2013;21(1):28-34.

98. Beaudreuil J, Bendaya S, Faucher M, Coudeyre E, Ribinik P, Revel M, et al. Clinical practice guidelines for rest orthosis, knee sleeves, and unloading knee braces in knee osteoarthritis. Joint Bone Spine. 2009;76(6):629-36.

99. Raja K, Dewan N. Efficacy of knee braces and foot orthoses in conservative management of knee osteoarthritis: a systematic review. Am J Phys Med Rehabil. 2011;90(3):247-62.

100. Ajemian S, Thon D, Clare P, Kaul L, Zernicke RF, Loitz-Ramage B. Cane-assisted gait biomechanics and electromyography after total hip arthroplasty. Arch Phys Med Rehabil. 2004;85(12):1966-71.

101. Simic M, Bennell KL, Hunt MA, Wrigley TV, Hinman RS. Contralateral cane use and knee joint load in people with medial knee osteoarthritis: the effect of varying body weight support. Osteoarthritis Cartilage. 2011;19(11):1330-7.

102. Jones A, Silva PG, Silva AC, Colucci M, Tuffanin A, Jardim JR, et al. Impact of cane use on pain, function, general health and energy expenditure during gait in patients with knee osteoarthritis: a randomised controlled trial. Ann Rheum Dis. 2012;71(2):172-9.

103. Crossley KM, Marino GP, Macilquham MD, Schache AG, Hinman RS. Can patellar tape reduce the patellar malalignment and pain associated with patellofemoral osteoarthritis? Arthritis Rheum. 2009;61(12):1719-25.

104. Hinman RS, Crossley KM, McConnell J, Bennell KL. Efficacy of knee tape in the management of osteoarthritis of the knee: blinded randomised controlled trial. BMJ. 2003;327(7407):135.

105. Warden SJ, Hinman RS, Watson MA, Avin KG, Bialocerkowski AE, Crossley KM. Patellar taping and bracing for the treatment of chronic knee pain: a systematic review and meta-analysis. Arthritis Rheum. 2008;59(1):73-83.

106. Handbook of Non Drug Intervention Project T. Taping for knee osteoarthritis. Aust Fam Physician. 2013;42(10):725-726.Also available online at: http://www.racgp.org.au/afp/2013/october/taping-for-knee-osteoarthritis/.

107. Rutjes AW, Nuesch E, Sterchi R, Juni P. Therapeutic ultrasound for osteoarthritis of the knee or hip. Cochrane Database Syst Rev. 2010;(1): CD003132.

108. Loyola-Sanchez A, Richardson J, MacIntyre NJ. Efficacy of ultrasound therapy for the management of knee osteoarthritis: a systematic review with meta-analysis. Osteoarthritis Cartilage. 2010;18(9):1117-26.

109. Hochberg MC, Altman RD, April KT, Benkhalti M, Guyatt G, McGowan J, et al. American College of Rheumatology 2012 recommendations for the use of nonpharmacologic and pharmacologic therapies in osteoarthritis of the hand, hip, and knee. Arthritis Care Res (Hoboken). 2012;64(4):465-74.

110. Nelson AE, Allen KD, Golightly YM, Goode AP, Jordan JM. A systematic review of recommendations and guidelines for the management of osteoarthritis: the chronic osteoarthritis management initiative of the U.S. bone and joint initiative. Semin Arthritis Rheum. 2014;43(6):701-12.

111. Laufer Y, Dar G. Effectiveness of thermal and athermal short-wave diathermy for the management of knee osteoarthritis: a systematic review and meta-analysis. Osteoarthritis Cartilage. 2012;20(9):957-66.

112. Manheimer E, Cheng K, Linde K, Lao L, Yoo J, Wieland S, et al. Acupuncture for peripheral joint osteoarthritis. Cochrane Database Syst Rev. 2010;(1): CD001977.

113. McAlindon TE, Bannuru RR, Sullivan MC, Arden NK, Berenbaum F, Bierma-Zeinstra SM, et al. OARSI Guidelines for the Non-Surgical Management of Knee Osteoarthritis. Osteoarthritis Cartilage. 2014;22(3):363-88.

114. Daigle ME, Weinstein AM, Katz JN, Losina E. The cost-effectiveness of total joint arthroplasty: a systematic review of published literature. Best Pract Res Clin Rheumatol. 2012;26(5):649-58.

115. Bhandari M, Smith J, Miller LE, Block JE. Clinical and economic burden of revision knee arthroplasty. Clinical medicine insights. Arthritis and musculoskeletal disorders. 2012;5:89-94.

116. Lane NE, Thompson JM. Management of osteoarthritis in the primary-care setting: an evidence-based approach to treatment. Am J Med. 1997;103(6A):25S-30S.

117. Cabana MD, Rand CS, Powe NR, Wu AW, Wilson MH, Abboud PA, et al. Why don't physicians follow clinical practice guidelines? A framework for improvement. JAMA. 1999;282(15):1458-65.

118. Cochrane LJ, Olson CA, Murray S, Dupuis M, Tooman T, Hayes S. Gaps between knowing and doing: understanding and assessing the barriers to optimal health care. J Contin Educ Health Prof. 2007;27(2):94-102.

119. Theis JC. Musculoskeletal undergraduate curriculum: what is required? N Z Med J. 2011;124(1335):10-2.

120. Woolf AD, Walsh NE, Akesson K. Global core recommendations for a musculoskeletal undergraduate curriculum. Ann Rheum Dis. 2004;63(5):517-24.

121. Queally JM, Kiely PD, Shelly MJ, O'Daly BJ, O'Byrne JM, Masterson EL. Deficiencies in the education of musculoskeletal medicine in Ireland. Ir J Med Sci. 2008;177(2):99-105.

122. Schmale GA. More evidence of educational inadequacies in musculoskeletal medicine. Clinical Orthopaedics and Related Research. 2005(437):251-9.

123. Hunter DJ. Lower extremity osteoarthritis management needs a paradigm shift. British Journal of Sports Medicine. 2011;45(4):283-8.

124. Wisloff U, Nilsen TI, Droyvold WB, Morkved S, Slordahl SA, Vatten LJ. A single weekly bout of exercise may reduce cardiovascular mortality: how little pain for cardiac gain? 'The HUNT study, Norway'. Eur J Cardiovasc Prev Rehabil. 2006;13(5):798-804.

125. Manson JE, Greenland P, LaCroix AZ, Stefanick ML, Mouton CP, Oberman A, et al. Walking compared with vigorous exercise for the prevention of cardiovascular events in women. N Engl J Med. 2002;347(10):716-25.

126. Hu FB, Sigal RJ, Rich-Edwards JW, Colditz GA, Solomon CG, Willett WC, et al. Walking compared with vigorous physical activity and risk of type 2 diabetes in women: a prospective study. JAMA. 1999;282(15):1433-9.

127. Sigal RJ, Kenny GP, Wasserman DH, Castaneda-Sceppa C, White RD. Physical activity/exercise and type 2 diabetes: a consensus statement from the American Diabetes Association. Diabetes Care. 2006;29(6):1433-8.

128. Battersby M, Von Korff M, Schaefer J, Davis C, Ludman E, Greene SM, et al. Twelve evidence-based principles for implementing self-management support in primary care. Jt Comm J Qual Patient Saf. 2010;36(12):561-70.

129. March L, Amatya B, Osborne RH, Brand C. Developing a minimum standard of care for treating people with osteoarthritis of the hip and knee. Best Pract Res Clin Rheumatol. 2010;24(1):121-145.

130. National Institute for Health and Clinical Excellence. Obesity: guidance on the prevention, identification, assessment and management of overweight and obesity in adults and children. NICE clinical guideline 2006;43.

131. Brosseau L, Wells GA, Tugwell P, Egan M, Dubouloz CJ, Casimiro L, et al. Ottawa Panel evidence-based clinical practice guidelines for the management of osteoarthritis in adults who are obese or overweight. Physical Therapy. 2011;91(6):843-61.

132. Messier SP, Loeser RF, Miller GD, Morgan TM, Rejeski WJ, Sevick MA, et al. Exercise and dietary weight loss in overweight and obese older adults with knee osteoarthritis: the Arthritis, Diet, and Activity Promotion Trial. Arthritis Rheum. 2004;50(5):1501-10.

133. Ravaud P, Flipo RM, Boutron I, Roy C, Mahmoudi A, Giraudeau B, et al. ARTIST (osteoarthritis intervention standardized) study of standardised consultation versus usual care for patients with osteoarthritis of the knee in primary care in France: pragmatic randomised controlled trial. BMJ. 2009;338:b421.

134. DeHaan MN, Guzman J, Bayley MT, Bell MJ. Knee osteoarthritis clinical practice guidelines--how are we doing? J Rheumatol. 2007;34(10):2099-105.

135. Jordan KM, Sawyer S, Coakley P, Smith HE, Cooper C, Arden NK. The use of conventional and complementary treatments for knee osteoarthritis in the community. Rheumatology. 2004;43(3):381-4.

136. Chapple CM, Nicholson H, Baxter GD, Abbott JH. Patient characteristics that predict progression of knee osteoarthritis: a systematic review of prognostic studies. Arthritis Care & Research. 2011;63(8):1115-25.

137. Jessep SA, Walsh NE, Ratcliffe J, Hurley MV. Long-term clinical benefits and costs of an integrated rehabilitation programme compared with outpatient physiotherapy for chronic knee pain. Physiotherapy. 2009;95(2):94-102.

138. Pinto D, Robertson MC, Hansen P, Abbott JH. Cost-effectiveness of Non-pharmacologic, Non-surgical Interventions for Hip and/or Knee Osteoarthritis: Systematic Review. Value in Health. 2012;15(1):1-12.

139. Trueman P, Haynes SM, Felicity Lyons G, Louise McCombie E, McQuigg MS, Mongia S, et al. Long-term cost-effectiveness of weight management in primary care. Int J Clin Pract. 2010;64(6):775-783.

140. Kersten P, McPherson K, Lattimer V, George S, Breton A, Ellis B. Physiotherapy extended scope of practice-who is doing what and why? Physiotherapy. 2007;93:235-42.

141. Brand CA, Amatya B, Gordon B, Tosti T, Gorelik A. Redesigning care for chronic conditions: improving hospital-based ambulatory care for people with osteoarthritis of the hip and knee. Intern Med J. 2010;40(6):427-36.

142. Blackburn MS, Cowan SM, Cary B, Nall C. Physiotherapy-led triage clinic for low back pain. Aust Health Rev. 2009;33(4):663-70.

143. Maddison P, Jones J, Breslin A, Barton C, Fleur J, Lewis R, et al. Improved access and targeting of musculoskeletal services in northwest Wales: targeted early access to musculoskeletal services (TEAMS) programme. BMJ. 2004;329(7478):1325-7.

144. Oldmeadow LB, Bedi HS, Burch HT, Smith JS, Leahy ES, Goldwasser M. Experienced physiotherapists as gatekeepers to hospital orthopaedic outpatient care. Med J Aus. 2007;186(12):625-8.

145. Hattam P, Smeatham A. Evaluation of an orthopaedic screening service in primary care. Clinical Performance & Quality Health Care. 1999;7(3):121-4.

146. Rabey M. Orthopaedic physiotherapy practitioners: surgical and radiological referral rates. Clinical Governance: An International Journal. 2009;14(1):15-9.

147. Pearse EO, Maclean A, Ricketts DM. The extended scope physiotherapist in orthopaedic out-patients - an audit. Annals of the Royal College of Surgeons of England. 2006;88(7):653-5.

148. MacKay C, Davis AM, Mahomed N, Badley EM. Expanding roles in orthopaedic care: a comparison of physiotherapist and orthopaedic surgeon recommendations for triage. Journal of Evaluation in Clinical Practice. 2009;15(1):178-83.

149. Abbott JH, Harcombe H. The Joint Clinic: programme evaluation of a clinical service delivered by the Orthopaedic Outpatient Department, Dunedin Hospital. Dunedin, New Zealand: Centre for Musculoskeletal Outcomes Research; 2014.

Hamstring Strain

Timothy L Vidale

ABSTRACT

The hamstrings are a group of three muscles located at the posterior thigh. The biceps femoris, semimembranosus and semitendinosus are two-joint muscles that function to extend the hip and flex the knee. The most often injured muscle of the hamstring group is the largest of the three muscles, the biceps femoris. Hamstring strain injuries (HSIs) are among the most common injuries in the active population, and they are notorious for their high reinjury rate. In the American National Football League, HSIs have been reported to account for 12% of all primary injuries sustained, and their recurrence rate is alarming, at 32%.

A strain of the biceps femoris generally resolves more rapidly than an injury incurred at the semimembranosus, and the two usually have different mechanisms of injury. Neuromuscular control, core strengthening and eccentric hamstring strengthening have all been researched as successful methods of rehabilitation of hamstring strains with the added benefit of decreased reinjury rates and relatively short return to sport times.

▨ INTRODUCTION

The hamstrings are commonly injured muscle group, and the ability to identify and appropriately treat the injury is paramount to returning the person to their prior level of function. Understanding the different types of muscle injuries and having an appreciation for the recovery period is also important when dealing with the hamstrings, as there is much to be considered.

Anatomy

The hamstrings are a group of three muscles located at the posterior thigh. The biceps femoris, semimembranosus and semitendinosus (Fig. 1) are two-joint muscles that function to extend the hip and flex the knee. They share a common origin at the ischial tuberosity but have distinct insertion sites. The semimembranosus and semitendinosus insert on the medial proximal tibia and therefore have the capacity to internally rotate the distal leg. The biceps femoris, however, which also has a short head originating at the posterolateral shaft of the femur, converges with the long head and inserts on the head of the fibula. Thus the biceps portion of the hamstrings may externally rotate the distal leg. The most often injured muscle of the hamstring group is the largest of the three muscles, the biceps femoris. It is important to note that the two heads of the biceps femoris have different neural innervations, and this has been identified as a possible contributor to injury.[1,2] The semitendinosus, semimembranosus and long head of the biceps femoris receive their innervation from the tibial nerve; while,

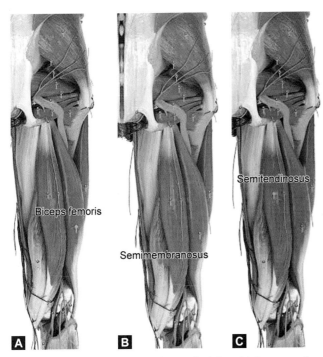

FIGS 1A TO C: Posterior view of right thigh prosection, locations of hamstrings musculature—(A) Biceps femoris; (B) Semimembranosus; (C) Semitendinosus

the short head of the biceps femoris is innervated by the common fibular nerve.[1]

Epidemiology

Hamstring strain injuries (HSIs) are among the most common injuries in the active population, and they are notorious for their high reinjury rate. In the American National Football League, HSIs have been reported to account for 12%[3] of all primary injuries sustained, and their recurrence rate is alarming, at 32%.[2] According to multiple studies, the best predictor for a hamstring injury is a prior hamstring injury.[4-6] There are other risk factors involved in predicting if someone is vulnerable to a hamstring injury but none have proven more consistent. This is not to say that if one suffers a hamstring injury that they will definitely suffer another one. However, the probability of reinjuring the same hamstring in the future becomes considerably higher.

This injury has been the topic of research for many years in attempts to discover why they occur, how to predict them, and how to prevent and to treat them. Through these studies, predisposing factors have been identified. Researchers have determined that the most consistent non-modifiable factors for HSIs are age and

the history of a prior hamstring injury.[4-6] Modifiable risk factors for this injury have been shown to be hamstring weakness, fatigue, decreased flexibility and muscular imbalance between the quadriceps and hamstrings.[6] Additional factors that may also have merit for the predisposition of HSI are limited quadriceps flexibility and deficient strength and coordination of pelvic and trunk muscles.[7,8]

Hamstring injury can occur in either a high-speed state, where the muscle is overstrained, or in a slow-speed state where the muscle is overstretched. The two mechanisms of injury contrast one another and generally occur in different locations. The most common mechanism of injury to the hamstring is during high-speed running and is believed to occur during the terminal swing phase of the gait cycle.[9,10] Biomechanically, during the second half of the swing phase, the hamstrings are actively lengthening (eccentrically contracting) and absorbing energy from the decelerating limb to prepare for ground contact.[11-13] The biceps femoris is required to contract forcefully while lengthening to decelerate the extending knee and flexing hip.[12,13] At this point, the long head of the biceps femoris is placed under the greatest amount of muscle-tendon stretch, reaching almost 110%[14] of its length during upright standing, often causing the muscle belly to be the site of injury for this kind of insult.[15] In contrast, HSIs that occur during slow movements such as dancing or stretching involve simultaneous hip flexion and knee extension, placing the hamstrings in a position of extreme stretch.[16] The proximal semimembranosus is most frequently insulted tissue in this situation and is therefore often the site of injury.[17,18] Although this mechanism of injury is less painful at onset, it tends to require a longer recovery period than a HSI incurred in a high-speed state.[17-19]

Simply put, physiologic healing of HSI depend upon the mechanism of injury, the locations and severity of the injury, and size of the injury.[16] For instance, a hamstring strain located proximally at the semimembranosus tendon that is incurred while stretching will require a longer recovery period than an injury incurred while sprinting, located distally in the biceps femoris muscle belly. These components have a direct effect on healing time for this injury and should be considered heavily when providing a diagnosis and prognosis.

Prognosis

Providing a patient with a precise prediction of when they can return to sport is a difficult task. Prognoses

are generally given in ranges to account for variation in individual responses to treatment. However, with the highly variable nature of a hamstring strain injury from person to person, ranges may tend to be wider, depending on severity of the injury. Following an optimal physical therapy regimen, ranges generally present:

- Grade I: Mild strain of the tissue with mild to moderate pain—1–3 weeks[20,21]
- Grade II: Partial rupture of the muscle tissue with mild to moderate pain and moderate to severe pain—4–8 weeks[20,21]
- Grade III: Full rupture of the muscle tissue, significant weakness and minimal pain—3-6 months[20]

Grade II and grade III injuries are not all the same, and return to sport is very much dependent on the physical demands that the sport places on the hamstring. For more severe injuries, where the injury site is at the ischial tuberosity attachment, the median time for return to sport is 31 weeks.[19] Grade III strains may require surgical intervention.[19]

Magnetic resonance imaging (MRI) is a useful tool in providing a realistic prognosis. MRI makes it possible to measure the actual size of the injury in length and cross-sectional area.[22] Length and cross-sectional area of the injury have been found to be directly proportional to the time away from sport necessary for recovery.[23,24] Although MRI, does provide this brilliant bit of information, it is of no value in predicting reinjury.[24,25]

The most recent research suggests that the following factors require longer recovery periods (greater than 3 weeks):

- Injury to the proximal semimembranosus[17-19]
- Close proximity of the injury to the ischial tuberosity[26]
- Increased length and cross-sectional area of the injury.[20,22,23,27]

Although injuries involving the long head of the biceps femoris present with greater initial starkness, the recovery period is generally much shorter than one involving the semimembranosus.[17]

CLINICAL PRESENTATION

Hamstring strain injury symptoms are few but generally consistent. Patients normally exhibit pain, edema, decreased range of motion (ROM), and weakness of the hamstrings.[16] Patients with more severe injuries will also present with a palpable gap in the muscle tendon proximally. In some cases, patients may present with ecchymosis or even pain with sitting.[21] The onset of symptoms may differ depending on the type and

location of the injury the patient incurs. For instance, a person experiencing a slow state HSI may feel and/or hear a pop at the posterior thigh but not experience any immediate pain.[19] In contrast, a patient who suffers a high-speed HSI may not have any audible presentation, but instead is likely to feel a sharp pain shooting down the posterior thigh that may cause them to cease activity immediately. This is generally followed by difficulty with normal walking. The severity and location of the injury are determined via examination and/or MRI.[28]

Hamstring strain injuries are classified into three grades according to degree of pain, weakness and loss of motion.[21] Grade I is considered a mild injury with mild to moderate pain and weakness as well as minimal damage to the muscle fibers.[21] Grade II is deemed moderate with tendon damage being more pronounced, weakness being evident and moderate to severe pain.[21] Grade III is classified as severe and presents with a complete rupture or tear of the tendon, with severe pain at the time of injury but minimal pain and notable weakness thereafter.[21] This grading system can be used to prognosticate the recovery period for the injury as well as design the appropriate rehabilitation regimen.[29] If a patient presents with a Grade I strain, neural testing to the sciatic nerve should be performed, as the cause for the posterior thigh pain may be of neural origin (Table 1).

CLINICAL EXAMINATION

High examination aptitude enables the clinician to provide a realistic prognosis for the amount of time the athlete should plan to miss from activity. The capacity to discern the severity and location of a HSI increases the clinician's ability to provide the appropriate treatment as well. A strong understanding of how this injury presents and what differences in location of injury can mean to the convalescent period, will provide a solid foundation for the rehabilitation process.

While a gold standard for HSI diagnosis has not been established, the most reliable method of confirming a hamstring strain is MRI. Ultrasound is often used as a diagnostic tool but is only comparable to MRI in the acute stage of injury.[21] As the healing process progresses, its sensitivity in detecting an insult decreases.[22] An MRI is also useful in showcasing edema and determining accurate cross-sectional measurement of the affected area.[22] Barring an MRI, clinical examination is a strong diagnostic tool for this injury. Clinical testing should include ROM testing, discerning palpation, strength testing and neural tension testing (Table 2).

TABLE 1: Differentiating HSI from referred neural pain in the posterior thigh[30]

Symptom/Sign	Hamstring strain injury	Referred to posterior thigh
Onset	Sudden	Sudden or gradual
Pain	Minimal to severe	Minimal to moderate pain. Patient may describe feeling of tightness or cramping
Function	Difficulty walking or running	Able to walk or run with minimal change in symptoms during the activity; may even reduce symptoms during the activity but increase after
Local hematoma, bruising	Likely with more severe injuries	None
Palpation	Substantial local tenderness. Possible defect at site of injury	Minimal to none
Decrease in strength	Substantial	Minimal to none
Decrease in flexibility	Substantial	Minimal
Slump test	Negative	Frequently positive
Gluteal trigger points	Palpation does not influence hamstring symptoms	Palpation may reproduce hamstring symptoms
Lumbar/sacroiliac exam	Occasionally abnormal	Frequently abnormal
Local ultrasound or MRI	Abnormal except for very mild strains	Normal

Source: Adapted from McGraw-Hill with permission.

TABLE 2: Characteristics of hamstring strain injuries[18,26]

Injury mechanism	Ecchymosis	SLR* deficit (compared to non-injured limb)	Knee flexion strength deficit (compared to non-injured limb)	Level of pain	Site of maximum pain from ischial tuberosity (cm)	Length of painful area (cm)	Median time to pre-injury level (weeks)
Running at maximal or near maximal speed	Minimal	40%	60%	Moderate	12±6 (range 5–24)	11±5 (range 5–24)	16 (range 6-50)
Movement involving extreme hip flexion and knee extension	None	20%	20%	Mild	2±1 (range 1–3)	5±2 (range 2–9)	50 (range 30-76)

*Straight leg raises.
Source: Adapted from SAGE with permission.

Range of Motion and Flexibility

The hamstrings are biarticular muscles, so ROM measurements and tests should be conducted at both the hip and knee joints. This assessment will normally take place acutely postinjury, so it is important to note that the extent of available motion may be limited by discomfort, stiffness or pain, leading to a deficient measurement. For this reason, testing should be done bilaterally.

Active Knee Extension Test[8,20]

The patient is positioned in supine with the clinician standing on the test side. The test side lower extremity is then passively flexed at the hip to end range with the knee flexed. The patient is then asked to actively extend the knee to end range. Once the knee meets restriction, this measurement should be taken at the knee, as this would be a true reflection of hamstring length. The knee should be able to extend to at least 20°.[31]

Fingertip to Foot

The patient is positioned in long sitting. Instructions are given for the patient to flex forward from the hip and reach for their toes as far as possible. The distance between the edge of the patient's fingertip and the dorsum of their foot is measured. This is used as an outcome measure to assess progress. The shorter that distance becomes without compensation denotes positive progress.

Palpation

This is one of the most important tools that any clinician has in their tool kit. The ability to discern differences in muscle tissue aids in making a proper diagnosis of this injury. Although not every patient with a HSI will present with a palpable defect in the muscle, tenderness and pain to the touch should also be documented.[16]

Hamstrings

In order to help locate the different muscles in the group, light resisted knee flexion with the patient in prone can be performed. Be mindful that this may be painful for the patient. Once muscles have been identified, palpation should begin distally and work toward the proximal attachment. This will allow for the clinician to feel consistency along the muscle fibers, making it easier to identify a defect. If the defect is distal, the clinician should notice an immediate to early change in tissue consistency, or the patient is likely to report pain during palpation. *Clinical pearl*: The location and severity of pain from the ischial tuberosity can provide insight about the potential length of the recovery period.[16] The more distal pain is located from the ischial tuberosity, the better the prognosis (Table 2).[16]

Hip Adductors

It is important to examine the adductors due to their proximity to the hamstrings, as adductor strains are also very common in the athletic population.[16] Adductor strains typically occur during movements involving quick acceleration or change of direction, as well as motions requiring extreme hip abduction and external rotation.[32] Due to its anatomic alignment, the posterior portion of the adductor magnus is sometimes considered functionally as a hamstring.[33] Injuries to the adductor magnus can be misidentified by the patient or clinician as a hamstring strain. The posterior adductor magnus originates at the ischial tuberosity, adjacent to the semimembranosus and can be palpated medial to the semimembranosus during the examination. A defect would also be palpable in this muscle tissue, if present. Furthermore, pain with palpation and isometric adduction resistance testing are positive indicators of injury to the adductor magnus.

Strength Testing

Isometric muscle testing should be conducted as part of a HSI examination to get a baseline postinjury measurement. These tests should be carried out bilaterally to gauge how deficient the affected limb has become. The hamstrings are two-joint muscles, so testing should be conducted in multiple test positions to account for changes that arise with hip and knee relative positioning.[16]

Knee Flexion

The patient should be positioned in the prone position with the hip in 0° of extension. While stabilizing the hip, the clinician's opposite hand should be placed just proximal to the medial and lateral malleoli, on the posterior shaft of the tibia. Knee flexion should then be resisted at both 15° and 90° (Fig. 2).[16] By internally or externally rotating the tibia, bias can be applied to the medial or lateral hamstrings.[16]

Hip Extension

With the patient positioned in prone and the knee flexed to 90°, resistance should be applied to the posterior distal thigh. This position biases the hamstring and pain or

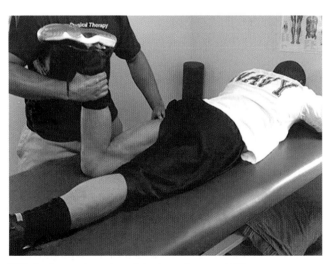

FIG. 2: Strength testing of the knee flexors at 90°

inability here would indicate a hamstring injury. Extension should also be assessed with the knee at 0° of flexion and resistance applied to the posterior shaft of the tibia just proximal to the medial and lateral malleoli, as this position incorporates the gluteals. Pain with resistance in this posture and not with the knee flexed would be more indicative of a gluteal injury. Pain provocation is a relevant finding during this test.[16]

Neural Tension Testing

Testing to clear the sciatic nerve should be conducted, as symptoms of a neural origin can be the cause of posterior thigh pain. This can be tested through the implementation of a slump test. The reproduction of symptoms from a positive slump test indicates a more proximal cause for the posterior thigh pain.[20,34] There has been a correlation found between positive neural tension and recurrent hamstring injuries, due to residual inflammation and scar tissue that is suspected to affect normal sciatic nerve mobility.[35]

Slump Test

The patient should be positioned in sitting with legs dangling and asked to place their hands behind their back. The patient would then passively be brought into neck and trunk flexion to their perceived limit. The clinician will then have the patient extend the knee and passively dorsiflex the foot. If pain presents in the posterior thigh, the patient is asked to extend the neck. If the pain in the thigh is alleviated with this maneuver, the test is positive for neural tension.

Clinical pearl: Neural tension could be the simple explanation for patients who present with posterior thigh pain without a mechanism of injury (Table 2).[36]

Passive Straight Leg Raise Test[8,28]

The patient is positioned in supine with the clinician standing on the test side. The lower extremity is held in knee extension and the hip passively flexed until restriction occurs. Attention must also be paid to the contralateral limb for hip or knee flexion as compensation to achieve greater hip flexion on the test side. The normal range for hip flexion with the knee extended is 80°–140°.[37] A measurement of less than 80° is considered deficient in ROM. Patients with adverse neural tension will likely report lower extremity or lumbar pain with this maneuver. The pain may occur in a region where it could be confused with a localized hamstring injury. Sensitization maneuvers, similar to those performed in the slump test, can be used to help differentiate between discomfort brought on by hamstring muscle tension and that of impaired sciatic neural mobility.

■ PHYSICAL THERAPY TREATMENT

The main goal of physical therapy treatment for a HSI is to return the athlete to sport at their prior level of function, pain free and with minimal risk of re-injury.[16] Recurrence is of serious concern with this particular injury due to its alarmingly high rate. The highest risk of recurrence is within the first 2 weeks of returning to sport.[38] Many elements of this injury and recovery have been found to contribute to the rate of reinjury.[39] Factors such as persistent weakness in the injured muscle, reduced extensibility of the muscle due to adaptive changes in the biomechanics and motor patterns of sporting movements following the original injury.[39] Consideration should also be given to why the original injury occurred when prescribing a treatment program.

Due to the fact that HSIs generally occur during eccentric contraction of the muscle, rehabilitation involving eccentric strength training of the hamstrings has been encouraged. Research suggests that residual scar tissue present at the muscle attachment site contributes to a shorter optimum length for active tension than in the previously injured muscle.[40,41] This is because scar tissue is tauter than the contractile tissue of the hamstring musculature and may alter the biomechanical function of the muscle by decreasing the peak muscle-tendon length.[16] Eccentric strength training has been shown to assist in shifting the peak force development to longer muscle-tendon lengths, thus reducing the risk of reinjury.[42]

Another proposed treatment of HSIs is to promote increased coordination of the lumbopelvic region. Doing so would allow the hamstrings to operate at safe lengths during sport motions, thus reducing the risk of reinjury.[8,16,38] These theories have been supported by recent research and appear to show the most promise with speedy return to sport, as well as prevention of recurrent injury. Many more interventions are presented and discussed in this chapter with the aim of optimizing treatment for HSIs. Typical progressions are provided, but each treatment program should be tailored to the individual patient.

TABLE 3: Phases of rehabilitation progression[16]

Phase I	
Goals	**Criteria for progression**
• Protect scar development • Minimize atrophy	• Normal walking stride without pain • Very low speed jog without pain • Pain free isometric contraction against submaximal (50–70%) resistance during prone knee flexion at 90° manual strength test
Phase II	
Goals	**Criteria for progression**
• Regain pain-free hamstring strength, beginning in mid-range and progressing to a longer hamstring length • Develop neuromuscular control of trunk and pelvis with progressive increase in movement speed	• Full strength (5/5 manual muscle test) without pain during prone knee flexion at 90° manual strength test • Pain free forward and backward jog, moderate intensity
Phase III	
Goals	**Criteria for return to sport**

• Symptom free during all activities
• Normal concentric and eccentric hamstring strength through full range of motion and speeds
• Improve neuromuscular control of trunk and pelvis
• Integrate postural control into sport-specific movements
	• Full strength without pain
	  ○ Four consecutive reps of maximum effort manual strength test in prone knee flexion position at 90° and at 15°
	  ○ Less than 5% bilateral deficit in eccentric hamstrings (30°/s): concentric quadriceps (240°/s) ratio during isokinetic testing
	  ○ Bilateral symmetry in knee flexion angle of peak isokinetic concentric knee flexion torque at 60°/s
	• Full pain free range of motion
	• Replication of sport specific movements near maximal speed without pain (e.g. incremental sprint test for running athletes)

Source: Adapted with permission from Journal of Orthopaedic & Sports Physical Therapy.

Rehabilitation of a HSI is broken down into three phases, each with goals and progression criteria for phase advancement and return to sport (Table 3).[16] Phase one focuses on minimizing pain and edema while protecting the healing area, especially immediately following insult.[29] Low intensity, pain-free activity encompassing the entire leg and core region are initiated through the pain free range to reduce atrophy and increase neuromuscular control in this phase.[16] ROM and intensity of the interventions as well as eccentric strengthening are increased according to the patient's tolerance, and progression of these variables continues in phase two of rehabilitation.[16] Phase three is when return to sport activities begin, incorporating more sport specific treatment interventions through the full, pain free ROM.[16] At this point the patient should be ready to begin assimilating back into their sport with gradually lessening restrictions.

Phase I

In this phase, where the injury is the most acute, there are two main goals. Treatment here must protect scar development and minimize atrophy. The following are examples of exercises that can be used as interventions in this phase that would adhere to safety guidelines yet help to meet the criteria for progression.

Stationary Bike

This activity is beneficial for a patient recovering from a hamstring strain as a component of an active warm-up. It is a non-impact, low stress method of actively warming up the muscle in preparation for the upcoming treatment. Biking promotes increased circulation, increases extensibility to the tissues, and should be guided by the clinician to an appropriate threshold for the patient.

Tissue Mobilization

The patient will lay prone on the treatment table with the entire hamstring area exposed. The location of treatment is to be focused and will vary dependent on where the site of injury. If the injury is proximal, at the semimembranosus near the ischial tuberosity (Fig. 3A), a palpable gap will be present indicating inconsistency in the muscle tissue.[21] Cross-friction massage to the area will aid in encouraging proper, perpendicular alignment of the muscle fibers and promote blood flow. If the injury is distal in the muscle belly of the biceps femoris (Fig. 3B), the same rules apply with respect to the delivery of cross-friction massage. However, there may be a palpable gap or lump with the presence of injury.[21]

Hamstring Stretching

Stretching of the hamstring postinjury can be dangerous in the acute phase, and should be carried out gently as it is a precaution. The purpose of the early stretching is to avoid dense scar formation in the area of the injury, which can prohibit muscle regeneration.[29] Hamstring stretching should be performed lightly in the early stages (starting more than 5 days postinjury), to tolerance and without pain.[16,29] Protection of the healing tissue in this regard holds true regardless of the location of the injury.[29] There are various methods of stretching the hamstring, but an easy method of allowing the patient control in stretching is in the half-seated position (Fig. 4A). The starting position is with the injured limb on the treatment table with the knee extended while the contralateral foot is on the floor. The patient should be told to begin sitting upright with the knee fully extended and the foot in dorsiflexion. The patient is then instructed to lean the trunk forward at the hip to tolerance. The degree of hip flexion may vary significantly from person to person. Prolonged stretching can have a positive effect here. Have the patient extend their upper extremity as far as they can without pain and measure the distance from their fingertip to the top of their foot. Periodically measuring their progress to show tangible improvement in flexibility and can be a good barometer of progress, as well as aid with patient morale. Other methods of hamstring stretching can also be employed (Fig. 4B).

Dynamic Stretching

Walking knee to chest[43]

The patient will walk forward pulling their knee toward their chest to the point of feeling a light stretch at the ipsilateral proximal posterior thigh, alternating legs as they advance (Figs 5A to C). This exercise places the patient in hip and knee flexion creating a light stretch at the proximal hamstring at its end range. It also encourages stabilization to through the stance limb and the core.

Inch worms[43]

The patient will begin in the plank position and inch their feet forward toward their hands to tolerance (Figs 6A to C). At this point they will then walk their hands back out towards the plank position. This exercise gradually stretches both hamstrings dynamically and aids in preparing the muscle for activity.

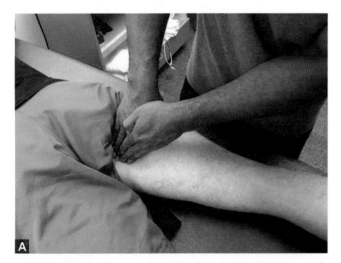
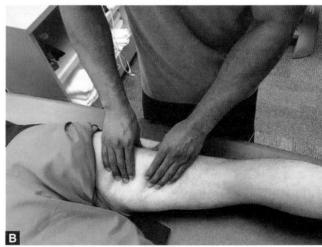

FIGS 3A AND B: Tissue mobilization by location: (A) Semimembranosus proximal to ischial tuberosity attachment; (B) Muscle belly of biceps femoris

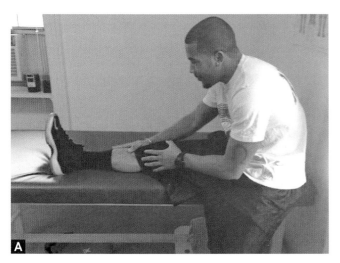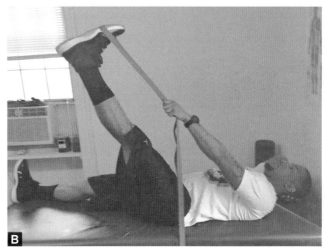

FIGS 4A AND B: Hamstring stretching in different positions: (A) Half-sitting trunk flexion; (B) Supine with hip flexed and knee extended with strap

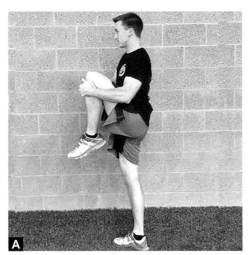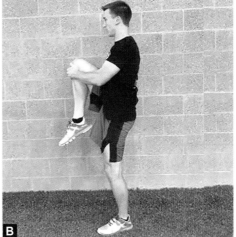

FIGS 5A AND B: Walking knee to chest—(A) Left hip and knee flexed; (B) Right hip and knee flexed

Frankensteins[43]

The patient begins standing with their shoulders flexed to 90° and elbows fully extended. The patient will walk forward alternately kicking each leg up towards their hands, or through a tolerable range (Figs 7A to C). This exercise should be performed under control and not for speed, but with proper form to aid in the dynamic stretch of the hamstring muscles.

Resistance Exercises

Isometric resisted hamstring curls

The patient is positioned in prone with the injured limb in knee flexion. This exercise should be conducted at 15°

and 90° (Fig. 8). The clinician places his hand at the distal tibia proximal to the ankle to apply resistance. The patient is then asked to resist extension with the command "don't let me move you" as the clinician applies enough force to generate an isometric contraction. If patient reports pain, resistance should be decreased.

Stool Pulls[43]

The patient begins by sitting on a wheeled stool with the heel of the affected limb planted into the ground (Figs 9A to D). The patient will use their hamstring to propel forward by flexing the involved knee. This enhances strength of the hamstring through concentric contraction. This activity can be progressed by adding distance or advancing to the use of only one leg.

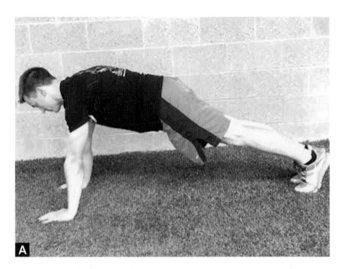

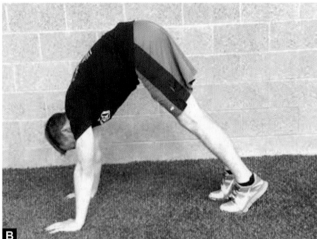

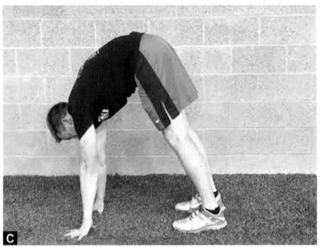

FIGS 6A TO C: Inchworms—(A) Plank position; (B) Feet moving towards hands into pike position; (C) End range of exercise

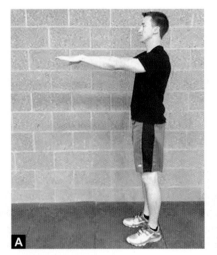

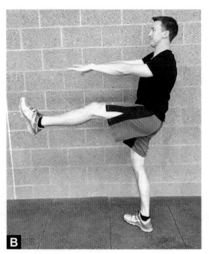

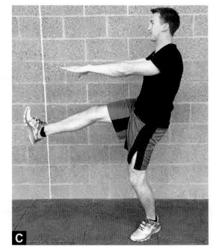

FIGS 7A TO C: Frankensteins: (A) Standing with arms flexed to 90°; B) Left hip flexed to 90° with knee fully extended; (C) Right hip flexed to 90° with knee fully extended

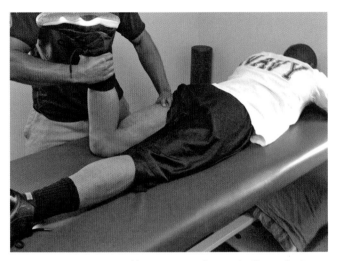

FIG. 8: Isometric resisted hamstring curls at 90° of knee flexion.

Standing hamstring curls[43]

This exercise is a progression of the isometric hamstring curls mentioned earlier. The patient stands at the edge of a table so they have something to help stabilize them while they have an ankle weight attached to the affected limb (Figs 10A and B). The patient then flexes the knee moving the foot toward the buttocks. This aids in improvement of both concentric and eccentric hamstring strength and should be introduced later in Phase I as a progression from isometric exercise.

Prone leg drops[43]

The patient lies prone with the involved foot in the air. The clinician will start moving the foot back and forth passively (Figs 11A and B) before suddenly dropping

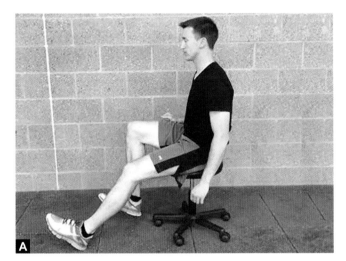
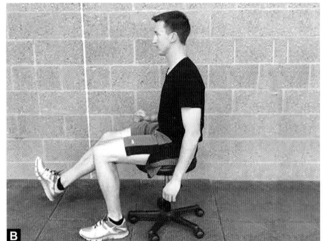
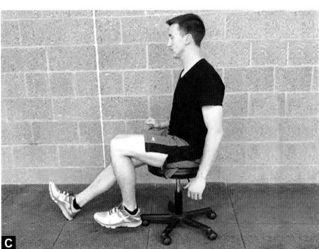
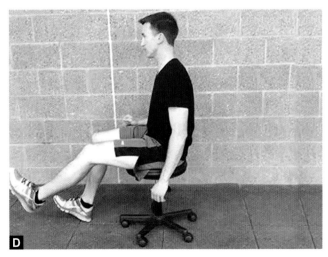

FIGS 9A TO D: Stool pulls—(A) Affected limb planted in the ground; (B) Affected limb pulling stool forward; (C) Unaffected limb planted in the ground; (D) Unaffected limb pulling stool forward

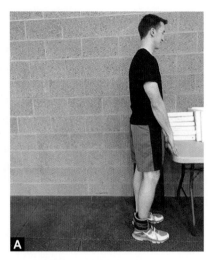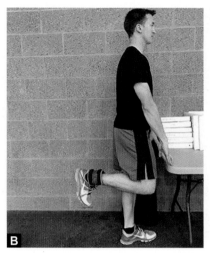

FIGS 10A AND B: Standing hamstring curls: (A) Starting position with weight attached at ankle; (B) Knee flexed moving toward buttocks

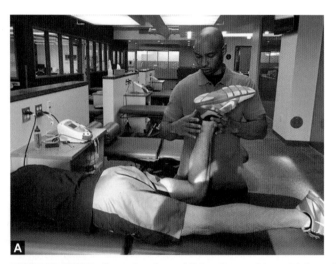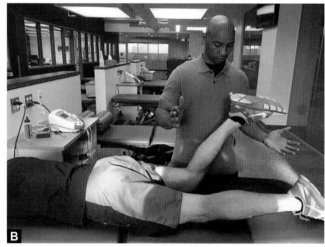

FIGS 11A AND B: Prone leg drops: (A) Starting position with knee flexed to approximately 90°; (B) Suddenly drop leg toward table

the foot toward the table. The patient is to catch the foot as soon as they feel it begin to drop. This activity aids in increasing proprioception as well as uses concentric contractions to strengthen the hamstring.

Exercise Progressions

Grapevines[16]

This exercise is a component of an active warm-up. The patient should be placed in an open space and positioned so that they can move laterally for approximately 30 feet. The patient is instructed to step laterally (for example to the left) placing the right foot over the front of the left foot and then continuing the motion laterally taking a

step left with the left foot as the right foot is then placed behind the left foot (Fig. 12). This is to be repeated for the assigned distance then the opposite motion is to be performed moving laterally in the opposite direction. The speed of this exercise should be started as a walk through to very light jog and can be increased as both the patient's performance of the motion and the condition of their hamstrings improve.

Basketball slides

The patient should be placed in an open area and positioned so that they can move laterally for approximately 30 feet. A resistance band loop should be placed around both ankles with the patient standing

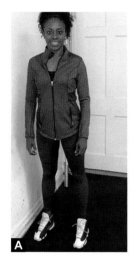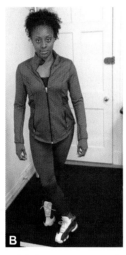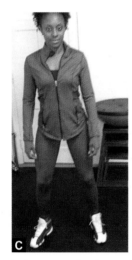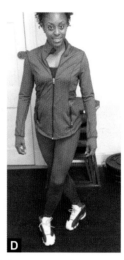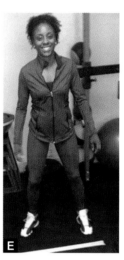

FIGS 12A TO E: Grapevines: (A) Start position; (B) Right leg crossed in front of left; (C) Neutral stance position; (D) Right leg crossed behind left; (E) Neutral stance position

with their feet shoulder width apart (Fig. 13) and in a squat stance reflective of a basketball defensive stance. The patient will then move laterally (for example to the left) leading with the left foot and bringing the right foot to meet the left. Patient must be instructed to control the hind leg (right leg in this case) and not let the tension of the resistance band loop pull their leg inward too fast. The eccentric control of the hip abductors will be called on to achieve this task. Prescription for basketball slides should be individualized to the patient. Progression of this exercise could be the addition of a second resistance band loop placed just above the knees. Further progression would be to move up the resistance band matrix in color thereby increasing the resistance. The extra resistance causes the patient to have to fire the targeted muscles more intensely.

Inverted hamstrings

This activity requires a component of balance that may increase the difficulty level for some patients. Guarding by the clinician to begin with may be helpful for the patient to successfully carry out the motion. The patient start position is in standing. They are advised to slightly flex the knee of the affected limb prior to beginning the motion (Fig. 14). The amount of flexion, which should be approximately 20°, is to be maintained for the duration of the movement and not increased as the patient begins to move. The patient is instructed to flex the trunk at the hip, reaching for the ground with the contralateral upper extremity so that the hamstring becomes lengthened. The contralateral leg should be brought into extension to counteract the forward flexion of the upper trunk and aid

with balance. The patient should be instructed to maintain a neutral pelvis and not to rotate toward the stance limb as a compensation for poor balance. Clinician guarding and facilitation of desired balance strategies will aid in decreasing this. The exercise should first be performed with a light-weight, to acclimate the muscle to this type of stress as well as to aid the patient with balance. This intervention should be individualized to the patient, as weight can be increased as tolerated for progression. Anecdotally, in the clinic bilateral performance of this intervention has been found to be beneficial.

Phase II

This phase aims at regaining pain free hamstring strength and the development of neuromuscular control of the trunk and pelvis. In order to be progressed to this phase, the patient must be able to walk with a normal stride and lightly jog pain free, as well as complete a sub-maximal isometric hamstring contraction pain free.[16] All of the interventions mentioned in Phase I should now be progressed and combined with the following activities to keep the patient moving smoothly toward a healthy return to sport. Phase II focuses more on eccentric strengthening of the hamstrings, as evidence has shown this to be favorable to a successful recovery regimen.

Fast Feet[16]

The patient starts in quiet standing and is instructed to begin jogging in place only picking the feet up off the ground a few inches (Fig. 15). The speed at which the

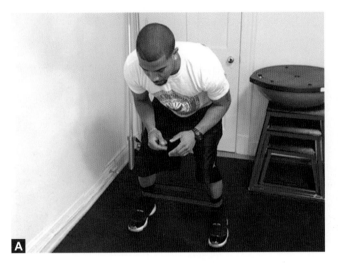

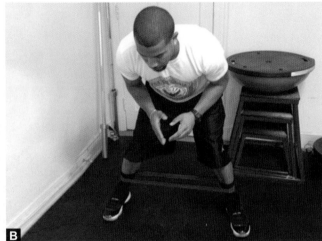

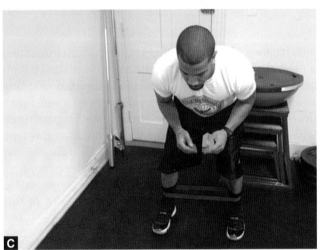

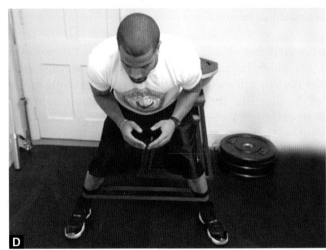

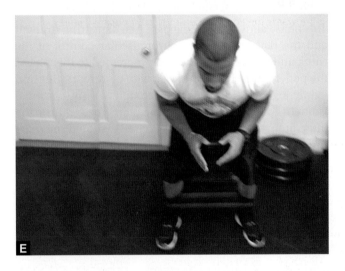

FIGS 13A AND E: Basketball slides: (A) Start position; (B) Lateral step left shifting weight onto left foot; (C) Lateral step bringing right foot toward left foot controlling band resistance; (D) Lateral step left shifting weight onto left foot; (E) Lateral step with right foot toward left foot

patient churns their feet should be moderate to start and increased with every round.[16] Lengthening the amount of time that the patient must carry out this task will increase difficulty.

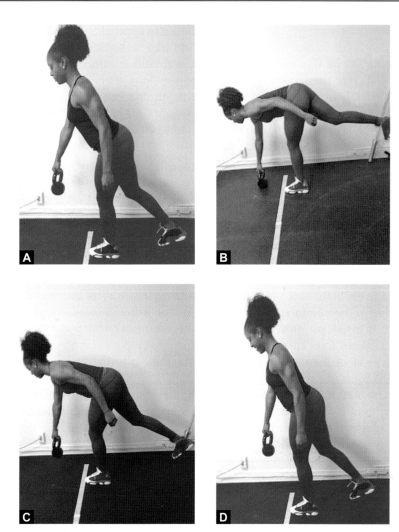

FIGS 14A TO D: Inverted hamstrings: (A) Start position with slightly bent stance knee; (B) Trunk flexed with slightly bent knee maintained and contralateral arm reaching towards the floor; (C) Return to start position while maintaining balance; (D) Start position

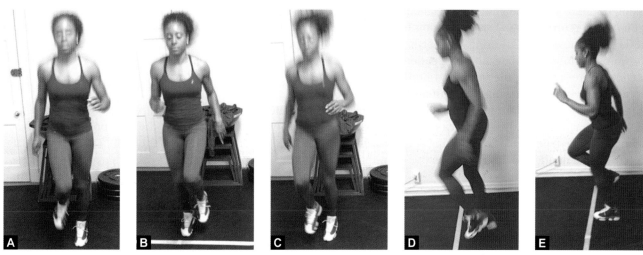

FIGS 15A TO E: Fast feet: (A) Frontal view quick right foot lift; (B) Frontal view left quick foot lift; (C) Frontal view right quick foot lift; (D) Lateral view left quick foot lift; (E) Lateral view right quick foot lift

Bridge Walkouts[16]

The start position for the patient in this exercise is the elevated bridge position (Fig. 16). The patient will then slowly walk their feet away from them to the limit of where they are able to support their body. Once in that position, the patient will then walk their feet back toward their body and pelvis returned to the floor for a brief (1–3 seconds) break before beginning the next repetition. Prescription of this activity should be tailored to the patient.

Hamstring Bridges[16]

The patient is positioned supine on the floor with a platform placed beneath both ankles to place the knees in 75°–100° of flexion (Fig. 17). The patient is then told to lift the pelvis off of the floor in the manner of a bridge. The patient will then flex the hip of the uninjured leg toward the chest and then return it to the platform before the pelvis is to be returned to the floor. This causes the patient to have to support the weight of their trunk with the affected limb by contracting the hamstring and engaging the core. This exercise can be prescribed according to the patient's deficits but may be modified as necessary. To progress this exercise, the platform can be moved further away from the patient increasing the demand placed on the hamstring.

Swiss Ball Hamstring Curls

The starting position of this intervention is with the patient in supine with their ankles placed on top of an exercise ball (Fig. 18). The patient assumes a bridge position and then pulls the ball towards their buttocks by flexing both knees. At the end of the available ROM, the patient then returns to the bridge position by extending the knees, followed by lowering the pelvis to the start position. Attention must be paid to the patient's attempts to compensate by using the uninjured limb to perform the activity without involving the injured limb, as well as lowering the hips before fully extending the knees at the end of the task. Hamstring curls can be progressed by having the patient perform the task using only the injured limb while the unaffected limb is held in the air.

Windmill Touches[16]

The patient begins in a single leg stance position on the injured limb with light dumbbells or weight plates in each hand held overhead (Fig. 19). The stance knee should be flexed to approximately 20° and maintained at this angle. The patient will then reach diagonally across the body toward the ground, aiming at touching the dumbbell to the floor, then return to the start position. Following this, the patient will then perform the same motion to the opposite side with the contralateral upper extremity, while still standing on the injured lower extremity.

Nordic Hamstrings[44]

This is a partner activity, so the clinician will have an active role in the performance of this exercise.[44] The starting position for the patient is kneeling on the floor with the body rigidly held straight from the knees upward (Fig. 20). The clinician will then apply a downward force at the ankles to stabilize the patient through the activity.[45] The patient will be instructed to resist a forward falling motion using the hamstrings to maximize loading during an eccentric contraction.[45] The patient is told to break the forward fall for as long as possible using the hamstrings.[45] The patient is instructed to use their arms and hands to buffer the fall, before reaching the floor with the chest, and to immediately push back up into the starting position using their hands to minimize concentric loading.[44]

Alternate Quick Lunges

A line of some sort is required as a point of reference for this exercise. This can be a line in the design of the floor, or a strip of tape placed on the floor. The patient is instructed to stand in a lunge stance with one foot in front of the line and one behind the line (Fig. 21). The activity involves moving laterally alternating the foot that is in front of the line for the assigned distance and speed can be tailored to the patient for variable levels of difficulty. This activity should be introduced at a low to moderate speed and then progressed to higher speeds.

Foot Catches[6]

The patient stands next to a wall, using the upper extremity on the wall side for stability. The start position is with the lower extremity further from the wall in 90° of hip flexion and 90° of knee flexion (Fig. 22). The patient begins by simulating the swing phase of walking or running. During this motion the patient extends the knee by performing a quick quadriceps contraction. The purpose of this exercise is for the patient to then catch, or stop, the lower leg before reaching full knee extension by performing a quick hamstring contraction.[6]

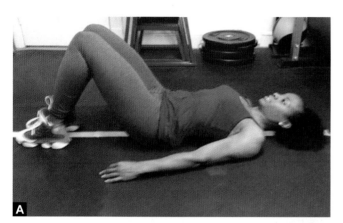

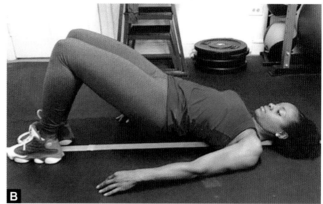

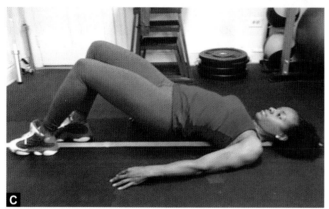

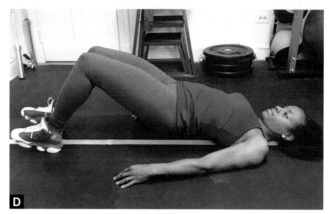

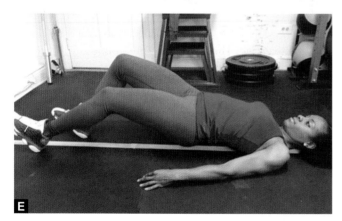

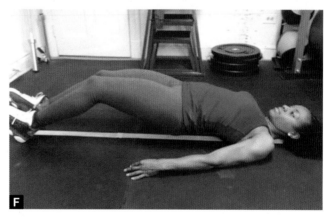

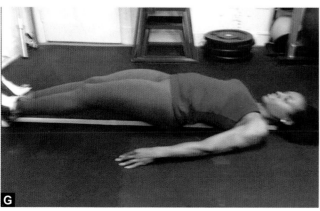

FIGS 16A TO G: Bridge walkouts: (A) Start position, supine hooklying; (B) Bridge position; (C) Walkout with left foot; (D) Walkout with right foot; (E) Walkout with left towards flat position; (F) Walkout with right foot toward flat position; (G) Flat position

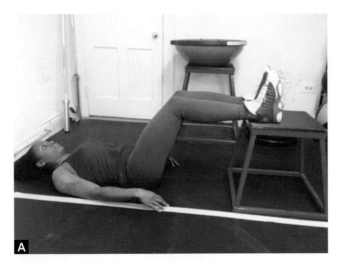

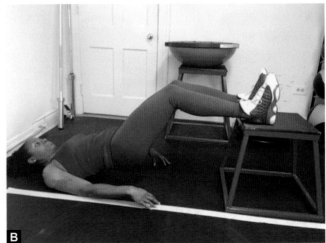

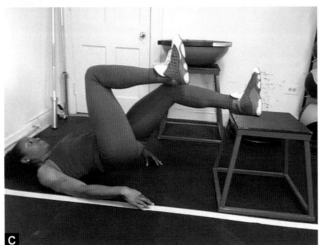

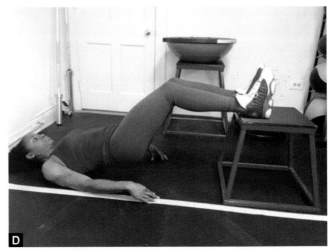

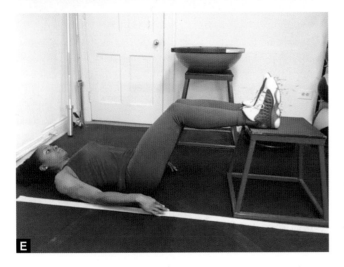

FIGS 17A TO E: Hamstring bridges: (A) Start position, supine with feet propped on platform; (B) Lifting hips off floor; (C) Lift left knee towards chest; (D) Return left leg to platform; (E) Return hips to floor

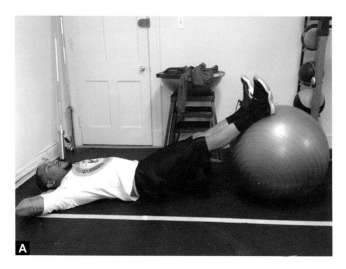

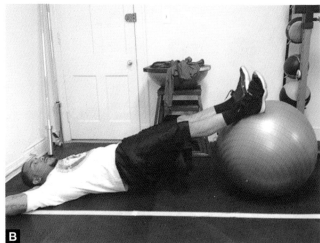

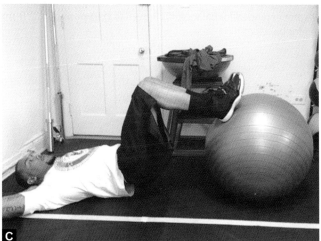

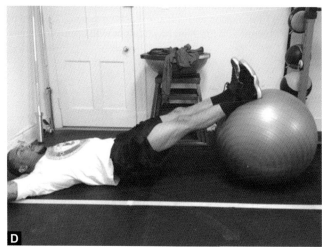

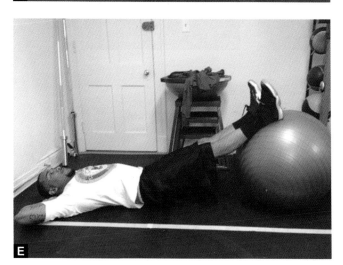

FIGS 18A TO E: Swiss ball hamstring curls: (A) Start position, supine with feet on exercise ball; (B) Pelvis lifted off floor with legs extended; (C) Ball pulled towards buttocks with pelvis elevation; (D) Ball rolled back out and returned to legs extended position; (E) The finish position is with the pelvis returned to floor

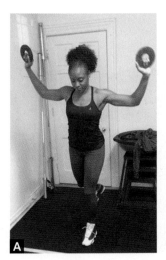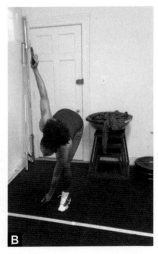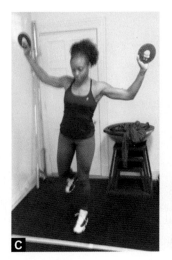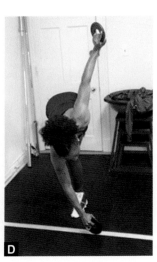

FIGS 19A TO D: Windmill touches: (A) Start position, single leg stance with slight knee flexion and arms lifted overhead with weights in hands; (B) Trunk flexion with left arm reaching toward floor and opposite arm extended for balance; (C) Return to start position; (D) Trunk flexed with right arm reaching toward floor with opposite arm extended for balance

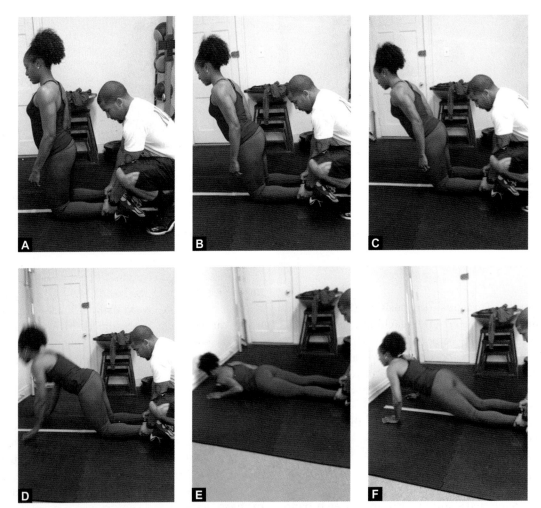

FIGS 20A TO F: Nordic hamstrings: (A) Start position, patient kneeling with clinician holding legs down at ankles; (B) Patient leaning forward from knees; (C) Patient continuing to lean forward from trunk; (D) Falling forward and catching herself on hands; (E) Lowering to let chest tough the ground; (F) Pushing back up to starting position to minimize concentric load on hamstrings

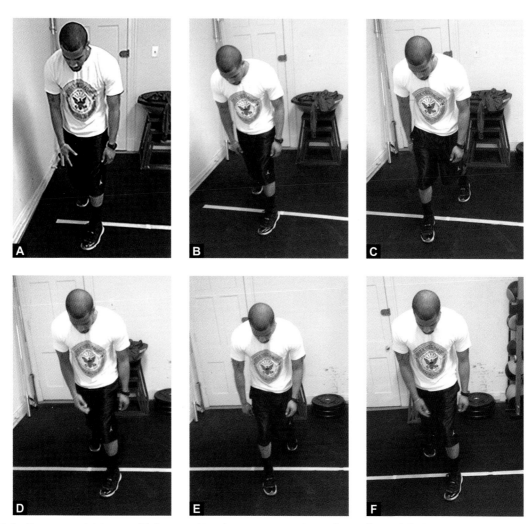

FIGS 21A TO F: Alternate quick lunges: (A) Start position, lunge stance with one foot in front of the line and the other behind; (B) Quick alternating of foot position; (C to F) Progression of alternating movement of feet down the line

Sunrisers

The patient begins in a push-up position (Fig. 23) and picks one hand up off the ground, reaching up toward the ceiling while rotating the upper trunk. Once the patient achieves the "sunrise" position, they are to pause for three seconds while engaging the core, then return to the start position. The patient will then repeat the same motion to the opposite side. Adding a weight to the motion will increase difficulty of this exercise when the patient is appropriate for progression.

Stretch-Band Backpedaling

The patient is positioned standing inside of a stretch-band with the clinician holding the opposite end of the band for

resistance. The patient is instructed to assume a squatted position, sitting into the band (Fig. 24). The patient then begins to walk backward using a back-pedaling motion while the clinician holds the band for resistance. This exercise should be prescribed according to patient tolerance over the available or allotted distance. Moving up to a harder stretch-band would progress this exercise.

Phase III

Once patients make it to this phase of rehabilitation, return to sport is in sight and activities preparing for a return should be implemented. Goals in this phase are for the patient to be symptom free with all activities, to have normal concentric and eccentric hamstring strength through the full ROM and to demonstrate the

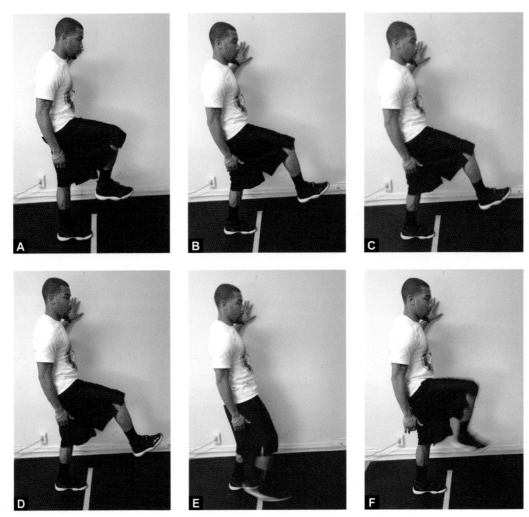

FIGS 22A TO F: Foot catches: (A) Start position, standing with hip and knee flexed to 90° with one arm on the wall for support; (B to D) Quick quadriceps contraction extending knee; (E) Catching the foot before reaching full leg extension; (F) Return to start position

ability to integrate postural control into sport specific movements.[16] Based on the best available evidence, athletes can be cleared to return to unrestricted sporting activities once full ROM, strength and functional abilities (running, jumping, cutting) can be performed pain free.[16] Despite this guideline, pain and stiffness often resolve within 1–2 weeks, while the underlying injury may persist for several more weeks.[21] Return to sport can occur anywhere from 3 weeks to 6 months.[20] Given the variation in muscle demand by different sports, treatment should become sport specific and demands of activity are at the discretion and guidance of the clinician. In addition to progressive versions of treatment presented in earlier phases, interventions at this phase may include the following.

Marching[42]

Marching is a walking exercise simulating the task of proper form running. High knee lift, contralateral arm swing, and reciprocation (Fig. 25) are the components of this movement. This is a method to gradually prepare your patient for return to sport.

A-Skips[16]

The A-skip is a running drill that resembles marching in that it focuses on the proper form of running in a simplified task (Fig. 26). The main difference between a march and an A-skip is the time interval when both feet are off of the ground, which adds a component of fast

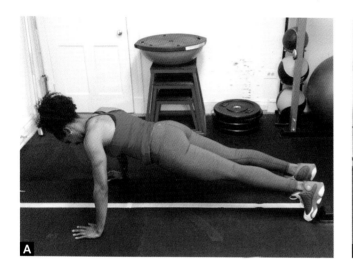

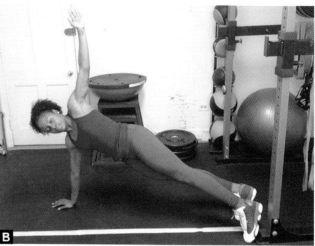

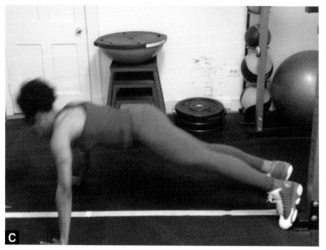

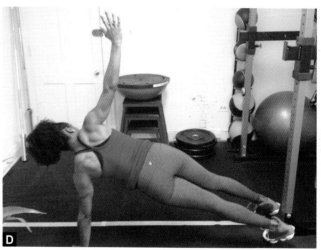

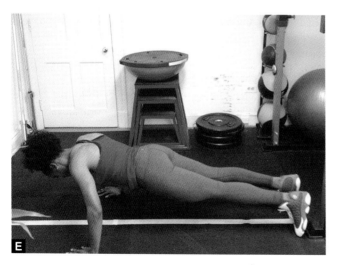

FIGS 23A TO E: Sunrisers: (A) Start position is a plank position; (B) One hand off the ground, rotating trunk upward toward ceiling; (C) Return to start position; (D) Opposite hand off the ground rotating trunk upward toward ceiling; E) Return to start position

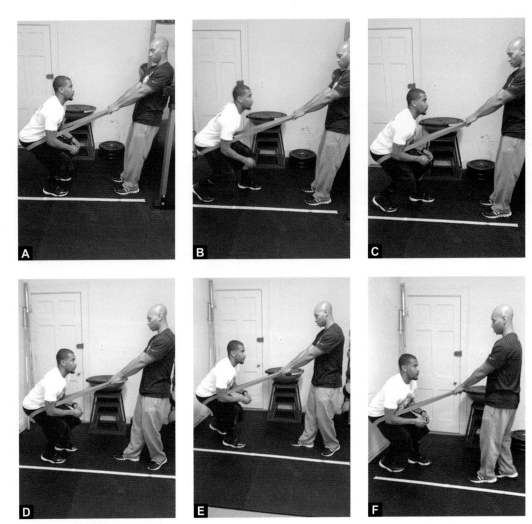

FIGS 24A TO F: Stretch-band backpedaling: (A) Start position, squatted as of sitting into the band; (B) Step backward with one foot while maintaining weight posteriorly into band; (C) Step backward with opposite foot while maintaining weight posteriorly; (D to F) Repeating movement and weight distribution along distance to be covered

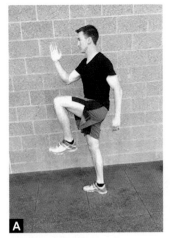
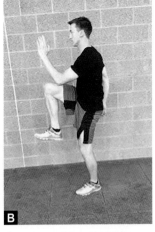

twitch muscle activation and light impact loading to the exercise.

B-Skips[16]

This exercise is the progression from an A-skip. The activity begins the same as with A-skip with a high knee lift in a skipping motion (Fig. 27) but at the top of the knee lift, the patient is to extend the knee in a kick-out motion and snap it to the ground quickly.

Straight Leg Jogging[43]

This activity is jogging with the knees extended (Fig. 28), keeping the legs stiff to prepare the patient for the impact of running.

FIGS 25A AND B: Marching: (A) High knee lift with high arm swing; (B) Reciprocal of movement with contralateral limbs

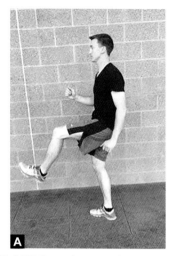 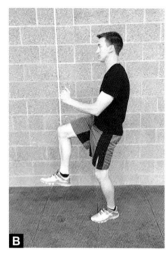 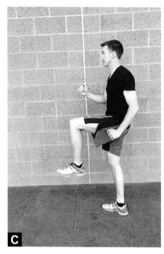

FIGS 26A AND B: A-skips: (A) Skip into knee lift and arm swing; (B and C) Reciprocation of skip into knee lift and arm swing

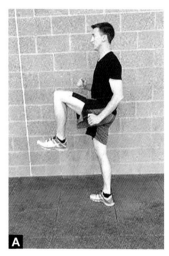 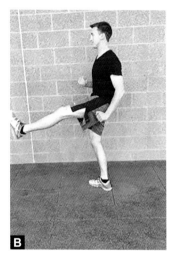 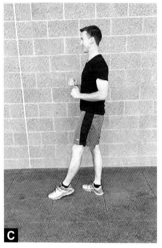

FIGS 27A TO C: B-skips: (A) Skip into high knee lift; (B) Knee extended during skip; (C) Extended leg snapped down towards ground

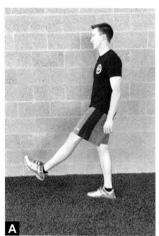 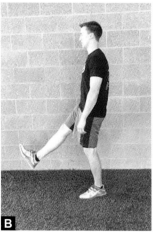 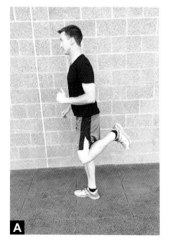 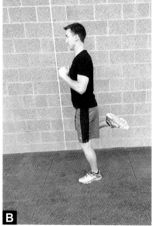

FIGS 28A AND B: Straight leg jogging: (A) Leg extended with hip flexed to begin motion; (B) Reciprocation during jog with opposite leg extended

FIGS 29A AND B: Butt kicks: (A) Neutral hip with knee bent and heel moving toward buttocks; (B) Reciprocation of movement with contralateral limb

Butt Kicks[42]

The patient will jog while bringing the heels toward the buttocks (Fig. 29). This will actively train the hamstrings to contract concentrically to successfully perform the drill.

High Knees[43]

The patient will jog while flexing the hip and knee as high as possible (Fig. 30).

The patient may be instructed to use the hands as a target for their knees to aid in a higher knee lift.

Box Jumps[43]

The patient will begin in a squatted position in front of the box (Fig. 31). The goal is for the patient to explode in an upward jump landing on the box.

Other activities that can be implemented in this phase to a successful promote return to sport are:
- Jogging
- Change of direction drills (for example, forward-backward acceleration)
- Cutting (for example, cone drills)
- Jumping
- Bounding

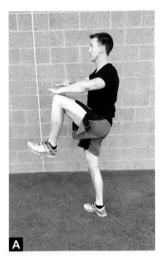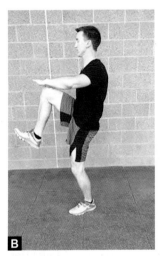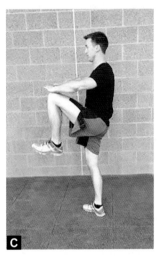

FIGS 30A TO C: High knees: (A) Hip flexed to highest point with knee flexed; (B and C) Reciprocal movement of contralateral lower extremity repeated over distance

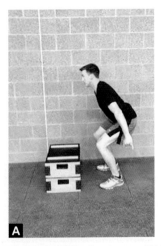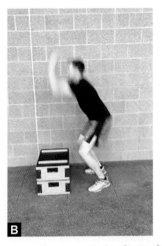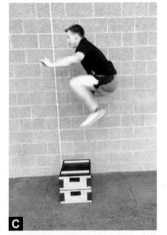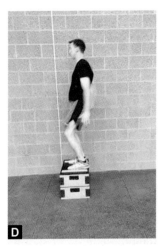

FIGS 31A TO D: Box jumps: (A) Start position, squatted in front of box preparing for jump; (B) Extending through trunk to prepare for explosion off the ground upwards; (C) Mid-jump; (D) Landing with both feet onto box simultaneously

Alternative Treatments

In addition to traditional physical therapy-based interventions, some patients and clinicians may seek to employ alternative methods. Some of these methods may be performed by physical therapists, whereas others fall outside their scope of practice. Alternative treatments have varied efficacy and, in some cases, little is known about how they may influence injury recovery from a research standpoint. The following are some of the more prominent and current treatment options that patients may receive in lieu of, or as adjuncts to, exercise-based interventions.

Instrument-assisted Soft Tissue Mobilization Techniques

There are various methods of instrument-assisted soft tissue mobilization, also known as scraping techniques. Graston[TM], Fibroblaster[TM], ASTYM[TM], The Edge[TM] and Gua Sha are some of the more popular methods and tools (Fig. 32). The belief behind scraping techniques is that they alter the soft tissue beneath the skin to decrease scar tissue, dysfunction and restrictive properties. This change in the soft tissue is said to stimulate proper healing and increase pain free ROM in muscles where there was restriction. Consequently, this method can be used to improve hamstring extensibility and improve soft tissue consistency both proximally, at the attachment site and distally, in the muscle belly. Scraping techniques have been shown to increase blood flow and microvascular morphology in the vicinity of healing tissue.[46] Handheld instrumentation like this is said to enable the clinician to topically locate underlying dysfunctional tissue and transfer pressure and appropriate shear forces to that tissue.[47,48] For instance, ASTYM[TM], is thought to activate a regenerative response in soft tissues via the induction of leakage from dysfunctional capillaries, which lead to fibroblast activation, phagocytosis and local release of growth factors.[47,49] There has been much anecdotal praise of these techniques, but there is very little in the way of quality research to support their use. This is not to say that there is no efficacy because some success has been seen clinically with these methods, but simply that more quality research needs to be done.

Dry Needling

If the treating clinician is trained in this technique, dry needling can be beneficial to a patient with a hamstring strain (Fig. 33). Dry needling involves the application of a fine filiform needle to soft tissues to treat the muscles.[50] Needling mechanically disrupts taut bands of muscle tissue found in areas of muscular dysfunction, allowing for normalized ROM.[51] It also decreases pain and excessive muscle tension.[51] Since this intervention requires advanced training, a specific description of how to treat a hamstring strain is beyond the scope of this text.

Modalities

Modalities such as ultrasound, electrical stimulation, ice and heat have traditionally been used as a form of treatment for hamstring strains.[6,16,29] However, these interventions have produced conflicting evidence about

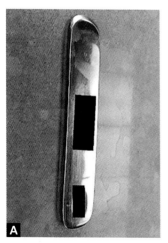 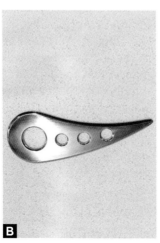 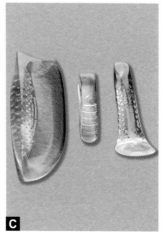 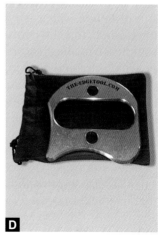

FIGS 32A TO D: Scraping tools: (A) Graston[TM]; (B) Fibroblaster[TM]; (C) ASTYM[TM]; (D) The Edge[TM]

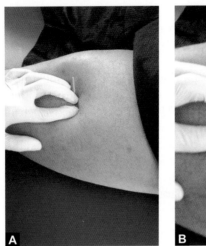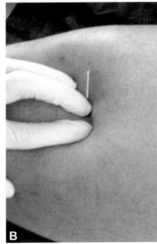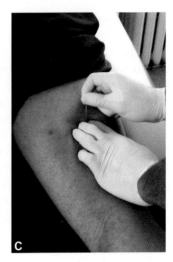

FIGS 33A TO C: Dry needling: (A) Needle in hamstring tissue; (B) Close up of filiform needle in hamstring tissue; (C) Hamstring tissue being treated with dry needling during pistoning of needle

their respective efficacy, and there is not much research to support their use.[52] Ultrasound has been recommended to relieve pain following injury and to enhance the initial stages of muscle regeneration, but its use has not been shown to have a beneficial influence on muscle healing.[53,54]

Medical Interventions

Steroid Injections

A form of medical intervention for HSI is corticosteroid injections. Corticosteroids are cortisol-like compounds. Cortisol is a hormone made by the adrenal glands, and injectable cortisone is a synthetic variation of this hormone. The injection is delivered directly to the site of injury, which is typically identified by MRI or ultrasound, and the cortisone is released immediately superficial to the hamstring tendons.[55] Care is taken to avoid intratendinous injection due to the likelihood of weakening the tendon.[55] Cortisone injections are believed to limit chronic inflammation that may lead to tendon scarring and adhesion formation.[55] This generally leads to pain relief in the area and may decrease the amount of time required for the rupture to heal. A drawback to this method of treatment is the side effects associated with long-term use of steroids, as the treatment may need to be repeated multiple times. The tendon can also be weakened leading to another rupture due to compromised vascularity associated with repeated use of this treatment.

Platelet Rich Plasma

Platelet rich plasma (PRP) is a form of injection therapy. The procedure begins with the collection of blood from the patient, which is then centrifuged to separate and harvest the plasma.[56] PRP is extracted and implanted into the posterior thigh at the insertion site of the hamstring at the injury site.[56] It is used to strengthen weakened muscle or connective tissue, alleviate pain and aid in healing ruptured tendons.[56] No adverse event related to PRP application has been reported, but the intervention's utility in treating soft tissue pathology remains under investigation.[56]

Surgery

Surgical intervention is widely considered as a last option for HSI, unless there has been a complete tendon avulsion. The surgical procedure reattaches the proximal tendon to the ischial tuberosity. Studies indicate that surgical intervention for an acute (less than 4 weeks) complete rupture have better outcomes and return to sport than surgery for chronic (greater than 4 weeks) complete ruptures.[57] Surgery to a chronic rupture tends to be more demanding for the surgeon, but typically occurs when a complete rupture is misdiagnosed and/or conservative treatments fail.

■ CONCLUSION

Hamstring strain injuries are one of the most nagging injuries a person can incur, due to the complex nature of hamstring tissue healing. The mechanism of injury and location of the injury are important factors in determining an accurate prognosis for HSI.[16] Injury to the biceps femoris generally recovers more rapidly than an injury incurred in the semimembranosus, and the two usually have different mechanisms of injury. Neuromuscular control, core strengthening and eccentric hamstring strengthening have all been researched as successful methods of rehabilitation of hamstring strains, with the added benefit of decreased reinjury rates and relatively short return to sport times. Alternative therapies may also augment exercise-based rehabilitation protocols, however, no consensus in the literature exists in this regard. Reinjury and prevention are matters that are of the greatest interest regarding hamstring strains, as these are the keys to making this injury less prevalent. However, more research needs to be conducted on this topic, as it still stands as one of the most common injuries in the active population.

■ REFERENCES

1. Woods C, Hawkins RD, Maltby S, Hulse M, Thomas A, Hodson A. The football association medical research programme: an audit of injuries in professional football. Analysis of hamstring injuries. Br J Sports Med. 2004;38(1):36-41.
2. Heiser TM, Weber J, Sullivan G, Clarke P, Jacobs RR. Prophylaxis and management of hamstring muscle injuries in intercollegiate football players. Am J Sports Med. 1984;12(5):368-70.
3. Feeley BT, Kennelly S, Barnes RP, Muller MS, Kelly BT, Rodeo SA, et al. Epidemiology of national football league training camp injuries from 1998 to 2007. Am J Sports Med. 2008;36(8):1597-603.
4. Foreman TK, Addy T, Baker S, Burns J, Hill N, Madden T. Prospective studies into the causation of hamstring injuries in sport: a systematic review. Physical Therapy in Sport. 2006;7:101-9.
5. Gabbe BJ, Bennell KL, Finch CF. Why are older Australian football players at greater risk of hamstring injury? J Sci Med Sport. 2006;9:327-33.
6. Worrell TW. Factors associated with hamstring injuries. An approach to treatment and preventative measures. Sports Med. 1994;17:338-45.
7. Cameron ML, Adams RD, Maher CG, Mission D. Effect of HamSprint drills training programme on lower limb neuromuscular control in Australian football players. J Sci Med Sport. 2007;12:24-30.
8. Sherry MA, Best TM. A comparison of 2 rehabilitation programs in the treatment of acute hamstring strains. J Ortho Sports Phys Ther. 2004;34:116-25.
9. Garrett WE. Muscle strain injuries. Am J Sports Med. 1996;24:S2-8.
10. Orchard J. Biomechanics of muscle strain injury. New Zealand J Sports Med. 2002;30:92-8.
11. Chumanov ES, Heiderscheit BC, Thelen DG. The effect of speed and influence of individual muscles on hamstring mechanics during the swing phase of sprinting. J Biomech. 2007;40:3555-62.
12. Thelen DG, Chumanov ES, Best TM, Swanson SC, Heiderscheit BC. Simulation of biceps femoris musculotendon mechanics during the swing phase of sprinting. Med Sci Sports Exerc. 2005;37:1931-8.
13. Yu B, Queen RM, Abbey AN, Liu Y, Moorman CT, Garrett WE. Hamstring muscle kinematics and activation during overground sprinting. J Biomech. 2008;41:3121-6.
14. Thelen DG, Chumanov ES, Hoerth DM, Best TM, Swanson SC, Li L, et al. Hamstring muscle kinematics during treadmill sprinting. Med Sci Sports Exerc. 2005;37:108-14.
15. Opar DA, Williams MD, Shield AJ. Hamstring strains: factors that lead to injury and re-injury. Sports Med. 2012;42(3):209-26.
16. Heiderscheit BC, Sherry MA, Slider A, Chumanov ES, Thelen DG. Hamstring strain injuries: recommendations for diagnosis, rehabilitation and injury prevention. J Ortho Sports Phys Ther. 2010;40(2):67-81.
17. Askling C, Saartok T, Thorstensson A. Type of acute hamstring strain affects flexibility, strength, and time to return to pre-injury level. Br J Sports Med. 2006;40:40-4.
18. Askling CM, Tengvar M, Saartok T, Thorstensson A. Acute first-time hamstring strains during slow-speed stretching: clinical, magnetic resonance imaging, and recovery characteristics. Am J Sports Med. 2007;35:1716-24.
19. Askling CM, Tengvar M, Saartok T, Thorstensson A. Proximal hamstring strains of stretching type in different sports: injury situations, clinical and magnetic resonance imaging characteristics, and return to sport. Am J Sports Med. 2008;36:1799-804.
20. Schneider-Kolsky ME, Hoving JL, Warren P, Connell DA. A comparison between clinical assessment and magnetic resonance imaging of acute hamstring injuries. Am J Sports Med. 2006;34:1008-015.
21. Cohen S, Bradley J. Acute proximal hamstring rupture. J Am Acad Orthop Surg. 2007;15:350-5.
22. Connell DA, Schneider-Kolsy ME, Hoving JL, Malara F, Buchbinder R, Koulouris G, et al. Longitudinal study comparing sonographic and MRI assessments of acute and healing hamstring injuries. Am J Roentgenol. 2004;183:975-84.
23. Slavotinek JP, Verrall GM, Fon GT. Hamstring injury in athletes: using MR imaging measurements to compare extent of muscle injury with amount of time lost from competition. Am J Roentgenol. 2002;179:1621-8.
24. Koulouris G, Connell DA, Brukner P, Schneider-Kolsky M. Magnetic resonance imaging parameters for assessing risk of recurrent hamstring injuries in elite athletes. Am J Sports Med. 2007;35:1500-6.
25. Verrall GM, Slavotinek JP, Barnes PG, Fon GT, Esterman A. Assessment of physical examination and magnetic resonance imaging findings of hamstring injury as predictors for recurrent injury. J Ortho Sports Phys Ther. 2006;36:435-9.
26. Askling CM, Tengvar M, Saartok T, Thorstensson A. Acute first time hamstring strains during high-speed running: a longitudinal study including clinical and magnetic resonance imaging findings. Am J Sports Med. 2007;35:197-206.
27. Gibbs NJ, Cross TM, Cameron M, Houang MT. The accuracy of MRI in predicting recovery and recurrence of acute grade one hamstring muscle strains within the same reason in Australian rules football players. J Sci Med Sport. 2004;7:248-58.
28. `Silder A, Heiderscheit BC, Thelen DG, Enright T, Tuite MJ. MR observations of long-term musculotendon remodeling following a hamstring strain injury. Skeletal Radiol. 2008;37:1101-9.
29. Jarvinen TA, Jarvinen TL, Kaariainen M, Aärimaa V, Vaittinen S, Kalimo H, et al. Muscle injuries: optimizing recovery. Best Pract Res Clin Rheumatol. 2007;21:317-31.
30. Brukner P, Khan, K. Clinical sports medicine. Sydney: McGraw-Hill Professional; 2006.
31. Magee DJ. Orthopedic Physical Assessment, 5th edition. St. Louis: Saunders; 2008.

32. Maffery L, Emery C. What are the risk factors for groin strain injury in sport? A systematic review of the literature. Sports Med. 2007;37:881-94.

33. Dutton M. Orthopaedic Examination, Evaluation and Intervention, 3rd edition. China. McGraw-Hill Medical; 2012.

34. Orchard JW, Farhart P, Leopold C. Lumbar spine region pathology and hamstring and calf injuries in athletes: is there a connection? Br J Sports Med. 2004;38:502-4.

35. Turl SE, George KP. Adverse neural tension: a factor in repetitive hamstring strain? J Ortho Sports Phys Ther. 1998;27:16-21.

36. Kornberg C, Lew P. The effect of stretching neural structures on grade on hamstring injuries. J Ortho Sports Phys Ther. 1989;10:481-7. http://dx.doi.org/10.2519/jospt.1989.10.12.481

37. Kendall FP, McCreary EK, Provance PG, Rodgers MM, Romani WA. Muscles: testing and posture with function and pain, 5th edition. Baltimore: Lippincott, Williams & Wilkins; 2005.

38. Lorenz D, Reiman M. The role and implementation of eccentric training in athletic rehabilitation: tendinopathy, hamstring strains, and ACL reconstruction. Int J Sports Phys Ther. 2011:6(1):27-44.

39. Orchard J, Best TM. The management of muscle strain injuries: an early return versus the risk of recurrence. Clin J Sport Med. 2002;12:3-5.

40. Brockett CL, Morgan DL, Proske U. Predicting hamstring strain injury in elite athletes. Med Sci Sports Exerc. 2004;36:379-87.

41. Proske U, Morgan DL, Brockett CL, Percival P. Identifying athletes at risk of hamstring strains and how to protect them. Clin Exp Pharmacol Physio. 2004;31:546-50.

42. Brockett CL, Morgan DL, Proske U. Human hamstring muscles adapt to eccentric exercise by changing optimum length. Med Sci Sports Exerc. 2001;33:783-90.

43. University of Delaware. (2011). Preventive exercise progression for hamstring strain. [online] Available from http://www.udel.edu/PT/PT%20Clinical%20Services/RehabGuidelines/HAMSTRING_EXERCISE_PROGRESSION.pdf. [Accessed January, 2015].

44. Mjolsnes R, Arnason A, Osthagen T, Raastad T, Bahr R. A 10-week randomized trial comparing eccentric vs. concentric hamstring strength training in well trained soccer players. Scand J Med Sci Sports. 2004;14:311-7.

45. Petersen J, Thorborg K, Nielsen MB, Budtz-Jorgensen E, Holmich P. Preventive effect of eccentric training on acute hamstring injuries in men's soccer: a cluster randomized controlled trial. Am J Sports Med. 2011;39:2296-303.

46. Loghmani, MT, Warden SJ. Instrument assisted crossfiber massage increases tissue perfusion and alters microvascular morphology in the vicinity of healing knee ligaments. BMC Complementary and Alternative Medicine. 2013;13:240-9.

47. McCormack J. The management of bilateral high hamstring tendinopathy with ASTYM® treatment and eccentric exercise: a case report. 2012;20(3):142-6.

48. Davies CC, Brockopp DY. Use of ASTYM treatment on scar tissue following surgical treatment for breast cancer: a pilot study. Rehabil Oncol. 2010;28(3):3-12.

49. Slaven EJ, Mathers J. Management of joint ankle pain using joint mobilization and ASTYM treatment: a case report. J Man Manip Ther. 2011;19(2):108-12.

50. Kietrys DM, Palombaro KM, Azzaretto E, Hubler R, Schaller B, Schlussel JM, et al. Effectiveness of dry needling for upper quarter myofascial pain: a systematic review and meta-analysis. J Ortho Sports Phys Ther. 2013;43:620-34.

51. Dembowski SC, Westrick RB, Zylstra E, Johnson MR. Treatment of hamstring strain in a collegiate pole-vaulter integrating dry needling with an eccentric training program: a resident's case report. Int J Sports Phys Ther. 2013;8(3):328-39.

52. Mason DL, Dickens V, Vail A. Rehabilitation for hamstring injuries. Cochrane Database Syst Rev. 2012;12:CD004575.

53. Markert CD, Merrick MA, Kirby TE, Devor ST. Nonthermal ultrasound and exercise in skeletal muscle regeneration. Arch Phys Med Rehabil. 2005;86:1304-10.

54. Rantanen J, Thorsson O, Wollmer P, Hurme T, Kalimo H. Effects of therapeutic ultrasound on the regeneration of skeletal myofibers after experimental muscle injury. Am J Sports Med. 1999;27:54-9.

55. Zissen MH, Wallace G, Stevens KJ, Fredricson M, Beaulieu CF. High hamstring tendinopathy: MRI and ultrasound imaging and therapeutic efficacy of percutaneous corticosteroid injection. Am J Roentgenol. 2010;195(4):993-8.

56. Karli DC, Robinson BR. Platelet rich plasma for hamstring tears. Pract Pain Manag. 2010;10(5):10-4.

57. Harris JD, Griesser MJ, Best TM, Ellis TJ. Treatment of proximal hamstring ruptures-a systematic review. Int J Sports Med. 2011;32 (7);490.

CHAPTER 11

Patellofemoral Pain Syndrome

Ross M Nakaji

ABSTRACT

Patellofemoral pain syndrome is a common and frequently frustrating condition for clinicians and patients alike. Patellofemoral pain syndrome is that it is one of the most common diagnosis in the knee, representing 25% of all diagnoses in the knee. Patellofemoral pain syndrome is a common complaint following anterior cruciate ligament or meniscal injury, as well as the primary reason for total knee arthroplasty. About 75–90% of patients improve with conservative management, by using sound clinical reasoning during the evaluation, by utilization of the classification system for patellofemoral disorders and by implementation of an ongoing progressive training program of the entire lower extremity. This chapter discusses the treatment of patellofemoral pain syndrome, with focus on evidence-based practices.

INTRODUCTION

Patellofemoral pain syndrome (PFP) is a common and frequently frustrating condition for clinicians and patients alike. It has been referred to as the "The Low Back Pain of the Lower Extremity" by Christopher Powers due to its enigmatic and perplexing presentation. Dr. Scott Dye has also been quoted as describing PFP as the "Blackhole of Orthopedics". What is known about PFP is that it is one of the most common diagnoses in the knee, representing 25% of all diagnoses in the knee.[1,2] PFP is a common complaint following anterior cruciate ligament or meniscal injury,[3] as well as the primary reason for total knee arthroplasty.[4] Patellofemoral problems are also common in tennis players, runners and in military basic training.[5-8] PFP is one of the most common soft tissue syndromes referred to rheumatology specialists and can be problematic in patients with cerebral palsy.[9-10]

Patellofemoral pain syndrome has numerous names, terms and diagnoses. The following list is a summary of common terms used for PFP:

- Chondromalacia patella
- Patellofemoral maltracking
- Malalignment of the patella
- Compression overload of the patellofemoral joint
- Arthrosis of the patellofemoral joint
- Chondrosis
- Arthralgia
- Anterior knee pain syndrome
- Excessive lateral pressure syndrome
- Extension subluxation

The common use of such ambiguous and nonspecific terms only adds to the confusion regarding optimal care for these patients. The dilemma for the clinician attempting to manage PFP occurs because there is no clear consensus on PFP treatment in the medical literature. Many conservative treatments have been advocated and numerous surgical techniques have been described simply because the pathophysiology is not well understood. Rehabilitation and treatment programs developed for the patients with PFP must match the specific disorder and dysfunction.

According to several sources, conservative care is preferred with successful short-term outcomes.[11-13] However, long-term outcomes have not proven quite as successful.[14,15] A couple of predictors and risk factors to PFP have been identified including quadriceps weakness and some specific anthropomorphic measures.[16,17] Current consensus on rehabilitation continues to support quadriceps strengthening as the primary factor in successful rehabilitation programs, with mixed results utilizing other interventions including taping, bracing, foot orthosis and hip strengthening.[18] The success of nonoperative treatment has been reported to be as high as 75–90%.[19-28]

The key to treating PFP is to treat the cause, not the symptoms, because PFP is vague and lacks a systematic approach to rehabilitation. The need for a more algorithmic approach to treatment prompted Wilk et al. to formulate a classification system for patellofemoral disorders (Table 1).[29]

The emphasis of the following material is a biomechanical approach and a thought process. It is important to identify the forces that break down or overload tissue. The lower body functions as a linkage system where each component influences and is influenced by other components thus, examining above or below sites of pain is critical. The goal of the clinician

should be to identify optimal loading of involved tissues, restore joint stability and regain full range of motion (ROM). An understanding of the basic anatomy, kinesiology and muscle training principles is paramount in this evaluation process.[30,31]

Functional Anatomy

A review of the anatomy is essential, with understanding of the mechanics and potential for pain generation. On the medial side of the patella there are two types of restraints. The primary dynamic medial restraint is the vastus medialis oblique (VMO). The VMO does not extend the knee, however, provides medial dynamic stability to patella and selectively atrophies post-surgery and/or injury. In contrast, the Vastus lateralis fibers extend the knee as well as provide lateral dynamic stability. Vastus medialis oblique dysplasia predisposes the patella to lateral displacement. The secondary static medial restraint is the medial retinaculum. The medial retinaculum opposes lateral patellar displacement at 20 degrees of knee flexion, contributing 60% of total restraining force.[32] There are dynamic and static patellofemoral lateral restraints as well. Dynamically, the Vastus lateralis opposes the medial displacement of patella. Statically, the lateral retinaculum with deep and superficial fibers as well as the ITB limit medial tilt and glide of the patella (Fig. 1).[33]

The patellar cartilage in the central portion is the thickest cartilage in the body, measuring approximately 5 mm thick. It allows almost friction-free motion between patella and femur.[34] The primary function of quadriceps, according to the anatomy texts, is extension of the knee. However, functionally the quadriceps muscles' role in standing and walking is to eccentrically control knee flexion and to provide shock absorption. Arthrokinematically, patellofemoral joint reaction forces (PFJRF) are greatest between 60–90 degrees of knee extension, with a force of up to 3000 Newtons.[35] The forces imparted on the patella vary with different functional tasks (Table 2). Walking increases PFJRF by 1.5 times body weight, climbing stairs by 3 times body weight, squatting to 90 degrees by 7–8 times body weight and running depending on angle of incline or decline, up to 4.6–7.7 times body weight respectively.[35-37]

Throughout most of the flexion-extension cycle, one part or another of patellar cartilage is loaded, except in full extension to early flexion. Patellofemoral contact surface area changes with the angle of the knee (Fig. 2). Patellofemoral contact area of the patella increases in area

TABLE 1: Classification system for patellofemoral disorders[29]

- Patellar compressive syndromes:
  - Excessive lateral pressure syndrome
  - Global patellar pressure syndrome
- Patellar instability
- Biomechanical dysfunction
- Direct patellar trauma
- Soft tissue lesions:
  - Plica, Iliotibial band (ITB) friction, Fat pad syndrome, Medial patellofemoral ligament injury
- Overuse syndromes:
  - Osgood-Schlatter, Sindig-Larsen-Johansson
- Osteochondral dessicans
- Neurologic disorders

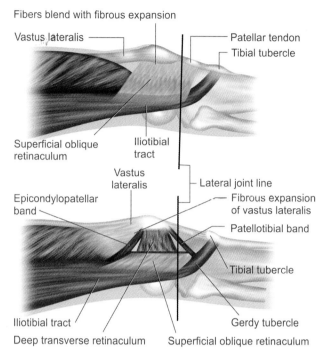

FIG. 1: Lateral anatomical structures of the knee[33]
Source: Reproduced with permission from Manske RC.

TABLE 2: Patellofemoral joint reaction forces[35-37]

Patellofemoral joint reaction forces	Activity
1.5 x BW	Walking
3.3 x BW	Stair climbing
7.5 x BW	Squatting
5.6 x BW	Running

BW, body weight.

with flexion and moves from distal to proximal (Fig. 3 and Table 3).[34]

CLINICAL PRESENTATION

Patellofemoral pain syndrome symptoms can be vague, difficult to localize and frustrating for the patient and clinician. However, anterior knee pain is the primary complaint, with reports of the joint "giving way" into flexion due to reflex inhibition, swelling or weakness of the quadriceps muscle group. Effusion from a synovial response has been reported as well. PFP has been associated with crepitus. It appears that the majority of patients' pain may originate from the surrounding soft tissues and not from the osseous or articular cartilage structures.[38-40] Pain is often associated with functional

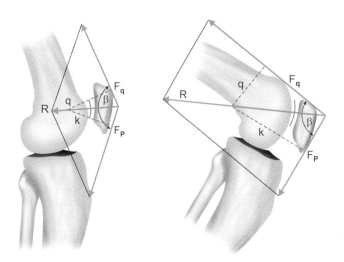

FIG. 2: Illustrated PFJRF at differing angles of knee flexion[33]
Source: Reproduced with permission from Manske RC.

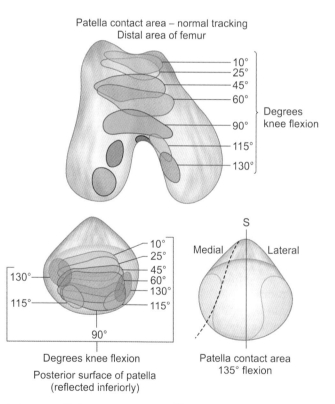

FIG. 3: Patellofemoral contact area[33]
Source: Reproduced with permission from Manske RC.

activities like climbing or descending stairs, or after prolonged sitting—also known as the "Movie Sign" for pain arising from prolonged periods of time in a 90 degree angle of knee flexion. PFP signs are frequently described

TABLE 3: Patellofemoral contact surfaces[34]

Degree of flexion	Patellar articulation	Femoral articulation
0	Femoral sulcus	Minimal contact
20–30	Inferior patellar facets	Middle femoral sulcus
60	Middle patellar facets	Superior femoral notch (SFN)
90	Middle-superior lateral patellar facets	Superior femoral notch
120	Lateral middle-superior facets	SFN/lateral femoral condyle (LFC)
135	Lateral middle-superior facet/odd facet	LFC/lateral surface of medial femoral condyle

as patellar hypomobility, patellar hypermobility and sometimes referred to as malpositioning of the patella—specifically as alta, baja or tilt. An increased quadriceps angle, or Q-Angle, is often observed, but not always significant.[41] With patellar instability, a positive apprehension sign can be elicited with passive lateral movement of the patella in knee extension creating pain and fear of allowing the patella to be displaced in a position over the trochlear groove. Local tenderness to palpation, VMO atrophy and flexibility deficits of the lower extremity, particularly the hamstrings, gastrocnemius and quadriceps muscle groups have been associated with PFP. The Clarke's sign, which requires the clinician to provoke a compressive grind of the patellofemoral joint, has been found to be unreliable and invalid by Duberstein et al.[42]

CLINICAL EXAMINATION

Evaluation of the entire kinetic chain from the lumbar spine to the toes is essential for data collection and to formulate a treatment plan for PFP.

Standing Examination

In standing, a brief observation of the entire lower quadrant is performed, including assessing the patient's standing lumbar lordosis, with an ideal range of 25–30 degrees for articular health and load distribution.[43] Pelvic girdle kinetic tests assess the patient's ability to move in the sagittal, frontal and transverse planes, for optimal movement and efficient forward propulsion. The half squat test is performed to assess the patient's available hip and knee flexion as well as ankle dorsiflexion. The Frankfort angle is used to assess proper form and mechanics performing a squat. If the ankle is limited in dorsiflexion, a compensatory excessive pronation of the longitudinal medial arch of the foot may be present.[44,45] A heel raise test is used to assess gastrocnemius strength as well as the forefoot's ability to pronate or evert, while

the rearfoot supinates or inverts. The standing position allows the clinician to observe for genu recurvatum, valgus or varus deformities in weight bearing or, even more importantly, a loss of knee extension. Special tests in standing also include assessment for subtalar joint axis of inclination (in author's experience, ~45 degrees is desirable). Closed kinetic chain (CKC) mechanics evaluation is performed via a single leg squat.

Seated Examination

The J-sign for abnormal patellar tracking pattern is assessed in open kinetic chain (OKC). For muscle strength and density, the author uses the Albert/Kendall/Worthingham VMO Test using a zero to five (0–5) scale. As the patient performs a quadriceps set (Fig. 4), the examiner looks for a 7–8 mm superior glide of the patella to qualify for a 3/5 manual muscle testing equivalent, in addition to palpation of the distal quadriceps and VMO using 30 pounds of pressure directed deep toward the femur.

Using a handheld dynamometer (Fig. 5), hip external rotator and internal rotator muscle strength is assessed. Several sources have suggested a weakness of the hip joint musculature may lead to uncontrolled hip internal rotation, excessive foot pronation and an increased Q-Angle in CKC activity, like a single leg squat.[44-47]

Supine Examination

In supine, measurements of knee active and passive ROM can be assessed; however, ROM is usually pain-free and full, similar to the other knee. Girth measurements are recorded at 6 inches above the knee to assess muscle atrophy, 3 inches above the patella to assess for effusion or distal quadriceps atrophy, mid-patella for swelling and joint effusion, and mid-calf to assess for differences in calf muscle mass. Lower extremity flexibility is also assessed in the supine position. Hamstring length is assessed with

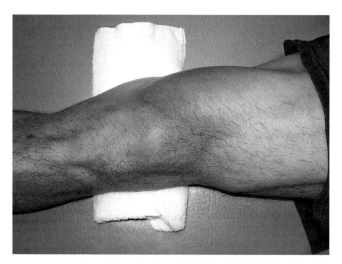

FIG. 4: Quadriceps set with towel under the knee

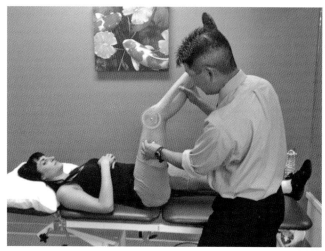

FIG. 6: Measuring hamstring flexibility

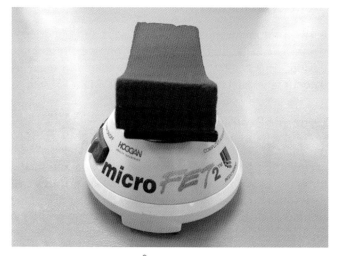

FIG. 5: Hoggan MicroFET2® Manual muscle tester

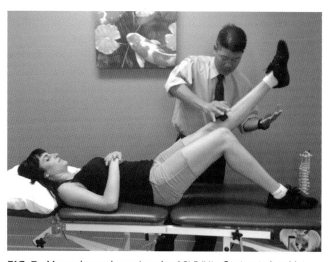

FIG. 7: Manual muscle testing the ASLR/Hip flexion in hooklying

the hip and knee started in a 90/90 position of flexion then extended at the knee only to the first tissue barrier or presence of resistance. The angle is then measured with an inclinometer or a goniometer. In author's experience, the goal is to achieve 30 degrees from full knee extension (Fig. 6).

Gastrocnemius flexibility is assessed with the ankle in maximal dorsiflexion, with a goal angle of 10 and 15 degrees, which, in author's experience, has been found to allow for efficient walking and running, respectively. Gluteus maximus flexibility is measured by performing hip flexion, with a desired angle of 120 degrees. While a ROM of 65 degrees is desired with the combined motion of flexion, abduction and external rotation (FABER)

about the hip.[44,45] Strength testing of the proximal lower extremity is assessed in a hooklying position, with one leg in full knee extension and the other flexed with the foot planted on the table. The patient is instructed to perform an active straight leg raise (ASLR), maintaining full knee extension and resisting against the examiner's force, with the handheld dynamometer placed just distal to the tibial tubercle. This method is used to assess the involved hip flexion strength compared to the uninvolved side (Fig. 7).

The supine examination is concluded with special tests to the knee, including knee ligament stability, especially if the history suggests macrotrauma. One significant ligament to examine is the posterior cruciate ligament (PCL), as up to 48% of chronic PCL deficient knees have reported a positive "Movie Sign". In case of PCL laxity, the pain and stiffness in the anterior compartment after prolonged sitting is attributed to increased PFJRF created by a posterior displacement of the tibial tuberosity.[48] Lastly, palpation and joint mobility of several landmarks are performed in the supine examination position.

To assess patellofemoral joint mobility, the examiner must manipulate the patella in a superior and inferior (cranial and caudal, respectively) direction as well as assess medial glide and tilt. Superior glide assesses the patella's ability to move cranially with a limiting structure of the infrapatellar fat pad or the patellar tendon. Inferior glide assesses the patella's passive ability to move caudally, which, if restricted, would be limited by the quadriceps tendon or muscle. Medial glide is the patella's passive ability to move toward the midline with the knee in 30 degrees of flexion, which would be limited by tight lateral retinacular tissues. Whereas medial tilt is the patella's passive ability to tilt the anterior facing portion of the patella to face medially in full extension, and would be limited by the deep retinacular fibers of the lateral retinaculum. Lateral glide of the patella could be assessed jointly with the apprehension test to determine if there is a laxity in medial retinacular tissues or patellar instability. Much has been made of assessing a patient's patellofemoral alignment; however, tests for intra- and inter-tester reliability using visual and goniometric examination of patellar orientation has been proven low.[49,50] For the purpose of this chapter, patellofemoral orientation will simply be referred to as a glide, tilt and rotation. But as stated earlier, assessment of these positions is highly unreliable, and therefore the author does not advocate using the terms for any other reason than for identifying directional components of taping, discussed later under physical therapy treatment.

Side-Lying Examination

The evaluation continues in side-lying, a position in which hip abduction strength can be assessed (Fig. 8). A handheld dynamometer can again be used for bilateral comparison with relationship to single leg frontal plane stability in a single leg stance position. Ireland et al. demonstrated 26–36% less hip abduction and external rotation strength in females with PFP compared to matched controls.[51] Assessment continues with lateral hip and leg structures for ITB tightness using the Ober's test.

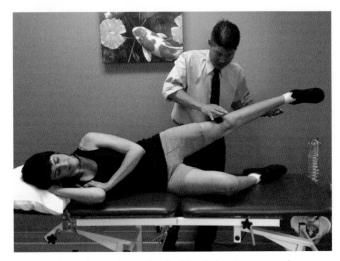

FIG. 8: Manual muscle testing for hip abduction strength

Prone Examination

Lastly in prone, evaluation of hip flexor and quadriceps tightness can be assessed by performing a prone knee flexion. Anecdotally, a value greater than 125 degrees, without increased hip flexion, are desired.

Dynamic Examination

A dynamic gait evaluation is crucial in patellofemoral examination for dynamic and real time loading of the lower extremity. About the knee, variances in valgus and varus thrusts can be observed at initial contact to loading response. At the hip, excessive hip adduction moments or Trendelenberg's sign may indicate gluteus medius weakness in single leg stance. Abnormal lower kinetic chain dynamics also can be observed with excessive pronation or supination of the medial longitudinal arch. However, gait evaluations are purely a part of the data collection and must not be used in isolation. When gait deviations are matched with other objective measurable findings, as mentioned above in the comprehensive evaluation of the lower extremity, they are most useful. Dynamic evaluations should include activities that the patient or athlete may need to perform: examples are running, jumping and/or cutting maneuvers.

Role of Imaging

Imaging is used to compliment all the clinical findings. The clinician should obtain all relevant diagnostic items, such as X-rays or magnetic resonance imaging results, if available. This enables the clinician to determine if there are other pathologies within or about the knee that may mimic pain generators or complicate treatment strategies. In the presence of articular cartilage lesions, it can be useful to know where the lesions are located, and which angles to avoid during flexion or loading activities.

Differential Diagnosis

Peripatellar dysfunctions can confuse the examiner in making a solid clinical decision in the management of PFP. Other dysfunctions that have also been termed "patellofemoral pain syndrome" simply due to the location and ambiguity of anterior knee pain are patellar tendinosis (degeneration of tendon with limited inflammatory response), retinacular pain, plica syndrome, Hoffa's syndrome (scarring of fat pad), meniscus tears, osteochondral defects, ITB syndrome, popliteal tendinitis, neuromas and L3 radicular symptoms.

■ PHYSICAL THERAPY TREATMENT

Once data collection during the subjective and objective portion of the evaluation is completed, the clinician must next formulate a working hypothesis. The hypothesis must be in regards to the stage of the condition, the irritability of the condition and the anatomical structures involved. Once these elements are established, treatment interventions can be selected. When selecting the physical therapy interventions, the initial strategy should focus on educating the patient. An understanding of the physical therapy diagnosis, prognosis and treatment plan will help the patient understand his or her role in self-management strategies and responsibility in the course of treatment. The clinician must next select methods in which to stretch, strengthen, functionally retrain and foster independence of the patient before initiating treatment. As treatment begins, several factors must be addressed:

- Prioritizing the treatment
- Treatment strategy
- The frequency and dosage of the treatment
- Monitoring if the patient is improving (positive), regressing (negative), static (same) or oscillating (improving, then not improving)
- Measuring the rate at which the patient is responding to the treatment.

To discern if goals are being met, the clinician should use outcome measures to determine change or functional improvement periodically once treatment commences. Examples of helpful, valid and reliable outcome measures

for the clinician are the Lysholm knee rating score[52-54] and Lower Extremity Functional Scale.[55]

Upon initiation of treatment, several "Clinical Pearls" must be considered. First, when treating PFP, the age old "No pain, No gain" theory generally does not apply. With minimal pain during treatment intervention, the clinician can minimize quadriceps inhibition and increase patient compliance, since many patients can be avoidant to activity that recreates their pain. Pain complaints can be reduced using cryotherapy, taping techniques, bracing and education. Keen observation of any passive knee extension loss is important. Restoration of extension prior to flexion is fundamental to knee rehabilitation.[56] Sachs and Daniels reported an extension deficit of 5 degrees or greater promotes minimal strength gain and can cause increased irritability with performing an ASLR exercise.[57]

Treatment of PFP can be categorized into the phase concept for rehabilitation initially presented by Davies and Gould.[58]

Phase I

In the acute phase, the focus is to decrease swelling and pain. DeAndrade et al. reported that fluid joint distention resulted in quadriceps muscle inhibition.[59] They also noted a decrease in quadriceps activity as the knee exhibited increased distention. Spencer et al. also found a similar decrease in quadriceps activation with joint effusion. They reported the threshold for inhibition of the vastus medialis to be approximately 20–30 mL of joint effusion and 50–60 mL for the rectus femoris and vastus lateralis.[60] Reducing knee joint swelling is crucial to restoration of normal quadriceps activity. Several favorable treatment options for swelling reduction include cryotherapy, high-voltage stimulation and joint compression using a knee sleeve or compression wraps.

As the patient progresses, McConnell patellar taping techniques may also be used to quickly reduce pain[61-67] and possibly normalize patellar tracking through mechanical shift of patella.[68] The taping technique described by Jenny McConnell is unique to each patient, and must address each component (glide, tilt and rotation)—with the most significant abnormality addressed first. Taping should improve symptoms immediately. If not, it should be reapplied, and the order of taping should be reconsidered. McConnell taping has been shown to provide greater pain relief than sham taping,[69-71] as well as to restore timing of the VMO and vastus lateralis activation.[72] In addition to reducing pain, taping has been reported to assist neuromotor control of vasti musculature.[73] Taping is less effective for patients with high body mass index, larger lateral patellofemoral angle and smaller Q-angle.[74] Whittingham et al. conducted a randomized controlled trial with 30 patients with PFP, who were categorized into three groups: (1) taping with standard exercise, (2) placebo taping with exercise and (3) exercise alone. Significant improvement was shown in all groups with regard to pain and function. However, the best group was taped and performed exercise.[75]

Several McConnell taping techniques have been advocated in the literature. The traditional technique (Fig. 9) addresses all components of glide, rotation and tilt, with a medially directed pull.

The reverse technique of McConnell taping (Fig. 10) addresses glide, rotation and tilt; however, all components have a laterally directed pull. This technique is less common, but is most beneficial in patients with varus knees or those who have a dynamic varus thrust in gait.

McConnell taping techniques have also been described for soft tissue lesions, such as for the patellar tendon, using a "Tee Pee" taping method (Fig. 11), pulling medially over mid substance of patellar tendon.

Taping the infra patellar fat pad (Fig. 12) unloads the fat pad, pulling the tibial tubercle up toward joint line in both medial and lateral directions.

An additional taping technique used by the author to facilitate full knee extension, as well as quadriceps activation, is called the Nakaji-Thompson Screw Home technique (Fig. 13). The tape is applied from the tibial tubercle, pulling laterally behind knee around toward

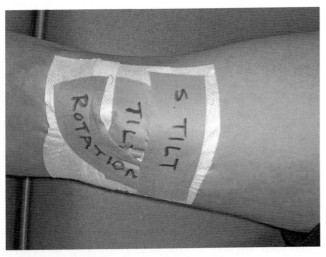

FIG. 9: Traditional McConnell patellofemoral taping

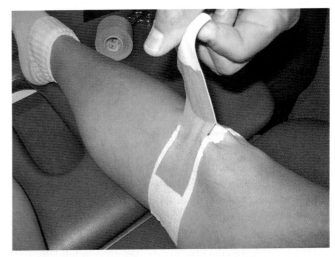

FIG. 11: Patellar tendon "Tee Pee" taping method

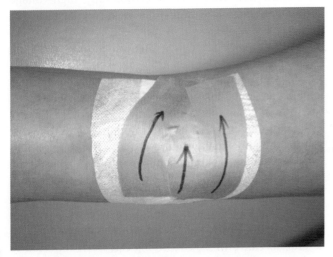

FIG. 10: Reverse McConnell patellofemoral taping

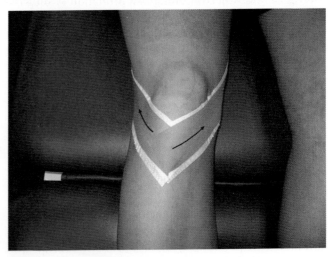

FIG. 12: Infrapatellar fat pad taping

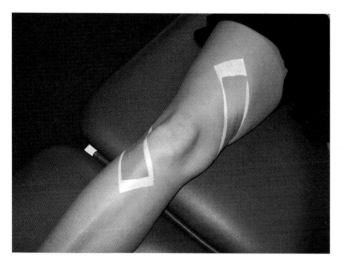

FIG. 13: Nakaji-Thompson screw home taping technique

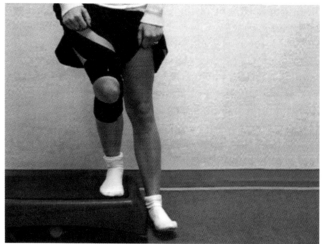

FIG. 14: SERF Strap®

the VMO in a distal to proximal manner. Upon active contraction of the quadriceps, the knee is pulled via the tape into extension. Taping is most successful with clean-shaven skin and for short periods of time of application. Care must be used with sensitive skin. If redness or a rash develops, the patient should discontinue use.

There are also arguments against the use of taping as an effective technique in treatment for PFP. Taping techniques should be utilized more as an adjunct and temporary modality, allowing the clinician to differentiate painful structures and tissues about the patellofemoral joint. Over the past decade, Dr. Powers has demonstrated that the hip places the patellofemoral joint in a mechanical disadvantage due to excessive hip adduction and internal rotation in the frontal and transverse planes. His research has advocated hip external rotation and abduction strengthening, and controlling foot pronation to keep the femur in a stable position relative to the patella.[76]

During the early phases of rehabilitation, external supports may be used for static as well as dynamic support to the patellofemoral joint (Figs 14 and 15).

Phase II

Phase II should emphasize restoring volitional muscle control and contraction of the quadriceps muscle group in addition to minimizing pain and swelling. Weakness and inhibition of the quadriceps is common in patellofemoral patients because of the presence of pain or swelling.[77,78] There have been many myths about focusing rehabilitation and strengthening on the VMO in PFP patients. There are inconclusive results in the literature with respect to being able to selectively recruit and strengthen the VMO.

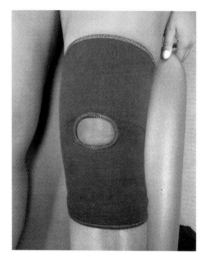

FIG. 15: Patellofemoral sleeve

There is no well-documented research on independently contracting the VMO. The author believes in a "back to basics" approach for quadriceps reeducation and training. This approach is highly patient-dependent, focusing on pain-free exercises and an acute awareness of other pathology within the knee, as well as the kinetic chain. Exercise that can strengthen quadriceps muscle group as a whole will likely positively affect VMO.

Progression of quadriceps and lower quadrant reeducation and strengthening requires an in-depth understanding of biomechanics, joint kinematics, arthro-kinematics, and strength and conditioning principles. Selection of exercises must allow the clinician to position the knee in angles, which minimize pain and PFJRF. Exercises can either be OKC or CKC, with respect to strengthening and training. An OKC activity is where the distal segment of the extremity is not fixed or non-weight bearing. Conversely, CKC activity is when the distal segment is fixed or weight bearing. CKC activity is thought to be more functional, in that it simulates activities of daily living. For example, a squat mimics a patient sitting down or raising from a seated position.[77] The literature supports use of both OKC and CKC exercises in patellofemoral joint rehabilitation. Witvrouw et al. found that in a 5-week training program, both CKC and OKC groups showed significant improvement in muscle characteristics, subjective pain symptoms and functional performance, with slightly better subjective and objective outcomes with the CKC group.[78] Steinkamp et al. measured PFJRF in 20 subjects performing leg press and knee extension exercises. They found that there was less PFJRF in CKC between 0–46 degrees of knee flexion, and that PFJRF was less in OKC between 50–90 degrees. Clinically speaking, CKC exercises (e.g. leg press) are safe in the range of 0–45 degrees and OKC exercises (e.g. knee extension) are safe in 90–45 degrees of knee flexion.[79] At 34–40 degrees, PFJRF peaks, and then it decreases past 50–60 degrees during OKC exercise. Therefore, OKC exercise is not recommended in 0–45 degrees of flexion, due to increased or larger articular cartilage stress[80,81] It can be logically concluded that OKC exercises such as quadriceps setting or isometric contractions in full extension (Fig. 4) are safe Phase I–II exercises. Isometrics can later be implemented at multiple pain-free joint angles based on PFJRFs and articular pathology.[82] The patient must hold the contraction for a minimum of 6 seconds for training effect of strength carry over, with a 60-second recovery in between repetitions.[83] To help motivate and educate the patient at the intensity and duration of the exercise, electromyography (EMG) biofeedback units or neuromuscular electrical stimulation units have been proven to be beneficial in early phases of rehabilitation.[84-86] Straight leg raise exercises (Fig. 16) can be performed in multiple positions, such as supine, long sitting and side-lying, with an emphasis on quadriceps control of the knee and isolated activity to the targeted proximal hip muscles.[87] Distefano et al. found that the highest EMG activity of the gluteus medius was observed with side-lying hip abduction against gravity.[88] Mascal et al. also advocated strengthening the hip musculature, particularly the gluteus medius in an OKC, non-weight bearing position and progressing to CKC weight bearing, with a focus on frontal plane pelvic control, in patients demonstrating excessive femoral adduction, internal rotation and knee valgus on a step down test.[89] Manual resistance can be applied to the lower extremity

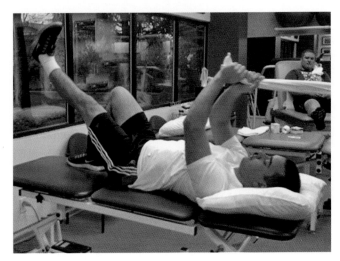

FIG. 16: Facilitated active straight leg raise

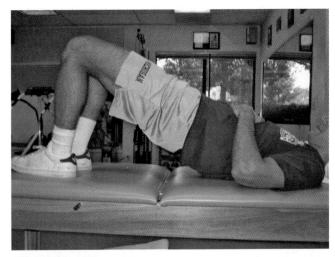

FIG. 17: Bridging

in strengthening as well as the use of proprioceptive neuromuscular facilitation patterns of the lower kinetic chain. Early CKC exercises include bridging (Fig. 17).

Phase III

Phase III or intermediate phase strengthening can be initiated when pain and swelling is absent, the patient demonstrates an understanding of joint angles which can be aggravating, and proximal hip strength measure a minimum 85% of the uninvolved side on tensiometer strength testing for hip flexion, abduction and external rotation. The emphasis begins to shift more toward CKC activity in this phase. The clinician should bear in mind that the PFJRF increases with deeper angles of knee flexion during CKC exercise. Also, the patellofemoral contact area increases as the knee reaches deeper flexion positions in a squat.[90] Maximum articular pressure in a squat occurs at 90 degrees of flexion.[91] The clinician should monitor for pain and increased joint irritability, as the patient progresses through this phase, especially between 50–90 degrees, where PFJRF is greatest.[92] The squat is a very functional activity with strong carry over to activities of daily living. It may be the most beneficial exercise for resistive purposes. However, instruction by the clinician in positioning and form is imperative while monitoring for joint symptoms. The squat (Fig. 18) is dictated by several key technical principles. This varies with differing sizes of the individual patient or athlete, however, as a general rule, the patient should start with shoulder width base of support, with wider stances emphasizing gluteus maximus contribution.[93] A common movement fault with the squat is the lack of optimal pelvic-femoral angle—or "stick butt out". Many youth athletes and patients shift their weight forward, posteriorly tilting the pelvis—or "tuck their butt", resulting in more perceived PFP. Keen awareness on equal weight distribution bilaterally due to quadriceps inhibition and avoidance[94] should be noted as well as vertical tibial alignment. Patients can be cued to maintain the knees behind their shoelaces and weight shifted toward the heels.[95,96] The squat progression can be incremental with multiple developmental exercises: leg press machines starting with the Total Gym® (Fig. 19) for less than full body weight, gradually progressing to full body weight: chair squat, wall ball squats (Fig. 20) to single leg ball squats (Fig. 21) to additional resistance exercise in addition to body weight using Smith Rack™ (Fig. 22).

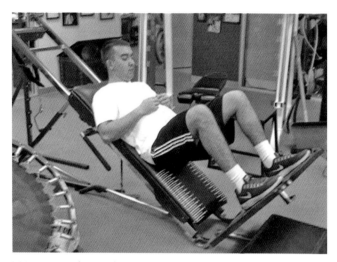

FIG. 19: Total Gym® leg press

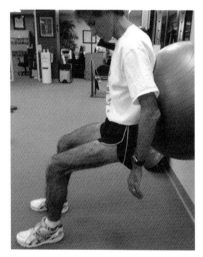

FIG. 20: Wall ball squats

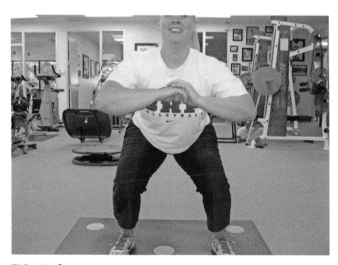

FIG. 18: Squats

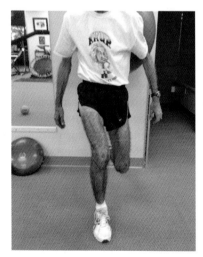

FIG. 21: Single leg ball squat

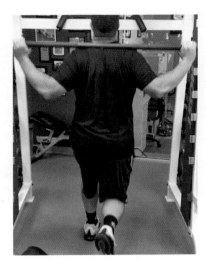

FIG. 22: Single leg Smith Rack™ squat

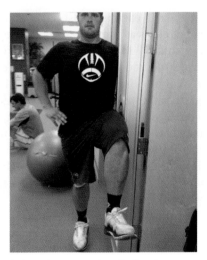

FIG. 24: Single leg gluteus medius facilitation

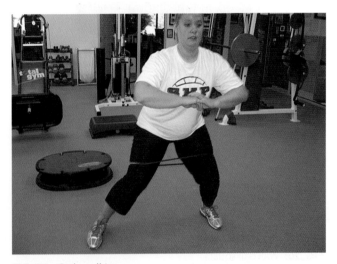

FIG. 23: Crab walking

Crab walking with the band (Fig. 23) is also helpful in facilitating hip abduction control in the frontal plane. The exercise can be executed in a straight leg position or a mini squat position, depending upon the patient's leg lengths and goal of target muscles. Anecdotally, the author has found that straight legged crab walking facilitates more gluteus medius activation and squat position crab walking facilitates more hip external rotators. Once the double leg squat is tolerated with adequate muscle facilitation, strength and without patellofemoral symptoms, a single leg squat progression can be initiated (Fig. 24). Again, key factors must be observed when instructing patients in single leg activity. The first priority is control of the pelvis in the frontal plane avoiding excessive hip adduction. The second is positioning the knee relative to the midline,

while controlling excessive valgus or varus movement. Thirdly, the patient should demonstrate adequate foot control of excessive pronation or supination, ideally with the foot in a subtalar neutral position. The step progression is utilized using an 8-inch step sequentially from stepping up, down backward, sideways, to laterally and eccentrically forward down. The lowest PFJRF has been observed with lateral step-ups and the greatest PFJRF observed with the forward step-downs.[97]

Intermediate rehabilitation proceeds with single leg progression and with a special focus on balance and proprioception, ensuring the patient can control the pelvis in the frontal plane. Single leg activity includes a progression of head movement, and upper and lower extremity reaching movement. For example, the use of the lower extremity functional reach test and/or star excursion balance test (Figs 25A and B) has been demonstrated to exhibit moderate test-retest reliability as well as inter- and intra-tester reliability.[98-100] Activities then increase in vigor, intensity and dynamic control by simulating running motions of reciprocal upper extremity movement, and by starting on a stable surface and progressing to unstable surfaces. Examples of unstable surfaces used clinically include: Airex® mats, TheraBand® foam pads (Fig. 26), Dyna-disc®, Duckwalkers, Rocker boards and Bosu® balls (Fig. 27).

As the patient progresses through the single leg dynamic stability and intermediate rehabilitation phase, the implementation of eccentric muscle training is introduced if the patient has low irritability of symptoms and good dynamic control of the knee in the frontal and transverse planes. Bennett and Stauber observed the

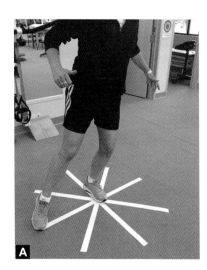

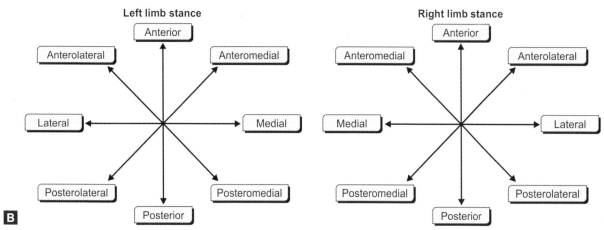

Left limb stance

Anterior

Anterolateral

Anteromedial

Lateral

Medial

Posterolateral

Posteromedial

Posterior

Right limb stance

Anterior

Anteromedial

Anterolateral

Medial

Lateral

Posteromedial

Posterolateral

Posterior

FIG. 25: (A) Star excursion—left limb stance medial reach; (B) Star excursion balance test[102]
Source: Reproduced with permission from Olmsted, LC.

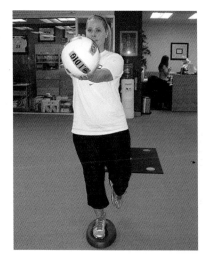

FIG. 26: Dynamic balance on foam pad

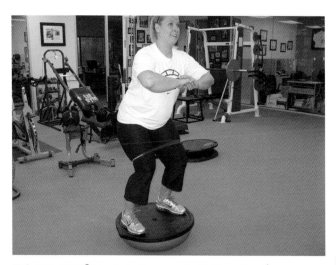

FIG. 27: BOSU® hip abduction squat with TheraBand®

ratio of eccentric quadriceps torque to concentric torque was not normal in a group with anterior knee pain. The expected eccentric torque was 130–300% of concentric torque, but those in the study were deficient. Bennet and Stauber also found that when performing squats, patient's anterior knee pain was relieved with eccentric training of the quadriceps within 2–4 weeks.[101] Using the Curwin-Stannish curve can be of assistance to the clinician in instruction and education to the patient for training purposes. The curve is a progressive eccentric strengthening program that uses three sets of ten repetitions, starting with a week-long progression at very slow speeds and gradually increasing the speed, if there is little to no lingering discomfort. If the week-long cycle is successfully completed, the speed of the progression is started over, however, adding resistance to the cycle.[102] Resistance can simply be added by concentrically rising from a squat on two legs, and lowering down on one. Likewise this technique can be implemented on a leg press or Smith Rack™. When utilizing the eccentric program, the patient must be educated on the potential side-effect of delayed onset muscle soreness. Similar to Bennet and Stauber, Jensen et al. found strength gains in a slightly longer time frame of training for 8 weeks, with pain being a primary limiting factor.[103]

Phase IV

Phase IV rehabilitation includes isotonic resistance terminal knee extensions in sitting and supine. Clinicians should avoid full arc of motion and keep the exercise and resistance within the safe ROM, while monitoring

for articular pathology and PFJRF. Quick kicking and perturbation training are also helpful in later phase, to ready the patient or athlete for unexpected contact or change of direction. Functional late phase rehabilitation can be considered only for patients requiring higher-level activity or sport specific demands. High-level exercises include pseudo hopping, lunges (Figs 28A and B), deeper squats, plyometrics and sports activities such as cutting and jumping. The author uses a clinical progression to simulate running (Appendix E), which prepares the patient for running in the next phase.

Phase V

Phase V, or return to play, criteria is assessed when the patient has concluded Phase IV with minimal pain complaints, no evidence of swelling and demonstrable good motor control in higher level activity. Again, this stage may never be broached with many general orthopedic population patients, but primarily with higher-level athletes. Additional criteria utilized by the author is greater than 90% score on Lysholm knee scale for the patient's perceived level of function. A minimal detectable change for functional improvement using the Lysholm scoring is 10 percentage points.[52,53] Jump and hop tests are also valuable tools in the clinic to determine sport readiness. The standing long jump is useful as a measure of bilateral power and deceleration.[104] Single leg hop for distance is helpful for measuring involved side hop strength and shock absorption with landing in comparison to the uninvolved side. A distance of 85% of the uninvolved side is considered as a good score for advancement in

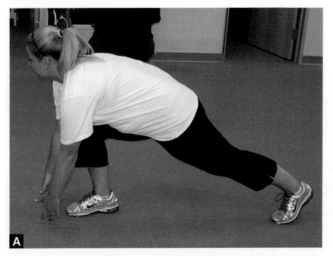
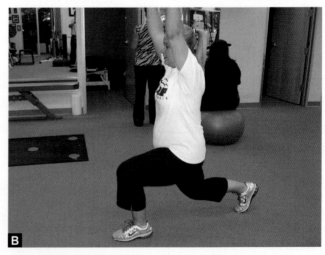

FIG. 28: (A) Lunge forward reach to facilitate gluteal muscles; (B) Lunge overhead reach to facilitate quadriceps muscles

activity.[105-109] The Lower Extremity Functional Test or LEFT (Appendix F) is very helpful in assessing athletic readiness by measuring the time to complete a series of running tests including sprints, backward running, crossover or cariocas and cutting angles of 45 and 90 degrees. The test provides an excellent insight to the patient's ability to perform sport specific activity in an intense and timed environment.[110] Safe, progressive and gradual return to running is advocated for runners with PFP. The author uses as systematic, timed interval type training and return to running progression (Appendix G).

Alternative Treatments

Acupuncture has shown promise with a decrease in pain better than a sham intervention in the treatment of PFP.[70,111,112] The use of custom molded foot orthotics also has been demonstrated in the literature to assist in the long-term management of PFP, yielding better results than flat foot insoles, but with little difference with or without physical therapy intervention.[18,113]

Medical and Surgical Considerations

Injection therapy can be an adjunct and considered to be one of the last non-operative modalities in the management of PFP.[114] Examples of intra-articular injection therapy include corticosteroids and hylan GF20 or hyaluronic acid. While not studied extensively in patients with PFP, a 2006 Cochrane Review found that corticosteroid injections provided short-term benefit, of up to 26 weeks, and was effective in reducing pain in patients with knee osteoarthritis.[115,116] Hyaluronic acid injections have had mixed results for effectiveness in the treatment of mild knee osteoarthritis, and might provide pain up to 24 weeks. However, these injections maybe cost-prohibitive to certain patients.[114,117] Clinically, the author has found that hyaluronic acid injection therapy for PFP is at best unremarkable, but can improve a patient's pain and function with medial or lateral knee compartment osteoarthritis.

Common surgical treatments for management of PFP performed by orthopedic surgeons include the lateral retinacular release, medial retinacular release, tibial tubercle transfers and chondroplasty. Success rates for the above listed PFP related surgeries are considered poor when compared to other orthopedic procedures; however, success rates can be greatly enhanced with good communication and progressive post surgical rehabilitation catered to the specific surgical procedure.[19, 118,119]

CONCLUSION

Patellofemoral pain syndrome is a common, complicated and chronic disorder which presents to physical therapists on a regular basis.[76, 120,121] While 75-90% improve with conservative management, the success rate can be enhanced by sound clinical reasoning during the evaluation, by utilization of the classification system for patellofemoral disorders and by implementation of an ongoing progressive training program of the entire lower extremity. Employing a combination of McConnell taping and exercise, the clinician should see significant improvement within the first 6-8 visits. The information obtained by the evaluation and through taping trials should allow the clinician to determine the primary pain generator and next course of treatment by visits 10-12. Depending on the patient's progress, a decision to discharge the patient to a home exercise program or refer back to the referring physician may need to be made. In the past, McConnell taping kits have been sold to patients and the patient was instructed to tape the knee "indefinitely". Based on the author's experience and unpublished data, the taping technique is a Phase I–II adjunct designed to serve two purposes: (1) allow the clinician to glean the pain generator of the patellofemoral joint by alleviating and provoking the patient's pain and (2) assisting in pain reduction, allowing the patient to strengthen the quadriceps inhibiting the muscle function and feeding into the patient's fear avoidance to exercise.[122] When referring the patient back to the doctor, the clinician should have a conclusion as to why the patient failed conservative rehabilitation. Additionally, the clinician should be able to provide an insight into potentially helpful surgeries, and/or advise the doctor on pain controlling injections or bracing, which may benefit the patient's function. Careful, systematic and precise rehabilitation can demonstrate functional improvement using functional measures like the Lysholm, objective functional tests like the step up-down, stair climbing and running. If the clinician is able to apply a sound clinical evaluation and treatment approach in conjunction with current and past relevant evidence from the medical literature, many previously difficult patients will improve and return to full function.

REFERENCES

1. Deveraux MD, Lachman SM. Patellofemoral arthralgia in athletes attending a sports injury clinic. Br J Sports Med. 1984;18(1):18-21.
2. Malek MM, Mangine RE. Patellofemoral pain syndromes: a comprehensive and conservative approach. J Orthop Sports Phys Ther. 1981;2(3):108-16.

3. Fulkerson JP, Hungerford DS. Disorders of the Patellofemoral Joint, 2nd edition. Baltimore, MD: William and Wilkins; 1990.

4. Brick GW, Scott RD. The patellofemoral component of total knee arthroplasty. Clin Ortho Relat Res. 1988;(231):163-78.

5. Restrom AF. Knee pain in tennis players. Clin Sports Med. 1995;14(1): 163-75.

6. Taunton JE, Ryan MB, Clement DB, McKenzie DC, Lloyd-Smith DR, Zumbo BD. A retrospective case-control analysis of 2002 running injuries. Br J Sports Med. 2002;36(2):95-101.

7. Jordaan G, Schwellnus MP. The incidence of overuse injuries in military recruits during basic military training. Mil Med. 1994;159(6):421-6.

8. Finestone A, Radin EL, Lev B. Treatment of overuse patellofemoral pain. Prospective randomized controlled trial in military setting. Clin Orthop Relat Res. 1993;293:208-10.

9. Grady EP, Carpenter MT, Koenig CD, Older SA, Battafarano DF. Rheumatic findings in Gulf War veterans. Arch Intern Med. 1998;158(4):367-71.

10. Samilson RL, Gill KW. Patellofemoral problems in cerebral palsy. Acta Orthop Belg. 1984;50:191-7.

11. McConnell J. The management of chondromalacia patellae: a long term solution. Aust J Physiol. 1986;2:215-23.

12. Gerrard B. The patellofemoral pain syndrome in young, active patients: a prospective study. Clin Orthop. 1989;179:129-33.

13. Kannus J, Nittymaki S. Which factors predict the outcome in the non-operative treatment of patellofemoral pain syndrome? A prospective follow-up study. Med Sci in Sport Exerc. 1994;26:289-96.

14. Whitelaw GP, Rullo DJ, Markowitz HD, Marandola MS, DeWaele MJ. A conservative approach to anterior knee pain. Clin Orthop Relat Res. 1989;(246):234-7.

15. Natri A, Kannus P, Jarvinen. Which factors predict the long term outcome in chronic patellofemoral pain syndrome? A 7-year prospective follow-up study. Med Sci Sport Exerc. 1998;30(11):1572-7.

16. Pappas E, Wong-Tom WM. Prospective Predictors of patellofemoral pain syndrome: a systematic review with meta-analysis. Sports Health: A Multidisciplinary Approach. 2012;4(2):115-20.

17. Lankhorts NE, Bierma-Zeinstra SM, van Middlekoop M. Risk factors for patellofemoral pain syndrome: a systematic review. J Orthop Sports Phys Ther. 2012;42(2):81-94.

18. Bolgla L, Boling M. An update for the conservative management of patellofemoral pain syndrome: a systematic review of the literature from 2000 to 2010. Int J Sports Phys Ther. 2011;6(2):112-25.

19. Grelsamer RP, McConnell J. The Patella: A Team Approach. Gaithersburg, MD; Aspen Publishers; 1998. pp. 109-18.

20. Busch MT, DeHaven KE. Pitfalls of the lateral retinacular release. Clin Sports Med. 1989;8(2):279-90.

21. Dehaven KE, Dolan WA, Mayer PJ. Chondromalacia patellae in athletes. Clinical presentation and conservative management. Am J Sports Med. 1979;7(1):5-11.

22. Fulkerson JP, Hungerford DS. Disorders of the Patellofemoral Joint, 2nd edition. Baltimore, MD: Williams and Wilkins; 1990.

23. Insall J. Current concepts review: patellar pain. J Bone Joint Surg Arm. 1982;64(1):147-52.

24. Mitcheli LJ, Stanitski CL. Lateral patellar retinacular release. Am J Sports Med. 1981;9(5):189-94.

25. Radin EL. A rational approach to the treatment of patellofemoral pain. Clin Orthop Relat Res. 1979;(144):107-9.

26. Sandow MJ, Goodfellow JW. The natural history of anterior knee pain in adolescents. J Bone Joint Surg Br. 1985;67:36-8.

27. Stougard J. Chondromalacia of the patella. Physical signs in relation to operative findings. Acta Orthop Scand. 1975;46(4):685-94.

28. Yates C, Grana WA. Patellofemoral pain: a prospective study. Orthopedics. 1986;9(5):663-7.

29. Wilk KE, Davies GJ, Mangine RE, Malone TR. Patellofemoral disorders: a classification system and clinical guidelines for non operative rehabilitation. J Orthop Sports Phys Ther. 1998;28(5):307-22.

30. Jackson, R. Functional Relationships of the Lower Half. 1995. Course notes and personal communication.

31. Powers C, Bolgla L, Callaghan M, Collins N, Sheehan F. Patellofemoral pain: proximal, distal, and local factors—Second International Research Retreat, August 31–September 2, 2011, Ghent, Belgium. J Orthop Sports Phys Ther. 2012;42(6):A1-A54.

32. Desio SM, Burks RT, Bachus KN. Soft tissue restraints to lateral patellar translation in the human knee. Am J Sports Med. 1998;26(1):59-65.

33. Manske RC. Post-Surgical Rehabilitation of the Knee and Shoulder. St. Louis, MO: Mosby; 2006.

34. Grelsamer RP, Weinstein DH. Applied biomechanics of the patella. Clin Orthop Rel Res. 2001;(389):9-14.

35. Huberti HH, Hayes WC, Stone JL, Shybut GT. Force ratios in the quadriceps tendon and ligamentum patella. J Orthop Res. 1984;2(1):49-54.

36. Percy EC, Strother RT. Patellalgia. Phys Sports Med. 1985;13(7): 43-6, 49-51, 55-6, 58-9.

37. Reilly DT, Martens M. Experimental analysis of the quadriceps muscle force and patello-femoral joint reaction force for various activities. Acta Orthop Scand. 1972;43(2):126-37.

38. Chrisman OD. The role of articular cartilage in patellofemoral pain. Orthop Clin North Am. 1986;17(2):231-4.

39. Dye SF, Boll DA. Radionuclide imaging of the patellofemoral joint in young adults with anterior knee pain. Orthop Clin North Am. 1986;17(2):249-62.

40. Fulkerson JP, Shea KP. Disorders of the patellofemoral joint. J Bone Joint Surg Am. 1990;72(9):1424-9.

41. Grelsamer RP, Weinstein CH. Applied biomechanics of the patella. Clin Orthop Relat Res. 2001;389: 9-14.

42. Doberstein ST, Romeyn RL, Reineke DM. The diagnostic value of the Clarke sign in assessing chondromalacia patella. Journal of Athletic Training. 2008;43(2):190-6.

43. Adams MA, Hutton WC. The effect of posture on the role of the apophysial joints in resisting intervertebral compressive forces. J Bone Joint Surg. 1980;62(3):358-62.

44. Irrgang et al. Closed Kinetic Chain for the Lower Extremity Theory & Application. Sports Physical Therapy Section home study course Current Concepts in Rehabilitation of the Knee. 1994.

45. Tiberio D. The effect of excessive subtalar joint pronation on patellofemoral mechanics: a theoretical model. J Orthop Sports Phys Ther. 1987; 9(4):160-5.

46. Pease et al. Anterior Knee pain: Differential Diagnosis and Physical Therapy management. American Physical Therapy Association Home Study Course. 1992.

47. Ireland ML, Wilson JD, Ballantyne BT, Davis IM. Hip strength in females with and without patellofemoral pain. J Orthop Sports Phys Ther. 2003;33(11):671-6.

48. Parolie JM, Bergfeld JA. Long-term results of nonoperative treatment of isolated posterior cruciate ligament injuries in the athlete. Am J Sports Med. 1986;14(1):35-8.

49. Tomsich DA, Nitz AJ, Threlkeld AJ, Shapiro R. Patellofemoral alignment: reliability. J Orthop Sports Phys Ther. 1996;23(3):200-8.

50. Fitzgerald GK, McClure PW. Reliability of measurements obtained by four tests of patellofemoral alignment. Phys Ther. 1993;75(2):84-92.

51. Ireland ML, Wilson JD, Ballantyne BT, Davis IM. Hip strength in females with and without patellofemoral pain. J Orthop Sports Phys Ther. 2003;33(11):671-6.

52. Briggs KK, Kocher MS, Rodkey WG, Steadman JR. Reliability, validity, and responsiveness of the Lysholm knee score and Tegner activity scale for

patients with meniscal injury of the knee. The Journal of Bone & Joint Surgery. 2006;88(4):698-705.

53. Tegner Y, Lysholm J. Rating systems in the evaluation of knee ligament injuries. Clin Orthop Relat Res. 1985;198:43-9.

54. Marx RG, Jones EC, Allen AA, Altchek DW, O'Brien SJ, Rodeo SA, et al. Reliability, validity, and responsiveness to change of four knee outcome scales for athletic patients. The Journal of Bone & Joint Surgery. 2001;83(10):1459-69.

55. Binkley JM, Stratford PW, Lott SA, Riddle DL. The lower extremity functional (LEFS): scale development, measurement properties, and clinical application. Phys Ther. 1999;79(4):371-83.

56. Greenfield BH. Rehabilitation of the Knee: A problem solving approach Contemporary Perspectives in Rehabilitation. F.A. David Company. 1993.

57. Sachs RA, Daniel DM, Stone ML, Garfein RF. Patellofemoral problems after anterior cruciate ligament reconstruction. Am J Sports Med. 1989;17(6):760-5.

58. Gould J, Davies G. Orthopedic and Sports Physical Therapy. St. Louis, MO: Mosby; 1985.

59. DeAndrade JR, Grant C, Dixon AS. Joint distension and reflex muscle inhibition in the knee. J Bone Joint Surg Am. 1965;47(2):313-22.

60. Spencer JD, Hayes KC, Alexander IJ. Knee joint effusion and quadriceps inhibition in man. Arch Phys Med Rehabil. 1984;65(4):171-7.

61. Aminaka N, Gribble PA. Patellar taping, patellofemoral pain syndrome, lower extremity kinematics, and dynamic postural control. Journal of Athletic Training. 2008;43(1):21-8.

62. Bockrath K, Wooden C, Worrell T, Ingersoll CD, Farr J. Effects of patella taping on patella position and perceived pain. Med Sci Sports Exerc. 1993;25(9):989-92.

63. Pfeiffer RP, DeBeliso M, Shea KG, Kelley L, Irmischer B, Harris C. Kinematic MRI assessment of McConnell taping before and after exercise. Am J Sports Med. 2004;32(3):621-8.

64. Herrington L, Payton CJ. The effects of corrective taping of the patella on patients with patellofemoral pain. Physiotherapy. 1997; 83(12):686.

65. Cerny K. Vastus medialis oblique/vastus lateralis muscle activity ratios for selected exercises in persons with and without patellofemoral pain syndrome. Phys Ther. 1995;75(8):672-82.

66. Conway A, Malone T, Conway P. Patellar alignment/tracking alteration: effect on force output and perceived pain. Isokinetics and Exercise Science. 1992;2(1):9-18.

67. Powers CM, Landel R, Sosnick T, Kirby J, Mengel K, Cheney A, et al. The effects of patellar taping on stride characteristics and joint motion in subjects with patellofemoral pain. J Orthop Sports Ther. 1997;26(6):286-91.

68. McConnell J. The management of chondromalacia patellae: a long term solution. Aust J Physiother. 1986;32(4):215-23.

69. Cowan SM, Hodges PW, Bennell KL, Crossley KM. Altered vastii recruitment when people with patellofemoral pain syndrome complete a postural task. Arch Phys Med Rehab. 2002; 83(7):989-95.

70. Crossley K, Bennell K, Green S, Cowan S, McConnell J. Physical therapy for patellofemoral pain: a randomized, double-blinded, placebo-controlled trial. Am J Sports Med. 2002;30(6):857-65.

71. Handfield T, Kramer J. Effect of McConnell taping on perceived pain and knee extensor torques during isokinetic exercise performed by patients with patellofemoral pain syndrome. Physiother Can. 2000;39-44.

72. Cowan SM, Bennell KL, Hodges PW. Therapeutic patellar taping changes the timing of muscle activation in people with patellofemoral pain syndrome. Clin J Sports Med. 2002;12(6):339-47.

73. Bennell K, Duncan M, Cowan S. Effect of patellar taping on vasti onset timing, knee kinematics, and kinetics in asymptomatic individuals with a delayed onset of vastus medialis oblique. Journal of Orthopaedic Research. 2006;24(9):1854-60.

74. Lan TY, Lin WP, Jiang CC, Chiang H. Immediate effect and predictors of effectiveness of taping for patellofemoral pain syndrome: a prospective cohort study. Am J Sports Med. 2010;38(8):1626-30.

75. Whittingham M, Palmer S, Macmillan F. Effects of taping on pain and function in patellofemoral pain syndrome: a randomized controlled trial. J Ortho Sports Phys Ther. 2004;34(9):504-10.

76. Powers CM, Bolgla LA, Callaghan MJ, Collins N, Sheehan FT. Patellofemoral pain: proximal, distal, and local factors 2nd International Research Retreat. J Ortho Sports Phys Ther. 2012;42(6):A1-54.

77. Palmitier RA, An KN, Scott SG, Chao EY. Kinetic chain exercise in knee rehabilitation. Sports Med. 1991;11(6):402-13.

78. Witvrouw E, Lysens R, Bellemans J, Peers K, Vanderstraeten G. Open versus closed kinetic chain exercise for patellofemoral pain. A prospective randomized study. Am J Sports Med. 2000;28(5):687-94.

79. Steinkamp LA, Dillingham MF, Markel MD, Hill JA, Kaufman KR. Biomechanical considerations in patellofemoral joint rehabilitation. Am J Sports Med. 1993;21(3):438-44.

80. Reilly DT, Martens M. Experimental analysis of the quadriceps muscle force and PF joint reaction forces for various activities. Acta Orthop Scand. 1972;43(2):126-37.

81. Hungerford DS, Barry M. Biomechanics of the patellofemoral joint. Clin Orthop Relat Res. 1979;144:9-15.

82. Davies GJ. A Compendium of Isokinetics in Clinical Usage. Lacrosse, WI: S&S Publishers; 1984.

83. Ariki PK, Davies GJ, Siewert M, Powinski M. Optimum rest interval between isokinetic velocity spectrum rehabilitation sets. Physical Therapy. 1985;65(5):733-4.

84. Snyder-Mackler L, Delitto A, Bailey S, Stralka SW. Quadriceps femoris muscle strength and functional recovery after anterior cruciate ligament reconstruction: a prospective randomized clinical trial of electrical stimulation. J Bone Joint Surg. 1995;77-A:1166-73.

85. Koh TJ, Grabiner MD, DeSwart FR. In vivo tracking of the human patella. J Biomech. 1992;25:637-43.

86. Bohannon RW. Effect of electrical stimulation to the vastus medialis muscle in a patient with chronically dislocating patellae. A case report. Phys TherJ. 1983;63(9):1445-7.

87. Peters JSJ, Tyson NL. Proximal exercises are effective in treating patellofemoral pain syndrome: a systematic review. Int J Sports Phys Ther. 2013;8(5):689-700.

88. Distefano LJ, Blackburn JT, Marshall SW, Padua DA. Gluteal muscle activation during common therapeutic exercises. Journal of Orthopaedic & Sports Physical Therapy. 2009;39(7):532-40.

89. Mascal CL, Landel R, Powers C. Management of patellofemoral pain targeting hip, pelvis, and trunk muscle function: 2 case reports. J Ortho Sports Phys Ther. 2003;33(11):647-60.

90. Cohen ZA, Roglic H, Grelsamer RP, Henry JH, Levine WN, Mow VC, et al. Patellofemoral stresses during open and closed kinetic chain exercises: an analysis using computer simulation. Am J Sports Med. 2001;29(4):480-7.

91. Huberti HH, Hayes WC. Patellofemoral contact pressures: the influence of q-angle and tendofemoral contact. J Bone Joint Surg (Am). 1984;66-A:715-24.

92. Grelsamer RP, McConnell J. The Patella: A Team Approach. Gaithersburg, MD; Aspen Publishers; 1998.

93. Paoli A, Marcolin G, Petrone N. The effect of stance width on the electromyographical activity of eight superficial thigh muscles during back squat with different bar loads. Journal of Strength. 2009;23(1):246-50.

94. Neitzel JA, Kernozek TW, Davies GJ. Loading response following anterior cruciate ligament reconstruction during the parallel squat exercise. Clinical Biomechanics. 2002;17(7):551-4.

95. Fry AC, Smith JC, Schilling BK. Effect of knee position on hip and knee torques during the barbell squat. J Strength Cond Res. 2003;17(4):629-33.

96. Escamilla R. Knee biomechanics of the dynamic squat exercise. Med Sci Sports Exerc. 2001;33(1):127-41.

97. Chinkulprasert C, Vachalathiti R, Powers CM. Patellofemoral joint forces and stress during forward step-up, lateral step-up, and forward step-down exercises. Journal of Orthopaedic & Sports Physical Therapy. 2011;41(4):241-8.

98. Manske RC, Andersen J. Test-retest reliability of the lower extremity functional reach test. J Orthop Sports Phys Ther. 2004;34(1):A52-3.

99. Hertel J, Miller SJ, Denegar CR. Intratester and intertester reliability during Star Excursion Balance Tests. J Sports Rehabil. 2009;9:104-16.

100. Olmsted LC, Carcia CR, Hertel J, Shultz SJ. Efficacy of the Star Excursion Balance Tests in detecting reach deficits in subjects with chronic ankle instability. J Athl Train. 2002;37(4):501-6.

101. Bennet JG, Stauber WT. Evaluation and treatment of anterior knee pain using eccentric exercise. Med Sci Sports Exerc. 1986;18(5):526-30.

102. Albert, MA et. al. Eccentric Muscle Training in Sports and Orthopedics 2nd Edition. Churchill Livingstone; 1991.

103. Jensen K, DiFabio RD. Evaluation of eccentric exercise in treatment of patellar tendinitis. PhysTher J. 1989;69(3):211-6.

104. Nakata H, Nagami T, Higuchi T, Sakamoto K, Kanosue K. Relationship between performance variables and baseball ability in youth baseball players. Journal of Strength and Conditioning Research. 2013;27(10):2887-97.

105. Bandy WD, Rusche KR, Tekulve FY. Reliability and limb symmetry for five unilateral functional tests of the lower extremities. Isokin Ex Sci. 1994;4:108-11.

106. Bogla LA, Keskula DR. Reliability of lower extremity functional performance tests. J Orthop Sports Ther. 1997;26(3):138-42.

107. Booher LD, Hench KM, Worrell TW, Strikeleather J. Reliability of three single leg hop tests. J Sports Rehabil. 1993;2:165-70.

108. Greenberger HB, Paterno MV. The test-retest reliability of a one legged hop distance in healthy young adults. J Orthop Sports Ther. 1994;1:62.

109. Manske RC, Smith B, Wyatt F. Test-retest reliability of the lower extremity functional tests after a closed kinetic chain isokinetic bout. J Sports Rehabil. 2003;12:119-32.

110. Tabor MA, Davies GJ, Kernozek TM. A multicenter study of the test-retest reliability of the lower extremity functional test. J Sports Rehabil. 2002;11:190-201.

111. Jensen R, Gøthesen O, Liseth K, Baerheim A. Acupuncture treatment of patellofemoral pain syndrome. J Altern Complement Med. 1999;5(6):521-7.

112. Cao L, Zhang XL, Gao YS, Jiang Y. Needle acupuncture for osteoarthritis of the knee. A systematic review and updated meta-analysis. Saudi Med J. 2012;33(5):526-32.

113. Collins N, Crossley K, Beller E, Darnell R, McPoil T, Vicenzino B. Foot orthoses and physiotherapy in the treatment of patellofemoral pain syndrome: randomised clinical trial. British Journal of Sports Medicine. 2009;43(3):163-8.

114. Ayhan E, Kesmezacar H, Akgun I. Intraarticular injections (corticosteroid, hyaluronic acid, platelet rich plasma) for the knee osteoarthritis. World Journal of Orthopedics. 2014;5(3):351-61.

115. Bellamy N, Campbell J, Robinson V, Gee T, Bourne R, Wells G. Intraarticular corticosteroid for treatment of osteoarthritis of the knee. Cochrane Database Syst Rev. 2006;(2):CD005328.

116. Arroll B, Goodyear-Smith F. Corticosteroid injections for osteoarthritis of the knee: meta-analysis. BMJ. 2004;328(7444):869.

117. Van Jonbergen H-PW, Poolman RW, van Kampen A. Isolated patellofemoral osteoarthritis. Acta Orthop. 2010;81(2):199-205.

118. Ford DH, Post WR. Open or arthroscopic lateral release: indications, techniques, and rehabilitation. Clin Sports Med. 1997;16(1):29-49.

119. Gambardella RA. Technical pitfalls of patellofemoral surgery. Clin Sports Med. 1999;18(4):897-903.

120. Roush JR, Bay CR. Prevalence of anterior knee pain in 18-35 year old females. Int J Sports Phys Ther. 2012;7(4):396-401.

121. Boling M, Padua D, Marshall S, Guskiewicz K, Pyne S, Beutler A. Gender differences in the incidence and prevalence of patellofemoral pain syndrome: epidemiology of patellofemoral pain. Scandinavian Journal of Medicine & Science in Sports. 2010;20(5):725-30.

122. Hart DL, Werneke MW, George SZ, Matheson JW, Wang YC, Cook KF, et al. Screening for elevated levels of fear-avoidance beliefs regarding work or physical activities in people receiving outpatient therapy. Physical Therapy. 2009;89(8):770-85.

CHAPTER 12

Patellar Tendinopathy

Luis A Feigenbaum

ABSTRACT

Anterior knee pain, in the form of patellar tendinopathy, is a condition that is difficult to manage and a major cause of decreased participation in sports activities. Reported cases of patellar tendinopathy have increased in recent years and are likely to be multifactorial. The incidence of patellar tendinopathy among elite athletes is relatively high, with special consideration given to sports that require repetitive, ballistic activities such as basketball and volleyball.

The mechanism of injury for patellar tendinopathy remains controversial, although there is agreement that inappropriate or excessive loading of the musculotendinous junction of the extensor apparatus of the knee is likely the primary cause. Management of patellar tendinopathy requires proper anatomical identification, evaluation of the potential causes and risk factors that may be predisposing to the injury, proper differential diagnosis, a global assessment of potential treatment options and execution of an evidence-based rehabilitation program.

◾ INTRODUCTION

Anterior knee pain, in the form of patellar tendinopathy, is a condition that is difficult to manage and a major cause of decreased participation in sports activities.[1-8] Patellar tendinopathy was first observed in volleyball players due to the high volume of jumping.[1] The term "jumper's knee", is often used to describe patellar tendinopathy as a result of its high incidence in athletes whose sports involved repetitive, sudden, ballistic movements.[2,4] Other names have been associated with this condition in the literature: patellar tendinitis, patellar tendinosis, patella tendon disorder, insertional tendinitis of the patellar tendon, partial rupture of the patellar tendon and patellar apicitis.[6-7] Classification of the stages of patellar tendinopathy was first described by Blazina.[2] These stages are based on the patient's ability to perform sport-related activities with respect to pain levels (Table 1).[2]

TABLE 1: Blazina's stages of patellar tendinopathy

Stage	Symptoms
1	Pain occurs only after activity
2	Pain starts at the beginning of activity; dissipates after warm-up, and recurs with fatigue
3	Pain occurs at rest and with activity and affects performance
4	The patellar tendon completely ruptures

The theoretical causes of the pathology behind tendinopathies have evolved in recent years. While historically such conditions were regarded as inflammatory, current research suggests the lack of histological signs of an acute inflammatory process with tendinopathies.[1,2,6,7] More recently it has been proposed that tendinopathy is due to a failed healing response.[1,2,6,7] The mechanism of injury for patellar tendinopathy also remains controversial, although there is agreement that inappropriate or excessive loading of the musculotendinous junction of the extensor apparatus of the knee is likely the primary cause.[1-8]

Epidemiology

Reported cases of patellar tendinopathy have increased in recent years and are likely to be multifactorial.[7] Jumping athletes are undergoing more strenuous activities over prolonged periods of training and competition, causing excessive loading of the musculotendinous unit. Additionally improvements have been made in the clinical examination of this condition by health care professionals.[5,7,9-12] The prevalence of patellar tendinopathy among elite athletes across different sports is approximately 14%, with an additional 8% reporting a previous bout of symptoms.[11] Sports that require repetitive, ballistic activities, such as basketball and volleyball, tend to have the highest incidence of patellar tendinopathy.[5,7,9-12]

Anthropometric factors including gender, taller heights, heavier weights and larger waist-to-hip ratios have been associated with abnormal patella tendon imaging, which may be indicative of patellar tendinopathy.[9,10,13-18] The prevalence of unilateral and bilateral patellar tendinopathy among the sexes differs.[11,13] Unilateral patellar tendinopathy is twice as common in males, with bilateral patellar tendinopathy equally present in both sexes. Higher waist-to-hip ratios (indicative of larger distribution of abdominal fat relative to gluteofemoral fat deposits), a higher body mass index (BMI), lower arch height, and increased leg length are present in both unilateral and bilateral cases of patellar tendinopathy.[15]

Additional clinical features have been identified that also discriminate between patients with unilateral or bilateral patellar tendinopathy.[14,15] Increases in the volume of sports hours of participation per week and greater amounts of posterior thigh flexibility are risk factors for bilateral tendinopathy. Poorer posterior thigh flexibility and functional measures (hop for distance and six-meter hop test), and strength deficits (normalized peak knee extensor torque) are predominately seen in unilateral cases.[15]

Higher vertical jumps, drop jumps, countermovement jumps, rebound jumps and standing jumps, in both males and females, are also risk factors and should be noted during preseason screening.[13,17,18] Herein lies the paradox of patellar tendinopathy, in that higher levels of jumping performance correspond to a higher incidence of developing clinically significant symptoms.

Anatomy and Etiology

The patellar tendon is considered to be an extension of the common tendon of the quadriceps femoris muscle group. The portion of the tendon that begins at the inferior pole of the patella and inserts into the tibial tuberosity composes the patella tendon. The dimensions are approximately 3 cm wide in the coronal plane and 4–5 mm deep in the sagittal plane. Histologically, it appears as a white, glistening and stringy tendon body.[7]

Blood is supplied through the anastomotic ring, which is found in the thin layers of loose connective tissue layers, which cover the more dense fibrous expansion of the rectus femoris muscle. Contributions of blood supply come from the medical inferior genicular, lateral superior genicular, lateral inferior genicular and the anterior tibial recurrent artery. The blood supply to the patella tendon is considered to enter through the proximal and posterior aspect of the tendon, which happens to be the area most commonly affected with tendinopathy.

The causes of pain in patellar tendinopathy are largely unknown, but may include changes in innervations, neovascularity, apoptosis and excessive mechanical loading leading to tissue failure.[6,19-25] Histological findings in biopsied specimens from tendinopathic patellar tendons have demonstrated a scarcity of inflammatory cells.[20,21] However, there are several changes in the innervation patterns and in tendon vascularity that occur.[6,19,22,23] Chronic, painful, patellar tendinopathy exhibits an increased occurrence of non-vascular, sensory, substance P-positive nerve fibers and a decreased occurrence of vascular sympathetic nerve fibers and thyroxin hydroxylase (a marker for noradrenaline). The altered sensory-sympathetic innervation may suggest a role in the pathophysiology of patellar tendinopathy.[19]

Biopsied tendinopathic patellar tendons have been found to have a significantly higher number of apoptotic cells per unit area, and a significant higher apoptotic index, compared with controls.[21] Apoptosis, also referred to as "programmed cell death", is a specific response to both physiological and stressful stimuli characterized by distinctive morphological and biochemical changes, which may be compatible with the degenerative process of tendon and/or late-stage remodeling at the level of the tenocyte.

The presence of neovascularization through mast cells and an expansion of the extracellular matrix may be a potential source of pain in abnormal patellar tendons.[22-25] Under ultrasound imaging, patellar tendons with neovascularization have lower functional scores on the Victorian Institute of Sports Assessment

(VISA-P) questionnaire, and higher pain scores while performing a deep squat than abnormal tendons without neovascularization.[22] The process of mediating neovascularization has also been linked to increased mast cell numbers.[24] A higher prevalence of mast cells associated with vascular hyperplasia has been identified in chronic patellar tendinopathy.[24] An expansion of the extracellular matrix and microvessel density through distribution of the large aggregating proteoglycan, versican, is seen in patellar tendinopathy.[25]

The patella tendon undergoes sufficient tensile forces during sporting activity to cause stresses that are high enough to cause fiber failure. The stress-strain curve is used to describe the characteristics of loading physiology and the impact of the tensile forces acting on tendons. The crimped configuration of the collagen fibers and fibrils at rest disappears when the tendon is stretched by about 2%. With further stretch to about 5% elongation, tendon fibers become more parallel, and the tendon has a relatively linear response to stress. Sports-related activities, such as jumping, cause an elongation of 5% or more. Beyond 5% elongation, tendon micro-failures occur, through failure of the collagenous fiber cross-links. Macroscopic damage will occur with further strain, causing tensile failure of the fibers themselves. In the patella tendon, a force of 0.5 kN is experienced in level walking, 8 kN during landing from a jump, up to 9 kN during fast running and 14.5 kN during competitive weight lifting (about 17 times body weight).[6] Basketball players jump an average of 70 times per game and the vertical component of each ground reaction force in a jump is around 6–8 times body weight.[6]

CLINICAL PRESENTATION

Patellar tendinopathy is typically localized over the patella tendon, specifically at the inferior pole of the patella. In general, the cardinal signs of inflammation are not clinically present, as there is no acute inflammatory response. Pain will be exacerbated with sports, negotiating stairs (ascending and/or descending), and prolonged knee flexion. Pain will have an insidious onset, which will likely correlate to a period of increased ballistic activity volume, frequency, intensity and/or duration.[2] Symptoms are initially a dull ache in the anterior knee following a bout of strenuous activity.[2] Continued participation will further painful symptoms during activity. Eventually, pain levels will interfere with performance and will result in time loss from participation.[6]

CLINICAL EXAMINATION

Clinical examination and diagnostic ultrasound imaging are key in evaluating for patellar tendinopathy.[4,26-35] Evaluation should begin with a lower-quarter screen to rule out lumbar and hip pathology. Subjectively, a description of the mechanism of injury, significant medical history, age, history of a growth spurt, and location of pain are all important in guiding objective testing. Special testing of the ankle, hip and knee should be performed for the purposes of differential diagnosis. Anthropometric measurements, palpation, imaging, flexibility and strength testing, foot arch posture measurement and jump assessments should all be a part of the clinical examination. Finally, an overall assessment of extrinsic and intrinsic factors should be included.

Anthropometry

Anthropometric measurements including leg length differences, BMI and waist-to-hip ratio should all be measured at the time of the initial evaluation.[13-15] Leg length can be measured in supine and in several different ways (Figs 1 and 2). Measurement of the waist-to-hip ratio is done with measuring tape to record the circumference. The waist measurement is taken at the natural waist, usually just above the navel. The hips are measured at the widest part of the buttocks. To determine the ratio, the waist measurement is divided by the hip measurement. Waist-to-hip ratios of more than 0.8 for women, and more than 1.0 for men are considered to be at increased health risk due to their fat distribution.[15]

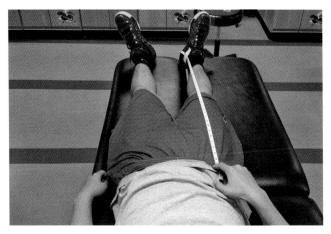

FIG. 1: Leg length measurement: anterior superior iliac spine to the tip of the medial malleolus (medial measure)

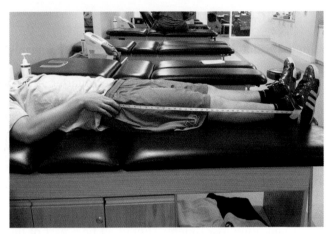

FIG. 2: Leg length measurement: lateral prominence of the greater trochanter to the lateral malleolus (lateral measure)[15]

Palpation

Tenderness on palpation is referred to as the "hallmark" sign of patellar tendinopathy, and is an important component in its clinical diagnosis.[28] The patellar tendon is easily palpated as it lies immediately beneath the skin and has no substantial peritendon. It can be exposed by tilting the inferior pole of the patella anteriorly.[29] It is only when the inferior pole of the patella is exposed, that palpation of the central, medial, and lateral aspects of the patella tendon is possible.[29] Tenderness over the patellar tendon may be found in full knee extension or full knee flexion.[4] When the patellar tendon is tender with both knee extension and flexion, the condition is thought to originate in the posterior portion of the patellar tendon at the patellar insertion.[4] Tenderness over the patella tendon in full knee extension may arise from the infrapatellar fat pad (IFP).[4] However, flexing the knee to 90 degree, places the patella tendon under tension and as a result tenderness may decrease, and, in certain cases, may disappear. The decrease in tenderness is a result of the anterior tendon fibers acting as a barrier to the potentially tendinopathic posterior fibers to applied pressure.[29]

Sensitivity and specificity of tendon palpation in clinically painful patellar tendons is 68% and 9%, respectively.[29] It has been found that moderate and severe tenderness (positive predictive value 36% and 38%, respectively) are better predictors of patellar tendinopathy than none or mild tenderness (positive predicted value less than 20%).[29] Clinicians should not attach undue significance to mild tenderness at the patellar tendon attachment site. Specificity and sensitivity

of ultrasonography are also low in the evaluation of patients with mild symptoms of patellar tendinopathy.[35]

Radiological Findings

Imaging is used as a compliment to palpation in evaluating for patellar tendinopathy. Abnormal ultrasound and magnetic resonance imaging (MRI) correlate well with the presence of tendinopathy. Ultrasonography has been used as a preparticipation screening tool, to assess the severity of tendinopathy, to monitor the progress of tendon healing, to provide objective indications for surgery, and to assess tendon vascularity.[7,34] MRI has been used to detect length of the lower patellar pole, as higher lengths have been associated with patellar tendinopathy.[31] However, clinically asymptomatic tendons have imaging abnormalities that have been shown in athletes playing volleyball, basketball, soccer, and track and field.

Typically, abnormal ultrasound appearance is considered to represent abnormal tendon tissue, which may be symptomatic. An abnormal ultrasound would reveal swelling of the tendon and a loss of fasicular continuity. These findings correspond histologically to collagen degeneration with increased ground substance and vascularity. Ultrasound abnormalities have been found to have a relative risk of developing patellar tendinopathy that is 4.2 times greater than normal tendon baseline.[33] Ultrasonographic tendon abnormality is also 3 times as common as clinical symptoms.[32]

However, imaging appearance of an asymptomatic tendinopathy is indistinguishable from that of symptomatic tendinopathy. Degenerative tendon pathology could remain asymptomatic for a period of time.[30] In cases of spontaneous patellar tendon ruptures, 97% had histopathological evidence of degeneration; however, only 34% of these tendons were symptomatic before rupture.[30]

Flexibility Testing

Decreased flexibility of the quadriceps and hamstring muscles are significantly associated with the development of patellar tendinopathy.[36] Limited flexibility of the quadriceps may often be described by patients as having "stiffness" or "achiness". Assessing quadriceps flexibility can be done by using the Ely and Modified-Thomas Tests (Figs 3 and 4), posterior thigh and hamstring flexibility can be assessed using the Sit-and-Reach Test and the Active Knee Extension Test (Figs 5 and 6).

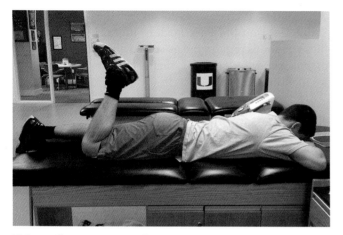

FIG. 3: Ely test: position for assessing quadriceps flexibility in prone

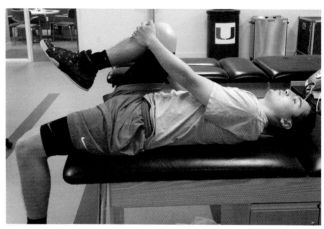

FIG. 4: Modified Thomas test: starting position for assessing hip flexor flexibility in supine

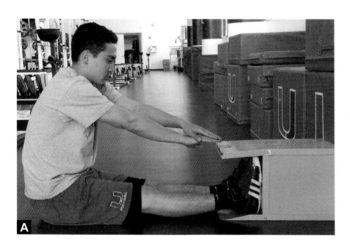

FIGS 5A AND B: Sit-and-Reach test. (A) Starting and (B) Ending position to assess posterior thigh flexibility in sitting

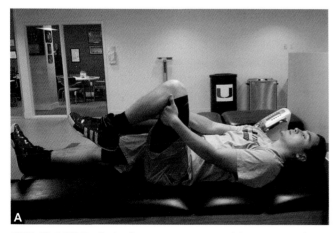

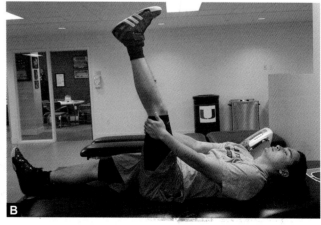

FIGS 6A AND B: Active knee extension test. (A) Starting and (B) Ending position to assess posterior thigh flexibility in supine

Strength Testing

Quadriceps strength can be measured either through manual muscle testing, or the use of an isometric dynamometer, and/or an isokinetic dynamometer (Fig. 7). Isometric dynamometer testing for peak torque should be set with the knee at 60 degree of flexion. Isokinetic strength of the quadriceps should be tested at 180 degree per second.[14]

Additional muscle groups of the lower extremity and trunk should be tested as well. These muscles include the lumbo-pelvic-hip complex, the posterior thigh and leg.

Foot Arch Posture

Several methods are available to classify and measure foot arch posture.[37-43] Measurements include the longitudinal arch angle (Fig. 8), foot mobility assessment through

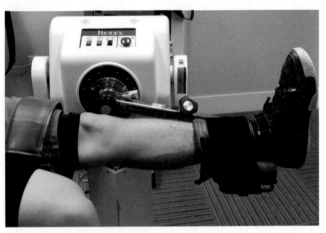

FIG. 7: Isokinetic dynamometer setup for testing peak torque of the quadriceps

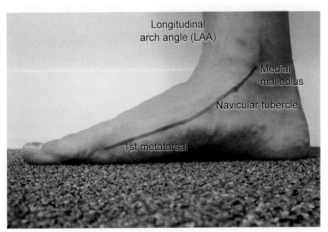

FIG. 8: Landmarks for measurement of the longitudinal arch angle

digital imaging, changes in dorsal arch height with the Sit-Stand Test and the Foot Posture Index.[37,42,43] Several of these methods require the use of a digital gauge, modified digital caliper, videotaping, digital imaging and platforms for measurement.[37,41-43]

Jump Assessment

Functionally, it is important to identify characteristics associated with jumping that may be contributors to patellar tendinopathy.[9,10,13,16-18] Functional leg strength can be measured using vertical and drop jumps.[13] When assessing jumping, landing technique should also be taken into consideration. If a landing technique that avoids loading through the lower extremity is observed, it may be associated with acute symptoms of patellar tendinopathy.[9,10,13,16-18]

Extrinsic and Intrinsic Factors

Extrinsic factors are commonly cited for their role in the pathogenesis of patellar tendinopathy.[44] The most frequently reported extrinsic factor is mechanical overload.[44] However, there are athletes who have been exposed to the same levels of mechanical overload who do not develop patellar tendinopathy. As a result, it is important to identify intrinsic factors which may play a role in the pathogenesis of the condition. The following intrinsic conditions may lead to the development of patellar tendinopathy: impingement of the inferior pole of the patella, altered patella anteroposterior tilt, a long inferior pole, malalignment of the lower quarter, patella alta, abnormal patellar laxity, muscular tightness and strength imbalances.[44]

Differential Diagnosis

Differential diagnosis is important in ruling out other pathologies of the anterior knee complex, including Osgood-Schlatter lesions, Sinding-Larsen-Johansson lesions, IFP pathology and tibial tuberosity avulsions.[5,27]

Osgood-Schlatter lesions are typically seen in 10–15 year-old males as a result of repetitive microtrauma, creating a traction apophysitis of the tibial tuberosity, with subsequent patellar tendinopathy.[5] Osgood-Schlatter lesions typically occur in sports that require jumping, squatting and kicking. Clinical presentation includes tenderness of the tibial tuberosity, swelling, pain, and at times a visible and palpable bump due to heterotopic bone formation at the tibial tuberosity. Radiographs and MRI can be used to diagnose Osgood-Schlatter lesions;

however, MRI is the test of choice due to its ability to detect soft tissue swelling.

Sinding-Larsen-Johansson lesions are related to repetitive microtrauma in prepubescent athletes between the ages of 10–13.[5] Repetitive traction forces due to sport cause a calcification in the proximal attachment of the patella tendon at the inferior pole. The mechanism of injury is associated with running, jumping and kicking sports. Patients will present with localized tenderness at the inferior pole of the patella. Diagnostically, plain radiographs, MRI and ultrasound imaging can all be used to view the calcification that forms as a result of the traction on the tendon.

Infrapatellar fat pad pathology is typically seen as a result of direct trauma to the anterior knee. Trauma to the IFP can be as a result of a direct blow to the knee or as a result of surgery that penetrates the joint capsule. The IFP, also known as Hoffa's fat pad, is located in the anterior knee, lying within the extrasynovial portion of the joint capsule. The IFP has numerous attachments that include: the proximal portion of the patellar tendon, inferior pole of the patella, transverse meniscal ligament, medial and lateral horns of the menisci, transverse meniscal ligament and the periostium of the tibia. The IFP is very richly innervated and highly vascularized, making it a potential source of pain if injured. The function of the IFP is not fully understood; however, studies have shown that it may play a role in the biomechanics of the knee as well as store reparative cells after injury.[45] Patients with IFP pathology will present with a burning or aching in the anterior knee, a potential loss of range of motion, and symptom reproduction through impingement maneuvers.[45]

Tibial tuberosity avulsions occur mostly in the 12–16 year old age group, as a result of a violent active extension or passive flexion against resistance at the knee. Patients will present with the cardinal signs of inflammation, tenderness over the tibial tuberosity and splinting of the knee in flexion. A plain radiograph will show the displacement of the tibial tuberosity. MRI can also be used and will show increased signal intensity over the avulsion site.

Outcome Tool

Symptoms of patellar tendinopathy should be measured as a means of grading its level of severity and to track patient progress through their course of rehabilitation. The VISA-P is a simple, practical questionnaire-based index of severity. The questionnaire assesses symptoms, simple tests of function and the ability to undertake physical activity. Six of the eight questions

are scored on a visual analog scale (VAS) from 0–10, with a 10 representing optimal health. The maximal VISA-P score for an asymptomatic, fully performing individual is 100 points and the theoretical minimum is 0 points (Appendix H).[26] An absolute change greater than 13 points on the VISA-P score based off baseline is considered to be the minimum threshold for a clinically important change.[26]

■ PHYSICAL THERAPY TREATMENT

Therapeutic exercise should be the primary intervention for the conservative management of patellar tendinopathy.[46-60] Drop squats, leg extensions and curls, eccentric exercises, heavy slow resistance exercises, concentric-eccentric single-leg squatting and static stretching may all provide a benefit in the management of patellar tendinopathy.[46-60] Varying opinions exist relative to the management of patellar tendinopathy with respect to exercising through pain, the use of a decline board for squatting, the depth of knee flexion during squatting, the frequency of exercising and the total training volume.[46-56] However, there is consensus that the depth of knee flexion for all exercises must be at least to 60 degree, which is the joint angle which places the maximal load on the patellar tendon.[46] Conservative treatment of patellar tendinopathy can be divided into three distinctive phases, which progressively increase the volume of work for the patient (Table 2).

Phase I: Protective Phase

As in most tendinopathies, controlled rest, immobilization/splinting and cryotherapy are important during the acutely painful stage. However, cessation from activity is controversial and not universally accepted.[57] Clinicians must be mindful that the patients maintain a degree of activity so that deconditioning is mitigated. An effective way to combat deconditioning is through cross-training, especially if the limb can be unweighted, as in a pool or a lower body positive pressure treadmill.[61,62] However, premature increases in intensity, frequency or volume of training at this phase should be avoided. For an uneventful recovery, abstaining from jumping and deep squatting prematurely is critical.

It is recommended that exercises in this phase are performed in pain-free ranges and with controlled loading of the knee. Static stretching of the quadriceps, hamstrings and calf for bouts of up to 2 minutes, produce gains in flexibility and can help to improve the attenuation of shock experienced during jumping and landing.[36,58]

TABLE 2: Phase progressions for conservative management of patellar tendinopathy

Intervention	Phase 1	Phase 2	Phase 3
Warm up	• Upper body ergometer • Lower body positive pressure treadmill	• Bicycle • Elliptical	Sports-specific
Tissue preparation	• Low intensity pulsed ultrasound • Extracorporeal shockwave therapy (ESWT)	Pro re Nata (PRN)	PRN
Tissue mobilization	• Patellar mobilizations • Fascial manipulation • Cross friction massage	PRN	PRN
Flexibility	Static stretching • Hamstrings • Quadriceps • Calf	Proprioceptive neuromuscular facilitation stretching • Hamstrings • Quadriceps • Calf	Self stretching • Hamstrings • Quadriceps • Calf
Strengthening	• Isotonic hip • Isotonics foot/ankle • Trunk stabilization	Protocol • Purdam[46] • Stanish/Curwin[48] Heavy slow resistance exercises[55] • Leg extensions • Hamstring curls	Maintenance program
Power/speed/agility	Rest	• Gravity-eliminated plyometrics	Plyometrics
Functional activity	• Movement screening • Extrinsic and intrinsic assessment	Sports-specific	Sports-specific
Endurance	Aquatic therapy	Sports-specific	Sports-specific
Cool down	Cryotherapy	Cryotherapy (PRN)	Cryotherapy (PRN)

Fascial manipulation to restore normal gliding between the intrafascial fibers and cross-friction mobilization are beneficial in properly orienting damaged collagen tissue during the early stages of healing.[59]

The use of infrapatellar straps, or counterforce bracing, is commonplace in the treatment of patellar tendinopathy (Fig. 9). Infrapatellar straps have been shown to increase the patella-patellar tendon angles and decrease patellar tendon length, allowing for less strain through the tendon.[52] Decreases in localized tendon strains is potentially a factor in lower perceived pain-levels through the use of the straps.

During the acute stage, modalities can be used to help modulate pain levels. Extracorporeal shockwave therapy (ESWT), low intensity pulsed ultrasound, pulsed ultrasound and dry needling have all been cited as treatments for patellar tendinopathy.[60,63-72] Of those,

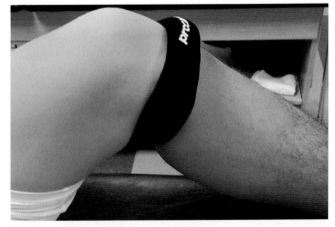

FIG. 9: Surround® Patella Strap DJO, LLC, which is indicated for use with patellar tendinopathy, chondromalacia patella, Osgood-Schlatter's lesions

ESWT has shown the most promising results.[63-71] ESWT uses pressure waves, either focused shockwaves or radial shockwaves. ESWT has been applied as an adjunct to conservative management, as a solitary intervention, and in combination with an eccentric exercise program.[63-71] Results are varied; however, no complications have been identified and most report improvements in VISA-P scoring.[63-71]

Phase 2: Intermediate Phase

The criteria to begin Phase 2 of rehabilitation should include reduced pain levels, full active range of motion, normalized gait, and tolerance to the exercises performed in the previous phase. This phase of rehabilitation should focus on normalizing flexibility and strength, correcting deficiencies in neuromuscular coordination, power, speed, strength and continued conditioning involving increasing loads on the knee. Progression principles should be applied when prescribing the rehabilitation during this phase. Loading can be progressed from modified weight bearing positions, such as exercising in a pool or in gravity-modified positions using a Shuttle®, Total Gym® and/or a leg press (Fig. 10), and finally to an upright stance. Additional considerations would include progression from level surfaces to a 25 degree decline board and increasing the amount of knee flexion during the eccentric portion of the drop squat (Fig. 11).[46-57]

Closed-chain strengthening is a proven and effective intervention in treating patellar tendinopathy.[46-57] The primary closed chain exercise used in the treatment of patellar tendinopathy is the drop squat, otherwise known as the single-leg squat. The drop squat can be performed on a flat surface or on a 25 degree decline board, with varying levels of acceptable pain, and with a combination of concentric and eccentric movements.[46-57] Several effective strength training protocols exist with respect to training prescription (Table 3). These training protocols should not be performed simultaneously during early implementation, rather clinicians should use their judgment as to which may be most appropriate for each patient.

Two hypotheses exist as to why exercising through pain may be of benefit. The first hypothesis states that eccentric loading of the patella tendon disrupts the non-vascular, sensory, substance P-positive nerve fibers. The second hypothesis is that eccentric tendon loading is associated with better tissue responses in terms of tissue repair mechanisms.[53] Patients can be instructed to exercise despite pain and to stop only if the pain becomes disabling using the VAS. When subjective pain levels decrease to less than 3/10, the patient can add additional load in a backpack in 5-kg increments. If pain increased to greater than 5/10, the participant is instructed to perform the exercise with less weight.[46]

Isotonic open-chain exercises, as in seated leg extensions and prone hamstring curls, can be an effective way of treating the pain associated with patellar tendinopathy (Figs 12 and 13).[56] Pain with open chain concentric contraction of the quadriceps may be present during exercising; however, if the pain levels are not debilitating, the patient should proceed as tolerated. Typically, concentric contractions of the hamstrings are pain free and can be easily performed. Prescription of an open chain program can be as intensive as 3 sets of 10 repetitions for 5 days per week.[56]

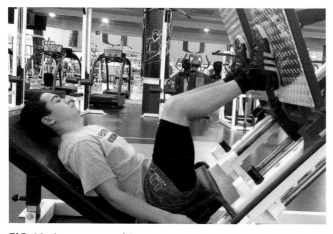

FIG. 10: Leg press machine

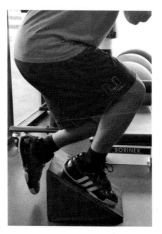

FIG. 11: Single limb drop squat on a decline board

TABLE 3: Strength training protocols for patellar tendinopathy

Purdam and Colleagues Eccentric Quadriceps Decline Board Program[46]

This protocol calls for sole use of an eccentric contraction of the affected limb to 90 degree of knee flexion with the trunk in an upright position. The eccentric training is performed twice daily, with 3 sets of 15 repetitions, for 12 weeks. Load is progressed by putting weights in a backpack once the exercises can be completed without pain. A return to the starting position is performed only using the non-injured side to avoid concentric quadriceps activity; in cases with bilateral patellar tendinopathy, the arms were used to return to the start position. Patients are not allowed to continue their competitive sporting activity for 8 weeks after treatment has begun. After 4 weeks, patients are allowed to cycle, jog on a flat surface, or to exercise in water if these activities could be done without pain.

Stanish and Curwin Program for Patellar Tendinopathy[48]

Start with a general, whole-body warm-up exercise not involving knee extension. Warm-up is followed by static stretching of the quadriceps and hamstrings for 3 times for 30 seconds. Squatting is then performed with a primary focus on the rapid deceleration phase between the downward and upward movements. Squats are progressed in the following manner: no added resistance on days 1 and 2 (slow) and increased speed on days 3–7. In week 2, resistance is added (10% of body weight). In weeks 3–6, 4.5–13.5 kg is added progressively. Instructions are to do 3 sets of 10 repetitions once daily. It is then reduced after 6 weeks, to 3 sets of 10 repetitions, 3 times a week. Every session ends with the same static stretching exercises as in the warm-up phase. The program concludes with ice on patellar tendon for 5 minutes.

Heavy Slow Resistance Protocol[55]

The Heavy Slow Resistance protocol consists of 3 weekly sessions of 3 bilateral, concentric and eccentric exercises (squats, leg press, and hack squats), for 12 weeks. The training volume consists of 4 sets of 6–15 repetitions, with a 2–3 minute rest between sets. The repetitions prescription is: 15 repetition maximum (RM) for week 1; 12 RM for weeks 2–3; 10 RM for weeks 4; 8 RM for weeks 6–8; and 6 RM for weeks 9–12. The exercises are performed from complete extension to 90 degree of knee flexion and back again. Each eccentric and concentric phase should take 3 seconds to complete. Pain during exercises is acceptable. However, pain and discomfort is not to increase following cessation of the treatment.

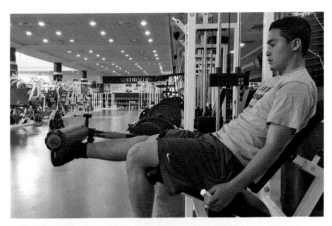

FIG. 12: Seated leg extensions

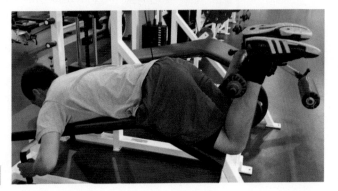

FIG. 13: Prone hamstring curls

Phase 3: Advanced Phase

The final phase of rehabilitation begins when the patient resumes sports-specific activities, all objective measures are normalized, and factors related to movement performance have been addressed. The primary goal of this phase is a concentration of higher-level skills and reconditioning for return to activities of daily living, work and recreational activities. While advanced strengthening exercises should continue, plyometrics should constitute the majority of therapeutic rehabilitation.

Careful progression with plyometric activity should be adhered to so that the chance of re-injury is lessened (Table 4).[73,74] Clinicians should avoid increasing the

TABLE 4: Plyometric training progressions[74]

Variable	Progression
Height	Jumps-in-place < Standing jumps < Multiple hops and jumps < Box < Depth
Landing	Two leg landings < One leg landings
Direction	Vertical < Lateral < Backward < Forward
Speed	Increased speed = Increased intensity
Distance	Increased height = Increased intensity
Resistance	Modified Bodyweight < Full < Added

TABLE 5: Vertical jump training progression[73]

Low level	Medium level	High level
Skipping	Tuck jump	Double-leg hops on-off 3 consecutive boxes
Ankling	Drop jump	Depth jumps to hurdles
Hip-twist ankle hop	Bounding	Medicine ball jumps
Side-side ankle hop	Double-leg hops	Box jumps series
Standing vertical w/o arms	Box jumps	Same-leg hops
Standing long jump	Lateral cone hops	Single-leg depth jump
Trampoline jumps		Depth jump to basketball dunk

TABLE 6: Guidelines for proper mechanics of the drop jump[74]

1. Drop jumps should have a maximum hip and knee flexion angle of ~130 degree and ~110 degree respectively when landing
2. Landing should be with legs partially flexed to produce the briefest contact time
3. Contact time should be brief to allow for a rapid switch between eccentrics to concentric
4. The heels should not contact the floor during the drop
5. The arms should be pulled behind the body during the drop to ensure their correct position and immediate availability to jump again after landing

volume and intensity of the plyometrics program simultaneously. A basic consideration in structuring such a program involves an analysis of the activity, specifically, the amount of knee flexion in sports.

Vertical jumping is a common movement across multiple sports. For those patients that have lost vertical jump height, this limitation should be properly addressed. A progression from low-level to high-level activity needs to be addressed during this phase (Table 5).[73] Because of the complexity and intensity of the depth jump, it is critical that standardized guidelines be implemented to obtain maximal results (Table 6).[74]

Alternative Treatment

Topical Therapy

Topical glyceryl trinitrate (GTN) has been found to have a healing effect with its use on the Achilles tendon, wrist extensors and supraspinatus tendon due to its ability to increase blood flow by widening the blood vessels over a transdermal patch. As a result of the increase in blood flow there is a decrease in pain and promotion of the healing process.[75] The active ingredient GTN, belongs to the drug group of nitrates. Nitrates are also used to help prevent attacks of angina (chest pain). Twelve weeks of treatment with continuous topical GTN (Minitran™ 6 GTN patch) in patients with chronic patellar tendinopathy has been recommended.[75] Application of the patch follows

a dosing regimen which calls for one-quarter of the transdermal patch be applied daily to the patellar tendon. Each application is to be left for 24 hours and then replaced with a new quarter patch. The patches are to be applied over the site of maximal tenderness and within a region of 1–2 cm around this point.[75] At this time, there is not enough evidence to support wide use of GTN for patellar tendinopathy.

Injection Therapy

Platelet-rich plasma (PRP)

These injections have become a common intervention for patellar tendinopathy due to its autologous nature and potential benefits.[76-82] PRP injections have a more pronounced physiologic effect on tendon healing if applied within the first 14 days of symptoms.[81] Multiple injections of PRP have also shown promising results.[82] However, there is minimal scientific support for widespread implementation of this treatment. PRP injections have been hypothesized to improve the mechanical properties of tendon and increase the time to failure, ultimate tensile stress and stiffness.[81] All studies describing the use of PRP to treat patellar tendinopathy have shown VISA-P score improvements.[76-82]

Aprotinin

It is a broad spectrum proteinase inhibitor, which affects the plasmin-activation pathway of metalloproteinases.

329

Increases in matrix metalloproteinases in tendinopathic tissue causes an excess in collagenases, potentially delaying recovery in patients. As a result, aprotinin injections have been incorporated in the treatment of patellar and Achilles tendinopathy.[83] Mid-Achilles tendinopathy proved to have a higher success rate (84%) than patellar tendinopathy (69%) after aprotinin injections.[83] However, because of the limited amount of studies, it is unclear whether aprotinin injections would be of benefit.

Sclerosing

The link between neovascularization and tendon pain in patients with chronic patellar tendinopathy has been established.[84-87] Injections of the sclerosing agent polidocanol, a chemical irritant that targets the neovessels, have been used for the treatment of patellar tendinopathy.[84-87] It has been hypothesized that by destroying the neovessels and their accompanying nerves chemically, tendon pain can be cured. The results tend to show an overall improvement in those who have received sclerosing injections on their symptoms in the short-term; however, many still had reduced function and substantial pain after 24 months of follow-up and as many as one-third of subjects resorted to arthroscopic surgery.[84-87]

High volume

A disruption of the neovascularization associated with patellar tendinopathy can also be achieved by injecting large volumes of fluid (high volume injections) into the area where the neovessels penetrate the tendon. This interface is found between the posterior aspect of the paratenon of the patellar tendon and Hoffa's body. However, only one study has investigated using high volume injections for patellar tendinopathy.[88] The injection used in this study contained a combination of bupivacaine, hydrocortisone and normosaline. Power Doppler ultrasound revealed an immediate disappearance of neovascularization after injection. The results of the injection were an associated improvement in the VAS for both pain and function.[88] However, several confounding variables, including using small amounts of local anesthetics and corticosteroids to relieve immediate pain and prevent an inflammatory reaction, were added and therefore cannot be overlooked for their potential therapeutic effects.

Hyaluronan

These injections are used as a viscosupplementation to treat conditions of knee. Hyaluronan injections have been used in competitive athletes with stage 2 or 3 patellar tendinopathy, and who have not responded to standard conservative treatment for a 2-month period. Hyaluronan is injected into the interface between the patellar tendon and the IFP at the proximal insertion or into the region of maximal tenderness. Fifty-four percent of the cases who received an Hyaluronan injection rated themselves as having excellent outcomes (resumption of previous athletic activities with little difficulty), while 40% of the cases were rated as having a good outcome (able to return to their previous sporting activities with some degree of limitation).[4]

Steroids

Local peritendinous injections with long-acting steroids have been used for the treatment of patellar tendinopathy.[89-91] Advances in ultrasonography in recent years have allowed physicians to administer local steroid injections more prescisely.[89-91] Steroid treatment can normalize the ultrasonographic pathological lesions in patellar tendons and have dramatic clinical effects in pain reduction. However, relapses in symptoms are fairly common, with one reported case of a complicated patient having ruptured bilateral patellar tendons due to steroid-induced changes in the tendon.[89,91] In studies monitoring outcome measures with steroid injections, all show improvements in the short term, yet appear to deteriorate in the 4–6 month range.[89-91]

Surgical Interventions

Surgical treatment of chronic patellar tendinopathy has been cited as a means of inducing modulation of the tendon cell-matrix environment and promoting either a renewal of the wound-repair cycle or in the removal of abnormal tissue.[30] Additionally, the majority of studies promote surgery only if conservative management has failed for a period of 6 months or more.[92-104] The results of both open and arthroscopic appear to have a positive result in symptom reduction, despite differing approaches with both the surgical technique and postoperative care.[92-104]

After either open or arthroscopic patellar tenotomy, most patients with stage 3 or 4 tendinopathy, report an improvement in symptomatic relief.[92-104] However, the ability to return to their previous level of sporting activity has been as low as 40%.[101] Long-term prognosis is highly dependent on symptoms within the first 12 months postoperatively.[101] Furthermore, patients undergoing patellar tenotomy can expect little improvement in symptoms beyond 12 months postoperatively and may thus need a repeat surgery if symptoms persist for 12 months.[101] Although there are no statistically significant differences in the long-term outcomes between an open or arthroscopic surgical procedure, the patients who underwent arthroscopy, typically returned to their pre-injury level of sports participation 4-months earlier than those who had the open procedure.[95-99,101,104]

Open Surgical Technique

A common open surgical technique involves longitudinal splitting of the patella tendon, excising of any abnormal tissue identified, and resection with drilling of the inferior patellar pole.[92] Open surgical technique has promising long-term results. At a minimum of 5 years, 82% of the competitive athletes returned to pre-injury sporting levels, with 63% of those patients being totally symptom-free after surgery. Shelbourne and colleagues[94] reported that return to intense sports participation was possible at a mean of 8.1 months following surgical removal of necrotic tissue, surgical stimulation of remaining tendon and aggressive rehabilitation. A systematic review of surgical management of chronic patellar tendinosis revealed improved results when no patella bony work was performed and no postoperative immobilization, as compared to the opposite conditions.[93]

Arthroscopic Surgical Technique

Several studies examining results after arthroscopic treatment of patellar tendinopathy have been published.[92-104] A majority of these studies have concluded with positive outcomes for the patients, despite having differing surgical protocols.[92-104] It is reported that 97% of patients obtain excellent or good functional outcomes with a mean follow-up of 4.4 years.[96]

Arthroscopic management of chronic patellar tendinopathy involves excision or resection of the distal pole of the patella with debridement of the surrounding areas.[97-104] Additional sites that have been targeted arthroscopically include the deep proximal patella tendon, debridement of adipose tissue of the Hoffa's body posterior to the patella tendon, and the peritenon.[97,99,104] Arthroscopy using a bipolar cautery system to release the paratenon and denervated bone at the inferior pole of the patella, including the tendon insertion site has also been identified.[95]

Arthroscopic surgery typically allows for a more aggressive rehabilitation program. Patients who undergo arthroscopic surgery should have the ability to return to sports by 3 months, and improvements can be maintained for as long as 10 years.[99]

CONCLUSION

The management of patellar tendinopathy requires proper anatomical identification, evaluation of the potential causes and risk factors that may be predisposing to the injury, proper differential diagnosis, a global assessment of potential treatment options, and execution of an evidence-based rehabilitation program. The incidence of patellar tendinopathy among elite athletes is relatively high, with special consideration given to sports that require repetitive, ballistic activities such as basketball and volleyball.[5,7,9-12]

Clinical presentation for patellar tendinopathy will be typical in most cases. Pain and tenderness to palpation will be localized over the patella tendon, specifically at the inferior pole of the patella. The cardinal signs of inflammation are typically not clinically present, due to the chronic degeneration of the tendon, which therefore lack an acute inflammatory response. Pain will be exacerbated with sports, negotiating stairs (ascending and/or descending), and prolonged knee flexion.

Clinical examination and diagnostic ultrasound imaging are key in evaluating for patellar tendinopathy.[4,26-35] Lower-quarter screening to rule out lumbar and hip pathology, subjective medical information, differential diagnosis and identification of the anthropometric factors including gender, taller heights, heavier weights and larger waist-to-hip ratios are all essential at arriving at the medical diagnosis of patellar tendinopathy.[9-10,13-18]

The preponderance of research points to conservative management as the primary focus for management of patellar tendinopathy. Most importantly, an evidence-based therapeutic exercise program should be considered as the primary intervention.[46-60] Drop squats, leg extensions and curls, eccentric exercises, heavy slow resistance exercises, concentric-eccentric single-leg squatting, and static stretching may all provide a benefit in the management of patellar tendinopathy.[46-60]

Patient education is also vital in treating patellar tendinopathy, as it is a degenerative and not an acute inflammatory condition. Adjunct therapies such as injections have demonstrated some promising results, while surgery is indicated if a prolonged trial of conservative management fails. Should the course of care warrant the need for surgical management, results are relatively encouraging, whether the procedure is open or arthroscopic. In which case, similar rehabilitation principles should be applied for the postoperative patient as described in the conservative management.

REFERENCES

1. Maurizio E. La tendinite rotulea del giocarte di pallavolo. Arch Soc Tposco Umbra Chir. 1963;24:443-7.
2. Blazina M, Kerlan RK, Jobe FW, Carter VS, Carlson GJ. Jumper's knee. Orthop Clin North Am. 1973;4(3):665-78.
3. Larsson ME, Käll I, Nilsson-Helander K. Treatment of patellar tendinopathy—a systematic review of randomized controlled trials. Knee Surg Sports Traumatol Arthrosc. 2012;20(8):1632-46.
4. Muneta T, Koga H, Ju YJ, Mochizuki T, Sekiya I. Hyaluronan injection for athletic patients with patellar tendinopathy. J Orthop Sci. 2012;17(4):425-31.
5. Maffuli N, Wong J, Almekinders LC. Types and epidemiology of tendinopathy. Clin Sports Med. 2003;22(4):675-92.
6. Khan KM, Cook JL, Bonar F, Harcourt P, Astrom M. Histopathology of common tendinopathies. Update and implications for clinical management. Sports Med. 1999;27(6):393-408.
7. Khan KM, Maffulli N, Cook JL, Taunton JE. Patellar tendinopathy: some aspects of basic science and clinical management. Br J Sports Med. 1998;32(4):346-56.
8. Hyman GS. Jumper's knee in volleyball athletes: advancements in diagnosis and treatment. Curr Sports Med Rep. 2008;7(5):296-302.
9. Bisseling RW, Hof AL, Bredeweg SW, Zwerver J, Mulder T. Are the take-off and landing phase dynamics of the volleyball spike jump related to patellar tendinopathy? Br J Sports Med. 2008;42(6):483-9.
10. Bisseling RW, Hof AL, Bredeweg SW, Zwerver J, Mulder T. Relationship between landing strategy and patellar tendinopathy in volleyball. Br J Sports Med. 2007;41(7):e8.
11. Lian OB, Engebretsen L, Bahr R. Prevalence of jumper's knee among elite athletes from different sports: a cross-sectional study. Am J Sports Med. 2005;33(4):561-7.
12. Ferretti A. Epidemiology of jumper's knee. Sports Med. 1986;3(4):289-95.
13. Cook JL, Kiss ZS, Khan KM, Purdam CR, Webster KE. Anthropometry, physical performance, and ultrasound patellar tendon abnormality in elite junior basketball players: a cross sectional study. Br J Sports Med. 2004;38(2):206-9.
14. Gaida JE, Cook JL, Bass SL, Austen S, Kiss ZS. Are unilateral and bilateral patellar tendinopathy distinguished by differences in anthropometry, body composition, or muscle strength in elite female basketball players. Br J Sports Med. 2004;38(5):581-5.
15. Crossley KM, Thancanamootoo K, Metcalf BR, Cook JL, Purdam CR, Warden SJ. Clinical features of patellar tendinopathy and their indications for rehabilitation. J Orthop Res. 2007;25(9):1164-75.
16. Richards DP, Ajemian SV, Wiley JP, Brunet JA, Zernicke RF. Relation between ankle joint dynamics and patellar tendinopathy in elite volleyball players. Clin J Sport Med. 2002;12(5):266-72.
17. Lian Ø, Refsnes PE, Engebretsen L, Bahr R. Performance characteristics of volleyball players with patellar tendinopathy. Am J Sports Med. 2003;31(3):408-13.
18. Lian O, Engebretsen L, Ovrebø RV, Bahr R. Characteristics of the leg extensors in male volleyball players with jumper's knee. Am J Sports Med. 1996;24(3):380-5.
19. Lian Ø, Dahl J, Ackermann PW, Frihagen F, Engebretsen L, Bahr R. Pronociceptive and antinoceptive neuromediators in patellar tendinopathy. Am J Sports Med. 2006;34(11):1801-8.
20. Khan KM, Bonar F, Desmond PM, Cook JL, Young DA, Visentini PJ, et al. Patellar tendinosis(jumper's knee): findings of histopathologic examination, US, and MR imaging. Victorian Institute of Sport Tendon Study Group. Radiology. 1996;200(3):821-7.
21. Lian Ø, Scott A, Engebretsen L, Bahr R, Duronio V, Khan K. Excessive apoptosis in patellar tendinopathy in athletes. Am J Sports Med. 2007;35(4):605-11.
22. Cook JL, Malliaras P, De Luca J, Ptasznik R, Morris ME, Goldie P. Neovascularization and pain in abnormal patellar tendons of active jumping athletes. Clin J Sport Med. 2004;14(5):296-9.
23. Cook JL, Malliaras P, De Luca J, Ptasznik R, Morris M. Vascularity and pain in the patellar tendon of adult jumping athletes: a 5 month longitudinal study. Br J Sports Med. 2005;39(7):458-61.
24. Scott A, Lian Ø, Bahr R, Hart DA, Duronio V, Khan KM. Increased mast cell numbers in human patellar tendinosis: correlation with symptom duration and vascular hyperplasia. Br J Sports Med. 2008;42(9):753-7.
25. Scott A, Lian Ø, Roberts CR, Cook JL, Handley CJ, Bahr R, et al. Increased versican content is associated with tendinosis pathology in the patellar tendon of athletes with jumper's knee. Scand J Med Sci Sports. 2008;18(4):427-35.
26. Hernandez-Sanchez S, Hidalgo MD, Gomez A. Responsiveness of the VISA-P scale for patellar tendinopathy in athletes. Br J Sports Med. 2012;48(6):453-7.
27. Rutland M, O'Connell D, Brismée JM, Sizer P, Apte G, O'Connell J. Evidence-supported rehabilitation of patellar tendinopathy. N Am J Sports Phys Ther. 2010;5(3):166-78.
28. Duri ZA, Aichroth PM, Wilkins R, Jones J. Patellar tendonitis and anterior knee pain. Am J Knee Surg. 1999;12(2):99-108.
29. Cook JL, Khan KM, Kiss ZS, Purdam CR, Griffiths L. Reproducibility and clinical utility of tendon palpation to detect patellar tendinopathy in young basketball players. Victorian Institute of Sport Tendon Group. Br J Sports Med. 2001;35(1):65-9.
30. Leadbetter WB, Mooar PA, Lane GJ, Lee SJ. The surgical treatment of tendinitis. Clinical rationale and biologic basis. Clin Sports Med. 1992;11(4):679-712.
31. Lorbach O, Diamantopoulos A, Kammerer KP, Paessler HH. The influence of the lower patellar pole in the pathogenesis of chronic patellar tendinopathy. Knee Surg Sports Traumatol Arthrosc. 2008;16(4):348-52.
32. Cook JL, Khan KM, Kiss ZS, Griffiths L. Patellar tendinopathy in junior basketball players: a controlled clinical and ultrasonographic study of 268 patellar tendon in players aged 14-18 years. Scand J Med Sci Sports. 2000;10(4):216-20.
33. Cook JL, Khan KM, Kiss ZS, Purdam CR, Griffiths L. Prospective imaging study of asymptomatic patellar tendinopathy in elite junior basketball players. J Ultrasound Med. 2000;19(7):473-9.
34. Cook JL, Ptasznik R, Kiss ZS, Malliaras P, Morris ME, De Luca J. High reproducibility of patellar tendon vascularity assessed by colour Doppler ultrasonography: a reliable measurement tool for quantifying tendon pathology. Br J Sports Med. 2005;39(10):700-3.
35. Lian O, Holen KJ, Engebretsen L, Bahr R. Relationship between symptoms of jumper's knee and the ultrasound characteristics of the patellar tendon among high level male volleyball players. Scand J Med Sci Sports. 1996;6(5):291-6.
36. Witvrouw E, Bellemans J, Lysens R, Danneels L,Cambier D. Intrinsic risk factors for the development of patellar tendinitis in an athletic population: a two-year prospective study. Am J Sports Med. 2001;29(2):190-5.
37. Cornwall MW, McPoil TG. Relationship between static foot posture and foot mobility. Journal Foot and Ankle Res. 2011;4:4.
38. Jonson SR, Gross MT. Intraexaminer reliability, interexaminer reliability, and mean values for nine lower extremity skeletal measures in Naval midshipmen. J Orthop Sports Phys Ther. 1997;25(4):253-63.
39. McPoil TG, Cornwall MW. Prediction of dynamic foot posture during running using the longitudinal arch angle. JAPMA. 2007;97(2):102-7.

40. McPoil TG, Cornwall MW, Medoff L, Vicenzino B, Forsberg K, Hilz D. Arch height change during sit-stand: an alternative for the navicular drop test. J Foot Ankle Res. 2008;1:3.

41. McPoil TG, Vicenzino B, Cornwall MW, Collins N, Warren M. Reliability and normative values for the foot mobility magnitude: a composite measure of vertical and medial-lateral mobility of the midfoot. J Foot Ankle Res. 2009;2:6.

42. Nilsson MK, Friis R, Michaelsen MS, Jakobsen PA, Nielsen RO. Classification of the height and flexibility of the medial longitudinal arch of the foot. J Foot Ankle Res. 2012;5:3.

43. Rathleff MS, Nielsen RG, Simonsen O, Olesen CG, Kersting UG. Perspectives for clinical measures of dynamic foot function-reference data and methodological considerations. Gait Posture. 2010;31(2):191-6.

44. Warden SJ, Metcalf BR, Kiss ZS, Purdam CR, Bennell KL, Crossley KM. Low-intensity pulsed ultrasound for chronic patellar tendinopathy: a randomized, double-blind, placebo-controlled study. Rheumatology. 2008;47(4):467-71.

45. Dragoo JL, Johnson C, McConnell J. Evaluation and treatment of disorders of the infrapatellar fat pad. Sports Med. 2012;42(1):51-67..

46. Purdam CR, Jonsson P, Alfredson H, Lorentzon R, Cook JL, Khan KM. A pilot study of the eccentric decline squat in the management of painful chronic patellar tendinopathy. Br J Sports Med. 2004;38(4):395-7.

47. Young MA, Cook JL, Purdam CR, Kiss ZS, Alfredson H. Eccentric decline squat protocol offers superior results at 12 months compared with traditional eccentric protocol for patellar tendinopathy in volleyball players. Br J Sports Med. 2005;39(2):102-5.

48. Visnes H, Bahr R. The evolution of eccentric training as treatment of patellar tendinopathy (jumper's knee): a critical review of exercise programmes. Br J Sports Med. 2007;41(4):217-23.

49. Bahr R, Fossan B, Løken S, Engebretsen L. Surgical treatment compared with eccentric training for patellar tendinopathy (Jumper's knee): a randomized, controlled trial. J Bone Joint Surg Am. 2006;88(8):1689-98.

50. Visnes H, Hoksrud A, Cook J, Bahr R. No effect of eccentric training on jumper's knee in volleyball players during the competitive season: a randomized clinical trial. Clin J Sport Med. 2005;15(4):227-34.

51. Frohm A, Saartok T, Halvorsen K, Renström P. Eccentric treatment for patellar tendinopathy: a prospective randomised short-term pilot study of two rehabilitation protocols. Br J Sports Med. 2007;41(7):e7.

52. Lavagnino M, Arnoczky SP, Dodds J, Elvin N. Infrapatellar straps decrease patellar tendon strain at the site of the Jumper's knee lesion: a computational analysis based on radiographic measures. Sports Health. 2011;3(3):296-302.

53. Jonsson P, Alfredson H. Superior results with eccentric compared to concentric quadriceps training in patients with Jumper's knee: a prospective randomised study. Br J Sports Med. 2005;39(11):847-50.

54. Peers KH, Lysens RJ. Patellar tendinopathy in athletes: current diagnostic and therapeutic recommendations. Sports Med. 2005;35(1):71-87.

55. Kongsgaard M, Qvortrup K, Larsen J, Aagaard P, Doessing S, Hansen P, et al. Fibril morphology and tendon mechanical properties in patellar tendinopathy: effects of heavy slow resistance training. Am J Sports Med. 2010;38(4):749-56.

56. Cannell LJ, Taunton JE, Clement DB, Smith C, Khan KM. A randomized clinical trial of the efficacy of drop squats or leg extension/leg curl exercises to treat clinically diagnosed Jumper's knee in athletes: pilot study. Br J Sports Med. 2001;35(1):60-4.

57. Saithna A, Gogna R, Baraza N, Modi C, Spencer S. Eccentric exercise protocols for patella tendinopathy: should we really be withdrawing athletes from sport? A systematic review. Open Orthop J. 2012;6:553-7.

58. Dimitros S, Manias P, Kalliopi S. Comparing the effects of eccentric training with eccentric training and static stretching exercises in the treatment of patellar tendinopathy. A controlled clinical trial. Clin Rehabil. 2012;26(5):423-30.

59. Pedrelli A, Stecco C, Day JA. Treating patellar tendinopathy with fascial manipulation. J Bodyw Mov Ther. 2009;13(1):73-80.

60. Stasinopoulos D, Stasinopoulos I. Comparison of effects of exercise programme, pulsed ultrasound and transverse friction in the treatment of chronic patellar tendinopathy. Clin Rehabil. 2004;18:347-52.

61. Grabowski AM. Metabolic and biomechanical effects of velocity and weight support using a lower-body positive pressure device during walking. Arch Phys Med Rehabil. 2010;91(6):951-7.

62. Raffalt PC, Hovgaard-Hansen L, Jensen BR. Running on a lower-body positive pressure treadmill: VO2max, respiratory response, and vertical ground reaction force. Res Q Exerc Sport. 2013;84(2):212-22.

63. Vetrano M, Castorina A, Vulpiani MC, Baldini R, Pavan A, Ferretti A. Platelet-rich plasma versus shock waves in the treatment of Jumper's knee in athletes. Am J Sports Med. 2013;41(4):795-803.

64. Rodriguez-Merchan EC. The treatment of patellar tendinopathy. J Orthop Traumatol. 2013;14(2):77-81.

65. van der Worp H, van den Akker-Scheek I, van Schie H, Zwerver J. ESWT for tendinopathy: technology and clinical implications. Knee Surg Sports Traumatol Arthrosc. 2013;21(6):1451-8.

66. van der Worp H, Zwerver J, van den Akker-Scheek I, Diercks RL. The TOPSHOCK study: effectiveness of radial shockwave therapy compared to focused shockwave therapy for treating patellar tendinopathy—design of a randomised controlled trial. BMC Musculoskelet Disord. 2011;12:229.

67. Zwerver J, Hartgens F, Verhagen E, van der Worp H, van den Akker-Scheek I, Diercks RL. No effect of extracorporeal shockwave therapy on patellar tendinopathy in jumping athletes during the competitive season: a randomized clinical trial. Am J Sports Med. 2011;39(6):1191-9.

68. Zwerver J, Dekker F, Pepping GJ. Patient guided Piezo-electric extracorporeal shockwave therapy as treatment for chronic severe patellar tendinopathy: a pilot study. J Back Musculoskelet Rehabil. 2010;23(3):111-5.

69. Zwerver J, Verhagen E, Hartgens F, van den Akker-Scheek I, Diercks RL. The TOPGAME-study: effectiveness of extracorporeal shockwave therapy in jumping athletes with patellar tendinopathy. BMC Musculoskelet Disord. 2010;11:28.

70. van Leeuwen MT, Zwerver J, van den Akker-Scheek I. Extracorporeal shockwave therapy for patellar tendinopathy: a review of the literature. Br J Sports Med. 2009;43(3):163-8.

71. Vulpiani MC, Vetrano M, Savoia V, Di Pangrazio E, Trischitta D, Ferretti A. Jumper's knee treatment with extracorporeal shock wave therapy: a long-term follow-up observational study. J Sports Med Phys Fitness. 2007;47(3):323-8.

72. James SL, Ali K, Pocock C, Robertson C, Walter J, Bell J, et al. Ultrasound guided dry needling and autologous blood injection for patellar tendinosis. Br J Sports Med. 2007;41(8):518-21.

73. Pate, TR. A conditioning program to increase vertical jump. J Strength Cond. 2000;22(2):7-11.

74. Chu DA. Jumping into Plyometrics, 2nd edition. Champaign, IL: Human Kinetics; 1998.

75. Steunebrink M, Zwerver J, Brandsema R, Groenenboom P, van den Akker-Scheek I, Weir A. Topical glyceryl trinitrate treatment of chronic patellar tendinopathy: a randomized, double-blind, placebo-controlled clinical trial. Br J Sports Med. 2013;47(1):34-9.

76. Bowman KF Jr, Muller B, Middleton K, Fink C, Harner CD, Fu FH. Progression of patellar tendinitis following treatment with platelet-rich plasma: case reports. Knee Surg Sports Traumatol Arthrosc. 2013;21(9):2035-9.

77. Gosens T, Den Oudsten BL, Fievez E, van't Spijker P, Fievez A. Pain and activity levels before and after platelet-rich plasma injection treatment

of patellar tendinopathy: a prospective cohort study and the influence of previous treatments. Int Orthop. 2012;36(9):1941-6.

78. Gaida JE, Cook J. Treatment options for patellar tendinopathy: critical review. Curr Sports Med Rep. 2011;10(5):255-70.

79. van Ark M, Zwerver J, van den Akker-Scheek I. Injections treatments for patellar tendinopathy. Br J Sports Med. 2011;45(13):1068-76.

80. Brown J, Sivan M. Ultrasound-guided platelet rich-plasma injection for chronic patellar tendinopathy: a case report. PMR. 2010;2(10):969-72.

81. Lyras DN, Kazakos K, Verettas D, Botaitis S, Agrogiannis G, Kokka A, et al. The effect of platelet-rich plasma gel in the early phase of patellar tendon healing. Arch Orthop Trauma Surg. 2009;129(11):1577-82.

82. Kon E, Filardo G, Delcogliano M, Presti ML, Russo A, Bondi A, et al. Platelet-rich plasma: new clinical application: a pilot study for treatment of Jumper's knee. Injury. 2009;40(6):598-603.

83. Orchard J, Massey A, Brown R, Cardon-Dunbar A, Hofmann J. Successful management of tendinopathy with injections of the MMP-inhibitor aprotinin. Clin Orthop Relat Res. 2008;466(7):1625-32.

84. Alfredson H, Ohberg L. Neovascularization in chronic painful patellar tendinosis—promising results after sclerosing neovessels outside the tendon challenge the need for surgery. Knee Surg Sports Traumatol Arthrosc. 2005;13(2):74-80.

85. Alfredson H. The chronic painful achilles and patellar tendon: research on basic biology and treatment. Scand J Med Sci Sports. 2005;15(4): 252-9.

86. Hoksrud A, Bahr R. Ultrasound-guided sclerosing treatment in patients with patellar tendinopathy (jumper's knee). 44-month follow-up. Am J Sports Med. 2011;39(11):2377-80.

87. Hoksrud A, Torgalsen T, Harstad H, Haugen S, Andersen TE, Risberg MA, et al. Ultrasound-guided sclerosis of neovessels in patellar tendiopathy: a prospective study of 101 patients. Am J Sports Med. 2012;40(3):542-7.

88. Crisp T, Khan F, Padhiar N, Morrissey D, King J, Jalan R, et al. High volume ultrasound guided injections at the interface between the patellar tendon and Hoffa's body are effective in chronic patellar tendinopathy: a pilot study. Disabil Rehabil. 2008;30(20-22):1625-34.

89. Clark SC, Jones MW, Choudhury RR, Smith E. Bilateral patellar tendon rupture secondary to repeated local steroid injections. J Accid Emerg Med. 1995;12(4):300-1.

90. Fredberg U, Bolvig L. Jumper's knee. Review of the literature. Scand J Med Sci Sports. 1999;9(2):66-73.

91. Fredberg U, Bolvig L, Pfeiffer-Jensen M, Clemmensen D, Jakobsen BW, Stengaard-Pedersen K, et al. Ultrasonography as a tool for diagnosis,

guidance of local steroid injection and, together with pressure algometry, monitoring of the treatment of athletes with chronic Jumper's knee and achilles tendinitis: a randomized, double-blind, placebo-controlled study. Scand J Rheumatol. 2004;33(2):94-101.

92. Ferretti A, Conteduca F, Camerucci E, Morelli F. Patellar tendinosis: a follow-up study of surgical treatment. J Bone Joint Surg Am. 2002; 84-A(12):2179-85.

93. Kaeding CC, Pedroza AD, Powers BC. Surgical treatment of chronic patellar tendinosis: a systematic review. Clin Orthop Relat Res. 2007;455:102-6.

94. Shelbourne KD, Henne TD, Gray T. Recalcitrant patellar tendinosis in elite athletes: surgical treatment in conjunction with aggressive postoperative rehabilitation. Am J Sports Med. 2006;34(7):1141-6.

95. Ogon P, Maier D, Jaeger A, Suedkamp NP. Arthroscopic patellar release for the treatment of chronic patellar tendinopathy. Arthroscopy. 2006;22(4):462.

96. Maier D, Bornebusch L, Salzmann GM, Südkamp NP, Ogon P. Mid- and long-term efficacy of the arthroscopic patellar release for treatment of patellar tendinopathy unresponsive to nonoperative management. Arthroscopy. 2013;29(8):1338-45.

97. Kelly JD 4th. Arthroscopic excision of distal pole of patella for refractory patellar tendinitis. Orthopedics. 2009;32(7):504.

98. Lorbach O, Diamantopoulos A, Paessler HH. Arthroscopic resection of the lower patellar pole in patients with chronic patellar tendinosis. Arthroscopy. 2008;24(2):167-73.

99. Pascarella A, Alam M, Pascarella F, Latte C, Di Salvatore MG, Maffulli N. Arthroscopic management of chronic patellar tendinopathy. Am J Sports Med. 2011;39(9):1975-83.

100. Cucurulo T, Louis ML, Thaunat M, Franceschi JP. Surgical treatment of patellar tendinopathy in athletes. A retrospective multicentric study. Orthop Traumatol Surg Res. 2009;95(8 Suppl 1):S78-84.

101. Coleman BD, Khan KM, Kiss ZS, Bartlett J, Young DA, Wark JD. Open and arthroscopic patellar tenotomy for chronic patellar tendinopathy. A retrospective outcome study. Victorian Institute of Sport Tendon Study Group. Am J Sports Med. 2000;28(2):183-90.

102. Griffiths GP, Selesnick FH. Operative treatment and arthroscopic findings in chronic patellar tendinitis. Arthroscopy. 1998;14(8):836-9.

103. Romeo AA, Larson RV. Arthroscopic treatment of infrapatellar tendonitis. Arthroscopy. 1999;15(3):341-5.

104. Santander J, Zarba E, Iraporda H, Puleo S. Can arthroscopically assisted treatment of chronic patellar tendinopathy reduce pain and restore function? Clin Orthop Relat Res. 2012;470(4):993-7.

CHAPTER 13

Achilles Tendinopathy

Lisa M Giannone

ABSTRACT

Although Achilles tendinopathy is a common condition among athletes and non-athletes alike, it particularly affects those engaged in running and jumping sports. Symptoms are usually mid-tendon and reflect a failed healing response, rather than chronic inflammation as previously thought. The etiology of Achilles tendinopathy is often due to an interaction of extrinsic and intrinsic factors, with research suggesting that training errors lead to the majority of tendon overuse injuries.

While Achilles tendinopathy can become chronic, conservative management with exercise is successful in the majority of cases. An exercise-based approach is overwhelmingly supported in the literature, so treatment should focus on strength building exercise for lower leg musculature. Of these elements, evidence is greatest for inclusion of eccentric exercise training for positive clinical outcomes in pain, function and return to activity.

At each step of the rehabilitation process, care should be taken not to rush through a phase until both the patient's symptoms and muscular readiness demonstrate a level appropriate to advancement. Too often, in the care of athletic or highly active individuals, there is the assumption that therapeutic exercise should immediately reproduce athletic movements without first ensuring that the patient has the requisite strength, ROM and muscle tone to start higher-level exercise.

◼ INTRODUCTION

Overuse injuries of the Achilles tendon are common among athletes, especially those who run and jump, because of the large and repetitive forces.[1] However, the sedentary are not immune, as cases are reported in those who do not exercise.[2] While incidence of Achilles tendinopathy increases with age, the typical age of those with Achilles disorders is between 30 and 50.[3-6] Despite the fact that the Achilles tendon is the largest tendon in the body, the repeated stresses placed on the tendon with locomotion and dynamic activity make it one of the more commonly injured sites of the body, affecting nearly 10% of runners, and resulting in 5% of the overall visits to sports medicine clinics.[7]

The condition is frequently divided into insertional and non-insertional/mid-portion types, with mid-portion Achilles tendinopathy, being the more common condition. For the purposes of this chapter, the rehabilitation principles presented apply to both types of the condition.

Pathophysiology

Traditionally, chronic injuries to the Achilles tendon have been referred to as tendonitis, assuming the condition

Acknowledgment: The author thanks Ian McMahan for his valuable contribution to this chapter.

is the result of an inflammatory process.[8] However, while trauma to the Achilles tendon can result in acute inflammation, histological analyses of chronic Achilles conditions do not demonstrate the classic hallmarks of tendon inflammation, but more typically show tendon substance degeneration and disorganization. Acute irritation of the Achilles tendon has been linked to inflammation of the paratenon.[9] Based on these findings, Achilles tendinopathy or tendinosis are now considered more accurate terms than tendonitis.

It has been proposed that Achilles tendon injury occurs along a continuum. Initial overload of the tendon results in reactive tendinopathy.[10] The subsequent non-inflammatory response thickens the tendon and increases stiffness in response to overload (Fig. 1). Further overload leads to tendon disrepair, highly disorganized tissue and, finally, degenerative tendinopathy (Fig. 2).[10] Degenerative tendon tissue shows little evidence of any biochemical markers of inflammation.[11,12] It is not known whether this tendon degeneration is the source of tendinopathy pain, as many asymptomatic tendons show the same degenerative changes. Those with symptomatic tendons do show an increase in sensory and sympathetic nerves in the highly innervated paratenon and fat pad.[13]

Over time, these chronic, degenerative changes associated with Achilles tendinopathy can lead to compromise in the integrity of the tendon and an increase in the risk of traumatic rupture of the tendon.[14] While Achilles tendinopathy is a common overuse injury, especially among runners and endurance athletes, treatment of these injuries can be clinically challenging. Of concern is the link between the frequently subclinical mechanical changes

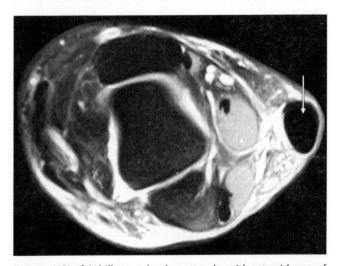

FIG. 1: MRI of Achilles tendon hypertrophy without evidence of tendinosis

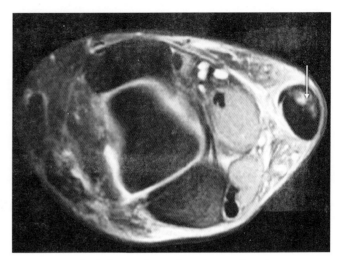

FIG. 2: MRI of Achilles tendon with evidence of tendinosis

in tendon stiffness and strength associated with chronic tendinopathy and, later, rupture of the tendon.[15]

Etiology and Epidemiology

Repetitive loading of the Achilles tendon during activity is thought to be the primary pathological stimulus.[16] Research on the cause of Achilles tendinopathy indicates that an interaction of factors is usually responsible for the development of chronic tendon disorders. With athletes, it is important to consider the influence of training factors such as volume, intensity and duration of exercise in the development of an overuse condition such as Achilles tendinopathy: training errors have been linked to 60–80% of runners with tendon overuse injuries.[17] Appreciation of these details is important in not only understanding the cause of Achilles tendinopathy, but also for the later return to functional activity and athletics.

Although abnormalities in the alignment and biomechanics of the lower quarter have been claimed as contributing factors in two-thirds of Achilles tendon disorders, the reason for this remains unclear.[18]

The intrinsic factors associated with Achilles tendinopathy are: age, gender, lower leg alignment and biomechanical abnormalities, leg length discrepancy and muscle weakness or imbalance.[1] Of the common malalignments of the ankle and foot, hyperpronation and a varus deformity of the foot are most associated with Achilles tendinopathy.[17,19-21] Increased hindfoot inversion and decreased ankle dorsiflexion are also associated with Achilles tendinopathy.[22,23]

Although the precipitating factors in the development of Achilles tendon disorders in an athletic population can be complex and multifactorial, the influence of muscle weakness and imbalance in the development of Achilles tendon disorders is a critical piece to consider.[23] Muscular strength, power and endurance are essential parts of athletic performance and are critical factors in the prevention of injury, notably tendon injury.[23] The impact-absorbing capacity of the whole muscle-tendon unit is reduced when the muscle is weak or fatigued, leaving the tendon unprotected from strain injury and subsequent inflammation and pain.[18]

CLINICAL PRESENTATION

Pain is the primary symptom that leads a patient to seek medical attention and is used to grade the significance of the condition.[24] Typically, pain is present 2–6 cm from the calcaneal insertion of the tendon, which coincides with a region of tendon hypovascularity.[25] As with other overuse tendon conditions, the initial phase of Achilles symptoms is characterized by pain after activity. As severity of the condition increases, pain becomes apparent throughout the provocative activity and with activities of daily living (ADL).

Other physical characteristics of Achilles tendinopathy include palpable tendon nodules, areas of swelling or crepitation, increased erythema and local heat. A thorough examination of the ankle and lower leg should include inspection and palpation of all these areas. Commonly, patients report tendon soreness and difficulty with the first several steps out of bed in the morning or after other periods of immobility.

In the majority of acute patients, tendon thickening and swelling are diffuse, and tenderness is most notable in the middle portion of the Achilles. Occasionally, palpation of the tendon will elicit crepitus.

With chronic sufferers of Achilles tendinopathy, exercise-induced pain is the primary complaint. Swelling and crepitus are often less apparent, and a more localized tender nodule is usually present.

CLINICAL EXAMINATION

The clinical examination is a critical factor in determining the presence of Achilles tendinopathy and its severity. Prior to objective assessment, a history is obtained.

History

A comprehensive history should include the following components:

- Onset, duration and intensity of symptoms.

Achilles tendon pain is usually characterized by discomfort after prolonged inactivity: for example, the first step out of bed in the morning or after prolonged sitting. Additionally, the chronology of symptoms can indicate severity, as early phase injuries are usually sore only after activity, while more advanced cases are symptomatic with all activity and ADLs.

- Changes in activity and training errors.
  Abrupt changes in frequency or duration of exercise can lead to maladaptive symptoms. Chronic overuse injuries are often the result of excessive volume, intensity or duration of exercise.
- Imaging studies (MRI, Ultrasound).
  If the diagnosis is unclear after a thorough history and physical examination, imaging studies can indicate the degree of Achilles tendon pathology.[9] Radiologic abnormalities have been found to correlate with histopathologic findings of tendinosis.[26] MRI and ultrasound studies can be effective in arriving at a diagnosis and grading the degree of tendinopathy when present.[27]
- Current and desired activity level.
  Activity level represents a variable that informs the clinician about the extent of therapeutic exercise and functional training needed to fully rehabilitate the injury.
- Activity history.
  Activities—including sports—that require significant amounts of repetitive load (such as running and jumping) are correlated with increased risk of Achilles injury.[28]
- Injury history.
  A previous history of Achilles or other distal lower extremity issues may provide clues as to biomechanical impairments or compensatory patterns.

Objective Examination

In addition to the subjective factors mentioned above, a number of physical factors need to be assessed.

Location of Tendon Pain (Insertional vs Non-insertional)

It is important to differentiate between the subtypes of Achilles conditions as the insertional variety of tendinopathy is generally more recalcitrant to treatment, and as such, the timeline for improvement may be longer. Additionally, research shows that insertional tendinopathies tend to be less responsive to eccentric exercise protocols.[29]

Appearance and Quality of Tendon (Swelling, Continuity of Tissue)

General swelling throughout the tendon is a frequent finding in acute Achilles tendinopathy. A palpable nodule or bump in middle of tendon is often found in more chronic cases.

Lower Leg Alignment (Pronation, Supination, External or Internal Rotation)

Runners with Achilles tendinopathy display greater pronation and calcaneal inversion.[23] However, while increased subtalar pronation has been associated with Achilles tendinopathy, a cause and effect relationship between pronation and Achilles tendinopathy has not been demonstrated.

Muscle Atrophy (Particularly Gastroc-soleus Complex)

A comparison of muscle girth to uninjured limb can imply a loss of calf strength and demonstrate reduced lower quarter muscle bulk.

Gait

Often a lack of toe push-off or active plantarflexion with gait is apparent with those suffering from Achilles tendinopathy.

Subtalar Range of Motion

Both increases and decreases in subtalar range of motion (ROM) have been linked to Achilles tendinopathy.[30]

Ankle Range of Motion

Abnormal increases or decreases in ankle dorsiflexion ROM are associated with the condition. Since normal ROM can vary greatly, assessment should consist of comparison to contralateral ankle dorsiflexion.

Lower Quarter Muscle Strength

Deficits in overall lower limb strength have been linked to a decrease in the ability to absorb impact, and a concurrent increase in the risk of overuse injury. Functional testing (e.g. single leg stance, squat, single leg squat, bilateral jump, single leg jump) for reproduction of symptoms or observable compensation can be used to assess this variable. As absolute normal values are difficult to quantify, assessment should be graded on performance of contralateral limb.

Plantar Flexion Strength and Endurance

Decreased plantar flexion strength has been linked to the development of Achilles pathology. Additionally, those with existing Achilles tendinopathy usually exhibit decreased levels of plantar flexion strength.[31] A bilateral or unilateral heel raise test can be used to assess plantarflexion strength and endurance. If able, a comparison of unilateral number of repetitions can be used to estimate relative strength. Ascertaining the location of muscle fatigue during calf testing or therapeutic exercise can help localize neuromuscular recruitment (NMR) of the calf complex. Often a patient with a chronic condition of the Achilles will demonstrate poor NMR and will report a feeling of fatigue in the peroneals or arch of the foot, rather than the calf.

Manual Strength Testing

The clinician must assess both neuromuscular control and recruitment of muscles responsible for the other ankle planes of movement. Testing for inversion (anterior tibialis, posterior tibialis), eversion (peroneals) and dorsiflexion (anterior tibialis, extensor hallucis, extensor digitorum) can help indicate overall muscular strength and stability of the ankle. Testing the foot intrinsic musculature, in particular, toe flexor strength[32] is also advocated.

Differential Diagnoses

Table 1 presents a number of conditions that can present in a manner similar to that of Achilles tendinopathy, as well as some of their distinguishing characteristics, which can aide the clinician in making the correct assessment.

■ PHYSICAL THERAPY TREATMENT

Rehabilitation Principles

Control of the mechanical and physiological stress to the tendon at each phase of rehabilitation, through manipulation of tendon load, should govern Achilles tendinopathy rehabilitation. In the case of tendon load, it is a tensile stress that has acutely or chronically resulted

TABLE 1: Differential diagnoses

Diagnosis	Differentiating clinical features
Retrocalcaneal bursitis	Findings of bursitis can be difficult to distinguish from insertional tendinopathy, as pain is near the insertion of the Achilles on the calcaneus, but bursitis can be differentiated, as pain is located anterior to the Achilles tendon and not on the tendon itself
Posterior tibialis tendon disorders	Posterior tibialis pain is generally localized medial to the Achilles tendon, closer to the medial malleolus. Discomfort can be reproduced with plantarflexion muscle testing, and tibialis posterior manual muscle testing. The location of pain is usually along the course of the tibialis posterior tendon and is more medial than typical Achilles tendon pain
Muscle strain of gastrocnemius-soleus complex	Discomfort is usually superior to the Achilles tendon and is located in the muscle belly of the soleus or gastrocnemius
Achilles rupture	On examination, a palpable gap is often found in the Achilles tendon. The Thompson test[33] can also be used to test integrity of the Achilles tendon
Posterior ankle impingement	Symptoms of posterior ankle impingement can refer to the posterior ankle joint, near the Achilles area, but can be differentiated from tendinopathy, as the tendon will not have any areas of tenderness or swelling. Additionally, plantar flexion will cause posterior discomfort, and, unlike Achilles tendinopathy, posterior ankle impingement is not symptomatic with ankle dorsiflexion
Sural nerve entrapment	Entrapment of the sural nerve can be characterized by numbness, pain or tingling along the nerve distribution and Achilles area (posterior calf and distally to the posterior lateral ankle and foot). The condition is usually the result of scar tissue, external compression by a boot or tight ankle wrap, or after a stretch injury such as an ankle sprain
Plantaris muscle injury	In a similar fashion to muscle strain of the gastrocnemius and soleus muscles, plantaris injury will result in pain and tenderness superior to the Achilles tendon. Plantaris muscle pain will be provoked by resisted plantarflexion with combined knee extension, and pain relieved when the same testing is done with the knee flexed

in tendon acute inflammation or degeneration. The factors influencing tendon load and those that need to be controlled during the rehabilitation process include ROM, tissue flexibility, joint mobility, neuromuscular function and muscular strength. Successful rehabilitation of Achilles tendinopathy will include manipulation of several or all of these factors during the process of full recovery. While the majority of eccentric exercise programs described in the literature use a 12-week protocol for treatment and evaluation of conservative outcomes the time frame for recovery can vary, and may often take up to year.[32]

Rehabilitating Achilles tendinopathy follows the same guidelines as other overuse conditions, meaning the rehabilitation progression is controlled through manipulating load—even limiting it with external devices such as a walking boot or the use of crutches, if necessary, ROM, muscle recruitment, type of muscle contraction and activity-specific rest. Precise manipulation of these variables allows the progression of therapeutic exercise and function until a complete return to activity is achieved.

An important consideration with athletic or highly active patients, which will likely be common given the injury's association with running and jumping, is the patient will not present with an obviously tight Achilles, nor weak gastrocnemius-soleus complex. Often the patient is exposed to too much, too sudden, or too long, a load in an otherwise normal appearing muscle, tendon and joint. Tendon overload and degeneration may occur due to a lack of readiness of the tissue to take this load or stress, resulting in the onset of the tendinopathy.

A good investigative, rehabilitation approach should be able to tell the story of how tendon overload occurred from a mechanical point of view. As the most relevant tools in the rehabilitation of tendinopathy are based in mechanics, the factor that must be managed is tendon load.

This load can be managed by controlling the various rehabilitation and exercise categories. Early in the treatment of acute or highly symptomatic patients, tensile load at the basic ADL level should be considered, in order to make a decision about how much unloading does the tendon require to control symptoms. Because the Achilles is subjected to load with activities as basic as standing and walking, a period of relative rest and load control may be necessary to address and diminish symptoms in those that continue to experience pain with simple ADLs.

This load control can come in the form of controlling tendon length (ankle ROM and subsequent tissue pull) by using a heel lift to shorten the Achilles in weight-bearing positions. Similarly, a walking boot can be used to reduce both tendon length and tendon contractile tension by eliminating the need for muscle action across the talocrural joint during gait. These devices can be used with both highly symptomatic and chronic patients.

Load can be conceptualized as an internal load specific to the structure and an external load that is applied to the structure from external conditions. Physiologically, internal load should be thought of as the load or tensile stress within the Achilles tendon. External load to the tendon is created through changes in actions that require muscle-tendon work, ankle position, type of movement and the forces that occur across the ankle joint (amount, volume, direction and angle of force).

Proper control and dosing of the external load is crucial to an effective and complete high-level recovery. When rehabilitating Achilles tendinopathy, load management and load application are controlled through the following categories.

Range of Motion

Range of motion includes the concepts of joint range, tissue length and joint mobilization. This is important as it relates to the concept of working the limb in non-lengthened ankle ranges. As Achilles tendon strain increases with larger angles of ankle dorsiflexion, initial treatment should aim to limit dorsiflexion during calf exercise. As symptoms subside, greater angles of dorsiflexion can be utilized with calf and general lower extremity concentric and eccentric exercise.

Neuromuscular Control

The targeted muscle's ability to contract normally and produce force without negative effect on the tendon is an essential component of neuromuscular control. This should be highlighted as the first criteria of any exercise (i.e. the patient should feel the exercise in the desired muscle and must be able to report sensation of fatigue and burn locally). An adept practitioner will closely look

at a patient's ability to actually activate and recruit each supportive muscle. Identifying whether this recruitment is limited by disuse versus limited by pain will determine pace and strategy for progression. Early in the recovery process, teaching the patient how to maximally recruit the gastrocnemius-soleus complex at a static length is critical to the success of a strengthening program and an eventual full return to activity.

Lower Quarter Exercise

More general exercises for the quadriceps, hamstrings and hip musculature are an important part of a comprehensive exercise program and can be used early in the treatment process where the calf and Achilles act as indirect stabilizers only. By targeting general NMR of the limb in functional exercise positions, the gastrocnemius-soleus complex can be indirectly utilized as a secondary mover, while direct Achilles tendons loads are kept low. Although non-specific to the calf and Achilles, general strengthening of the leg is also important in improving the overall shock absorptive capability of the limb. Exercise can progress to more direct calf strengthening as symptoms allow.

Muscle Force Production

Characteristics of muscle force production include not only the amount of force, but also the type of contraction (isometric, concentric and eccentric), and the role the muscle plays in the movement or joint action (primary or secondary contributor, stabilizer). The introduction of direct muscle work should be at a time and amount that is appropriate to the healing tendon. Early on, complicated, multi-joint, high force exercise must be avoided and less complex, low force isometrics substituted. Isometric contraction allows for focused isolation at variable loads at one controlled length of the muscle tendon complex. Isometric exercises do not introduce the more complicated step of coordinating a lengthening and shortening of a pathological muscle-tendon complex. This type of contraction can be considered as a higher stress load in the load-progression exercise continuum. In this way, early muscle work can be introduced safely. Once a patient has achieved good neuromuscular control of the calf, muscle strengthening exercise can progress from isometric to isotonic; then greater ranges of ankle dorsiflexion and plantarflexion; and eventually into more dynamic contractions.

General Mobility and Function

The level of outside force that is appropriate for tendon loading at any time during rehabilitation needs to be modulated with ADL and with the incremental reintroduction of more demanding activities. This is a supportive part of the overall rehabilitation and a step in the progression back to more vigorous levels of training for the more athletic patients. This area should be influenced by therapist in all phases of rehabilitation to guide patients in appropriate type, volume and frequency of standing, walking and cross training. Successful progression of this parameter will ultimately result in a return to the patient's prior level of function, including sports participation.

Treatment Progression

Treatment progression should be organized based on four distinct phases of rehabilitation: (1) early, (2) transition, (3) strength development and (4) dynamic (Table 2). In planning the rehabilitation process, each phase should have a specific purpose and should appropriately manipulate the components of load outlined in the rehabilitation principles. The criteria for progressing from one phase to the next will be dictated by improvement of symptoms and muscle function, and should not be based simply on time. This is largely because the factors that lead to Achilles tendinopathy, and likewise the timeline for recovery, can vary greatly from patient to patient. Additionally, the greater the amount of time an individual has suffered from the condition, the more likely that greater degrees of muscle dysfunction will be present (e.g. decreased gastroc-soleus NMR, calf muscle atrophy, loss of plantarflexion strength).

Early Phase

Goal: Symptom Control

Symptom control is achieved with relative rest from ADL, exercise and provocative activity. Strategies employed toward this end include anti-inflammatory measures, and controlling loads, if needed, through the use of crutches, a walking boot or heel lift.

Exercise Guidelines

Isometric, low-load gastrocnemius-soleus exercises for early neuromuscular control are emphasized locally. General, indirect lower quarter exercises and non-weight-bearing cardiovascular training can also safely be performed to maintain conditioning and enhance mechanics of the kinetic chain.

Key Components

Activity modification/relative rest

As an independent treatment, complete rest has not been shown to be an effective approach.[34] However, relative rest from athletic activity can be an important treatment strategy and may allow for control of a patient's symptoms. The timeline for relative rest is related to the severity of symptoms, the pain and the patient's level of activity.[35]

Modalities

Little support has been found for the utility of modalities such as heat, ice and ultrasound for the treatment of Achilles tendinopathy.[36,37] This may be due to the

TABLE 2: Rehabilitation phases and exercise progression

Phase	Load	ROM	Muscle	Type of contraction	Cardiovascular
Early	Non or partial weight bearing (WB)	Plantarflexion only	Indirect lower quarter early Progress to light direct	Isometric Progress to small range concentric and eccentric	Bike in boot Progress to bike in regular shoe
Transition	Partial or full WB	Dorsiflexion to neutral only	Direct	Concentric and eccentric. Partial WB calf, indirect full WB	Bike Progress to stair stepper or elliptical
Strength development	Full WB. Progress to functional loads	Full dorsiflexion with exercise	Direct, dynamic stabilizer	Concentric and eccentric Progress to dynamic eccentric and impact	Treadmill walk then jog Activity related functional drills
Dynamic, return to function	Full WB dynamic	Full dorsiflexion to plantarflexion	Eccentric absorptive	High velocity concentric and eccentric	Sport-specific conditioning

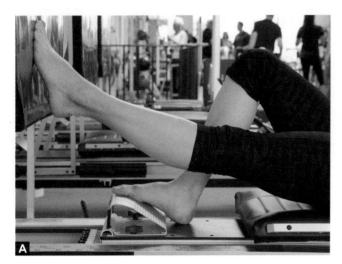 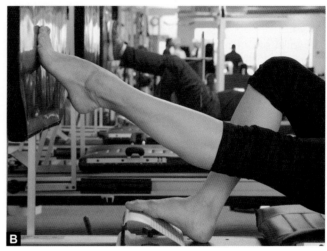

FIGS 3A AND B: Partial WB calf raise off of flat surface using sled. (A) Initial foot posture in neutral dorsiflexion. (B) End range foot posture in pain-free ankle plantarflexion

fact that chronic Achilles tendinopathy is the result of tissue degeneration and traditional modalities aimed at the reduction of inflammation are unlikely to yield a positive outcome. These modalities can be considered as an adjunct, but cannot alone be expected to yield much change or effect on the healing process. Promising outcomes have been found with the use of iontophoresis with dexamethasone in those with Achilles tendinopathy.[38]

Manual treatment

For some individuals, manual treatment, particularly manual joint mobilization, can be helpful in normalizing talocrural and subtalar ROM. As relative loss of ankle dorsiflexion has been cited as a risk factor for development of Achilles tendinopathy, manual ankle mobilization can be an important tool in regaining normal movement. Manual treatment can be performed in all phases of treatment but is likely most relevant in the early phase of recovery. Full ROM is important for progression to later phases of recovery, especially with increased strengthening and functional exercise demands.

Sample Exercises

Partial WB calf raise—from flat surface (Figs 3A and B)

Primary muscles: Gastrocnemius, soleus.
Muscle action: Isometric.
Equipment: Sled or leg press (Pilates™ Reformer, Shuttlet™, Total Gym™).
Purpose: Establishment of proper gastrocnemius-soleus muscle NMR with minimal tendon load.

Soleus press—from flat surface (Fig. 4)

Primary muscles: Soleus.
Muscle action: Isometric.
Equipment: Soleus machine or modified prone hamstring curl machine.
Purpose: Establishment of proper soleus muscle NMR with minimal tendon load.

Partial WB Leg Press (Fig. 5)

Primary muscles: Quadriceps.
Muscle action: Isometric (initial), concentric and eccentric (progression).

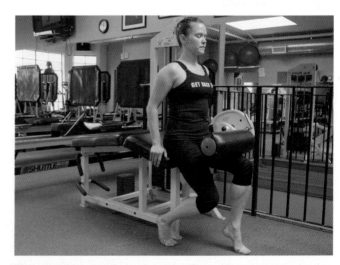

FIG. 4: Soleus strengthening from flat surface. Exercise can use soleus machine or adapted prone hamstring curl machine

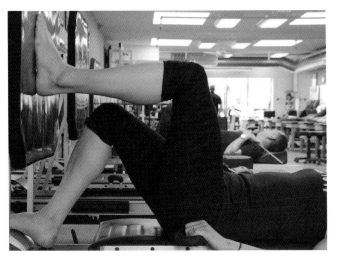

FIG. 5: Partial WB press on sled

Equipment: Sled or leg press (Pilates™ Reformer, Shuttle™, Total Gym™).
Purpose: Reconditioning of lower quarter, gross work of overall limb with ankle as secondary stabilizer.

Transition Phase

Goal: Curtail Protective Measures and Advance Neuromuscular Exercise

The patient is weaned from protective WB devices if used in the early phase, and a significant focus becomes neuromuscular control of the calf-increasing ability to recruit pain-free the gastrocnemius-soleus muscle group along with the secondary plantarflexors across the joint in a pain-free fashion.

Exercise Guidelines

Isometric exercises are progressed to controlled range concentric and eccentric exercises, with caution to avoid ranges that create a combination of greater tendon length and higher tension. Full WB work can be introduced but must create indirect action across Achilles itself (e.g. leg press or squat).

Key Components
Soft-tissue flexibility

While the supposition could be made that stretching induced tension within the Achilles tendon would result in a mechanically similar response as an eccentric loading of the Achilles tendon, it appears that physiological improvements are due to some other mechanism than loading tension, specifically force oscillations within the tendon during eccentric loading.[34] This may explain why stretching programs do not show the same clinical benefit as other treatment components, despite the fact of their common inclusion in treatment for Achilles tendon conditions.

Clinically, often an early aggressive dorsiflexion ROM and calf-stretching program can worsen symptoms and delay, or impede recovery. Stretching can be considered a negative stressor, potentially over-pulling a tissue that is already stressed as it is lengthened beyond its comfortable range. Often, patients may independently start a self-stretching program and may need to discontinue or modify this to allow for tendon healing. When symptoms subside, a gradual stretching program to normalize ROM can safely be implemented. This program should direct the patient to focus the stretch on the gastrocnemius-soleus muscle complex without a feeling of stretch or discomfort in the Achilles tendon itself.

Sample Exercises

Partial WB calf raise plus: "Big Toe-Little Toe"—allow for increased dorsiflexion ROM (Figs 6A to D)
Primary muscles: Gastrocnemius, soleus, posterior tibialis, peroneals.
Muscle action: Concentric and eccentric with combined inversion and eversion through increased range of plantarflexion and dorsiflexion.
Equipment: Sled or leg press (Pilates™ Reformer, Shuttle™, Total Gym™).
Purpose: Calf strengthening with involvement of ankle stabilizers and secondary plantarflexors. Patient is to emphasize pronation through the 1st ray and supination through the 5th.

Soleus—from raised surface (Figs 7A to D)
Primary muscles: Soleus.
Muscle action: Concentric and eccentric with combined inversion and eversion through increased range of plantarflexion and dorsiflexion.
Equipment: Soleus machine, modified prone hamstring curl machine.
Purpose: Establishment of proper soleus muscle NMR with minimal tendon load.

Standing posterior tibialis (Figs 8A and B)
Primary muscles: Tibialis anterior, posterior tibialis.

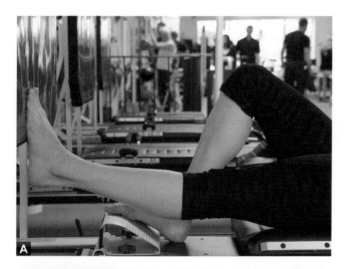
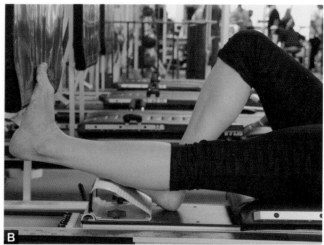
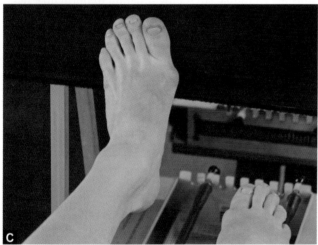
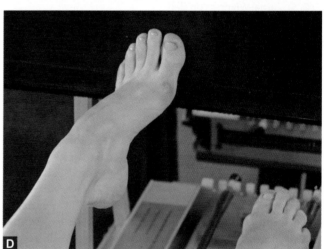

FIGS 6A TO D: Partial weight-bearing calf raise with "Big Toe-Little Toe" series. (A) Neutral ankle position. (B) Dorsiflexed ankle position. (C) Pronation through 1st ray. (D) Supination through 5th ray

Muscle action: Concentric and eccentric inversion, arch-forming

Equipment: Thera-Band™.

Resistance level: Variable by Thera-Band resistance/tension.

Purpose: Dynamic arch support, posterior tibialis strengthening.

Squat (Figs 9A and B)

Primary muscles: Quadriceps, hamstrings, gluteals.

Muscle action: Isometric (initial), concentric and eccentric (progression).

Equipment: None.

Resistance level: Body weight.

Purpose: Reconditioning of lower quarter, gross work of overall limb with ankle as secondary stabilizer.

Strength Development Phase

Goal: Optimizing calf and lower extremity strength

To progress to this phase, the patient must have achieved good neuromuscular function and have proven to be pain-free with all current exercise and ADL loads. Maximizing calf and lower quarter strength is target of phase.

Exercise guidelines

Direct calf exercise can progress from isometric partial WB to full WB concentric and eccentric loads. Exercise can progress into heavier work through full ranges of dorsiflexion (e.g. bilateral calf raise to single calf raise, from flat to ledge or slope). A cardiovascular exercise progression that aligns with patient's current strength, neuromuscular coordination, WB status and goals is an

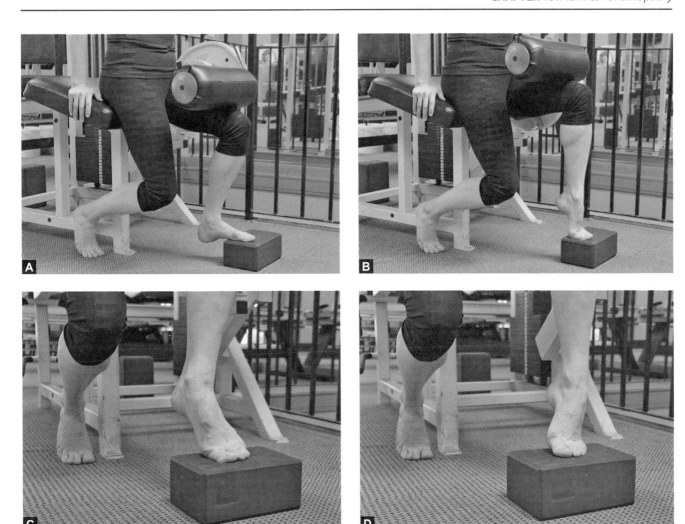

FIGS 7A TO D: Soleus calf raise with "Big Toe-Little Toe" series. (A) Ankle dorsiflexed beyond neutral. (B) Plantarflexed ankle position. (C) Pronation through 1st ray. (D) Supination through 5th ray

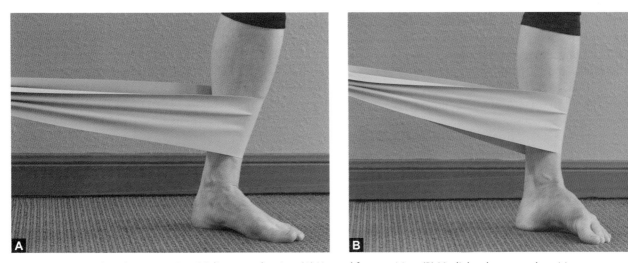

FIGS 8A AND B: Standing posterior tibialis strengthening. (A) Neutral foot position. (B) Medial arch engaged position

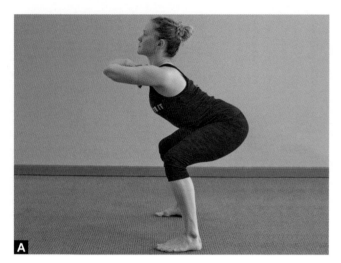

FIGS 9A AND B: Body weight squat. (A) Sagittal view. (B) Frontal view

integral part of general exercise progression. The WB load involved with each cardiovascular training step should be considered.

Key Components

Muscle strengthening

During activity, optimal muscular strength and flexibility can protect soft-tissue by acting as a shock absorber against impact forces. Muscle weakness, namely of the gastrocnemius-soleus complex, can contribute to the development of Achilles tendinopathy, as deficits in strength and muscular endurance can impair the muscular system's ability to protect itself and lead to overuse and acute injury.

Research indicates that the inclusion of eccentric gastroc-soleus exercise is a key part of successful tendinopathy rehabilitation. The majority of research protocols use the Alfredson protocol, in which patients perform 3 x 15 repetitions, twice daily.[37-39] These exercises are performed 7 days a week for a period of 12 weeks.[39] All studies that used this protocol found significant improvement.[40-42] While strengthening exercise, particularly eccentric exercise, may elicit discomfort or soreness in the Achilles during or after exercise, it is up to the clinician to determine if such symptoms will result in worsening of the condition or will ultimately be part of a productive strengthening program. Certainly discomfort that persists or significantly worsens after exercise may be considered counterproductive. Additionally, painful exercise may reduce compliance and may lead to decreased levels of muscle strength after a conservative treatment exercise program. Therefore, designing a program that minimizes pain may improve outcomes and likelihood of a successful result.[43]

While direct comparison of eccentric and concentric exercise programs suggests that eccentric exercises are more likely to produce a positive outcome in symptom reduction than concentric exercises, the improvements in symptoms and function are more evident than group differences in muscle performance.[44] The typical eccentric exercise protocol (3 × 15 repetitions, twice daily) cannot be considered an optimal strengthening program in isolation. After all, the mechanism by which eccentric exercise leads to positive improvement appears to be through changes in the mechanical loading profile, rather than just tendon loading or calf strengthening.[45] Eccentric strengthening can be considered one component of a comprehensive exercise program, one that is bolstered by the inclusion of concentric strengthening. This suggests that an eccentric only program may not be optimal for muscle strengthening, and that resistance training, and a sport-specific functional rehabilitation program should be included in a comprehensive program.[46]

In trained and elite athletes, muscle function may be graded as sufficient for basic demands, but inadequate for the specific high-level demands of muscle strength and endurance for the individual's sport. When dealing with this population, muscle function should be assessed on a scale that accounts for this sport-specific requirement.

Sample Exercises

Standing calf raise with "Big Toe-Little Toe" (Figs 10A to D)

Primary muscles: Gastrocnemius, soleus, posterior tibialis, peroneals.

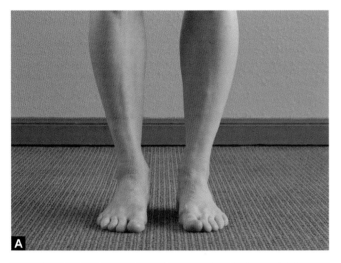
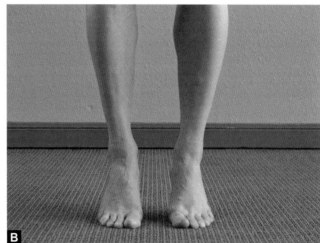
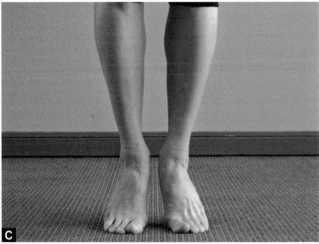
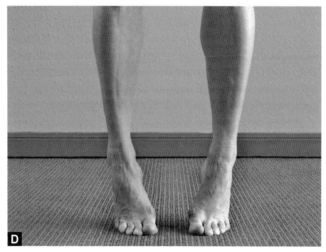

FIGS 10A TO D: Standing calf raise, with "Big Toe-Little Toe" series. (A) Neutral starting ankle position. (B) Plantarflexed ankle position. (C) Pronation through 1ˢᵗ ray. (D) Supination through 5ᵗʰ ray

Muscle action: Concentric and eccentric with combined inversion and eversion through increased range of plantarflexion and dorsiflexion.
Equipment: None.
Resistance level: Body weight.
Purpose: Full body weight calf strengthening with involvement of ankle stabilizers and secondary plantarflexors. Patient is to emphasize pronation through the 1ˢᵗ ray and supination through the 5ᵗʰ.

Turned out squat on toes (Figs 11A and B)

Primary muscles: Quadriceps, soleus.
Muscle action: Concentric and eccentric at knee and ankle.
Equipment: None.
Resistance level: Body weight.
Purpose: Reconditioning of lower quarter, gross work of overall limb with ankle as secondary stabilizer.

Standing Closed Chain Calf (Figs 12A to D)

Primary muscles: Gastrocnemius, soleus, quadriceps.
Muscle action: Concentric and eccentric at knee and ankle.
Equipment: Theraband™, multi-hip machine.
Resistance level: Theraband™.
Purpose: Functional calf strengthening through broad ankle and knee ROM.

Return to Function Phase

Goal: prepare for return to full function via increasingly dynamic activity

Exercises are devised and advanced to become increasingly dynamic, to prepare the patient for the demands of ensuing activity level. All activities are managed and controlled systematically to resume

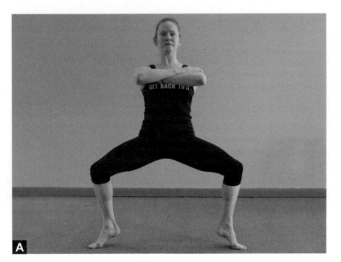
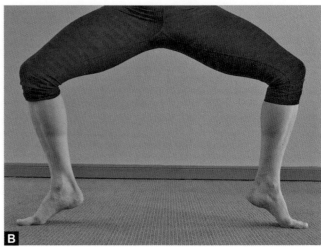

FIGS 11A AND B: Turned out body weight squat with ankle plantarflexion. (A) Frontal view. (B) Close-up of ankle position

full specific activity in this phase. The patient is discouraged from experimenting with attempting advanced progression without exercise, preparation and demonstrable adequate muscle-tendon function.

Exercise guidelines

The Achilles tendon is prepared for the full functional loads specific to the patient's activity goals by advancing absorption, lateral motion, acceleration and deceleration demands. Exercise and progression will be unique for each activity (e.g. exercises in preparation for a hiker will differ from those of a tennis player). As a leading cause of overuse injuries is abrupt changes in training variables (volume, intensity and frequency), a careful progression to full activity, and consideration of the magnitude of applied loads, is critical. A gradual rebuilding of daily tolerance is important when selecting the duration or dose of movement and endurance training, as well as recovery.

Key Components

Functional, sport-specific exercise

Therapeutic exercise that reproduces athletic movements should not be introduced without first ensuring that the patient has the requisite strength, ROM and muscle tone. If those criteria have been met, these exercises (including cardiovascular training) should be introduced in a progressive fashion, in which impact load and dynamic stress are added according to previously mentioned exercise principles, i.e. bilateral impact before single leg impact, full WB cardiovascular training (Stairmaster™, elliptical) before running. For those returning to sports,

once patients have shown a tolerance for the isolated components of their sports (lateral movement, impact, jumping, running) a safe progression should begin with on the field or court drills before scrimmaging or full play. Rushing through this critical point in the rehabilitation process can lead to later problems in the return to activity, especially with the increased risk of Achilles tears in those with Achilles tendinopathy.[15] For runners returning from Achilles tendinopathy, a running progression can be found in Appendix G.

Sample Exercises

Lateral step or jump (Figs 13A to C)

Primary muscles: Quadriceps, lateral hip, gastroc-soleus, peroneals.
Muscle action: Dynamic.
Equipment: N/A.
Resistance level: N/A.
Purpose: To retrain dynamic absorption of the lower quarter in order to prepare for activities and sports which require lateral movement.

Pseudo-Hop (Figs 14A to C)

Primary muscles: Gastrocnemius, soleus, quadriceps, gluteus complex.
Muscle action: Dynamic.
Equipment: N/A.
Resistance level: N/A.
Purpose: Sagittal plane impact absorption at knee and ankle in preparation for higher-level absorption such as running and jumping.

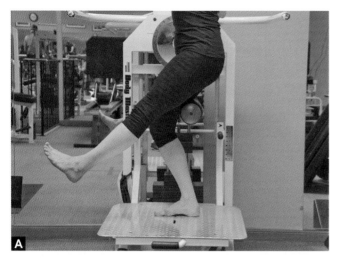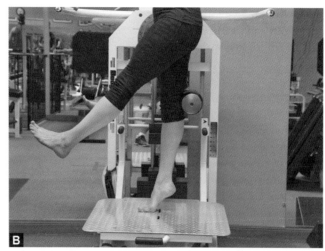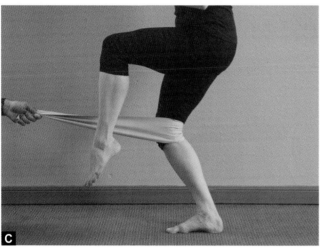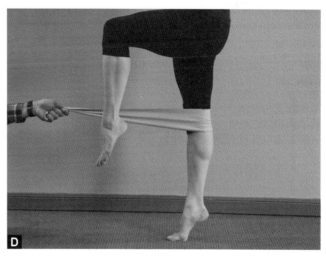

FIGS 12A TO D: Standing closed chain calf exercise. (A) Starting ankle and knee position using multi-hip machine. (B) Top plantar flexed ankle position using multi-hip machine. (C) Starting ankle and knee position using Thera-Band.™ (D) Top plantar-flexed position using Thera-Band™

Alternative Therapies

Research on the effectiveness of exercise based treatment for Achilles tendinopathy reports success from 60% to 90%, although with varying follow-up times.[4,29,47] Studies also suggest that if the patient has not recovered by 12 weeks, then other treatment options should be proposed, such as injections or surgery.[48]

Extracorporeal Shockwave Therapy (ESWT)

While the mechanism is not understood, the use of high-energy acoustic waves has been used for the treatment of sports related tendinopathies for over 10 years.[49] The evidence suggests that ESWT can be an effective alternative when conservative measures fail in the treatment of chronic Achilles tendinopathy. The long-term effects of ESWT are speculated to include an increase in blood flow and reduction of symptoms.[50] Research suggests its usefulness for treatment of patients with chronic insertional[51] and mid-substance Achilles tendinopathy.[52]

Instrument-assisted Soft Tissue Mobilization

A variety of instruments and techniques are used in clinical settings to influence soft tissue metabolism, structure and symptoms, but there is no consensus in the literature as to the efficacy of these techniques. ASTYM™ is one such technique. ASTYM™ is a form of specialized soft-tissue

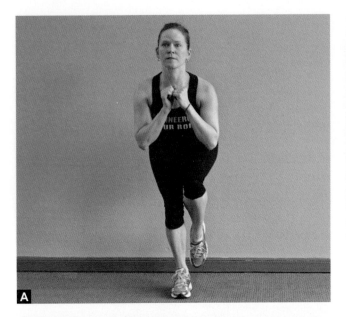

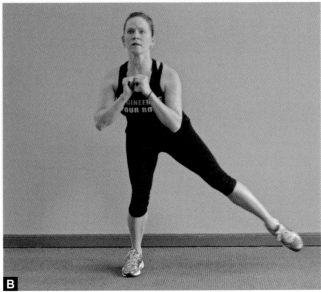

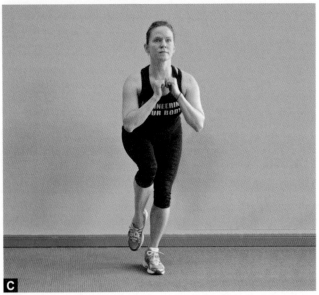

FIGS 13A TO C: Lateral step or jump. (A) Starting position showing ankle and knee absorption. (B) Step or hop transition. (C) Finishing position showing contralateral absorption

mobilization that uses patented instruments to transfer pressure and force to underlying dysfunctional structures. Research on ASTYM™ has shown increased fibroblast recruitment and activation in rat tendons, which could theoretically promote healing, but has not been studied in humans.[53] A recent case study showed a favorable result when ASTYM™ was used in conjunction with eccentric training.[54] Another technique widely used by clinicians is the Graston™ technique—a form of instrument-assisted soft-tissue mobilization with the goal of breaking down scar tissue and improving function. At present, there is no clinical research to evaluate the effectiveness of Graston™ treatment for Achilles tendinopathy.

Medical Interventions

Injections

A variety of substances can be injected into the Achilles tendon or the surrounding tissue, with equally varied objectives.

Corticosteroids

Historically, corticosteroids have been used to manage the hypothesized inflammatory process associated with Achilles tendinopathy and as such have been reported to reduce pain and swelling.[55] However, the efficacy

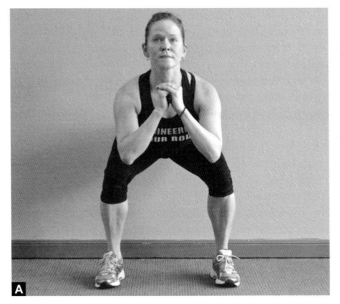
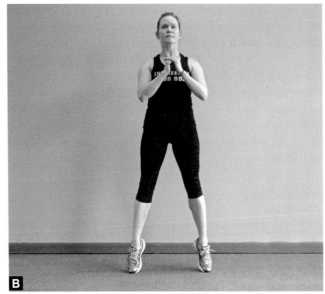
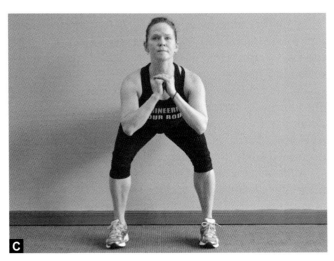

FIGS 14A TO C: Lateral step or jump. (A) Starting position showing ankle and knee. (B) Dynamic jump movement without leaving ground—peak of movement is full hip and knee extension and ankle plantar flexion. (C) Finishing position showing ankle and knee absorption

of peritendinous steroid injections depend on the underlying process behind the Achilles condition and despite a possible early benefit, adverse reactions have been found in 82% of clinical trials.[56] These include decreased tendon strength[57] and rupture.[58] The reason for this may be that painful Achilles conditions once thought to be characterized by a chronic inflammatory process are now believed to be the result of a degenerative process. Tissue markers of inflammation are found infrequently, suggesting that corticosteroid injections should relieve symptoms in few cases of Achilles tendinopathy. Given the potential risks and questionable utility of steroid injection, the benefit of steroid injection for the treatment of Achilles tendinopathy is outweighed by its risks.[59]

Platelet Rich Plasma

Platelet Rich Plasma (PRP) injections involve the extraction of a patient's blood with a subsequent reinjection of isolated platelets into the injury site. Theoretically, PRP induces tendon healing through a release of tissue regenerating growth factors. Following the injection, the area is then immobilized to allow healing. The use of PRP therapies has become widespread for a variety of different acute and chronic tendon disorders. For Achilles tendinopathy, the procedure has been used as an alternative to surgery and can be used in conjunction with physical therapy, or used when more conservative measures fail. PRP injection is an attractive alternative to surgery given its relatively low cost and morbidity. While MRI analysis of patients who have received PRP do not show changes in the MRI appearance of the Achilles tendon more than a year after the procedure, patients experienced a modest improvement in symptoms.[60] However, one study that compared PRP to saline injections found no significant difference in clinical outcome between the two groups, suggesting that the mere act of injecting fluid into a tendon achieves a degree of pain-relief.[61]

Prolotherapy

Prolotherapy is an injection treatment in which a formula of glucose and local anesthetic is injected into the tendon in order to incite inflammation and lead to collagen deposition. Achilles tendinopathy patients treated with prolotherapy experienced the greatest relief when the procedure was combined with eccentric exercise training.[62]

Surgical Intervention

For those who fail to respond to conservative treatment, a surgical intervention may be necessary. Conventional surgeries primarily consist of open release of adhesions with or without resection of the paratenon. Areas of tendinopathy are removed through a central longitudinal tenotomy, with further tendinopathies able to be performed on the surrounding tissue as needed to initiate healing. If greater than 50% of the tendon is involved in the debridement, augmentation with a tendon transfer may be required. Successful outcomes for open procedures vary between 75% and 100%.[63]

For those patients with isolated nodules of tendinopathy and without signs of paratendinopathy, percutaneous longitudinal tenotomies have been successfully undertaken, with results comparable with those observed after more invasive procedures. These procedures can be performed under local anesthesia on an outpatient basis, and are relatively safe, with less risk of complications.[64]

■ CONCLUSION

Achilles tendinopathy is a common condition affecting athletes and non-athletes alike. Athletes, particularly those engaged in running and jumping sports, are more likely to experience the condition.[9] Symptoms are usually mid-tendon and reflect a failed healing response, rather than chronic inflammation. Histological analysis of tendinopathy reveals evidence of tendon degeneration that may develop well before symptoms become apparent.[13] Tendinopathy can be described as a three-stage continuum: reactive tendinopathy, tendon disrepair and degenerative tendinopathy. The condition can be divided into mid-tendon and insertional types with the latter being more recalcitrant to treatment.[31] Of concern is link between tendon degeneration and tendon mechanical weakening.[14,15]

Most Achilles tendinopathy is located 2–6 cm from the calcaneus, which likely coincides with a region of hypovascularity.[27] Although tendon degeneration may reflect disruption of the normal collagen structure, pain is considered a consequence of increased vascularization and nerve in-growth. Although Achilles tendinopathy can become chronic, conservative management with exercise is successful in the majority of cases.[4,29,44]

While the etiology of Achilles tendinopathy is often due to an interaction of extrinsic and intrinsic factors, research suggests that training errors lead to the majority of tendon overuse injuries. Errors of this type include excessive volume, intensity and duration of training. The intrinsic factors most associated with Achilles tendinopathy include hyperpronation, calf muscle weakness, varus deformity, leg-length difference and decreased ankle dorsiflexion.[1]

Although the patient's history is usually enough to make the diagnosis of Achilles tendinopathy, a careful physical examination should be conducted to elucidate the possible factors that have led to development of the problem. The critical points of analysis should include; ankle dorsiflexion, plantarflexion strength and endurance, subtalar ROM, and pronation. Palpation of the tendon can reveal areas of tenderness, crepitation, possible defects and swelling.

As an exercise-based approach is overwhelmingly supported in the literature,[4,29,44] treatment should focus on concentric and eccentric strength building exercise. Of these elements, evidence is greatest for inclusion of eccentric exercise training for positive clinical outcomes in pain, function and return to activity.[42-45]

Clinically, control of the patient's symptoms is the initial priority of conservative care, and may require the use of immobilization and usually some measure of activity or sport limitation. Additional goals of this early phase of treatment include reestablishment of gastrocnemius-soleus NMR and general reconditioning of the lower quarter.

Once Achilles tendon symptoms are controlled, and the patient has demonstrated the ability to tolerate exercise without worsening of symptoms, then treatment can progress to the next phase of exercise, in which exercise WB loads can increase. Subsequent phases can progress to more functional and sport-specific exercise as symptoms decrease, and calf and lower quarter strength normalize.

Control of the rehabilitation process should include the final phases of returning to full activity. At each step, care should be taken to not rush through a phase until both the patient's symptoms and muscular readiness demonstrate a level appropriate to advancement. Too often, in the care of athletic or highly active individuals, there is the assumption that therapeutic exercise should immediately reproduce athletic movements without first ensuring that the patient has the requisite strength, ROM and muscle tone to start higher-level exercise. Skipping progressive steps or rushing through the rehabilitation process because a patient is generally fit, or because the patient's symptoms have decreased, can lead to later problems in more dynamic exercise or with a return to activity. Those with Achilles tendinopathy are at increased risk of Achilles tears.[15] therefore, extra caution should be observed.

Future research should concentrate on the utility of combined concentric and eccentric exercise programs that have the dual goal of improving symptoms and increasing plantarflexion strength. There is also currently a lack of scientific evidence for conservative therapies other than exercise, specifically emerging techniques in soft-tissue mobilization.

■ REFERENCES

1. Paavola M, Kannus P, Järvinen T, Khan K, Józsa L, Järvinen M. Achilles tendinopathy. J Bone Joint Surg. 2002;84(11):2062-76.
2. Kujala U, Sarna S, Kaprio J. Cumulative incidence of Achilles tendon rupture and tendinopathy in male former elite athletes. Clinical Journal of Sport Medicine. 2005;15(3):133-5.
3. Kannus P, Niittymäki S, Järvinen M, Lehto M. Sports injuries in elderly athletes: a three-year prospective, controlled study. Age Ageing. 1989;18(4):263-70.
4. Magnussen RA, Dunn WR, Thomson AB. Nonoperative treatment of midportion Achilles tendinopathy: a systematic review. Clinical Journal of Sport Medicine. 2009;19(1):54-64.
5. Petersen W, Welp R, Rosenbaum D. Chronic achilles tendinopathy: a prospective randomized study comparing the therapeutic effect of eccentric training, the AirHeel brace, and a combination of both. Am J Sports Med. 2007;35(10):1659-67.
6. Rompe J, Nafe B, Furia J, Maffulli N. Eccentric loading, shock-wave treatment, or a wait-and-see policy for tendinopathy of the main body of tendo Achillis: a randomized controlled trial. Am J Sports Med. 2007;35:374-83.
7. Lysholm J, Wiklander J. Injuries in runners. Am J Sports Med. 1987;15(2):168-71.
8. Courville XF, Coe MP, Hecht PJ. Current Concepts Review: Noninsertional Achilles Tendinopathy. Foot & Ankle International. 2009;30(11):1132-42.
9. Sorosky B, Press J, Plastaras C, Rittenberg J. The practical management of Achilles tendinopathy. Clinical Journal of Sport Medicine. 2004;14(1):40-4.
10. Cook JL, Purdam CR. Is tendon pathology a continuum? A pathology model to explain the clinical presentation of load-induced tendinopathy. British Journal Of Sports Medicine. 2009;43(6):409-16.
11. Alfredson H, Thorsen K, Lorentzon R. In situ microdialysis in tendon tissue: high levels of glutamate, but not prostaglandin E2 in chronic Achilles tendon pain. Knee Surg Sports Traumatol Arthrosc. 1999;7(6):378-81.
12. Järvinen T, Kannus P, Maffulli N, Khan K. Achilles tendon disorders: etiology and epidemiology. Foot Ankle Clin. 2005;10(2):255-66.
13. Forsgren S Danielson P, Alfredson H. Vascular NK-1 receptor occurrence in normal and chronic painful Achilles and patellar tendons: studies on chemically unfixed as well as fixed specimens. Regul Pept. 2005;126(3):173-81.
14. Tallon C, Maffulli N, Ewen S. Ruptured Achilles tendons are significantly more degenerated than tendinopathic tendons. Med Sci Sports Exerc. 2001;33(12):1983-90.
15. Kannus P, Jozsa L. Histopathological changes preceding spontaneous rupture of a tendon. A controlled study of 891 patients. Journal Bone Joint Surg. 1991;73(10):1507-25.
16. Xu Y, Murrell GAC. The Basic Science of Tendinopathy. Clinical Orthopaedics and Related Research. 2008;466(7):1528-38.
17. Kvist M. Achilles tendon injuries in athletes. Sports Med. 1994:18(3):173-201.
18. Kannus P. Etiology and pathophysiology of chronic tendon disorders in sports. Scan Med Sci Sports Exerc. 1997;7(2):78-85.
19. Nigg B. The role of impact forces and foot pronation: a new paradigm. Clin J Sports Med. 2001;11(1):2-9.
20. Clement D, Taunton J, Smart G. Achilles tendinitis and peritendinitis: etiology and treatment. Am J Sports Med. 1984;12(3):179-84.
21. Azevedo LB, Lambert MI, Vaughan CL, O'Connor CM, Schwellnus MP. Biomechanical variables associated with Achilles tendinopathy in runners. British Journal Of Sports Medicine. 2009;43(4):288-92.
22. Ryan M, Grau S, Krauss I, Maiwald C, Taunton J, Horstmann T. Kinematic analysis of runners with Achilles mid-portion tendinopathy. Foot & Ankle International. 2009;30(12):1190-5.
23. McCrory J, Martin D, Lowery R, Cannon D, Curl W, Read H. Etiologic factors associated with Achilles tendinitis in runners. Med Sci Sports Exerc. 1999;31(10):1374-81.
24. Schepsis A, Jones H, Haas A. Achilles tendon disorders in athletes. Am J Sports Med. 2002;30(2):287-305.
25. Chen TM, Rozen WM, Pan W, Ashton MW, Richardson MD, Taylor GI. The arterial anatomy of the Achilles tendon: anatomical study and clinical implications. Clinical Anatomy. 2009;22(3):377-85.
26. Åström M, Gentz C, Nilsson P, Rausing A, Sjöberg S, Westlin N. Imaging in chronic achilles tendinopathy: a comparison of ultrasonography, magnetic resonance imaging and surgical findings in 27 histologically verified cases. Skeletal Radiol. 1996;25(7):615-20.
27. Bleakney R, White L. Imaging of the Achilles tendon. Foot Ankle Clin. 2005:10(2):239-54.
28. Asplund CA, Best TM. Achilles tendon disorders. BMJ. 2013;346:f1262.
29. Wiegerinck JI, Kerkhoffs GM, van Sterkenburg MN, Sierevelt IN, van Dijk CN. Treatment for insertional Achilles tendinopathy: a systematic review. Knee Surgery, Sports Traumatology, Arthroscopy. 2013;21(6):1345-55.

30. Kaufman K, Brodine S, Shaffer R, Johnson C, Cullison T. The effect of foot structure and range of motion on musculoskeletal overuse injuries. Am J Sports Med. 1999;27(5):585-93.

31. Silbernagel K, Gustavsson A, Thomeé R, Karlsson J. Evaluation of lower leg function in patients with Achilles tendinopathy. Knee Surg Sports Traumatol Arthrosc. 2006;14(11):1207-17.

32. Soysa A, Hiller C, Refshauge K, Burns J. Importance and challenges of measuring intrinsic foot muscle strength. Journal of Foot and Ankle Research. 2012;5(1):29.

33. Thompson TC. A test for the rupture of tendo Achilles. Acta Ortha. 1962;32(1-4):461-5.

34. Rompe JD, Nafe B, Furia JP, Maffulli N. Eccentric loading, shock-wave treatment, or a wait-and-see policy for tendinopathy of the main body of tendo Achillis: a randomized controlled trial. Am J Sports Med. 2007;35(3):374-83.

35. Maffulli N, Longo UG, Petrillo S, Denaro V. Management of tendinopathies of the foot and ankle. Orthopaedics and Trauma. 2012;26(4):259-64.

36. Gam A, Johannsen F. Ultrasound therapy in musculoskeletal disorders: a meta-analysis. Pain. 1995;63(1):85-91.

37. Robertson V, Baker K. A review of therapeutic ultrasound: effectiveness studies. Phys Ther. 2001;81(7):1339-50.

38. Neeter C, Thomee R, Silbernagel K, Thomee P, Karlsson J. Iontophoresis with or without dexamethazone in the treatment of acute Achilles tendon pain. Scan Med Sci Sports Exerc. 2003;13(6):376-82.

39. Alfredson H, Pietilä T, Jonsson P, Lorentzon R. Heavy-load eccentric calf muscle training for the treatment of chronic Achilles tendinosis. Scan Med Sci Sports Exerc. 1998:26(3):360-6.

40. Stasinopoulos D, Manias P. Comparing two eccentric exercise programmes for the management of Achilles tendinopathy. A pilot trial. J Bodyw Mov Ther. 2013;17(3):309-15.

41. Stevens M, Tan C-W. Effectiveness of the Alfredson protocol compared with a lower repetition-volume protocol for midportion Achilles tendinopathy: a randomized controlled trial. J Orthop Sports Phys Ther. 2014;44(2):59-67.

42. Öhberg L, Lorentzon R, Alfredson H. Eccentric training in patients with chronic Achilles tendinosis: normalised tendon structure and decreased thickness at follow up. Br J Sports Med. 2004;38(1):8-11.

43. Silbernagel KG, Brorsson A, Lundberg M. The majority of patients with Achilles tendinopathy recover fully when treated with exercise alone: a 5-year follow-up. Am J Sports Med. 2011;39(3):607-13.

44. Grävare Silbernagel K, Thomee R, Thomee P, Karlsson J. Eccentric overload training for patients with chronic Achilles tendon pain—a randomised controlled study with reliability testing of the evaluation methods. Scan Med Sci Sports Exerc. 2001;11(4):197-206.

45. Rees JD, Lichtwark GA, Wolman RL, Wilson AM. The mechanism for efficacy of eccentric loading in Achilles tendon injury: an in vivo study in humans. Rheumatology (Oxford). 2008;47(10):1493-7.

46. Allison GT, Purdam C. Eccentric loading for Achilles tendinopathy—strengthening or stretching? Br J Sports Med. 2009;43(4):276-9.

47. Sayana M, Maffulli N. Eccentric calf muscle training in non-athletic patients with Achilles tendinopathy. J Sci Med Sport. 2007;10(1):52-8.

48. Rompe JD, Furia JP, Maffulli N. Mid-portion Achilles tendinopathy—current options for treatment. Disabil Rehabil. 2008;30(20-22):1666-76.

49. Wang C-J. Extracorporeal shockwave therapy in musculoskeletal disorders. J Orthop Surg Res. 2012;7:11.

50. Vulpiani M, Trischitta D, Trovato P, Vetrano M, Ferretti A. Extracorporeal shockwave therapy (ESWT) in Achilles tendinopathy. A long-term follow-up observational study. J Sports Med Phys Fitness. 2009;49(2):171-6.

51. Rompe JD, Furia J, Maffulli N. Eccentric loading compared with shock wave treatment for chronic insertional achilles tendinopathy. A randomized, controlled trial. J Bone Joint Surg Am. 2008;90(1):52-61.

52. Magnussen RA, Dunn WR, Thomson AB. Nonoperative treatment of midportion Achilles tendinopathy: a systematic review. Clin J Sport Med. 2009;19(1):54-64.

53. Gehlsen G, Ganion L, Helfst R. Fibroblast responses to variation in soft tissue mobilization pressure. Med Sci Sports Exerc. 1999;31(4):531-5.

54. McCormack J. The management of mid-portion Achilles tendinopathy with ASTYM and eccentric exercise: a case report. Int J Sports Phys Ther. 2012:7(6):672-7.

55. Fredberg U, Stengaard-Pedersen K. Chronic tendinopathy tissue pathology, pain mechanisms, and etiology with a special focus on inflammation. Scand J Med Sci Sports. 2008;18(1):3-15.

56. Hart L. Corticosteroid and other injections in the management of tendinopathies: a review. Clin J Sport Med. 2011;21(6):540-1.

57. Hugate R, Pennypacker J, Saunders M, Juliano P. The effects of intratendinous and retrocalcaneal intrabursal injections of corticosteroid on the biomechanical properties of rabbit Achilles tendons. J Bone Joint Surg. 2004:86(4):794-801.

58. Chen S-K, Lu C-C, Chou P-H, Guo L-Y, Wu W-L. Patellar tendon ruptures in weight lifters after local steroid injections. Arch Orthop Trauma Surg. 2009;129(3):369-72.

59. Shrier I, Matheson G, Kohl III H. Achilles tendonitis: are corticosteroid injections useful or harmful? Clinical Journal of Sport Medicine. 1996;6(4):245-50.

60. Owens R, Ginnetti J, Conti S, Latona C. Clinical and magnetic resonance imaging outcomes following platelet rich plasma injection for chronic midsubstance Achilles tendinopathy. Foot Ankle Int. 2011;32(11):1032-9.

61. De Vos RJ, Weir A, van Schie HT, Bierma-Zeinstra SM, Verhaar JA, Weinans H, et al. Platelet-rich plasma injection for chronic Achilles tendinopathy: a randomized controlled trial. JAMA. 2010;303(2):144-9.

62. Yelland MJ, Sweeting KR, Lyftogt JA, Ng SK, Scuffham PA, Evans KA. Prolotherapy injections and eccentric loading exercises for painful Achilles tendinosis: a randomised trial. Br J Sports Med. 2011;45(5):421-8.

63. Roche AJ, Calder JDF. Achilles tendinopathy: a review of the current concepts of treatment. Bone Joint J. 2013;95-B(10):1299-307.

64. Maffulli N, Testa V, Capasso G, Bifulco G, Binfield P. Results of percutaneous longitudinal tenotomy for Achilles tendinopathy in middle-and long-distance runners. Am J Sports Med. 1997:25(6):835-40.

CHAPTER 14

Medial Tibial Stress Syndrome

Daniel J Hass

ABSTRACT

Medial tibial stress syndrome (MTSS) is a common pathology in physically active individuals. The pathology is most likely due to bony overload of the posteromedial border of the tibia; however, it is unknown if this is due to excessive bending forces, soft tissue traction, some combination of the two, or other mechanisms that have not yet been identified. MTSS is a clinical diagnosis, but careful differential diagnosis is imperative. Conservative management is typical, and most athletes will return to prior level of activity with appropriate education and rehabilitation. The role of the physical therapist is to identify the causative factors and correct underlying movement impairments that may contribute to future occurrence or exacerbation. In addition to these interventions, the skilled practitioner can guide the patient through an appropriate progression of activity that will allow the patient to safely return to prior level of activity.

■ INTRODUCTION

Medial tibial stress syndrome (MTSS), as defined by Yates and White,[1] is pain along the posteromedial border of the tibia that occurs due to exercise, excluding pain from ischemic origin or signs of stress fracture. The authors add that pain must be diffuse and spread over a minimum of 5 cm.[1] This is considered to be the most thorough description of MTSS,[2] although no standardized definition exists in the literature. Shin splints has long been used as a catch all term to describe any leg injury (leg defined as below the knee, but above the ankle), such as MTSS, compartment syndrome, stress fractures, popliteal artery entrapment, tendonitis and muscle strains.[3-9] The term shin splints describes the location of pain, but does not describe the underlying pathology nor helps to guide treatment, rendering it an inappropriate term for

clinical diagnosis and treatment.[2,10] Lower leg pain can be a difficult area for clinicians to diagnose and treat, and part of the challenge revolves around confusion in the medical community regarding appropriate terminology and definitions of various pathologies that affect the lower leg.[2,3,10] Differential diagnosis is imperative for proper management and will be addressed in this chapter; however, the focus of the chapter will be on the most common pathology of the lower leg: MTSS.[5,11-13] A historical perspective over the past several decades can help to explain the evolving understanding of MTSS and the variable terminology associated with this condition.

In 1958, the first attempt to define what would now be characterized as MTSS was made by Devas, when he used the term shin soreness to describe what he considered an incomplete fracture of the tibial cortex.[14] In 1966, the American Medical Association (AMA) published an official definition of shin splints as "pain or discomfort in the leg from repetitive running on hard surfaces or forcible excessive use of the foot flexors; diagnosis should be limited to musculotendinous inflammations, excluding fracture or ischemic disorder".[15] Building on this description offered by the AMA, Clement theorized the shin pain described above was a periostitis of the medial tibia that resulted from muscle fatigue and led to increased stress on the bone, which he termed tibial stress syndrome in 1974.[16] Also in 1974, Puranen offered his theory that shin splints was an exercise-related ischemic condition of the deep flexor compartment of the lower leg, which he termed medial tibial syndrome.[17] The first documented use of the term medial tibia stress syndrome was in 1982 by Mubarak et al., who credited the origin of the term to D. Drez.[18] Mubarak agreed with Clement and believed that the shin splint condition most likely represented a periostitis of the distal posteromedial tibia. Also in 1982, Johnell proposed that shin splints was actually a bone stress injury, as evidenced by metabolic changes that he found in the tibia bone during surgical biopsies.[19] Clearly, at this time, no consensus existed in the medical community, as all of these authors appear to have been describing the same activity-related, diffuse posteromedial tibial pain, but with different conclusions as to the underlying cause and pathologic tissue. This lack of consensus remains evident to this day, despite the evolving theories as to the etiology of MTSS.

Epidemiology

Differentiating between causes of leg pain is of the utmost importance, as general exercise-related lower leg pain (ERLP) is very common in the active population. In fact, up to 68% of cross country runners report a history of ERLP, with the majority of athletes reporting bilateral symptoms localized to the medial aspect of the leg.[20] MTSS is a subset of ERLP and has been reported to be as low as 4%[3] to as high as 35%[1] in military studies. Bennett et al.[21] and Yates and White[1] have both shown that females are at greater risk with incidences of 3% in men, 19.1% in women; and 28% in men, 53% in women, respectively. The mean age for tibial stress syndrome has been reported as 30.7 years of age in the general running population.[22] The pathology most commonly affects runners and military personnel, but has also been reported in sports that require repetitive jumping such as basketball, volleyball and long jump.[2,9] Running is a popular form of exercise due to the multiple reported health benefits; however, anywhere from

19.4% to 79.3% of runners will sustain a running related injury every year.[23] During a 13-week running training program designed to reduce injury, the most commonly diagnosed injury was tibial stress syndrome.[24] Lopes et al. corroborated these findings in a systematic review, finding that the most frequently reported running-related musculoskeletal injury was MTSS, with an incident rate of 13.6–20.0% and an overall prevalence rate of 9.5%.[25] In a survey of community runners at a local race, 63.6% of participants reported a history of ERLP with 35.1% reporting ERLP in the 3 months leading up to the race.[13] Bilateral medial ERLP was the most common presentation, and 41.8% of the runners reported needing to alter their running because of the pain.[13]

Specific intrinsic and extrinsic risk factors for the development of MTSS have been studied by multiple authors in prospective and case-control studies.[26] Risk factor identification is imperative for developing prevention methods and guiding treatment for MTSS. Risk factors that have been prospectively identified by more than one study include increased navicular drop (a measure of pronation),[21,27-30] decreased hip internal rotation,[28,31] greater plantar flexion range of motion (ROM),[28,32] female sex,[1,12,21,33] increased body mass index (BMI),[12,31] a prior history of MTSS,[1,20,27,29,32] a prior history of any running-related injury,[12,29,30] and the use of orthotics at baseline (increased likelihood of developing MTSS with orthotics).[12,32] A recent systematic review concluded that female gender, previous history of MTSS, orthotic use, increased BMI, increased navicular drop and increased hip external rotation ROM in males were all significantly associated with the development of MTSS. Other extrinsic factors commonly thought to increase risk of running-related injury such as training distance, training intensity, running surfaces, type of shoes and cross-training have weak evidence, no evidence or conflicting evidence when assessing risk for development of MTSS.[13,20,21,29,31-34] The results of these studies remain far from conclusive; however, as identified potential risk factors from one series of studies are inevitably ruled out as contributory by conflicting research. For example, Moen et al.[28] and Yagi et al.[31] found *decreased* hip internal rotation as a risk factor, whereas Burne et al.[33] found *increased* hip internal rotation in men as a risk factor. Likewise, there are numerous authors who report markers of pronation as predictors of developing MTSS,[21,27-30] while several other authors fail to find a link between this factor and the development of MTSS.[12,31,32,34,35] This complicates clinical decision making and highlights the importance of performing a thorough examination and developing an individualized treatment algorithm specific to each patient.

Anatomical Considerations

The lower leg is considered the region between the knee and ankle joints and consists of the fibula and tibia bones

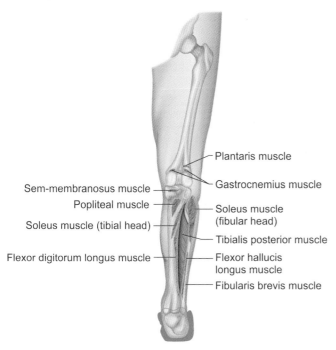

Plantaris muscle

Sem-membranosus muscle

Gastrocnemius muscle

Popliteal muscle

Soleus muscle (fibular head)

Soleus muscle (tibial head)

Tibialis posterior muscle

Flexor digitorum longus muscle

Flexor hallucis longus muscle

Fibularis brevis muscle

FIG. 1: Posterior view of the right lower extremity bony anatomy, demonstrating muscle insertion points and lower leg (area between knee and ankle joints)

(Fig. 1). The tibia is the second largest bone in the body and is responsible for absorbing greater than 90% of the load transmitted to the lower leg during weight bearing activities.[36] The anterior and medial borders of the tibia are subcutaneous making it easy to directly palpate during clinical examination. The lower leg is divided into four compartments (Fig. 2). The lateral compartment of the lower leg is innervated by the superficial fibular nerve and contains the peroneus longus and peroneus brevis muscles.[37] The anterior compartment is innervated by the deep fibular nerve and contains the tibialis anterior, extensor digitorum longus, extensor hallucis longus and the peroneus tertius muscles.[37] The posterior compartment of the leg, innervated by the tibial nerve, is subdivided into a superficial and a deep posterior compartment, and is the most pertinent compartment in MTSS.[37] The muscles of the superficial posterior compartment include the gastrocnemius, soleus and the smaller plantaris (Fig. 3), while the deep posterior compartment musculature consists of the tibialis posterior, flexor hallucis longus and the flexor digitorum longus (Fig. 4). The deep posterior muscles are particularly important for controlling excessive pronation at the subtalar and mid-tarsal joints as they cross these joints posteriorly and medially. The tibialis posterior, in particular, has multiple attachments along the foot, making it an important dynamic stabilizer of the medial longitudinal arch (MLA) (Fig. 5). The precise attachment sites of these muscles along the tibia as they travel distally down the posteromedial aspect of the lower leg are debated, but they are important to consider as they may relate to the pathomechanics of MTSS. The location of pain in subjects with MTSS can occur anywhere along the

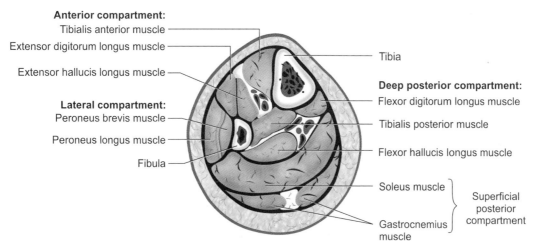

Anterior compartment:
Tibialis anterior muscle

Extensor digitorum longus muscle

Extensor hallucis longus muscle

Lateral compartment:
Peroneus brevis muscle

Peroneus longus muscle

Fibula

Tibia

Deep posterior compartment:
Flexor digitorum longus muscle

Tibialis posterior muscle

Flexor hallucis longus muscle

Soleus muscle

Gastrocnemius muscle

Superficial posterior compartment

FIG. 2: Cross-sectional anatomy of lower leg[40]
Source: Reproduced with permission from Elsevier.

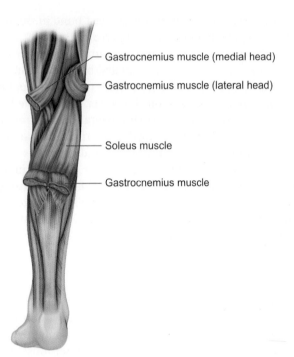

Gastrocnemius muscle (medial head)

Gastrocnemius muscle (lateral head)

Soleus muscle

Gastrocnemius muscle

FIG. 3: Superficial musculature of the posterior compartment of the lower leg, with gastrocnemius reflected

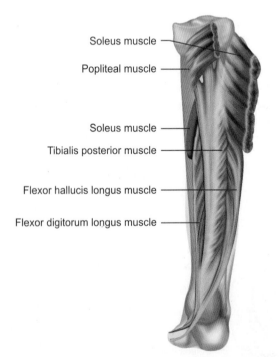

Soleus muscle

Popliteal muscle

Soleus muscle

Tibialis posterior muscle

Flexor hallucis longus muscle

Flexor digitorum longus muscle

FIG. 4: Deep musculature of the posterior compartment of the lower leg

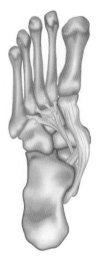

FIG. 5: The tibialis posterior tendon attaches to the medial tuberosity of the navicular (one main slip) and continues through the second slip to the plantar surface of the foot, where it arborizes and inserts into all three cuneiforms, the cuboid, and the bases of the first, second, third, fourth and fifth metatarsals[40]
Source: Reproduced with permission from Elsevier.

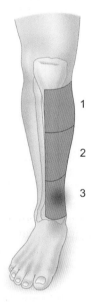

1

2

3

FIG. 6: Anteromedial view of the area most commonly affected by MTSS

Etiology and Pathomechanics

As noted in the historical review of the pathology, various theories—incomplete fracture,[14] tibial periostitis,[16,18] ischemic conditions,[17] periosteal-fascial avulsions[6] and bone stress reactions[19]—exist to describe what is now commonly known as MTSS. More recent research

posteromedial border of the tibia, but is most commonly located along the distal two-thirds (Fig. 6).[2,7,38,39]

provides a deeper understanding of underlying patho-mechanics and relevant anatomy contributing to MTSS. Deep posterior compartment syndrome is unlikely, as post-exercise compartment pressures have not proven significantly elevated over resting values in MTSS subjects.[18,41] The two predominant theories that exist today to explain the pathomechanics of MTSS are excessive soft-tissue traction and repetitive tibial microbending.[5]

Soft tissue traction on the tibia is theorized to occur due to excessive pronation caused by tight and/or fatigued plantar flexors, or due to biomechanical abnormalities causing excessive eccentric contraction of the muscles in the deep flexor compartment of the lower leg.[5] Soft tissue traction of the tibialis posterior,[42] flexor digitorum longus,[4,43] soleus[6,8] and deep crural fascia[5,44] have all been proposed to cause tibial periostitis in MTSS.[18] Saxena et al.[42] implicated the tibialis posterior as the culprit, but this study has been criticized for the low number of subjects,[9] and the proposed mechanism is unlikely, as the fibers have not been found to attach to the symptomatic area of the tibia in other anatomical studies.[4,8,44] In a recent anatomical study, Stickley et al.[44] found that very few specimens demonstrated fibers of the tibialis posterior, flexor digitorum longus or soleus attaching to the distal one half to one-third of the posteromedial border of the tibia.[44] The deep crural fascia was the only structure found to consistently attach to the distal one-third of the medial tibia, and inflammation of the fascia has been identified in histological studies of patient's undergoing surgery of MTSS.[7,18,19] Building on these findings, Bouche and Johnson tensioned the tendons of the soleus, flexor digitorum longus and tibialis posterior in cadavers and found an increase in linear strain on the deep crural fascia as measured with a strain guage.[5] Through these attachments, the authors suggest that excessive eccentric contractions due to overpronation may cause inflammation to the deep crural fascia.[5] Several histological, magnetic resonance and bone scan studies fail to demonstrate any evidence of inflammation of the periosteum[19,45-47] to indicate an inflammatory condition, making periostitis improbable. Although periostitis is unlikely, it is possible that soft tissue traction may cause a periosteal remodeling that can be a contributing factor to the pathology in MTSS.[44]

While soft tissue traction and periostitis have long been thought to be the mechanism and pathology in MTSS, tibial microbending is receiving increasing attention of late. Recent studies support Johnell and colleague's[19] original findings of increased bone porosity leading to a bone stress reaction in MTSS.[19,47] Magnuson et al.

reported that bone mineral density was 11% lower in the tibia of male athletes with MTSS compared to non-athlete asymptomatic male control subjects.[48] It has also been found that the symptomatic region of the tibia in MTSS is osteopenic on computed tomography (CT) scans.[11,49] It is interesting to note that subjects with MTSS demonstrate decreased tibial cross-sectional area compared to non-injured controls,[50] a finding that has been reported prospectively in military personnel who go on to develop tibial stress fractures.[51,52] Tibial bending occurs through weight bearing activity as a result of normal physiological loads applied to the bone,[53] and long bones with narrow diaphyses bend more than those with wider diaphyses.[10] Continued bending forces from repetitive activities, such as running and jumping, may cause a vicious cycle of osteoclastic activity that results in a hypermetabolic state in the bone.[54] Individuals with decreased bone cross-sectional area may not be able to withstand the stress transmitted to the bone during high-impact, repetitive activities, which causes a stress reaction of the tibia and subsequent pain and disability. Figures 7A to C illustrate

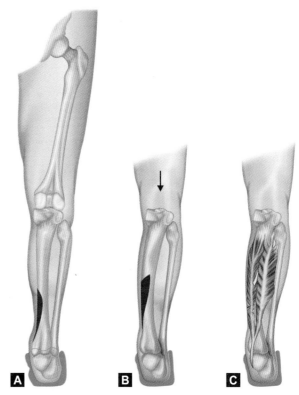

FIGS 7A TO C: Proposed mechanism for MTSS. (A) Posterior view of the lower leg identifying area of pain in MTSS. (B) Repetitive bending forces of the tibia associated with bony overload. (C) Overpronation and subsequent excessive eccentric contraction of the deep posterior compartment, theorized to cause excessive periosteal remodeling

the two proposed mechanisms leading to MTSS in a runner during stance phase of gait cycle.

Understanding the pathomechanics and pathology of a disease process is useful in developing a treatment strategy to decrease pain and disability. It seems that there is a stress reaction of the tibia bone, but whether this occurs due to microbending, soft tissue traction or a combination of the two is unknown. A skilled clinician must be able to ascertain the underlying deficits that lead to the pathology so that treatment measures can be taken to mitigate the offending cause. Both potential mechanisms described above need to be considered when treating a patient.

CLINICAL PRESENTATION

Medial tibial stress syndrome should be at the forefront of differential diagnosis when a patient describes a dull, aching pain along the medial aspect of the lower leg that occurs with activity and is commonly bilateral.[2,3,7,18,38,39,55] Patients are typically younger and report the pain occurs during some form of running or jumping activity.[2,9,22] The patient commonly describes pain that initially occurred near the beginning of activity, subsided with continued exertion, and was absent at rest.[2,3,7,39] With continued progression, the patient may describe more persistent and severe pain that eventually begins to hinder performance and is occasionally present with activities of daily living.[2,3,7,39] With true MTSS, the patient will deny any radicular symptoms, numbness or tingling, changes in sensation, significant weakness, systemic issues, night pain or weight loss.[39]

CLINICAL EXAMINATION

History

A thorough subjective history is the first step in a comprehensive examination and evaluation of a patient presenting with lower leg pain. Identification of the inciting activity and a description of the onset of symptoms will guide the clinician. Inquiring about potential training errors helps to identify correctable factors and educate the patient to prevent future occurrence. Training errors have been reported to account for up to 60% of MTSS cases.[7,56] The physical therapist should ask about recent changes in training, footwear, terrain, cross-training, use of orthotics and fitness level, all of which have been implicated as contributory to the onset of MTSS.[10,12,29,32,39,57] As MTSS

is most common in distance runners, a runner's profile should be used to identify years of running experience, miles run per week, days run per week, pace, warm-up and cool-down routines, and how these variables changed leading up to the injury. Past medical history is important to identify previous injuries: a well-accepted risk factor for development of MTSS is prior occurence.[1,12,13,20,27,29,30,32] A systematic review of risk factors for running injuries revealed strong evidence for running greater than 40 miles per week and a history of previous injuries.[58]

Physical Examination

Very few studies report on sensitivity and specificity of physical examination tests and measures for MTSS. Diagnosis is usually made based on subjective history, reported symptoms, palpation and other examination techniques to rule out other potential causes of lower leg pain. The most common physical finding in patients with MTSS is pain with palpation along the distal one half to one-third of the posteromedial border of the tibia.[2,7,38,39] This is reported by Moen et al. to be the most sensitive measure for MTSS.[2] The soft tissue of the posteromedial lower leg can be palpated, and pushed medially to palpate the posterior aspect of the tibia bone. Although rare, there may also be mild swelling or erythema over the posteromedial tibia.[2,3,38,39,59] The pain most often is diffuse, over an area of at least 5 cm.[1] The patient may also have pain with maximal stretch of the plantar flexors or with loading the plantar flexors during toe raises and/or hopping.[7] The most important aspect of the examination is to rule out other potential causes of lower leg pain, which serves to guide decisions on the need to refer for additional imaging or other tests and measures.

Differential Diagnosis

As implied by Yates and White's earlier definition of MTSS,[1] the two most common diagnoses which must be ruled out during examination are compartment syndrome and stress fracture. Other conditions which the clinician must rule out, but are beyond the scope of this chapter, include lumbar radiculopathy, peripheral nerve impingement, popliteal artery entrapment, intermittent claudication, neoplasm, infection, muscle strains, tendonitis and referred pain from proximal joints.[39]

Stress fractures usually develop insidiously, similar to MTSS, but the pain typically becomes more severe and occurs earlier during exercise.[2,39,60] The pain often continues after exertion, interfering with activities of daily living and causing night pain in some instances.[2,39] This is in contrast to MTSS, where less than 10% of the population experiences pain with activities of daily living.[13] The patient should be questioned about any gastrointestinal disorder, history of eating disorders, intake of calcium, vitamin D, protein, caffeine and alcohol, as well as menstrual function in females, that may predispose a patient to stress fracture.[60] A history of previous stress fracture is also a red flag that warrants further medical work up. On physical examination, the patient is tender in a much more focal region, and the pain is sharp and severe.[2,39,60] Percussion of the bone away from the site of fracture may also reproduce the pain.[2,39,60] When a stress fracture is suspected, the patient should be referred for appropriate medical management which may include, but is not limited to, serial radiographs, bone scan or magnetic resonance imaging (MRI), bone densitometry and metabolic panel.[60] Posteromedial tibial stress fracture is the most common type of tibial stress fracture, but the clinician should be especially concerned when the patient demonstrates symptoms of stress fracture over the anterior tibial diaphysis.[60] These stress fractures may require surgical intervention as they demonstrate poorer healing, risk for non-union and potential for progression to a complete fracture.[61,62]

Chronic exertional compartment syndrome (CECS) is caused by ischemia in one of the four compartments of the lower leg (anterior, lateral, superficial posterior, deep posterior) that occurs when a fascial compartment is unable to adequately contain the increase in swelling and volume that occurs from repetitive muscle contractions during activity[63] (Fig. 2). The most common compartments involved are the anterior and lateral compartments, and CECS is the second most common cause of lower leg pain, with a reported prevalence of 27–33%.[64] Symptoms are often bilateral and occur equally in males and females.[39] The key subjective finding is a sensation of fullness and pain that is described as burning, cramping, aching and/or tightness that occurs consistently at the same intensity and time duration with each exercise or activity bout, and dissipates quickly after a bout of exertion.[39,65-67] At rest, the clinician is unable to provoke the pain, and neurovascular examination is normal.[39,65-67] In this case, it is helpful for the clinician to have the patient perform his/her regular exercise until the symptoms are present and then re-examine the patient.[39,65] After the provocative exercise bout, palpable tenderness is present over the muscles of the involved compartment and there is increased fullness and swelling of the leg that can often be visualized.[39,65] The ultimate differential diagnosis is based on compartmental

pressure testing: pressures greater than 15 mm Hg at rest, greater than 30 mm Hg 1 minute after exercise or greater than 20 mm Hg 5 minutes after exercise are indicative of compartment syndrome.[67] When CECS is suspected, it is important to consult with a sports medicine physician to discuss implications for further diagnostic measures such as compartment testing, as many of these patients will require surgery to release the fascia that is constraining the compartment, rendering it unable to accommodate the increase in volume. Although non-operative treatment is successful in a number of patients, a recent 10-year cohort found an 81% success rate in patients who had a fasciotomy, and only a 41% success rate in the non-operative group.[66]

Role of Imaging

Advanced imaging is not helpful in making a diagnosis of MTSS; however, it is valuable when other causes of leg pain are suspected. Radiographs are almost always normal in subjects with MTSS, with only a few reports of callus formation or periosteal elevation.[2] Three-phase bone scans have shown diffuse uptake along posterior tibial cortex on delayed images in MTSS, but specificity has been reported to be 33%, leading to high number of false positives.[2,11,68,69] Tibial stress fractures demonstrate a more focal region and increased uptake on bone scan compared to MTSS where the diffuse uptake is indicative of a stress reaction of the bone (Figs 8 and 9).[70] In addition, changes can be identified on the first two sequences of the three-phase scan with stress fractures.[68,71] MRI

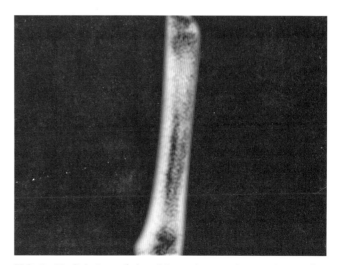

FIG. 8: Medial view of the tibia on isotope bone scintigraphy: tubular pattern characteristic of medial tibial syndrome[76]
Source: Reproduced with permission from Elsevier.

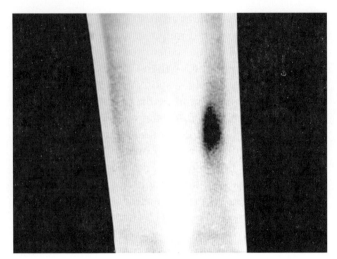

FIG. 9: Typical bone scan appearance of stress fracture of tibia[77]
Source: Reproduced with permission from Elsevier.

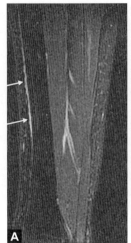
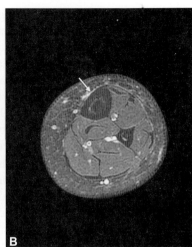

FIGS 11A AND B: A 26-year-old person with pain when running. (A) Sagittal short-tau inversion recovery image shows periosteal edema along the anterior tibia (arrows). (B) Axial fat-suppressed T2-weighted image confirms the high signal adjacent to the anteromedial tibia (arrow). Periosteal edema without marrow or cortical involvement is consistent with medial tibial stress syndrome or shin splints[78]
Source: Reproduced with permission from Elsevier.

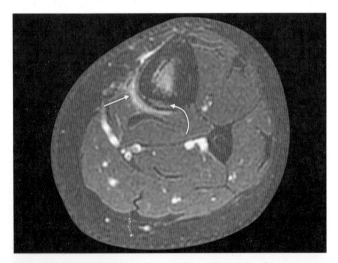

FIG. 10: A 24-year-old person with lower leg pain when running. Axial fat-suppressed T2-weighted image shows periostitis (straight arrow), marrow edema and abnormal signal within the tibial cortex (curved arrow), indicating a stress fracture[78]
Source: Reproduced with permission from Elsevier.

demonstrates a linear increase in signal intensity along the posteromedial tibia in MTSS, whereas an abnormally wide high signal can be seen in tibial stress fracture—often with a clear fracture line.[72] Figures 10 and 11 demonstrate the differences between MTSS and tibial stress fracture on MRI. When employed to identify tibial stress fractures, MRI demonstrates good sensitivity and specificity,[73] but similar to bone scan, specificity and likelihood ratios are low for MTSS, leading to little clinical value in making a diagnosis of MTSS.[2,68] High-resolution CT scan has the ability to pick up osteopenic changes, but again a large percentage of healthy subjects also demonstrate

CT abnormalities.[2,11,49] Because of these factors, the clinical evaluation is considered the gold standard for diagnosing MTSS.[2] The most common role for imaging is when there is suspicion for other pathology, such as infection, malignancy, tendinopathy, muscle strains and, most commonly, stress fracture. When diagnosing stress fractures, MRI and bone scan have similar sensitivities, but MRI has superior specificity and also has the advantage of identifying soft tissues.[74,75] CT scans are rarely used because sensitivity is lower than bone scan and MRI, and radiation exposure is high.[74]

Pertinent Tests and Measures

Once a clear diagnosis of MTSS has been established, further tests and measures are performed by the evaluating physical therapist to establish a baseline that will aid in setting goals, developing a plan for care, determining prognosis, and enable later comparative measures to determine treatment efficacy. In addition to patient goals, these measures will help to provide a complete clinical picture of the pathology and guide treatment.

Functional Outcome Measures

A standardized functional outcome measure provides a common language to gather baseline information on pain, impairments, functional limitations and disability to track changes over the course of treatment.[79] There is not a single functional outcome measure that has been validated in a subset of individuals with MTSS nor is there a standard measure utilized for research purposes.[80-82] The Lower Extremity Functional Scale (LEFS) has shown to be reliable, with good construct validity compared to the Medical Outcomes Study 36-Item Short-Form Health Survey (SF-36) in patients with a lower extremity musculoskeletal condition.[83] The University of Wisconsin Running Injury and Recovery Index (UWRI) is a relatively new outcome measure that has shown good test-retest reliability, internal consistency, and construct validity against the LEFS and Global Rating of Change (GROC).[84,85] This may be an especially useful tool as MTSS is a very common injury in runners.[24,25] The Numeric Pain Rating Scale (NRS), Visual Analog Scale (VAS), Pain Disability Index (PDI), short-form McGill Pain Questionnaire (SF-MPQ) have all been used to assess pain, functional limitations and disability in subjects with MTSS, and may be utilized in the clinical setting.[86-88]

Palpation

Because palpation plays such a key role in the diagnosis of MTSS, pressure algometry is an excellent tool to objectify pain and monitor progress in this population. A pressure algometer allows the application of a force to a specific area that measures the pain pressure threshold—the minimal amount of pressure necessary to cause pain.[89] A recent study showed moderate to excellent intra-rater reliability in asymptomatic patients, and significantly lower pain pressure thresholds in subjects with MTSS from three-ninths to four-ninths the distance from the medial malleolus to medial tibial condyle.[89] The physical therapist may decide to perform this along the entire medial border of the tibia in certain increments, or choose two to three locations of maximal palpable tenderness to test. The most important factor is to accurately document the location of measurements for repeatability on subsequent re-evaluations.

Posture Assessment

Postural and anatomical assessment can be utilized to identify any misalignment that may be contributing to, or a result of, the pathology. Anthropometric measurements, such as leg length discrepancy, tibiofemoral angle, intermalleolar or intercondylar angle, tibiofibular varum and quadriceps angle have not been implicated as risk

factors for development of MTSS;[21,30,31,33] however, compilation of these measurements may help the clinician to develop the complete picture of contributory biomechanics for an individual patient. The value of this consideration is evident in runners, where threshold for injury is based on three main constructs: (1) anatomical structure, (2) running mechanics and (3) dosage.[90] A runner who has poor mechanics and structure will not require a high dosage of exercise for an overuse injury to occur.[90] Understanding the structure and how it relates to function will allow the clinician to individualize a patient's plan of care, develop interventions and educate him/her on appropriate dosage. Excessive pronation has been suggested by several investigators to be a risk factor for MTSS.[21,27-30] However, accurately assessing foot structure and biomechanics in the clinical setting is challenging, and no consensus on an ideal method for classifying foot type exists.[91-93] The challenge stems in large part from the complexity of the foot structure and mechanics: 26 bones, 33 joints and 112 ligaments compose the foot, and the associated multiplanar and multi-joint kinematics are difficult to measure.[91-93] The most common ways to assess foot types are based on visual inspection, anthropometric measures and footprint characteristic evaluations.[93] Visual inspection attempts to qualify foot type based on the calcaneal angle in relation to the leg or floor, and/or by the height of the MLA.[93] An observational clinical rating system, the Foot Posture Index (FPI) was developed by Remdan et al. and has shown good concurrent validity with the Valgus Index, radiographs and a three-dimensional lower limb model using an electromagnetic motion tracking system.[94-96] This tool also demonstrates moderate to excellent intra- and inter-rater reliability, and has the added advantage of assessing multiple planes and foot regions.[96-98] Six clinical criteria are utilized in the FPI with a score ranging from -2 (clear signs of supination) to +2 (clear signs of pronation), with 0 representing neutral.[96] The six criteria are talar head palpation, supra and infra lateral malleolar curvature, calcaneal frontal plane position, prominence of the region of the talonavicular joint, congruence of the MLA, abduction or adduction of the forefoot on the rearfoot[96] (Fig. 12). All observational grades are made in relaxed double limb stance, and the index takes about 2 minutes to complete.[96] Higher scores represent a more pronated foot and lower scores represent a more supinated resting foot posture.[96] Yates and White reported a significantly higher FPI in a group of military recruits who went on to develop MTSS over the course of training, with the recruits being twice as likely to develop MTSS with a pronated foot

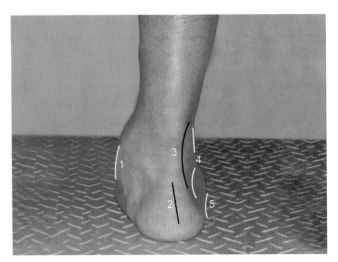

FIG. 12: Posterior view of a pronated foot, as defined by the foot posture index. (1) Talar navicular prominence; (2) calcaneal frontal plane position; (3) Helbing's sign; (4) inferior and superior lateral malleolar curves; (5) congruence of the lateral border[76]
Source: Reproduced with permission from Elsevier.

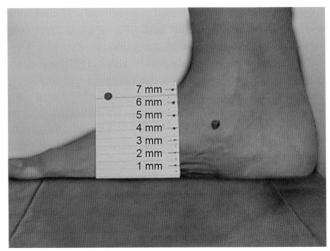

FIG. 13: Navicular drop[107]
Source: Reproduced with permission from Elsevier.

type.[1] Normative value for the FPI has been reported at +4 in the adult population, indicating the norm is a slightly pronated foot posture, with no difference identified based on gender or BMI.[99] The FPI screening form and URL for more detailed information can be found in Appendix I.

Another common measure used to indicate the degree of pronation (and very commonly used in the MTSS literature) is the navicular drop test.[100] With this technique, the clinician marks the most prominent point on the navicular tuberosity, and measures the distance from the ground to the navicular in subtalar neutral, with the subject standing on the leg to be tested and the opposite knee flexed.[92,93,101,102] The patient is then asked to relax with equal weight through the lower-extremities, and the difference in height of the navicular is measured with a ruler or card.[92,93,101,102] (Fig. 13). This gives the clinician a sagittal plane estimate of the amount of arch flattening, or pronation. Several authors have found significantly greater navicular drop in subjects who went on to develop MTSS.[21,27-30] The advantage of this measure is that it reflects a component of foot mobility in addition to structure. Normative values for this measure in the literature vary. Brody originally reported greater than 15 mm representing abnormal pronation, but the rationale for this number was not given.[100] Accepted normative data for navicular drop ranges from 6.0 to 8.1 mm,[101-106] and one author found that college cross country runners were seven times more likely to develop ERLP with a navicular drop greater than 10 mm.[27] It may be important

to compare this measure bilaterally, especially in those with unilateral symptoms where an increase in navicular drop may be considered more clinically relevant.

Ankle Mobility, Flexibility and Strength

Ankle ROM, flexibility and strength should be carefully measured in patients with MTSS. Increased plantar flexion ROM has been implicated by multiple authors to be a risk factor MTSS[28,32] and can be measured with a standard goniometer in supine, prone or short sitting. There is no agreement in the literature on how best to measure the ankle dorsiflexion angle, and a number of techniques exist.[108] Some authors suggest first finding subtalar neutral and then dorsiflexing the ankle, as it has been proposed that a more pronated foot will cause a greater dorsiflexion angle.[108] However, the reliability of identifying subtalar neutral has been questioned, which would in turn call into question the reliability of the ankle dorsiflexion measure.[109] Whatever method the clinician utilizes, he/she should be consistent with the measurement technique for reproducibility upon re-evaluation. Ankle dorsiflexion should be measured with the knee flexed and extended to differentiate between gastrocnemius inflexibility, soleus inflexibility and/or hypomobility of the talocrural joint.[108] Further joint mobility testing of the talocrural joint may be helpful to differentiate between a joint hypomobility or soft tissue restriction. Although ankle dorsiflexion ROM and plantar flexor inflexibility have not been shown to be a risk factor in MTSS, from a biomechanical perspective it is certainly feasible to rationalize how inadequate ankle motion may be contributory. For example, if dorsiflexion is limited during the mid-stance phase of gait, the subtalar joint may pronate excessively to allow for tibial advancement, subsequently leading to a greater bending force on the tibia or requiring greater eccentric contractions of the deep lower leg supinator muscle group. The single limb heel raise test is recommended to assess strength and endurance of the plantar flexors.[110] The patient is allowed to use finger tips for balance assist as the patient raises the heel up until the ankle is in full plantar flexion.[110] The total number of heel raises should be compared side to side, with a normative value reported as 25.[111] This can be performed with the knee extended and the knee flexed to test the gastrocnemius and the soleus respectively[110] (Fig. 14). In addition, calf girth may be assessed with a tape measure to give an indirect measurement of the cross-sectional area. Both decreased lean calf girth and decreased plantar flexor endurance have been noted in subjects with MTSS and may be important objective data for treatment and goal planning.[33,112] Inversion and eversion strength can be assessed manually or with a dynamometer, as it has been reported that subjects with MTSS demonstrate a reduced ratio of invertor to evertor strength.[113] Normal inversion: eversion strength ratios range from 1.10 to 1.33, when tested isokinetically at 30 degrees per second.[113] Those with MTSS have shown an average ratio of 0.95.[113] Decreased inversion strength could potentially cause an increased tendency to pronate, resulting abnormal stresses on the medial tibia or excessive eccentric contractions of the supinator muscles.

A thorough proximal examination is important in capturing various impairments that may be contributing

to pathology. Of special importance in MTSS, is hip rotation ROM measurements, which can be measured short-sitting or prone, with a large range of normative data, and greater total rotational ROM in prone.[110] Several authors have reported significant increases[33] and/or decreases[28,31] in hip rotation ranges that should be measured during physical examination. Hip abductor weakness has been shown to be a predictor of exertional medial tibial pain in college aged women,[114] and this may have significant rehabilitation implications. Decreased proximal strength may result in distal biomechanical impairments that lead to MTSS, and correction of the underlying cause may not only decrease current symptoms, but also decrease the risk of future occurrence.

Functional Assessment

The last, and probably the most important part of the examination, is a functional assessment. Walking gait, running gait, single limb stance, squat, single limb squat, hopping, drop jump landing and take-off or similar functional movements should all be examined during the physical examination. Movements relevant to the individual patient should be assessed to identify impairments that may be contributory to the injury. It has been demonstrated that strengthening exercises allow for increases in strength, but may not carry over to changes in specific neuromuscular movement patterns that are thought to be causing the underlying pathology.[115] Abnormal jumping and landing mechanics have been identified in large, prospective studies as risk factors that predispose subjects to lower extremity musculoskeletal injuries, such as anterior cruciate ligament tears and patellofemoral pain syndrome.[116,117] Recently, increased rotation of the hip and thorax during landing and push-off of a single-leg drop jump was identified as a prospective risk factor in college aged women who went on to develop MTSS.[118] As the lower extremity and deep stabilizing musculature of the trunk combine to create an integrated segment, one can speculate that abnormal rotations from proximal segments will travel distally down the chain, resulting in increased bending forces and/or eccentric traction forces on the posteromedial tibia. Two-dimensional video analysis of functional tasks has become a very useful clinical tool that is easy to perform, and has been shown to be a reliable tool for certain lower extremity biomechanical measures.[119,120] Video gait analysis is becoming more popular in physical therapy, as research regarding gait retraining in various

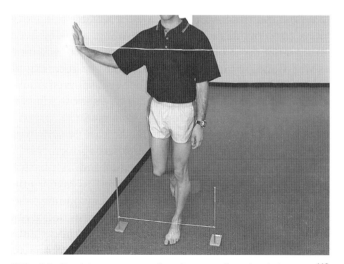

FIG. 14: Participant set-up for the standing heel-rise test[112]
Source: Reproduced with permission from Elsevier.

lower extremity pathologies has demonstrated promising results.[121-124]

PHYSICAL THERAPY TREATMENT

The demand for practicing evidence-based medicine has grown considerably in recent years.[125] Unfortunately, high quality research on the treatment of MTSS is lacking, as a recent systematic review revealed only eleven trials examining the effectiveness of various interventions.[82] Most of these studies demonstrated methodological flaws and high risk of bias, with no study being graded as higher than Level III evidence.[82] There is also no consistency in outcome utilization, as a standardized outcome measure for MTSS does not exist, which makes comparison of findings difficult between studies.[80-82] Several studies have examined the effectiveness of passive modalities, such as iontophoresis, phonophoresis, ice massage, ultrasound and laser treatment.[86,88,126,127] Smith et al. found that there was no difference between groups in pain perception in those who received heel cord stretching in conjunction with either ice massage, iontophoresis, phonophoresis and ultrasound.[126] There was, however, significantly less pain compared to a control group receiving only heel cord stretching,[126] leading one to conclude that some adjunct treatment may augment the benefits of stretching. Another randomized controlled trial (RCT) found no difference in time to completion of a graded running program in a group receiving only a six-phase graded running program versus two treatment groups receiving either compression stockings or strengthening and stretching exercises for the calf musculature, in addition to the graded running program.[81] The use of leg braces has also shown no additional benefit when paired with a graded running program.[87,128] Insight into the optimal treatment of MTSS does not appear to have improved in the past 40 years, when the first RCT was published, finding no significant differences in average days lost running between five different treatment interventions.[57] This presents a frustration for the clinician attempting to practice evidence-based medicine. But the critically thinking clinician will develop an awareness and understanding of the literature, and apply this knowledge, as well as clinical experience and incorporate creative, individualized interventions in conjunction with patient goals to develop an effective treatment plan.[125] A sound understanding of the relevant anatomy, biomechanics, etiology, tissue healing capacity and available literature will allow the physical therapist to develop an effective, individualized course of intervention.

The most important element in developing a treatment plan is determining the patient's goals and expectations. MTSS is most often activity-based, with the majority of patients participating in sports or exercise programs.[2,9] Very few patients present with pain during walking and every day activities.[13] Relative rest and cessation of activity is the most consistent treatment advice given by medical practitioners.[10,39,54,55,57,80,82] While relative rest is most likely an important component of treatment, it is not always necessary to stop activity altogether nor restrict athletic participation. Tibial stress fractures and MTSS are on the same bone-stress failure continuum, but opposite ends of the spectrum.[10,44,48] Multiple studies finding decreased bone mineral density on dual-energy X-ray absorptiometry, or DXA, scan, osteopenic findings on CT scans, and diffuse uptake on MRI and bone scans support this.[2,11,48,49,68,69,72] Therefore, MTSS should initially be treated as a bony injury with an understanding of the severity of symptoms. MTSS has been reported to progress to tibial stress fractures, but this is rare.[10] Certainly, if the patient is limping, having pain with walking and other activities of daily living, the clinician may recommend a walking boot or crutches for a short period of time, until symptoms are absent with these activities.[7] A patient with only activity-based, diffuse posteromedial tibial pain will be managed differently. Assuming a stress fracture has been ruled out, absolute rest from activity is typically not warranted. Instead, the patient should be educated on bony injuries and the healing process.[55] The patient must understand that the bone is breaking down faster than it can build back up, which leads to weakening of the bone and subsequent pain with activity.[55] Low impact activities, such as biking, swimming, upper body weight training and water running can all maintain a patient's fitness level while reducing tibial loading, allowing bone formation.[7,54,55] The initial physical therapy consultation is where the physical therapist identifies training errors, potential injurious workout routines or decreased fitness levels that may have predisposed the patient to injury.[55] Education on these factors is necessary to prevent recurrence of symptoms. A global decrease in activity of 50% has been suggested based on expert opinion,[7,10,54,80] but again, this needs to be individualized. A physical therapist has the advantage of being able to exercise the patient, and record the time it takes for symptom onset to occur. Moen et al. described a running test that can be utilized by physical therapists in the clinic to determine appropriate activity level.[81,128,129] The patient runs on the treadmill until the pain reaches a 4 out of 10 on the visual analog scale.[81,128,129] The time at which the patient rated the pain as 4/10 is recorded and the patient is then placed into a graded running program at an initial intensity that coincided with the running test.[81,128,129] This running test and graded running program has not been validated; however, it offers a more objective way to prescribe activity duration and intensity. Of note, if the patient had pain with walking, then he/she did not begin a graded running program until pain had ceased with walking.[81,128,129] Gradual bone loading is important for strengthening the tibial cortex, and should be progressed in a steady manner by about 10% a week,[7,39,55] depending on symptoms, to stimulate osteoblastic activity. Wolff's Law has established that repeated bone strain causes microdamage.[130] Normally, the bone has the capacity to repair the microdamage and increase the threshold for future stresses and strains.[130] However, repeated strains above the bone's recovery threshold can accumulate and lead to fatigue failure.[130] Non-weight bearing for any extended time beyond a few days is discouraged, as it has been shown that bone remodeling after microdamage is impaired without physiological loading.[131] In other words, the damaged bone needs to be loaded, but clearly to a lesser, therapeutic threshold. Because the tibia bone in a patient with MTSS is osteopenic, the load on the bone needs to be controlled, with adequate rest time to allow repair. The patient should be counseled not only on the gradual loading principle, but also on the importance of taking rest days, or relative rest days, where the patient performs non-impact activities as discussed above.[55] End-stage rehabilitation should also include some form of plyometric activity, as this has shown to cause high in vivo tibial strain rates, which, when gradually introduced and progressed, can result in improved bone strength.[131]

Mobility Restrictions

Identification of various musculoskeletal impairments should also be addressed early in the rehabilitation process. Managing ankle mobility deficits is a common area for clinicians to begin, and dorsiflexion ROM limitations can be addressed in a number of ways. It has been demonstrated that a 3-week intervention of gastrocnemius stretching of five repetitions for 30 seconds performed twice daily resulted in significant improvements in open and closed chain dorsiflexion ROM.[132] There was no difference based on whether the subject performed stretching interventions in weight-bearing versus non-weight bearing.[132] Although not covered in this chapter, talocrural mobilizations may also be utilized if the clinician feels there is a joint hypomobility that is limiting dorsiflexion ROM.

Strength, Endurance and Neuromuscular Activation

Muscular strength and endurance are important to dissipate and absorb forces through the lower extremity, and inadequate muscle performance can result in increased strain on the tibia bone.[133] Specifically, for a number of years decreased plantar flexor endurance has been speculated to result in increased forces on the bone, leading to MTSS.[16] Madeley et al. found that a group of athletes with MTSS had significantly decreased plantar flexor endurance compared to a group of healthy controls.[112] Milgrom et al. used percutaneous strain-gauge staples to measure tibial strain in vivo and found that tension and bending strain rates increased significantly after a marching fatigue protocol, in addition to a significant reduction in gastrocnemius isokinetic torque.[134] Various interventions can be utilized in the clinic to increase the strength and/or endurance of the plantar flexor muscle group. Depending on baseline strength and severity of symptoms, the patient can begin simply using an elastic band, then progress to double limb closed chain calf raises. This can either be performed with body weight, or the clinician can begin heel raises on a leg press to carefully monitor load. The patient can advance to single limb heel raises with upper extremity assist, progressing to no upper extremity assist. Performing the single limb heel raise on a stair or step allows the patient to work the plantar flexors in greater degrees of dorsiflexion. Lastly, additional dumbbells or weighted backpacks can be used to increase the intensity. Eccentric training of the plantar flexors is also a highly effective intervention to improve muscle and tendon strength, and has the advantage of overloading the muscle-tendon complex to a greater degree than concentric based exercise, while requiring less energy.[135-138] A solid strength base needs to be established, and then working into higher repetitions to establish endurance is recommended. The calf musculature should also be trained for power production with some form of plyometrics, as the muscles must overcome large eccentric forces with jumping and cutting activities. Figures 15A to G illustrates a heel raise progression sequence, with emphasis on the eccentric component.

Various extrinsic muscles have been discussed related to their importance in stabilizing the MLA, but special attention must also be paid to the intrinsic foot muscles. In particular, the abductor hallucis is considered an important dynamic stabilizer of the MLA, as it has been shown to elevate the arch when tensioned in isolation.[140] Building on this, Headlee et al. demonstrated navicular

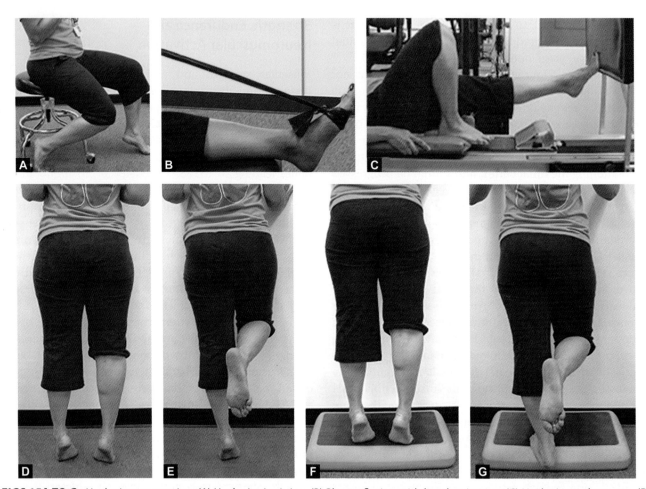

FIGS 15A TO G: Heel raise progression. (A) Heel raise in sitting. (B) Plantar flexion with band resistance. (C) Heel raise on leg press. (D) Double limb heel raise on level ground. (E) Single limb heel raise on level ground. (F) Double limb heel raise off step. (G) Single limb heel raise off step[139]

Source: Reproduced with permission from Elsevier.

drop significantly increased following a fatiguing protocol of the foot intrinsic muscles.[141] Common clinical interventions used to activate the foot intrinsics include towel curls and picking up objects with the toes. A more useful exercise may be the short foot isometric exercise. In this exercise, the patient attempts to lift the arch by pulling the metatarsal heads toward the calcaneus without flexing the toes. Jung et al. reported that the short foot exercise demonstrated significantly greater electromyography (EMG) activation of adductor hallucis, the most significant intrinsic arch stabilizer, and increased arch height compared to the towel curls. Performing the short foot exercise in standing further increased the activation of the abductor hallucis.[142] Undoubtedly, strength and endurance in these muscles provides an important foundation, but neuromuscular activation patterns are

equally important to retrain faulty biomechanics. To teach proper activation, the patient sits in the chair and the clinician instructs the patient to lift the arch of the foot up without curling the toes. The clinician may give tactile cues for intrinsic activation by holding at the metatarsal heads and posterior calcaneus and squeezing lightly (Figs 16A and B). In addition, a piece of paper may be placed under the toes to ensure there is minimal toe flexor activation. This exercise can be progressed to standing, then to single limb balance, and eventually into functional exercises such as the single limb squat and single limb Romanian dead lift (Fig. 17). These exercises can also be progressed to unstable surfaces to further challenge the stabilizing muscles. Certainly other extrinsic muscles, such as the posterior tibialis, peroneals, and tibialis anterior, will also be activated and trained with standing and more functional

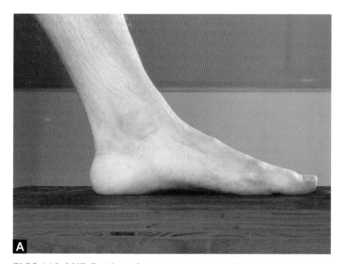
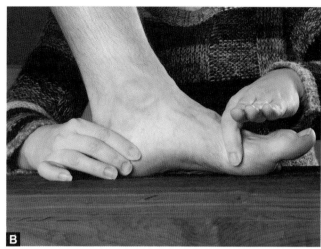

FIGS 16A AND B: Short foot isometric (A) without and (B) with tactile cueing

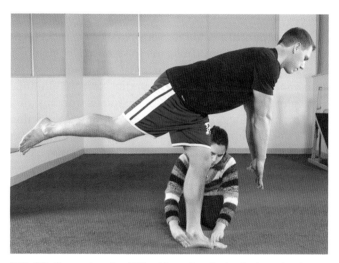

FIG. 17: Romanian dead lift with cueing for intrinsic activation

method to train dynamic stabilizers, the objective is not to train patients to perform voluntary arch activation during running or other sport-specific activities. More proximally based neuromuscular activation functional training program can teach the patient to incorporate these foot positions and lower extremity mechanics into full weight bearing dynamic activity, and will have positive carryover for distal biomechanics as well.

Proximal Considerations

A more proximal treatment approach addressing core strength and stability has been more recently advocated by several authors.[80,114,118] Although debated in the literature, the core will be defined as the lumbopelvic hip complex, which includes osseous and ligamentous structures, local and global stabilizing muscles of the lumbar spine, as well as the hip musculature.[145] Proximal stability is required for optimal biomechanics to avoid excessive motion and impact loading forces on distal segments.[114,118,146] Because all of the lower extremity joints are coupled, excessive proximal movement will transfer down the kinetic chain and cause excessive distal motion.[145] Attempts to control and stabilize this motion may result in greater eccentric contractions of the lower leg musculature and/or excessive tibial bending, both of which have been proposed as a pathomechanical cause of MTSS (Fig. 19). The literature is beginning to support this theory, as Verrelst et al. recently found that subjects who went on to develop MTSS had significantly less hip abduction strength[114] and greater trunk and hip rotation during a single-leg drop jump.[118] Historically, poorly controlled distal movements (i.e. excessive

single limb exercises listed above. Resisted closed chain foot adduction is a good beginning level exercise to activate the tibialis posterior muscle, as shown in Figures 18A and B.[143] The clinician may also have the patient squeeze a ball between the heels during a bilateral heel raise to increase the recruitment of the tibialis posterior. Once an adequate strength base has been established, proprioceptive, balance, single limb strengthening and plyometrics are utilized with an emphasis on appropriate lower extremity mechanics, which trains these muscles to fire in a more functional manner. Along these lines, a useful technique is to have patients remove his/her shoes for various neuromuscular re-education interventions, as this has been shown to increase postural sway and to increase activation of the foot and ankle muscles.[144] While specific activation of the foot intrinsic muscles serve as

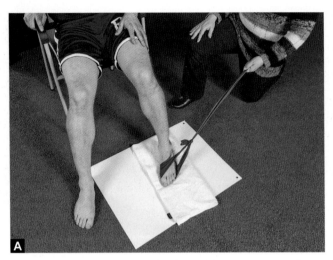 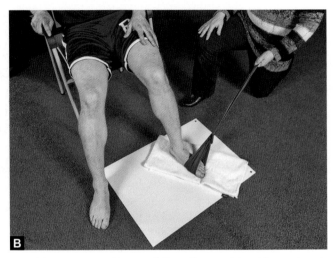

FIGS 18A AND B: Eccentric forefoot adduction exercise demonstrating (A) starting position and B) ending position. The patient is instructed to focus on slow, controlled eccentric contractions

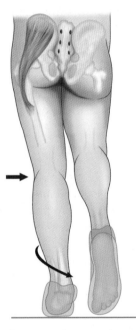

FIG. 19: A weak gluteus medius muscle can result in excessive hip adduction, knee valgus and pronatory collapse of the lower extremity. This movement impairment may result in excessive tibial bending or excessive eccentric contractions of the deep posterior lower leg muscles, both of which may lead to MTSS

pronation causing excessive movement up the chain) were theorized to cause the overload in MTSS. More recent research has begun to identify proximal strength impairments and movement dysfunctions as risk factors in common musculoskeletal pathologies.[115,124,145-149] As biomechanical experts, physical therapists have an

excellent opportunity to intervene and retrain movement patterns and thereby mitigate the causative factor(s). The musculature of the core most often targeted for proximal stabilization includes the deep abdominal and gluteal muscle groups. The gluteus medius and maximus each have portions that contribute to abduction and external rotation of the hip, and play an important role in lumbopelvic transverse and frontal plane stabilization.[150-152] Inadequate strength is not always the culprit, but rather a deficit in timing, coordination and activation patterns—even with adequate force production—can result in dysfunction and pathology. Initial interventions and exercises should focus on proper recruitment, and progress from less-challenging to more-challenging.[151] This may start very basically with gluteal isometrics, which have been shown to recruit the gluteus maximus to 81% of maximal voluntary isometric contraction (MVIC).[153] Additional open chain gluteal exercises demonstrated include: in Figures 20A and B, side-lying clam shells (53% MVIC gluteus maximus and 47% MVIC gluteus medius); in Figures 21A and B, side-lying hip abduction (51% MVIC gluteus maximus and 63% MVIC gluteus medius) and in Figures 22A and B, quadruped hip extension (60% MVIC gluteus maximus and 47% MVIC gluteus medius).[153-155] The clam shell specifically has demonstrated low tensor fascia lata to gluteus medius activation ratio.[152] The clinician may need to use verbal and tactile cueing for gluteal contraction, as an important criteria to progress is the ability to voluntarily contract the gluteals. The patient must understand basic activation patterns before progressing to more functional positions.

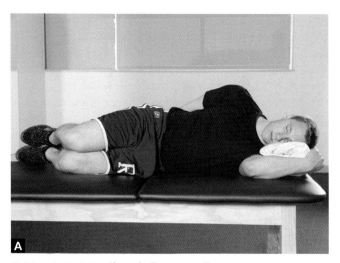
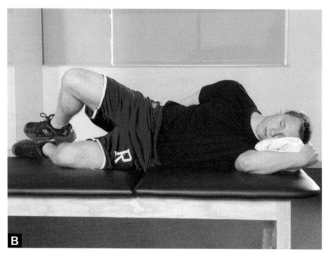

FIGS 20A AND B: Clam shell exercise illustrating (A) starting position and (B) ending position. Emphasis should be placed on gluteal activation while maintaining correct pelvic alignment

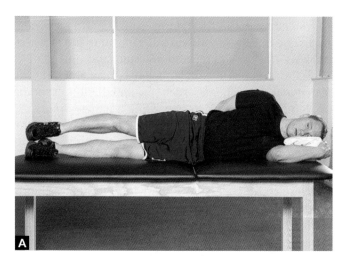
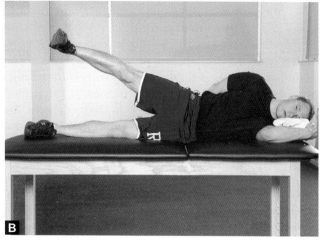

FIGS 21A AND B: Side lying hip abduction exercise illustrating (A) starting position and (B) ending position. Emphasis should be placed on gluteal activation with pelvis rolled forward slightly to put the leg in line with the fiber direction of the gluteus medius muscle

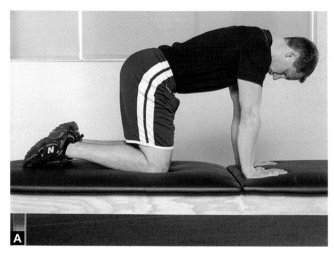
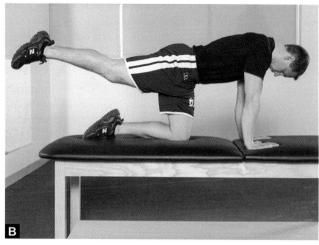

FIGS 22A AND B: Quadruped hip extension exercise illustrating (A) starting position and (B) ending position. Emphasis should be placed on maintaining a neutral spine while extending the hip and activating the gluteus maximus with tactile and verbal cueing for proper activation

Once recruitment patterns have been established, exercises can be progressed to closed chain, more functional movements. The body weight squat is a good starting point for many closed chain exercises. The patient can be taught appropriate lower extremity mechanics with the basic squat that can be carried over to a variety of single limb activities. Figures 23A to D illustrate the proper form for a body weight squat with common verbal cues for proper mechanics in all three cardinal planes. The hip hike exercise is an excellent tool not only to increase strength of the gluteus medius (58% MVIC)[153] but also to teach patients gluteal and pelvic control in the weight bearing position. The patient stands on the edge of a box and hikes the hip up on the non-stance limb while focusing on squeezing the gluteal muscles on the stance limb (Figs 24A and B). Once these two exercises have been mastered, a single limb squat progression can begin. The single limb squat has demonstrated greater than 70% MVIC for gluteus maximus and medius[153] and requires good lower extremity and trunk control. Figures 25A to F outline a progression for single limb squat, starting with a small 4 inch step, and progressing to squats with hand held weight. This exercise may be performed on a box (similar to the lateral step up) to avoid the patient having to flex the non-stance hip in front of them. The step height can also be increased strategically to control the depth of single limb squat. Although these exercises above report on EMG activity for the gluteal muscles, the abdominal and lumbar musculature are also active. Most of the literature on spinal stabilization focuses on

low back pain, and controversy exists regarding how to train these muscles. Some authors emphasize training the deep core muscles (transverse abdominis and multifidi), while others emphasize a more global stabilizing approach.[156] Whatever approach the clinician utilizes, the progression should begin with simple exercises and progress to more dynamic, complex exercises (similar to the single limb progression), where the core muscles must act as an integrated unit to maintain lumbopelvic stability.[157] Most importantly, the skilled clinician needs to provide appropriate cues and feedback to train optimal movement patterns.

Gait Retraining

Interest in the role of gait retraining in runners presenting with various musculoskeletal overuse injuries is on the rise. Physical therapists have the ability to analyze movement patterns to identify gait abnormalities and intervene to decrease abnormal loads on tissue.[158] Video analysis can be a helpful, simple tool to implement in the clinic to observe the patient's mechanics during functional movements, such as ambulation, running or jumping. The video recording enables frame by frame analysis which can aid not only in identifying impairments, but also in educating the patient.[159] Support for gait retraining is growing, as it has been shown that basic strengthening of specific muscles often does not result in a change in underlying mechanics that is suspected to lead to pathology.[115,160] Running kinematics,

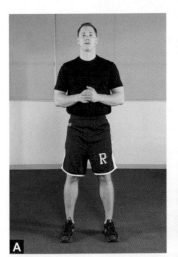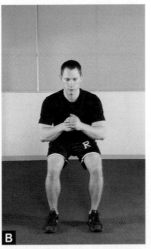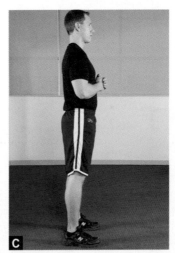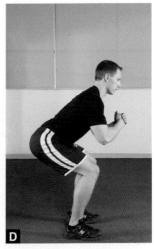

FIGS 23A TO D: Proper squat form is an important fundamental movement pattern to teach early on in the rehabilitation process. (A and B) These figures illustrate starting position from the frontal and sagittal perspective, respectively. (C and D) These figures illustrate the ending position from the frontal and sagittal perspective, respectively. The patient needs to be cued to keep the knees behind the toe, keep a neutral spine, and maintain good frontal and transverse plane alignment of the hips and knees

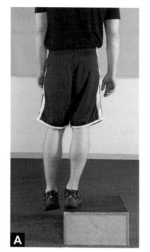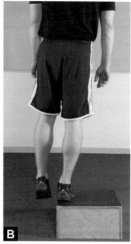

FIGS 24A AND B: Hip hike exercise illustrating the (A) beginning position and (B) ending position

kinetics and gait retraining have not been studied in the MTSS population specifically; however, there have been several studies examining these factors in relation to tibial stress fracture.[147,161-163] As previously noted, MTSS and tibial stress fracture lie on the same bone-stress injury continuum, with MTSS being a beginning level stress reaction,[5] therefore it is only logical to examine these more global movement considerations in managing patients with MTSS. Milner et al. found that a group of subjects with a history of tibial stress fracture had significantly greater impact loading rates and tibial shock as measured with motion analysis software, force plate, and tibial accelerometer.[162] In a follow-up study, Crowell and Davis attached an accelerometer to the distal tibia of uninjured subjects with high baseline peak positive tibial acceleration and then used real-time visual feedback to identify if these associated factors could be reduced with

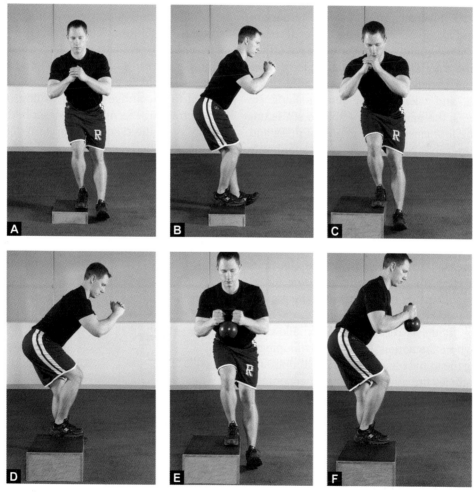

FIGS 25A TO F: Single limb squat progression, viewed from the frontal and sagittal planes, respectively, beginning with (A and B) 4 inch step, (C and D) 8 inch step and (E and F) 8 inch step with free weight. Frontal and transverse hip and knee control is emphasized, as is an appropriate hip hinge from the lateral view

gait retraining.[122] In eight sessions over 2 weeks with a reduced feedback model, subjects were able to reduce impact loading rates by 30% and tibial acceleration by 50%, and maintain these changes at 1 month follow-up.[122] Although the exact mechanism the runners used to reduce these variables was not investigated in this study, other studies have shed light on this area.[164]

In a small case series, subjects with patellofemoral pain syndrome altered their landing pattern with the use of a force transducer in the heel of the running shoe connected to an audible buzzer that would sound when initial contact was made with the heel.[165] With the same reduced feedback model as noted above, ground reaction forces measured on an instrumented treadmill revealed decreased impact loading rates with a non-heel first landing that subjects were able to maintain at 3 month follow-up.[165] A number of studies have identified a relationship between heel striking and higher ground reaction forces,[166-168] which may be an important variable to address in the MTSS population to decrease the loading, and, subsequently, the bending force on the tibia. The clinician may encourage a flatter foot strike pattern in the clinic by cueing the patient to land softly, avoid heel strike, and take shorter, quicker steps. By taking shorter steps, the patient is not able to stride out as far, keeping the foot closer to the center of mass and encouraging a flatter foot contact. A strategy commonly used and easily implemented clinically is modifying the runner's cadence.[169,170] Increasing the step rate by 5–10% alone has shown significant reductions in vertical loading rates and can be readily incorporated by the clinician with the use of a metronome.[159,170] For example, if a patient has a cadence of 160 steps per minute and the clinician would like to increase that cadence by 5% (to 168 steps per minute), the clinician can set a metronome for 84 beats per minute and cue the patient to strike the ground with the right foot every time he/she hears the beat. A reduced feedback model is recommended to allow for motor learning, where the patient has the metronome on at all times during the initial phases of gait retraining, and then gradually reduces the audible cueing to encourage integration over a period of 2–6 weeks.[121-124]

While the above strategy focuses on reducing lower extremity loading variables, another approach is to address abnormal mechanics in the frontal and transverse planes. This relates back to lumbopelvic stability and proximal to distal control of the lower extremity. An abnormal gait pattern that commonly presents involves excessive hip adduction, hip internal rotation, and contralateral pelvic drop, with apparent valgus collapse of the knee.[115,123,124] Although this pattern is most studied in patellofemoral pain, there may be gait retraining implications for MTSS, as coupled motion from proximal to distal may result in excessive pronation at the subtalar and midtarsal joints and/or excessive medial tibial bending.[114,118] Associations between increased hip adduction during stance phase of running gait and a history of tibial stress fracture have been identified,[147,161] lending support to this theory. Success in retraining these factors has been demonstrated in both the laboratory and clinical setting.[90,122,123] Before retraining commences, it is important to teach appropriate gluteal activation patterns as discussed in the lumbopelvic recruitment section above. The use of a full length mirror with verbal cues for gluteal recruitment during running has been successful in significantly reducing contralateral pelvic drop and hip adduction in subjects with patellofemoral pain syndrome.[124] Cues utilized by Willy et al. that may be used to improve lower extremity alignment include "squeeze your buttock muscles" and "keep your knee caps pointed straight ahead."[124] Figures 26A and B demonstrate pre-gait and post-gait retraining mechanical changes. Again, a reduced feedback model should be utilized to encourage motor learning. The two potential gait retraining techniques described above provide examples of interventions supported by the literature, but the specific type of gait retraining should be based on each individual presentation after a thorough physical

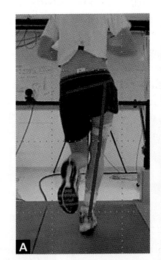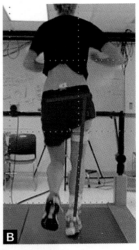

FIGS 26A AND B: Representative subject during treadmill running (A) Pre-gait and (B) Post-gait retraining. Note the reduction of contralateral pelvic drop and hip adduction in the post-condition. This subject demonstrated a 3.8°, 8.1° and 4.5° reduction in contralateral pelvic drop, hip adduction and thigh adduction, respectively[124]

Source: Reproduced with permission from Elsevier.

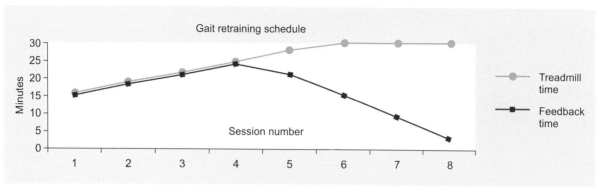

FIG. 27: The gait retraining schedule. Over the first four visits, run time and feedback time is increased from 15 minutes to 24 minutes. Over the last four visits, run time is increased to 30 minutes while feedback is faded to 3 minutes by the eighth visit[124]

Source: Reproduced with permission from Elsevier.

examination and video running analysis. Important parameters to remember in gait retraining include initially restricting running to in the clinic, to discourage resorting back to faulty mechanics, the use of a reduced feedback model, and with progression of run time as demonstrated in Figure 27. Advancing running volume gradually allows the body to adapt to new stresses, and the use of appropriate verbal cues as well as some type of biofeedback encourages appropriate changes.[90,122-124] Basic motor learning principles emphasize the difference between internally focused learning (patient's awareness of body movements) and externally focused learning (patient focusing on completion of an outside task). Research suggests that externally focused learning may be a more effective method for patients to successfully change movement patterns.[171,172] For example, a retraining technique to shorten stride length may be to provide an internal cue to the patient to land with a flatter foot. In contrast, setting a metronome to 5% above the patient's preferred cadence will also result in a flatter foot contact, and this external cue can be gradually reduced to allow motor learning.

Shoe Prescription and Orthotics

Excessive pronation has been identified as a risk factor by several investigators,[21,27-30] therefore, consideration of the role of orthotics and shoe prescription in those with MTSS is relevant. Orthotics are a very common intervention utilized in the clinic,[7,39] but minimal evidence to support this intervention can be found in scientific literature. Loudon and Dolphino reported that 15 of 23 subjects with MTSS prescribed off the shelf orthotics and calf stretching reported a 50% decrease in

symptoms.[173] The lack of control group for comparison and the follow-up of only 3 weeks, makes the conclusion somewhat suspect. In a prospective, RCT of 146 military conscripts, there was a significant reduction in shin splint incidence in subjects receiving custom foot orthoses compared to subjects receiving no intervention.[174] However, it must be noted that findings from military studies are not always generalizable to runners or other sport specific populations.[175] Contradictory evidence also permeates the research: two authors reported a significant increase in MTSS incidence in those who used orthotics at baseline testing.[12,32] Despite the inability to draw sound conclusions regarding orthotic effectiveness, many clinicians may utilize orthotics based on theoretical and biomechanical evidence. The rationale for orthotics is that by controlling excessive pronation, there will be decreased bending moments on the distal tibia and decreased demand and velocity of eccentric contractions for the subtalar and midtarsal supinators. Several authors have reported decreases in eversion excursion and velocity with kinematic analyses.[176-179] If orthotics are included in the plan of care, it may be wise to first trial off the shelf orthotics, which offer the advantage of reduced cost and faster implementation. Several investigators have found that off the shelf and semi-custom orthotics perform comparably to custom orthotics.[180-182] The clinician should also thoroughly investigate the patient's shoes for signs of abnormal or excessive wear. Older shoes have been shown to be associated with an increased rate of injury in runners,[24] and kinematic variables change considerably with increased wear.[183] Clinicians commonly prescribe running shoes based on foot shape and motion, with overpronators (low arch) prescribed motion control shoes, minimal pronators (normal arch) prescribed stability shoes and supinators (high arch) prescribed cushion shoes.[23,184,185] This is often accepted as the best practice; however, studies examining biomechanical factors and injury rates offer no evidence to warrant this approach.[185] In two large, military based, randomized controlled trials there was no difference in injury risk when assigning shoes based on plantar shape of the foot.[186,187] Similar findings have also been identified in female runners randomized to different shoe conditions.[184] Based on these findings, clinicians should avoid prescribing orthotics or a new type of shoes routinely to every individual with MTSS. The need for orthotics and shoe prescription can be incorporated into the plan of care, but should be based on an individual assessment and as an adjunct to other interventions. As is the case with most of the treatment options for MTSS, further research is needed in well-designed randomized controlled trials to identify effective interventions. Of particular importance, the clinician should identify if the pathology is stemming from the ground up or from the trunk down. In other words, is excessive pronation truly because the foot is abnormal and needs to be braced or are there proximal factors that can be addressed to decrease the overall medial collapse of the lower extremity.

Alternative Treatments and Medical Interventions

In the event conservative treatment fails, alternative treatments should be considered with the last consideration being surgery. One treatment intervention that has been growing in popularity is extracorporeal shockwave therapy (ESWT), which has shown promising results in two different studies examining pain and time required to complete a graded running program.[129,188] Evidence exists that MTSS is due to mechanical overloading of the bone, leading it to appear osteopenic on CT scans[11,49] and demonstrate decreased bone density on DEXA scans.[48] During ESWT, a high-intensity sound wave is delivered through a focused applicator head that causes a mechanical disruption in the tissue.[129,188] Several studies have shown improvements in bone healing by inducing microfractures that result in increased angiogenesis and delivery of growth-factors, ultimately promoting osteogenesis.[189-191] This is a potential modality that could be employed by physical therapists and deserves further research in large RCTs. Another treatment option that has been examined in a small case series with reported benefits is ultrasound guided subperiosteal prolotherapy injection, which may be a consideration

in chronic MTSS.[192] Corticosteroid injections have been utilized in the past, but concern for long-term weakening of tissue structures limit its appeal.[193] Platelet-Rich Plasma (PRP), autologous whole blood, and dry needling are all interventions that have shown promise in other musculoskeletal conditions and may be considered in the treatment of MTSS.[194,195] Surgical treatment is rarely indicated and is only considered for refractory cases that have failed all conservative treatment measures, but different procedures have been described in the literature with good outcomes.[41,196,197] These procedures include fasciotomy of the posteromedial tibia and/or removal of a periosteal strip along the tibia.[76]

CONCLUSION

Medial tibial stress syndrome (MTSS) is a common pathology in physically active individuals. The pathology is most likely due to bony overload of the posteromedial border, however, it is unknown if this is due to excessive bending forces, soft tissue traction, some combination of the two or other mechanisms that have not yet been identified. MTSS is a clinical diagnosis, but advanced imaging such as triple phase bone scintigraphy or MRI may be helpful when stress fracture is suspected. Conservative management is typical, and most athletes will return to prior level of activity with appropriate education and rehabilitation. The role of the physical therapist is to identify causative factors not only to manage current symptoms, but to also correct underlying movement impairments that may contribute to future occurrence or exacerbation. In addition to these interventions, the skilled practitioner can guide the patient through an appropriate progression of activity that will allow the patient to his/her prior level of activity in a safe and efficient process with relative, rather than absolute, rest. At present, there are minimal findings to support any form of treatment is better than rest alone, and high quality research is needed in the future.

REFERENCES

1. Yates B, White S. The incidence and risk factors in the development of medial tibial stress syndrome among naval recruits. Am J Sports Med. 2004;32(3):772-80.
2. Moen MH, Tol JL, Weir A, Steunebrink M, De Winter TC. Medial tibial stress syndrome: a critical review. Sports Med. 2009;39(7):523-46.
3. Andrish J. The leg. Orthopaedic Sports Medicine: Principles and Practice, 2nd edition. Pennsylvania: Saundors P; 2003. pp. 2155-9.
4. Beck BR, Osternig LR. Medial tibial stress syndrome. The location of muscles in the leg in relation to symptoms. J Bone Joint Surg Am. 1994;76(7):1057-61.

5. Bouche RT, Johnson CH. Medial tibial stress syndrome (tibial fasciitis): a proposed pathomechanical model involving fascial traction. J Am Podiatr Med Assoc. 2007;97(1):31-6.

6. Detmer DE. Chronic shin splints. Classification and management of medial tibial stress syndrome. Sports Med. 1986;3(6):436-46.

7. Kortebein PM, Kaufman KR, Basford JR, Stuart MJ. Medial tibial stress syndrome. Med Sci Sports Exerc. 2000;32(3 Suppl):S27-33.

8. Michael RH, Holder LE. The soleus syndrome. A cause of medial tibial stress (shin splints). Am J Sports Med. 1985;13(2):87-94.

9. Tweed JL, Avil SJ, Campbell JA, Barnes MR. Etiologic factors in the development of medial tibial stress syndrome: a review of the literature. J Am Podiatr Med Assoc. 2008;98(2):107-11.

10. Beck BR. Tibial stress injuries. An aetiological review for the purposes of guiding management. Sports Med. 1998;26(4):265-79.

11. Gaeta M, Minutoli F, Scribano E, Ascenti G, Vinci S, Bruschetta D, et al. CT and MR imaging findings in athletes with early tibial stress injuries: comparison with bone scintigraphy findings and emphasis on cortical abnormalities. Radiology. 2005;235(2):553-61.

12. Plisky MS, Rauh MJ, Heiderscheit B, Underwood FB, Tank RT. Medial tibial stress syndrome in high school cross-country runners: incidence and risk factors. J Orthop Sports Phys Ther. 2007;37(2):40-7.

13. Reinking M, Austin T, Hayes A. A survey of exercise-related leg pain in community runners. Int J Sports Phys Ther. 2013;8(3):269-76.

14. Devas MB. Stress fractures of the tibia in athletes or shin soreness. J Bone Joint Surg Br. 1958;40-B(2):227-39.

15. American Medical Association. Standard Nomenclature of Athletic Injuries Presented by Subcommittee on Classification of Sports Injuries. Illinois: AMA C; 1966. p. 122.

16. Clement DB. Tibial stress syndrome in athletes. J Sports Med. 1974;2(2):81-5.

17. Puranen J. The medial tibial syndrome: exercise ischemia in the medial fascial compartment of the leg. J Bone Joint Surg Br. 1974;56-B(4):712-5.

18. Mubarak SJ, Gould RN, Lee YF, Schmidt DA, Hargens AR. The medial tibial stress syndrome. A cause of shin splints. Am J Sports Med. 1982;10(4):201-5.

19. Johnell O, Rausing A, Wendeberg B, Westlin N. Morphological bone changes in shin splints. Clin Orthop Relat Res. 1982;167:180-4.

20. Reinking MF, Austin TM, Hayes AM. Exercise-related leg pain in collegiate cross-country athletes: extrinsic and intrinsic risk factors. J Orthop Sports Phys Ther. 2007;37(11):670-8.

21. Bennett JE, Reinking MF, Pluemer B, Pentel A, Seaton M, Killian C. Factors contributing to the development of medial tibial stress syndrome in high school runners. J Orthop Sports Phys Ther. 2001;31(9):504-10.

22. Taunton JE, Ryan MB, Clement DB, McKenzie DC, Lloyd-Smith DR, Zumbo BD. A retrospective case-control analysis of 2002 running injuries. Br J Sports Med. 2002;36(2):95-101.

23. Fields KB, Sykes JC, Walker KM, Jackson JC. Prevention of running injuries. Curr Sports Med Rep. 2010;9(3):176-82.

24. Taunton JE, Ryan MB, Clement DB, McKenzie DC, Lloyd-Smith DR, Zumbo BD. A prospective study of running injuries: the Vancouver sun run "in training" clinics. Br J Sports Med. 2003;37(3):239-44.

25. Lopes AD, Hespanhol Junior LC, Yeung SS, Costa LO. What are the main running-related musculoskeletal injuries? A systematic review. Sports Med. 2012;42(10):891-905.

26. Newman P, Witchalls J, Waddington G, Adams R. Risk factors associated with medial tibial stress syndrome in runners: a systematic review and meta-analysis. Open Access Jounral of Sports Medicine. 2013;4:229-41.

27. Bennett JE, Reinking MF, Rauh MJ. The relationship between isotonic plantar flexor endurance, navicular drop, and exercise-related leg pain in a cohort of collegiate cross-country runners. Int J Sports Phys Ther. 2012;7(3):267-78.

28. Moen MH, Bongers T, Bakker EW, Zimmermann WO, Weir A, Tol JL, et al. Risk factors and prognostic indicators for medial tibial stress syndrome. Scand J Med Sci Sports. 2012;22(1):34-9.

29. Reinking MF. Exercise-related leg pain in female collegiate athletes: the influence of intrinsic and extrinsic factors. Am J Sports Med. 2006;34(9):1500-7.

30. Raissi GR, Cherati AD, Mansoori KD, Razi MD. The relationship between lower extremity alignment and medial tibial stress syndrome among non-professional athletes. Sports Med Arthrosc Rehabil Ther Technol. 2009;1(1):11.

31. Yagi S, Muneta T, Sekiya I. Incidence and risk factors for medial tibial stress syndrome and tibial stress fracture in high school runners. Knee Surg Sports Traumatol Arthrosc. 2013;21(3):556-63.

32. Hubbard TJ, Carpenter EM, Cordova ML. Contributing factors to medial tibial stress syndrome: a prospective investigation. Med Sci Sports Exerc. 2009;41(3):490-6.

33. Burne SG, Khan KM, Boudville PB, Mallet RJ, Newman PM, Steinman LJ, et al. Risk factors associated with exertional medial tibial pain: a 12 month prospective clinical study. Br J Sports Med. 2004;38(4):441-5.

34. Reinking MF, Hayes AM. Intrinsic factors associated with exercise-related leg pain in collegiate cross-country runners. Clin J Sport Med. 2006;16(1):10-4.

35. Winters M, Veldt H, Bakker E, Moen M. Intrinsic factors associated with medial tibial stress syndrome in athletes: a large case-control study. South African Journal of Sports Medicine. 2013;25(3):63-7.

36. Takebe K, Nakagawa A, Minami H, Kanazawa H, Hirohata K. Role of the fibula in weight-bearing. Clin Orthop Relat Res. 1984(184):289-92.

37. Moore K, Dalley A, Agur A. Clinically Oriented Anatomy, 6th edition. Baltimore: Lippincott Williams & Wilkins; 2010.

38. Clanton TO, Solcher BW. Chronic leg pain in the athlete. Clin Sports Med. 1994;13(4):743-59.

39. Edwards PH Jr, Wright ML, Hartman JF. A practical approach for the differential diagnosis of chronic leg pain in the athlete. Am J Sports Med. 2005;33(8):1241-9.

40. Larkin B, Stewart J. Compartment syndrome testing. The sports medicine resource manual. In: Seidenberg P, Beutler A (Eds). Philadelphia, PA: Elsevier; 2008. pp. 561-7.

41. Wallensten R. Results of fasciotomy in patients with medial tibial syndrome or chronic anterior-compartment syndrome. J Bone Joint Surg Am. 1983;65(9):1252-5.

42. Saxena A, O'Brien T, Bunce D. Anatomic dissection of the tibialis posterior muscle and its correlation to medial tibial stress syndrome. J Foot Surg. 1990;29(2):105-8.

43. Garth WP Jr, Miller ST. Evaluation of claw toe deformity, weakness of the foot intrinsics, and posteromedial shin pain. Am J Sports Med. 1989;17(6):821-7.

44. Stickley CD, Hetzler RK, Kimura IF, Lozanoff S. Crural fascia and muscle origins related to medial tibial stress syndrome symptom location. Med Sci Sports Exerc. 2009;41(11):1991-6.

45. Allen MJ, O'Dwyer FG, Barnes MR, Belton IP, Finlay DB. The value of 99Tcm-MDP bone scans in young patients with exercise-induced lower leg pain. Nucl Med Commun. 1995;16(2):88-91.

46. Anderson MW, Ugalde V, Batt M, Gacayan J. Shin splints: MR appearance in a preliminary study. Radiology. 1997;204(1):177-80.

47. Bhatt R, Lauder I, Finlay DB, Allen MJ, Belton IP. Correlation of bone scintigraphy and histological findings in medial tibial syndrome. Br J Sports Med. 2000;34(1):49-53.

48. Magnusson HI, Ahlborg HG, Karlsson C, Nyquist F, Karlsson MK. Low regional tibial bone density in athletes with medial tibial stress syndrome normalizes after recovery from symptoms. Am J Sports Med. 2003;31(4):596-600.

49. Gaeta M, Minutoli F, Vinci S, Salamone I, D'Andrea L, Bitto L, et al. High-resolution CT grading of tibial stress reactions in distance runners. AJR Am J Roentgenol. 2006;187(3):789-93.

50. Franklyn M, Oakes B, Field B, Wells P, Morgan D. Section modulus is the optimum geometric predictor for stress fractures and medial tibial stress syndrome in both male and female athletes. Am J Sports Med. 2008;36(6):1179-89.

51. Giladi M, Milgrom C, Simkin A, Stein M, Kashtan H, Margulies J, et al. Stress fractures and tibial bone width. A risk factor. J Bone Joint Surg Br. 1987;69(2):326-9.

52. Milgrom C, Giladi M, Simkin A, Rand N, Kedem R, Kashtan H, et al. The area moment of inertia of the tibia: a risk factor for stress fractures. J Biomech. 1989;22(11-12):1243-8.

53. Lanyon LE, Hampson WG, Goodship AE, Shah JS. Bone deformation recorded in vivo from strain gauges attached to the human tibial shaft. Acta Orthop Scand. 1975;46(2):256-68.

54. Couture CJ, Karlson KA. Tibial stress injuries: decisive diagnosis and treatment of 'shin splints'. Phys Sportsmed. 2002;30(6):29-36.

55. Craig DI. Current developments concerning medial tibial stress syndrome. Phys Sportsmed. 2009;37(4):39-44.

56. Fredericson M, Bergman AG, Hoffman KL, Dillingham MS. Tibial stress reaction in runners. Correlation of clinical symptoms and scintigraphy with a new magnetic resonance imaging grading system. Am J Sports Med. 1995;23(4):472-81.

57. Andrish JT, Bergfeld JA, Walheim J. A prospective study on the management of shin splints. J Bone Joint Surg Am. 1974;56(8):1697-700.

58. Van Gent RN, Siem D, Van Middelkoop M, van Os AG, Bierma-Zeinstra SM, Koes BW. Incidence and determinants of lower extremity running injuries in long distance runners: a systematic review. Br J Sports Med. 2007;41(8):469-80.

59. Newman P, Adams R, Waddington G. Two simple clinical tests for predicting onset of medial tibial stress syndrome: shin palpation test and shin oedema test. Br J Sports Med. 2012;46(12):861-4.

60. Shindle MK, Endo Y, Warren RF, Lane JM, Helfet DL, Schwartz EN, et al. Stress fractures about the tibia, foot, and ankle. J Am Acad Orthop Surg. 2012;20(3):167-76.

61. Batt ME, Kemp S, Kerslake R. Delayed union stress fractures of the anterior tibia: conservative management. Br J Sports Med. 2001;35(1):74-7.

62. Beals RK, Cook RD. Stress fractures of the anterior tibial diaphysis. Orthopedics. 1991;14(8):869-75.

63. Paik RS, Pepple DA, Hutchinson MR. Chronic exertional compartment syndrome. BMJ. 2013;346.

64. Davis DE, Raikin S, Garras DN, Vitanzo P, Labrador H, Espandar R. Characteristics of patients with chronic exertional compartment syndrome. Foot Ankle Int. 2013;34(10):1349-54.

65. George CA, Hutchinson MR. Chronic exertional compartment syndrome. Clin Sports Med. 2012;31(2):307-19.

66. Packer JD, Day MS, Nguyen JT, Hobart SJ, Hannafin JA, Metzl JD. Functional outcomes and patient satisfaction after fasciotomy for chronic exertional compartment syndrome. Am J Sports Med. 2013;41(2):430-6.

67. Pedowitz RA, Hargens AR, Mubarak SJ, Gershuni DH. Modified criteria for the objective diagnosis of chronic compartment syndrome of the leg. Am J Sports Med. 1990;18(1):35-40.

68. Batt ME, Ugalde V, Anderson MW, Shelton DK. A prospective controlled study of diagnostic imaging for acute shin splints. Med Sci Sports Exerc. 1998;30(11):1564-71.

69. Holder LE, Michael RH. The specific scintigraphic pattern of "shin splints in the lower leg": concise communication. J Nucl Med. 1984;25(8):865-9.

70. Zwas ST, Elkanovitch R, Frank G. Interpretation and classification of bone scintigraphic findings in stress fractures. J Nucl Med. 1987;28(4):452-7.

71. Goldfarb CR, Ongseng F. Interpretation and classification of bone scintigraphic findings in stress fractures. J Nucl Med. 1988;29(6):1150-2.

72. Aoki Y, Yasuda K, Tohyama H, Ito H, Minami A. Magnetic resonance imaging in stress fractures and shin splints. Clin Orthop Relat Res. 2004;421:260-7.

73. Beck BR, Bergman AG, Miner M, Arendt EA, Klevansky AB, Matheson GO, et al. Tibial stress injury: relationship of radiographic, nuclear medicine bone scanning, MR imaging, and CT severity grades to clinical severity and time to healing. Radiology. 2012;263(3):811-8.

74. Patel DS, Roth M, Kapil N. Stress fractures: diagnosis, treatment, and prevention. Am Fam Physician. 2011;83(1):39-46.

75. Berger FH, de Jonge MC, Maas M. Stress fractures in the lower extremity. The importance of increasing awareness amongst radiologists. Eur J Radiol. 2007;62(1):16-26. 76. Reshef N, Guelich DR. Medial tibial stress syndrome. Clin Sports Med. 2012;31(2):273-90.

77. Brukner P, Bennell K. Stress fractures: there causes and principles of treatment. In: Baxter D, Porter D, Schon L (Eds). Baxter's the Foot and Ankle in Sport, 2nd edition. Elsevier; 2008. pp. 45-72.

78. Tuite MJ. Imaging of triathlon injuries. Radiol Clin North Am. 2010;48(6):1125-35.

79. Rothstein J, Campbell S, Echternach J, Jette A, Knecht H, Rose S. Standards for tests and measurements in physical therapy practice. Physical Therapy. 1991;71:589-622.

80. Galbraith RM, Lavallee ME. Medial tibial stress syndrome: conservative treatment options. Curr Rev Musculoskelet Med. 2009;2(3):127-33.

81. Moen MH, Holtslag L, Bakker E, Barten C, Weir A, Tol JL, et al. The treatment of medial tibial stress syndrome in athletes: a randomized clinical trial. Sports Med Arthrosc Rehabil Ther Technol. 2012;4:12.

82. Winters M, Eskes M, Weir A, Moen MH, Backx FJ, Bakker EW. Treatment of medial tibial stress syndrome: a systematic review. Sports Med. 2013;43(12):1315-33.

83. Binkley JM, Stratford PW, Lott SA, Riddle DL. The lower extremity functional scale (LEFS): scale development, measurement properties, and clinical application. North American Orthopaedic Rehabilitation research network. Phys Ther. 1999;79(4):371-83.

84. Nelson E, Trabulsi G, Ryan M, Heiderscheit B. Development of the university of wisconsin running injury and recovery index. American Physical Therapy Association Combined Sections Meeting. 2012.

85. Nelson E, Wille C, Chumanov E, Heiderscheit B. Reliability and validity of the university of Wisconsin running injury and recovery index: a pilot study. American Physical Therapy Association Combined Sections Meeting. 2013.

86. Robertson M. The relative effectiveness of periosteal pecking combined with therapeutic ultrasound compared to therapeutic ultrasound in the treatment of medial tibial stress syndrome type II. [Master's degree in technology: chiropractic]. Durban, South Africa: Faculty of Health at the Durban Institute of Technology. Available from URL: http://ir.dut.ac.za/bitstream/handle/10321/166/Robertson_2003.pdf?sequence=5. Accessed December 8, 2013.

87. Johnston E, Flynn T, Bean M, Breton M, Scherer M, Dreitzler G, et al. A randomized controlled trial of a leg orthosis versus traditional treatment for soldiers with shin splints: a pilot study. Mil Med. 2006;171(1):40-4.

88. Nissen LR, Astvad K, Madsen L. Low-energy laser therapy in medial tibial stress syndrome. Ugeskr Laeger. 1994;156(49):7329-31.

89. Aweid O, Gallie R, Morrissey D, Crisp T, Maffulli N, Malliaras P, et al. Medial tibial pain pressure threshold algometry in runners. Knee Surg Sports Traumatol Arthrosc. 2014;22(7):1549-55.

90. Davis I. Gait retraining in runners. Orthopaedic Practice. 2005;17(2):8-13.

91. Billis E, Katsakiori E, Kapodistrias C, Kapreli E. Assessment of foot posture: correlation between different clinical techniques. The Foot. 2007;17(2):65-72.

92. Menz HB. Alternative techniques for the clinical assessment of foot pronation. J Am Podiatr Med Assoc. 1998;88(3):119-29.

93. Razeghi M, Batt ME. Foot type classification: a critical review of current methods. Gait Posture. 2002;15(3):282-91.
94. Scharfbillig R, Evans AM, Copper AW, Williams M, Scutter S, Iasiello H, et al. Criterion validation of four criteria of the foot posture index. J Am Podiatr Med Assoc. 2004;94(1):31-8.
95. Keenan AM, Redmond AC, Horton M, Conaghan PG, Tennant A. The foot posture index: Rasch analysis of a novel, foot-specific outcome measure. Arch Phys Med Rehabil. 2007;88(1):88-93.
96. Redmond AC, Crosbie J, Ouvrier RA. Development and validation of a novel rating system for scoring standing foot posture: the foot posture index. Clin Biomech (Bristol, Avon). 2006;21(1):89-98.
97. Cornwall MW, McPoil TG, Lebec M, Vicenzino B, Wilson J. Reliability of the modified foot posture index. J Am Podiatr Med Assoc. 2008;98(1):7-13.
98. Evans AM, Copper AW, Scharfbillig RW, Scutter SD, Williams MT. Reliability of the foot posture index and traditional measures of foot position. J Am Podiatr Med Assoc. 2003;93(3):203-13.
99. Redmond AC, Crane YZ, Menz HB. Normative values for the foot posture index. J Foot Ankle Res. 2008;1(1):6.
100. Brody DM. Techniques in the evaluation and treatment of the injured runner. Orthop Clin North Am. 1982;13(3):541-58.
101. Allen MK, Glasoe WM. Metrecom measurement of navicular drop in subjects with anterior cruciate ligament injury. J Athl Train. 2000;35(4):403-6.
102. Mueller MJ, Host JV, Norton BJ. Navicular drop as a composite measure of excessive pronation. J Am Podiatr Med Assoc. 1993;83(4):198-202.
103. Nielsen RG, Rathleff MS, Simonsen OH, Langberg H. Determination of normal values for navicular drop during walking: a new model correcting for foot length and gender. J Foot Ankle Res. 2009;2:12.
104. Shrader JA, Popovich JM Jr, Gracey GC, Danoff JV. Navicular drop measurement in people with rheumatoid arthritis: interrater and intrarater reliability. Phys Ther. 2005;85(7):656-64.
105. McPoil TG, Cornwall MW. The relationship between static lower extremity measurements and rearfoot motion during walking. J Orthop Sports Phys Ther. 1996;24(5):309-14.
106. Sell KE, Verity TM, Worrell TW, Pease BJ, Wigglesworth J. Two measurement techniques for assessing subtalar joint position: a reliability study. J Orthop Sports Phys Ther. 1994;19(3):162-7.
107. Magrum E, Wilder RP. Evaluation of the injured runner. Clin Sports Med. 2010;29(3):331-45.
108. Gatt A, Chockalingam N. Clinical assessment of ankle joint dorsiflexion: a review of measurement techniques. J Am Podiatr Med Assoc. 2011;101(1):59-69.
109. Picciano AM, Rowlands MS, Worrell T. Reliability of open and closed kinetic chain subtalar joint neutral positions and navicular drop test. J Orthop Sports Phys Ther. 1993;18(4):553-8.
110. Hislop H, Montgomery J. Daniels and Worthingma's Muscle Testing: Techniques of Manual Examination, 8th edition. St. Louis, MO: Saunders Elsevier; 2007.
111. Lunsford BR, Perry J. The standing heel-rise test for ankle plantar flexion: criterion for normal. Phys Ther. 1995;75(8):694-8.
112. Madeley LT, Munteanu SE, Bonanno DR. Endurance of the ankle joint plantar flexor muscles in athletes with medial tibial stress syndrome: a case-control study. J Sci Med Sport. 2007;10(6):356-62.
113. Yuksel O, Ozgurbuz C, Ergun M, I legen C, Taskiran E, Denerel N, et al. Inversion/Eversion strength dysbalance in patients with medial tibial stress syndrome. J Sports Sci Med. 2011;10(4):737-42.
114. Verrelst R, Willems T, De Clercq D, Roosen P, Goossens L, Witvrouw E. The role of hip abductor and external rotator muscle strength in the development of exertional medial tibial pain: a prospective study. Br J Sports Med. 2014;48(21):1564-9.
115. Willy RW, Davis IS. The effect of a hip-strengthening program on mechanics during running and during a single-leg squat. J Orthop Sports Phys Ther. 2011;41(9):625-32.
116. Hewett TE, Myer GD, Ford KR, Heidt RS Jr, Colosimo AJ, McLean SG, et al. Biomechanical measures of neuromuscular control and valgus loading of the knee predict anterior cruciate ligament injury risk in female athletes: a prospective study. Am J Sports Med. 2005;33(4):492-501.
117. Boling MC, Padua DA, Marshall SW, Guskiewicz K, Pyne S, Beutler A. A prospective investigation of biomechanical risk factors for patellofemoral pain syndrome: the joint undertaking to monitor and prevent ACL injury (JUMP-ACL) cohort. Am J Sports Med. 2009;37(11):2108-16.
118. Verrelst R, Clercq D, Vanrenterghem J, Willems T, Palmans T, Witvrouw E. The role of proximal dynamic joint stability in the development of exertional medial tibial pain: a prospective study. Br J Sports Med. 2014;48(5):388-93.
119. McLean SG, Walker K, Ford KR, Myer GD, Hewett TE, van den Bogert AJ. Evaluation of a two dimensional analysis method as a screening and evaluation tool for anterior cruciate ligament injury. Br J Sports Med. 2005;39(6):355-62.
120. Munro A, Herrington L., Carolan M. Reliability of 2-dimensional video assessment of frontal-plane dynamic knee valgus during common athletic screening tasks. J Sport Rehabil. 2012;21(1):7-11.
121. Barrios JA, Crossley KM, Davis IS. Gait retraining to reduce the knee adduction moment through real-time visual feedback of dynamic knee alignment. J Biomech. 2010;43(11):2208-13.
122. Crowell HP, Davis IS. Gait retraining to reduce lower extremity loading in runners. Clin Biomech (Bristol, Avon). 2011;26(1):78-83.
123. Noehren B, Scholz J, Davis I. The effect of real-time gait retraining on hip kinematics, pain and function in subjects with patellofemoral pain syndrome. Br J Sports Med. 2011;45(9):691-6.
124. Willy RW, Scholz JP, Davis IS. Mirror gait retraining for the treatment of patellofemoral pain in female runners. Clin Biomech (Bristol, Avon). 2012;27(10):1045-51.
125. Jette DU, Bacon K, Batty C, Carlson M, Ferland A, Hemingway RD, et al. Evidence-based practice: beliefs, attitudes, knowledge, and behaviors of physical therapists. Phys Ther. 2003;83(9):786-805.
126. Smith W, Winn F, Parette R. Comparative study using four modalities in shinsplint treatments. J Orthop Sports Phys Ther. 1986;8(2):77-80.
127. Singh A, Sethy G, Sandhu J, Sinha A. A comparative study of the efficacy of iontophoresis and phonophoresis in the treatment of shin splint. Physiotherapy. The Journal of the Indian Association of Physiotherapists. 2002-2003;1(1):2013-17-20.
128. Moen MH, Bongers T, Bakker EW, Weir A, Zimmermann WO, van der Werve M, et al. The additional value of a pneumatic leg brace in the treatment of recruits with medial tibial stress syndrome; a randomized study. J R Army Med Corps. 2010;156(4):236-40.
129. Moen MH, Rayer S, Schipper M, Schmikli S, Weir A, Tol JL, et al. Shockwave treatment for medial tibial stress syndrome in athletes; a prospective controlled study. Br J Sports Med. 2012;46(4):253-7.
130. Frost HM. A 2003 update of bone physiology and wolff's law for clinicians. Angle Orthod. 2004;74(1):3-15.
131. Milgrom C, Miligram M, Simkin A, Burr D, Ekenman I, Finestone A. A home exercise program for tibial bone strengthening based on in vivo strain measurements. Am J Phys Med Rehabil. 2001;80(6):433-8.
132. Dinh NV, Freeman H, Granger J, Wong S, Johanson M. Calf stretching in non-weight bearing versus weight bearing. Int J Sports Med. 2011;32(3):205-10.
133. Radin EL. Role of muscles in protecting athletes from injury. Acta Med Scand Suppl. 1986;711:143-7.
134. Milgrom C, Radeva-Petrova DR, Finestone A, Nyska M, Mendelson S, Benjuya N, et al. The effect of muscle fatigue on in vivo tibial strains. J Biomech. 2007;40(4):845-50.
135. Alfredson H, Pietila T, Jonsson P, Lorentzon R. Heavy-load eccentric calf muscle training for the treatment of chronic achilles tendinosis. Am J Sports Med. 1998;26(3):360-6.

136. Langberg H, Ellingsgaard H, Madsen T, Jansson J, Magnusson SP, Aagaard P, et al. Eccentric rehabilitation exercise increases peritendinous type I collagen synthesis in humans with achilles tendinosis. Scand J Med Sci Sports. 2007;17(1):61-6.

137. Ohberg L, Lorentzon R, Alfredson H. Eccentric training in patients with chronic achilles tendinosis: normalised tendon structure and decreased thickness at follow up. Br J Sports Med. 2004;38(1):8-11.

138. Stanish WD, Rubinovich RM, Curwin S. Eccentric exercise in chronic tendinitis. Clin Orthop Relat Res. 1986;208:65-8.

139. Mulligan E. Lower leg, ankle, and foot rehabilitation. In: Andrews J, Harrelson G, Wilk K (Eds). Physical Rehabilitation of the Injured Athlete, 4th edition. Elsevier; 2012. pp. 426-63.

140. Wong YS. Influence of the abductor hallucis muscle on the medial arch of the foot: a kinematic and anatomical cadaver study. Foot Ankle Int. 2007;28(5):617-20.

141. Headlee DL, Leonard JL, Hart JM, Ingersoll CD, Hertel J. Fatigue of the plantar intrinsic foot muscles increases navicular drop. J Electromyogr Kinesiol. 2008;18(3):420-5.

142. Jung DY, Kim MH, Koh EK, Kwon OY, Cynn HS, Lee WH. A comparison in the muscle activity of the abductor hallucis and the medial longitudinal arch angle during toe curl and short foot exercises. Phys Ther Sport. 2011;12(1):30-5.

143. Kulig K, Burnfield JM, Requejo SM, Sperry M, Terk M. Selective activation of tibialis posterior: evaluation by magnetic resonance imaging. Med Sci Sports Exerc. 2004;36(5):862-7.

144. Landry SC, Nigg BM, Tecante KE. Standing in an unstable shoe increases postural sway and muscle activity of selected smaller extrinsic foot muscles. Gait Posture. 2010;32(2):215-9.

145. Chuter VH, Janse de Jonge XA. Proximal and distal contributions to lower extremity injury: a review of the literature. Gait Posture. 2012;36(1):7-15.

146. Lawrence RK 3rd, Kernozek TW, Miller EJ, Torry MR, Reuteman P. Influences of hip external rotation strength on knee mechanics during single-leg drop landings in females. Clin Biomech (Bristol, Avon). 2008;23(6):806-13.

147. Milner CE, Hamill J, Davis IS. Distinct hip and rearfoot kinematics in female runners with a history of tibial stress fracture. J Orthop Sports Phys Ther. 2010;40(2):59-66.

148. Dolak KL, Silkman C, Medina McKeon J, Hosey RG, Lattermann C, Uhl TL. Hip strengthening prior to functional exercises reduces pain sooner than quadriceps strengthening in females with patellofemoral pain syndrome: a randomized clinical trial. J Orthop Sports Phys Ther. 2011;41(8):560-70.

149. Fukuda TY, Rossetto FM, Magalhaes E, Bryk FF, Lucareli PR, de Almeida Aparecida Carvalho N. Short-term effects of hip abductors and lateral rotators strengthening in females with patellofemoral pain syndrome: a randomized controlled clinical trial. J Orthop Sports Phys Ther. 2010;40(11):736-42.

150. Hamstra-Wright KL, Huxel Bliven K. Effective exercises for targeting the gluteus medius. J Sport Rehabil. 2012;21(3):296-300.

151. Reiman MP, Bolgla LA, Loudon JK. A literature review of studies evaluating gluteus maximus and gluteus medius activation during rehabilitation exercises. Physiother Theory Pract. 2012;28(4):257-68.

152. Selkowitz DM, Beneck GJ, Powers CM. Which exercises target the gluteal muscles while minimizing activation of the tensor fascia lata? Electromyographic assessment using fine-wire electrodes. J Orthop Sports Phys Ther. 2013;43(2):54-64.

153. Boren K, Conrey C, Le Coguic J, Paprocki L, Voight M, Robinson TK. Electromyographic analysis of gluteus medius and gluteus maximus during rehabilitation exercises. Int J Sports Phys Ther. 2011;6(3):206-23.

154. Bolgla LA, Uhl TL. Electromyographic analysis of hip rehabilitation exercises in a group of healthy subjects. J Orthop Sports Phys Ther. 2005;35(8):487-94.

155. Distefano LJ, Blackburn JT, Marshall SW, Padua DA. Gluteal muscle activation during common therapeutic exercises. J Orthop Sports Phys Ther. 2009;39(7):532-40.

156. Standaert CJ, Herring SA. Expert opinion and controversies in musculoskeletal and sports medicine: core stabilization as a treatment for low back pain. Arch Phys Med Rehabil. 2007;88(12):1734-6.

157. Kibler WB, Press J, Sciascia A. The role of core stability in athletic function. Sports Med. 2006;36(3):189-98.

158. Heiderscheit BC. Gait retraining for runners: in search of the ideal. J Orthop Sports Phys Ther. 2011;41(12):909-10.

159. Schubert A, Kempf J, Heiderscheit B. Influence of stride frequency and length on running mechanics: a systematic review. Sports Health. 2013.

160. Wouters I, Almonroeder T, Dejarlais B, Laack A, Willson JD, Kernozek TW. Effects of a movement training program on hip and knee joint frontal plane running mechanics. Int J Sports Phys Ther. 2012;7(6):637-46.

161. Pohl MB, Mullineaux DR, Milner CE, Hamill J, Davis IS. Biomechanical predictors of retrospective tibial stress fractures in runners. J Biomech. 2008;41(6):1160-5.

162. Milner CE, Ferber R, Pollard CD, Hamill J, Davis IS. Biomechanical factors associated with tibial stress fracture in female runners. Med Sci Sports Exerc. 2006;38(2):323-8.

163. Zadpoor AA, Nikooyan AA. The relationship between lower-extremity stress fractures and the ground reaction force: a systematic review. Clin Biomech (Bristol, Avon). 2011;26(1):23-8.

164. Clansey AC, Hanlon M, Wallace ES, Nevill A, Lake MJ. Influence of tibial shock feedback training on impact loading and running economy. Med Sci Sports Exerc. 2013.

165. Cheung RT, Davis IS. Landing pattern modification to improve patellofemoral pain in runners: a case series. J Orthop Sports Phys Ther. 2011;41(12):914-9.

166. Shih Y, Lin KL, Shiang TY. Is the foot striking pattern more important than barefoot or shod conditions in running? Gait Posture. 2013;38(3):490-4.

167. Lieberman DE. What we can learn about running from barefoot running: an evolutionary medical perspective. Exerc Sport Sci Rev. 2012;40(2):63-72.

168. Lieberman DE, Venkadesan M, Werbel WA, Daoud AI, D'Andrea S, Davis IS, et al. Foot strike patterns and collision forces in habitually barefoot versus shod runners. Nature. 2010;463(7280):531-5.

169. Hobara H, Sato T, Sakaguchi M, Sato T, Nakazawa K. Step frequency and lower extremity loading during running. Int J Sports Med. 2012;33(4):310-3.

170. Heiderscheit BC, Chumanov ES, Michalski MP, Wille CM, Ryan MB. Effects of step rate manipulation on joint mechanics during running. Med Sci Sports Exerc. 2011;43(2):296-302.

171. Johnson L, Burridge JH, Demain SH. Internal and external focus of attention during gait re-education: an observational study of physical therapist practice in stroke rehabilitation. Phys Ther. 2013;93(7):957-66.

172. Wulf G, Hoss M, Prinz W. Instructions for motor learning: differential effects of internal versus external focus of attention. J Mot Behav. 1998;30(2):169-79.

173. Loudon JK, Dolphino MR. Use of foot orthoses and calf stretching for individuals with medial tibial stress syndrome. Foot Ankle Spec. 2010;3(1):15-20.

174. Larsen K, Weidich F, Leboeuf-Yde C. Can custom-made biomechanic shoe orthoses prevent problems in the back and lower extremities? A randomized, controlled intervention trial of 146 military conscripts. J Manipulative Physiol Ther. 2002;25(5):326-31.

175. Hume P, Hopkins W, Rome K, Maulder P, Coyle G, Nigg B. Effectiveness of foot orthoses for treatment and prevention of lower limb injuries: a review. Sports Med. 2008;38(9):759-79.

176. McMillan A, Payne C. Effect of foot orthoses on lower extremity kinetics during running: a systematic literature review. J Foot Ankle Res. 2008; 1(1):13.

177. Dixon SJ, McNally K. Influence of orthotic devices prescribed using pressure data on lower extremity kinematics and pressures beneath the shoe during running. Clin Biomech (Bristol, Avon). 2008;23(5):593-600.

178. Eslami M, Begon M, Hinse S, Sadeghi H, Popov P, Allard P. Effect of foot orthoses on magnitude and timing of rearfoot and tibial motions, ground reaction force and knee moment during running. J Sci Med Sport. 2009;12(6):679-84.

179. MacLean CL, an Emmerik R, Hamill J. Influence of custom foot orthotic intervention on lower extremity intralimb coupling during a 30-minute run. J Appl Biomech. 2010;26(4):390-9.

180. Finestone A, Novack V, Farfel A, Berg A, Amir H, Milgrom C. A prospective study of the effect of foot orthoses composition and fabrication on comfort and the incidence of overuse injuries. Foot Ankle Int. 2004;25(7):462-6.

181. Zifchock RA, Davis I. A comparison of semi-custom and custom foot orthotic devices in high- and low-arched individuals during walking. Clin Biomech (Bristol, Avon). 2008;23(10):1287-93.

182. Dixon SJ. Influence of a commercially available orthotic device on rearfoot eversion and vertical ground reaction force when running in military footwear. Mil Med. 2007;172(4):446-50.

183. Kong PW, Candelaria NG, Smith DR. Running in new and worn shoes: a comparison of three types of cushioning footwear. Br J Sports Med. 2009;43(10):745-9.

184. Ryan MB, Valiant GA, McDonald K, Taunton JE. The effect of three different levels of footwear stability on pain outcomes in women runners: a randomised control trial. Br J Sports Med. 2011;45(9):715-21.

185. Richards CE, Magin PJ, Callister R. Is your prescription of distance running shoes evidence-based? Br J Sports Med. 2009;43(3):159-62.

186. Knapik JJ, Brosch LC, Venuto M, Swedler DI, Bullock SH, Gaines LS, et al. Effect on injuries of assigning shoes based on foot shape in air force basic training. Am J Prev Med. 2010;38(1 Suppl):S197-211.

187. Knapik JJ, Trone DW, Swedler DI, Villasenor A, Bullock SH, Schmied E, et al. Injury reduction effectiveness of assigning running shoes based on plantar shape in marine corps basic training. Am J Sports Med. 2010;38(9):1759-67.

188. Rompe JD, Cacchio A, Furia JP, Maffulli N. Low-energy extracorporeal shock wave therapy as a treatment for medial tibial stress syndrome. Am J Sports Med. 2010;38(1):125-32.

189. Moretti B, Notarnicola A, Garofalo R, Moretti L, Patella S, Marlinghaus E, et al. Shock waves in the treatment of stress fractures. Ultrasound Med Biol. 2009;35(6):1042-49.

190. Wang L, Qin L, Lu HB, Cheung WH, Yang H, Wong WN, et al. Extracorporeal shock wave therapy in treatment of delayed bone-tendon healing. Am J Sports Med. 2008;36(2):340-7.

191. Taki M, Iwata O, Shiono M, Kimura M, Takagishi K. Extracorporeal shock wave therapy for resistant stress fracture in athletes: a report of 5 cases. Am J Sports Med. 2007;35(7):1188-92.

192. Curtin M, Crisp T, Malliaras P, Padhiar N. The effectiveness of prolotherapy in the management of recalcitrant medial tibial stress syndrome: a pilot study. Br J Sports Med. 2011;45(e1):2013.

193. Warriner AH, Saag KG. Glucocorticoid-related bone changes from endogenous or exogenous glucocorticoids. Curr Opin Endocrinol Diabetes Obes. 2013;20(6):510-6.

194. Moraes VY, Lenza M, Tamaoki MJ, Faloppa F, Belloti JC. Platelet-rich therapies for musculoskeletal soft tissue injuries. Cochrane Database Syst Rev. 2013;12:CD010071.

195. Thanasas C, Papadimitriou G, Charalambidis C, Paraskevopoulos I, Papanikolaou A. Platelet-rich plasma versus autologous whole blood for the treatment of chronic lateral elbow epicondylitis: a randomized controlled clinical trial. Am J Sports Med. 2011;39(10):2130-4.

196. Holen KJ, Engebretsen L, Grontvedt T, Rossvoll I, Hammer S, Stoltz V. Surgical treatment of medial tibial stress syndrome (shin splint) by fasciotomy of the superficial posterior compartment of the leg. Scand J Med Sci Sports. 1995;5(1):40-3.

197. Jarvinen M, Aho H, Niittymaki S. Results of the surgical treatment of the medial tibial syndrome in athletes. Int J Sports Med. 1989;10(1):55-7.

CHAPTER 15

Plantar Heel Pain

Kris B Porter

ABSTRACT

Plantar heel pain, a category of musculoskeletal disease that includes various anatomical structures, is an important public health concern because of the frequency, chronicity and disability associated with this condition. The average duration of a plantar heel pain episode is 6–12 months; however, 90% of cases are treated successfully with evidence-based conservative care. This common disorder is experienced by 10–15% of Americans, leads to 2 million patient visits per year and is the most common foot condition seen in physical therapy clinics. This chapter balances the best scientific evidence with a collaborative reasoning process that leverages the clinician's expertise with the patient's values and expectations, outlining a pathway for the patient and clinician to quickly and completely resolve the symptoms and disability associated with plantar heel pain.

■ INTRODUCTION

Plantar heel pain can originate from many different sources but often involves the plantar fascia, notably at its insertion near the medial calcaneal tubercle or in the mid-portion proximal to the metatarsal heads (Fig. 1). Most cases of plantar fasciitis may not be a true inflammatory condition, as histological findings do not typically produce inflammatory cells. Chronic cases are more accurately described as "plantar fasciosis", notably if the symptoms persist beyond what would be expected during the inflammatory stage of healing. Histological findings of chronic plantar fascia pathology typically include fascial thickening, fibrosis, collagen necrosis, angiofibroblastic hyperplasia, chondroid metaplasia, disorganized collagen and zones of avascularity.[1] Plantar fasciosis can be further classified as insertional versus non-insertional and can involve the lateral, central or medial parts of the plantar fascia (Fig. 1). Plantar fasciosis may be referred to as the

following: plantar fasciitis (plantar), heel pain syndrome, plantar heel pain and plantar fascial fibromatosis, among others. The differential diagnosis list for plantar heel pain is extensive and is discussed in more detail in the clinical examination section.

Plantar heel pain is an important public health concern because of the frequency, chronicity and disability associated with the condition. This common disorder is experienced by 10–15% of Americans which leads to 2 million patient visits per year, and 1% of all visits to orthopedic clinics.[2,3] Additionally, it is considered to be the most common foot condition seen in physical therapy clinics and the most common condition seen in podiatric clinics with a frequency of greater than 40%.[3,4] The average duration of a plantar heel pain episode is 6–10 months, and approximately 90% of cases are treated successfully with conservative care within 6–12 months of symptom onset.[5-7] This condition is experienced most commonly in middle age between 45–64, but is frequently seen in those

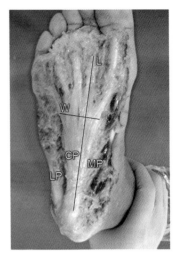

LP, lateral part; CP, central part; MP, medial part; L, length; W, width.

FIG. 1: Axial view of the plantar fascia
Source: Reproduced from an open-access article published by PLoS One.

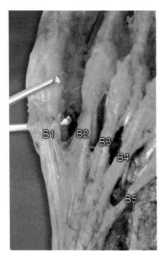

FIG. 2: : Five plantar fascia bundles of the central part of the plantar fascia. B1-5
Source: Reproduced from an open-access article published by PLoS One.

younger than 45 years of age. There is a higher incidence in females versus males and in the athletic population. For example, plantar heel pain accounts for up to 8–10% of all running-related injuries.[8]

Anatomy

The plantar fascia is a layer of connective tissue supporting the plantar aspect of the foot and consisting of five bundles (Fig. 2). Because of its relatively variable fiber orientation, it may be best referred to as fascia versus the more linear orientation commonly associated with the term aponeurosis. The insertion of the plantar fascia travels from the medial calcaneal tubercle to the deep transverse ligaments of the metatarsal heads and proximal phalanx of each toe, splitting around the metatarsal heads to form the fibrous flexor sheath on the plantar aspect of each toe. The plantar fascia is contiguous with the paratenon of the Achilles tendon and is firmly joined to the muscles of the arch of the foot. The fascia blends in with the associated skin and subcutaneous tissue forming a complex, multi-structural enthesis as it originates into the periosteum of the calcaneus.[9,10] The plantar heel pad (fat pad) is a viscoelastic multilobular fatty mass responsible for absorbing up to 110% of body weight during walking and 250% during running.[11] The fat pad naturally deforms during weight bearing, and shows increased deformation during barefoot walking versus shod walking illustrating its collaborative role in attenuating load in the plantar heel along with the plantar fascia.

In weight bearing, the foot may be described as a triangular truss (Fig. 3). During static weight-bearing, the

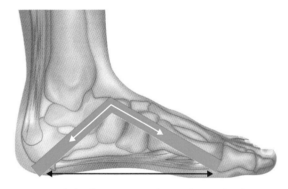

FIG. 3: Truss of the foot. The rearfoot (talus and calcaneus) can be likened to the posterior strut, and the 1st ray (the largest metatarsal along with the medial cuneiform and navicular) can be likened to the anterior strut, connected by the plantar fascia tie-rod (black arrow). In weight bearing, the anterior and posterior strut are compressed, which creates tension (black arrow) and foot stability via the plantar fascia and other soft tissues of the plantar aspect of the foot
Source: Reproduced with permission from Elsevier.

tibia loads the peak of the truss which creates tension in the plantar fascia. The tension created in the plantar fascia adds critical stability to a loaded foot with minimal muscle activity. Surgical release of the plantar fascia will generate forces through the foot that may lead to early onset of midfoot arthritis, lateral foot pain, ultimate rupture of the spring ligament, as well as other pathologies.[12-14] The medial collateral ligament (deltoid ligament), notably the spring ligament portion, contributes to formation of the medial longitudinal arch and, if sprained or weakened, will shift load to other structures such as the plantar fascia (Fig. 4).[15]

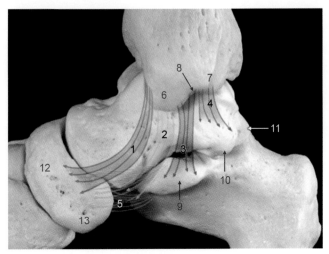

FIG. 4: Schematic representation of the main components of the medial collateral ligament. (1) Tibionavicular ligament; (2) tibiospring ligament; (3) tibiocalcaneal ligament; (4) deep posterior tibiotalar ligament; (5) spring ligament complex (plantar and superomedial calcaneonavicular ligaments); (6) anterior culliculus; (7) posterior culliculus; (8) intercullicular groove; (9) sustentaculum tali; (10) medial talar process; (11) lateral talar process; (12) navicular; (13) navicular tuberosity[16]

Source: Reproduced from an open-access article via Springerlink.

The plantar fascia is further tensioned via the windlass mechanism (Fig. 5). This mechanism creates plantar fascia tension (as well as tension in several intrinsic and extrinsic toe muscles) as the toes extend during terminal stance and preswing.[17] This tension not only creates compression of the anterior and posterior struts of the truss leading to elevation of the medial longitudinal arch, but also contributes to rearfoot supination and plantar flexion of the metatarsals as the foot itself shortens and narrows. This is most noticeable via 1st metatarsophalangeal (1st MTP) joint extension, in part because of the large diameter of this axis relative to toes 2 through 5, although all toes contribute to the windlass mechanism. During stance phase of the gait cycle, most humans shift their weight toward the 1st MTP from loading response toward preswing and toe-off, highlighting the importance of 1st ray stability during the gait cycle.

Intrinsic Muscles

The first layer of intrinsic muscles originates on the calcaneus and associated soft tissues. The flexor digitorum

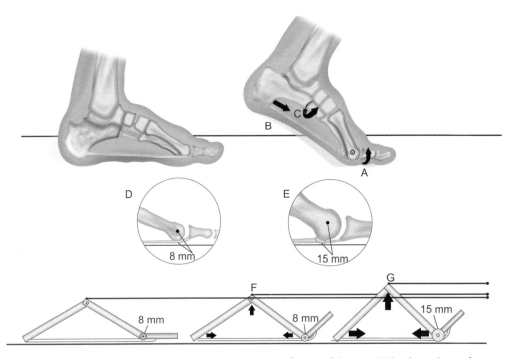

FIG. 5: The Windlass Mechanism. Between mid-stance and pre-swing, dorsiflexion of the toes (A) leads to plantar fascia tension (B) which leads to approximation of the forefoot and rearfoot and elevation of the arch (C). The average lesser metatarsal has 8 mm between the transverse axis and the plantar fascia (D) versus the first metatarsal average of 15 mm which is due to a larger metatarsal head and the presence of the sesamoids (E). Dorsiflexion of the lesser digits (F) creates less tension in the plantar fascia versus the great toe (G). Therefore, the lesser digits have less influence on arch height than the first metatarsal

Source: Reproduced with permission from Newton Biomechanics.

brevis (FDB) inserts onto the proximal phalanx of toes 2–5. The abductor hallucis (AH) inserts on the proximal phalanx of the 1st toe. The abductor digiti minimi (ADM) inserts on the proximal phalanx just on the 5th toe. In the second layer, the lumbrical muscles, like in the hand, will plantar flex the MTP and extend the distal interphalangeal (DIP) and proximal inerphalangeal joints of toes 2–5. In the third layer, the flexor hallucis brevis (FHB) inserts into the proximal phalanx from its origin around the midtarsal region on the 1st toe along with the adductor hallucis (Figs 6 and 7). There is some evidence that tension in the plantar fascia decreases concurrently with increasing tension in the intrinsic muscles of the foot, illustrating the role of these muscles in arch support and in protecting the plantar fascia.[18] Fatigue in the intrinsic muscles has been postulated to increase pronation and loss of medial longitudinal arch height.[19] Additionally, there is evidence of plantar intrinsic muscle atrophy in a plantar fasciitis population.[20] Although studies are limited, it has been suggested that 13–36% of body weight can be borne by the intrinsic muscles of the foot further highlighting the important role of the intrinsic muscles in stabilizing the foot.[21]

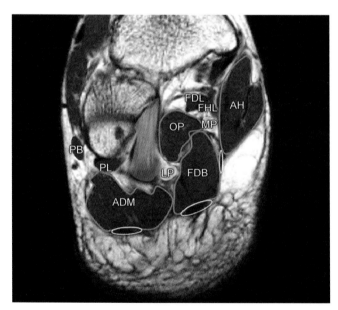

ADM, abductor digiti minimi; AH, abductor hallucis; FDB, flexor digitorum brevis; QP, quadratus plantae. The nerves: LP, lateral plantar nerve; MP, medial plantar nerve. The tendons: FDL, flexor digitorum longus; FHL, flexor hallucis longus; PB, peroneal brevis; PL, peroneus longus.

FIG. 6: Coronal T1-weighted image through the midfoot showing the important anatomical structures related to the central and lateral bands of the plantar fascia (ovals)

Source: Reproduced with permission from Thieme Medical Publishers, Inc.

Extrinsic Muscles

The primary plantar flexors reside in the superficial posterior compartment and play a critical role during nearly all weight bearing activities by controlling ankle dorsiflexion, knee flexion and hip flexion during antigravity closed chain movements.[22,23] The soleus muscle volume is larger than that of all other muscles in the leg, and the soleus is more active than the gastrocnemius (GN) during walking, squatting and running, notably in the intermediate and late stages of these movements, when the body is under the most load.[23] When the plantar flexors are fatigued, center of mass (COM) displacements increase, highlighting this muscle group's importance during balance-related tasks.[24,25] When the subtalar joint is in a pronated position, the triceps surae may contribute to pronation and when in a supinated position may contribute to supination.[23] This illustrates the variable and dynamic function of the superficial posterior compartment in supporting the foot.

The muscles of the deep posterior compartment have important roles in stabilizing the foot in various planes while also generating plantar flexion torque. Rupture of the posterior tibialis leads to acquired flat foot deformity and a variety of other pathologies such as: spring ligament rupture, plantar ligament rupture and plantar fasciitis indicating its role in stabilizing the foot and plantar heel structures.[13,14] The extrinsic toe flexors generate an important stabilizing force to maintain metatarsal head and phalange surface area contact with the ground, contributing to a stable platform for push off.

During gait from loading response to approximately mid-stance, the lateral hip muscles (gluteus medius, minimus and tensor fascia latae) function to eccentrically control adduction of the femur and to stabilize the pelvis in the frontal plane, important components of preventing excessive pronation. In the transverse plane, the deep hip external rotators, posterior fibers of the gluteus medius and the gluteus maximus assist with eccentrically controlling internal rotation of the femur and ultimately pronation. Experimentally, hip fatigue of the abductors has been shown to increase only medial-lateral postural sway, resulting in increased peroneus longus activity.[26] In contrast, fatigue of the hip extensors leads to increased postural sway velocity and variability in a single leg task in both the anterior/posterior and medial/lateral directions.[27] A recent study has shown that an increase in postural challenges in single leg stance lead directly to a coordinated intrinsic muscle activation—AH, FDB and quadratus plantae (QP)—notably with sway toward

SECTION 3: Lower Extremity

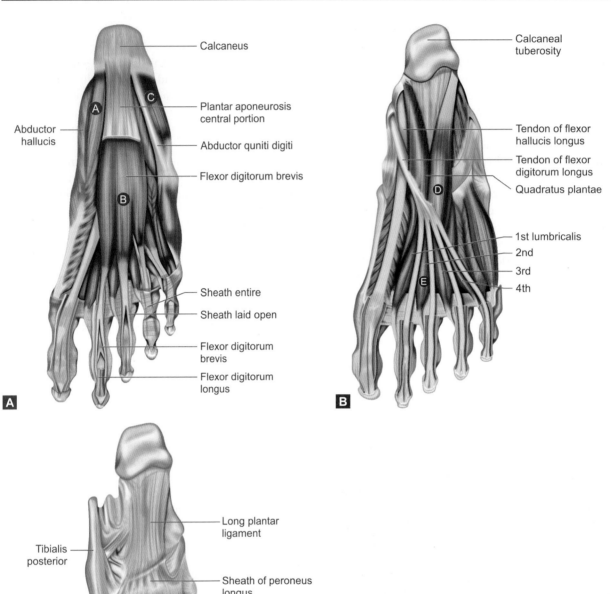

Calcaneus

Plantar aponeurosis
central portion

Abductor quniti digiti

Flexor digitorum brevis

Abductor
hallucis

Sheath entire

Sheath laid open

Flexor digitorum
brevis

Flexor digitorum
longus

Calcaneal
tuberosity

Tendon of flexor
hallucis longus

Tendon of flexor
digitorum longus

Quadratus plantae

1st lumbricalis
2nd
3rd
4th

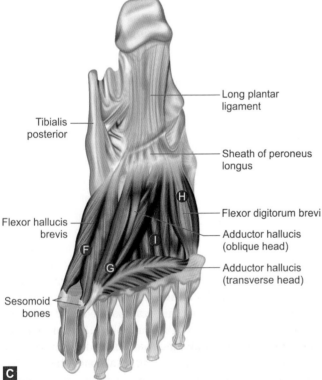

Long plantar
ligament

Tibialis
posterior

Sheath of peroneus
longus

Flexor digitorum brevi

Adductor hallucis
(oblique head)

Adductor hallucis
(transverse head)

Flexor hallucis
brevis

Sesomoid
bones

FIGS 7A TO C: Plantar intrinsic muscles of the foot. (A)
First Plantar Layer. Abductor Hallucis **A**, Flexor Digitorum
Brevis **B**, Abductor Digiti Minimi **C**. (B) Second Plantar Layer.
Quadratus Plantae **D**, Lumbricals **E**. (C) Third Plantar Layer. Flexor
Hallucis Brevis **F**, Adductor Hallucis oblique and transverse heads
G, Flexor digiti minimi brevis **H**, plantar interrosei in "fourth
plantar layer" **I**.

Source: Reproduced from Grey's Anatomy, 20th Edition, 1918.

the medial side of the foot.[28] These three studies indicate the close biomechanical relationship between the hip, extrinsic foot muscles and intrinsic foot muscles, which may help the clinician identify possible contributing factors in plantar heel pain.

Innervation

The plantar intrinsic muscles and the plantar fascia are innervated by branches of the medial and lateral plantar nerves.[10,21] Because of the presence of Pacini and Ruffini corpuscles in the plantar fascia and associated intrinsic musculature, the plantar fascia is theorized to have proprioceptive functions.[10] Several different entrapment neuropathies have been proposed that may generate plantar heel and arch pain as noted in Figures 8 and 9. For example, the first branch of lateral plantar nerve may get entrapped in the deep fascia of the AH muscle and the medial head of QP.[29] Clinical evidence suggests the medial calcaneal branch of the tibial nerve may be correlated with heel pain, as it has demonstrated a conduction latency and decreased sensory nerve action potential in nerve conduction testing in a plantar fasciitis population.[30]

■ CLINICAL PRESENTATION

Plantar fasciosis and fasciitis symptoms are typically of a gradual onset, often insidious, and may radiate proximally or distally from the attachment at the heel. Initial steps after a period of inactivity often provoke

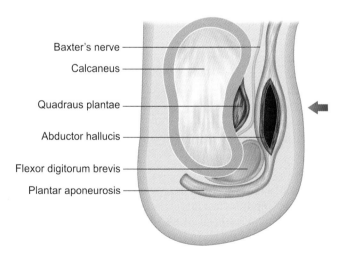

Baxter's nerve
Calcaneus
Quadraus plantae
Abductor hallucis
Flexor digitorum brevis
Plantar aponeurosis

FIG. 8: : Baxter's nerve and relative anatomy, also known as the 1st branch of lateral plantar nerve (1st B-LPN)
Source: Reproduced with permission from Elsevier.

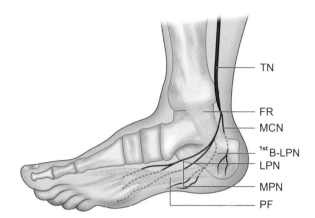

TN
FR
MCN
1st B-LPN
LPN
MPN
PF

FR, flexor retinaculum; MCN, medial calcaneal nerve; MPN, medial plantar nerve; PF, plantar fascia; TN, tibial nerve.

FIG. 9: Medial view of right foot demonstrating the relation of the tibial nerve and its branches to other structures. 1st B-LPN or the first branch of lateral plantar nerve
Source: Reproduced with permission from Churchill Livingstone.

TABLE 1: Risk factors for developing plantar heel pain[3,33-35]

- Decreased ankle dorsiflexion
- Leg length discrepancy
- Hallux limitus
- Tightness of the foot, calf, and hamstring musculature
- Pes cavus or pes planus deformities
- Excessive foot pronation
- Prolonged daily weight bearing
- Weight bearing endurance activity (e.g. dancing, running)
- BMI > 25 kg/m^2
- Recent changes in weight bearing frequency or exercise regimen
- Heel contusion or trauma
- Middle age
- Metabolic disorders (e.g. diabetes mellitus)
- Sickle cell disease
- Infection
- Vascular disorders (e.g. peripheral vascular disease)

symptoms (i.e. getting out of bed in the morning and/or rising after prolonged sitting). It is common for people to describe a reduction of symptoms with resumption of some activity, but prolonged periods of weight bearing usually exacerbate the condition. Subjective complaints may also include radiating pain and/or changes in sensation (hyperesthesia, anesthesia, paresthesia). In addition to biomechanical and neurological factors, there is evidence that progressive increases in vascular pressure are correlated with muscular fatigue and may contribute to increased symptoms associated with the duration of weight bearing.[31] Some common risk factors identified with plantar fasciosis and plantar heel pain are listed in Table 1, in no particular order. It is important to consider that the predictive value of these risk factors depends on the patient population and single variables taken in isolation may not always serve as reliable predictors of injury for every individual.[32]

Static foot posture has not been shown as a consistent predictor of plantar heel pain, although there is some evidence that overpronation correlates with plantar heel pain.[36] Pes cavus and pes planus foot types can both present with plantar heel pain. Static arch height has only a weak correlation with injury risk and dynamic function of the foot, and should not be used as the primary tool to guide treatment. More comprehensive measures of foot posture, such as the foot posture index (FPI) and/or the arch height index (AHI) may be used in lieu of static arch height measures. Literature suggests these tools can predict mobility of the foot to some degree, as well as dynamic function and injury risk.[37-39] High-arched and low-arched individuals may bias loading to different aspects of the plantar surface of the foot, which may contribute to plantar heel pain via different mechanisms. Normal- to low-arched military recruits, in loaded and unloaded conditions, have demonstrated load bias to the medial midfoot and great toe; whereas those with a high arch appear to selectively bias their load to the plantar heel and the first metatarsal head (Fig. 10).[40]

■ CLINICAL EXAMINATION

Medical Screening and Differential Diagnosis

The differential diagnosis and medical screening process for plantar heel pain are extensive and summarized below in Table 2. Possible red flags highlighted below may be indications for physician referral, if history and examination findings raise the index of suspicion that symptoms are not of musculoskeletal origin.

Imaging is generally not recommended for plantar heel pain suspected to be of a soft tissue origin unless differential diagnosis is a challenge, and the case is recalcitrant to conservative care. Radiographs frequently show a plantar calcaneal heel spur, but only somewhat greater in incidence than in an asymptomatic population, and therefore this finding should rarely drive treatment decisions. The FDB muscle is now thought to be the actual source of plantar heel spurs, not the plantar fascia,

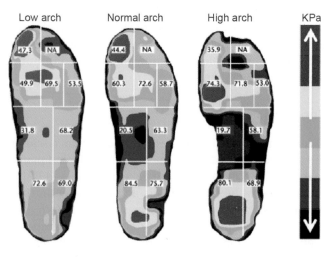

NA, not assessed.

FIG. 10: Arch types, as categorized by arch height index (AHI), had characteristic distributions of force-time integral (FTI). Normally-arched and low-arched feet displayed significantly higher FTIs in the great toe region, whereas high-arched feet demonstrated higher forces in the medial forefoot and the plantar heel. Low-arched feet demonstrated higher FTIs in the medial midfoot compared with normally arched and high-arched feet. The figure is from a composite pressure map of ten error-free steps from a representative participant for each arch type in the weight-bearing condition.[40] The data overprint is FTI (in newton-seconds) *Source:* Reproduced with permission from the American Physical Therapy Association.

which further highlights the important stabilizing force of the intrinsic muscles.[41] However, spurs may contribute directly to entrapment neuropathies or adjacent soft tissue irritation and should be noted when reviewing radiograph findings.[2]

Bone scans and/or magnetic resonance imaging (MRI) can be used to rule out occult fractures, stress fractures and other soft tissue lesions. Although typically deemed unnecessary in most plantar heel pain cases with a low index of suspicion for occult injury, MRI is sensitive for determining plantar fascia thickening (Fig. 11).[5] Additionally, MRI can detect Achilles tendon thickening, which is related to plantar fasciosis, perifascial edema, bone marrow edema of the calcaneus at the plantar fascia origin, as well as intrinsic muscle atrophy.[10,21] Ultrasound has been shown to have reasonable levels of reliability to detect plantar fascia thickening, a sign of plantar fasciosis.[10] Electromyography and nerve conduction velocity studies may be helpful if a peripheral nerve lesion is suspected (e.g. lumbar radiculopathy or tarsal tunnel syndrome).

TABLE 2: Other sources of plantar heel pain

Soft tissue related differentials	Differentiating clinical features
Calcaneal fat pad atrophy	+ fat pad sequestration test, + fat pad shearing test, + response to fat pad taping, displaced or thinned pad in WB
Subcalcaneal bursitis	Diagnosis of exclusion (lies between plantar fascia and the plantar fat pad)
Tibial nerve and its branches	Nerve symptoms diffusely in heel and/or plantar foot, + tinel's, + nerve tension, tenderness at entrapment site(s)
Plantar ligament strain	Arch collapse, deep foot pain, + stress testing
Intrinsic muscle strain	Pain with contraction, palpation and stretching
Skin shearing (blisters, ulcers, callous)	Visual skin wear and superficial tenderness
Lumbar radiculopathy (S1 or possibly S2)	+ neurological screening, + lumbar exam
Non soft tissue related differentials	**Differentiating clinical features**
Bone bruise of calcaneus	Pain with calcaneal weight bearing. Symptoms are dull, constant, boring and deep. History of trauma
Bone spur	Can visualize on X-ray, although common in asymptomatic population
Calcaneal apophysitis (Sever's disease)	Tenderness along active growth plate, pain with Achilles loads
Calcaneal fracture/stress fracture	Tenderness on the calcaneus, history of trauma, + imaging
Possible red flags	**Differentiating clinical features**
Bone neoplasm (cyst, tumor)	Deep bone pain, notably at rest. Other signs of neoplasm
Paget disease of bone	Cranial symptoms (e.g. hearing loss, headache), other bone pains, kyphosis, bowing of tibias
Neurological disease	Positive CNS and/or PNS findings
Systemic arthritis (RA, seronegative spondyloarthropathies)	History of autoimmune and/or other rheumatological diseases
Metabolic disease (e.g. peripheral neuropathy)	Impaired sensation of feet bilaterally
Infection	Vector borne disease history, low grade fever, and/or systemic symptoms

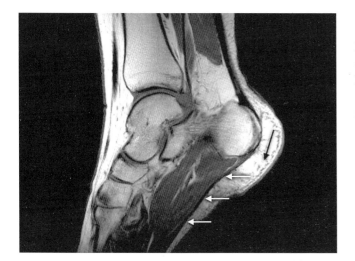

FIG. 11: Sagittal T1-weighted MRI. The fascia is low signal on most MR sequences demonstrating little of its internal structure. Plantar fascia (white arrows), calcaneal fat pad (black arrow)

Source: Reproduced with permission from Thieme Medical Publishers, Inc.

Movement and Postural Screen

During resting calcaneal stance posture (RCSP), the clinician should note calcaneal fat pad position, arch and leg musculature development, soft tissue contours (i.e. swelling, atrophy, defects), color of skin (i.e. ecchymosis, redness), presence of hair (e.g. vascular disease), gross structural faults to include, but are not limited to: lower extremity alignment, knee hyperextension/loss of ankle dorsiflexion, leg-length discrepancy and scoliosis. Excessive hip internal rotation is correlated with an anterior pelvic tilt and pronation, and therefore lower extremity and lumbopelvic posture must be viewed as a functional unit during the postural assessment process.[42] Foot shape and posture are also important at this stage of the examination, and some key clinical observations are highlighted efficiently with the FPI (Appendix I).[39,43] This efficient and nearly hands-off screen takes approximately 2 minutes to administer. Static and dynamic function of the foot is variable within the same person and could change depending on weight bearing activity within the same day.[44] Despite this limitation, it is helpful to follow static observation with a movement screen to assess the function of the ankle, midfoot, forefoot and MTP joints and related soft tissue structures while assessing for quantity, quality and symptoms (Table 3). Movement screens have drawbacks as they do not clearly implicate specific tissues, but they do provide insight into individual movement preferences that influence foot loading. Other relevant activities may also need to be observed in whole or component form, which include but are not limited to: gait, running, stair climbing and cutting or pivoting.

Palpation and Provocation

The clinician should palpate for general bony contours and deformity in the rearfoot, midfoot and forefoot, and should identify tenderness along the length of the plantar fascia and the plantar fat pad. If tenderness is found along a relaxed plantar fascia, the MTP joints should be dorsiflexed to end range and the palpation repeated over the now more superficially prominent plantar fascia. If structures deep to the plantar fascia are involved instead of the plantar fascia, the patient will notice a decrease in symptoms during the repeat palpation. Pain to palpation of the plantar surface of the

TABLE 3: Objective examination

Pronation/supination (movement screen)
There is evidence of a coupling effect between limb rotation and foot motion.[51,52] Simulate this coupling in standing by encouraging the patient to rotate their pelvis and lower limbs as far as is comfortable while keeping their heels and toes on the ground. Observe for pronation during limb internal rotation and supination during external limb rotation. If symptoms, impaired quality or reduced/excessive motion is noted, further biomechanical examination is warranted to determine the cause.

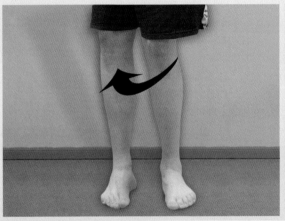 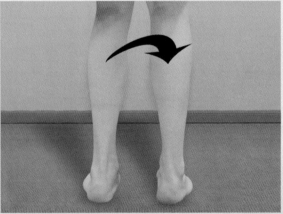

Heel raise (movement screen)
Ask the patient to perform a single leg heel rise (can perform with double leg) with fingertip support and a stable knee and trunk. Observe for supination of the rearfoot relative to a pronating forefoot and the tibia. Also make note of the height of the heel rise. Measurement with a ruler may be helpful to compare to the opposite side or to establish a baseline. Symptoms, insufficient rearfoot inversion or plantar flexion height warrants further biomechanical examination to determine the cause.

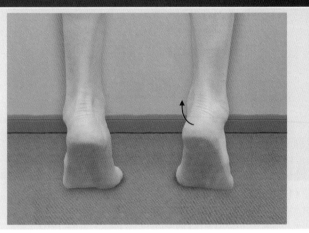

Continued

Continued

Squat: double and single leg (movement screen)

Encourage a squat to induce end range dorsiflexion of the ankle. Slight internal rotation of the tibia and foot pronation should occur. Also make note of knee, hip and trunk function. If symptoms are provoked, impaired quality is noted or motion is reduced or excessive, further biomechanical examination is warranted to determine the cause.

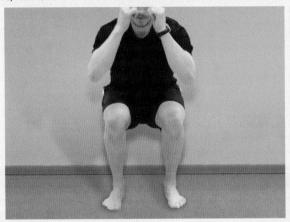
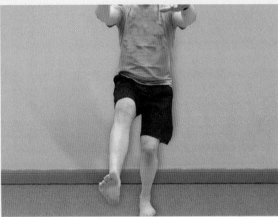

Closed chain dorsiflexion (movement screen and ROM)[45]

Zero an inclinometer on the wall and place just below the tibial tuberosity and instruct the participant to lunge forward, keeping the heel on the floor. Over 40 degrees of dorsiflexion with the knee flexed is normal, slightly less if performed with the knee straight.[48] Preventing tibial internal rotation (i.e. knee over second toe), forefoot abduction, navicular drop or rearfoot eversion will bias the talocrural component of dorsiflexion (instead of the rear, mid and forefoot) and expected values would reduce accordingly. The knee should be able to easily clear the foot. Other evidence based options include measuring the distance in centimeters the knee travels from the heel using tape on the floor.[53]

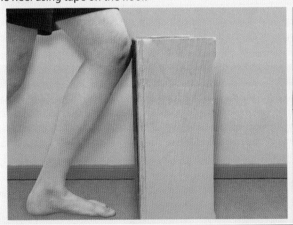
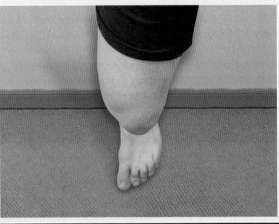

Windlass test (movement screen) and provocation[3,54]

Movement screen: With the patient in a relaxed stance and bearing weight evenly across the foot, dorsiflex the 1st MTP and observe for limitation and/or inadequate hallux dorsiflexion, rearfoot supination and elevation of the medial longitudinal arch. If motion is reduced, further biomechanical examination is warranted to determine the cause.

Provocation: Hold the ankle out of end range dorsiflexion and apply an end range load via MTP dorsiflexion of the 1st MTP to strain the central band, and then include all bands via dorsiflexion of toes 2–5. Concordant arch and/or heel pain may indicate plantar fascia strain and/or intrinsic muscle strain.

Continued

Continued

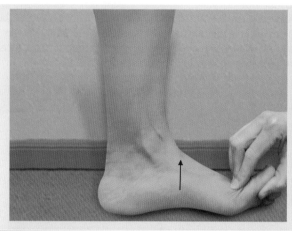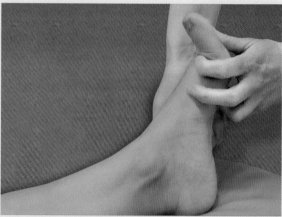

Navicular drop (movement screen)[39,55-57]

In sitting (top image), make a mark on the navicular prominence. Ensure that the talar head is neutral (lateral and medial borders are equally prominent). Next, measure the height of the navicular from the floor with a ruler. Ask the patient to stand (middle image) measure and then squat (bottom image) and re-measure.

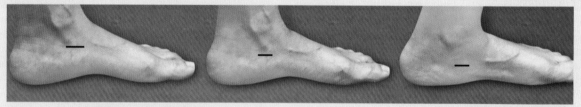

The differences between the three positions are indicators of midtarsal pronation. Approximately 5–8 mm of motion is considered normal. Other similar examination options exist such as measuring navicular drift (medial/lateral excursion) and dorsal arch height (vertical excursion) with a caliper are described elsewhere.[30]

Intrinsic and extrinsic toe flexion (strength)

There are various ways to test the strength of the intrinsic toe musculature; however, accurate and clinically feasible options have not been validated. Although hard to quantify, strength of toe flexion, abduction, adduction may all be estimated, with or without a handheld dynamometer, with loads being placed on the proximal phalanx and a relaxed leg to reduce the influence of the extrinsic toe flexors. To judge the strength of the extrinsic toe flexors, load should be placed on the distal phalanx combined with active ankle plantar flexion.

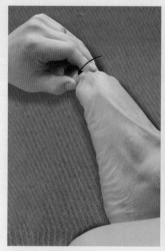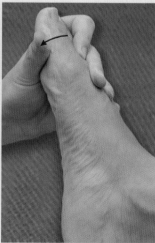

Continued

Continued

Plantar flexion (strength, endurance, and symptom screen)[58]

While using fingertips for balance, the patient performs a unilateral heel raise with the knee fully extended through the full available ROM at a pace of 1 repetition every 2 seconds until unable to complete a full repetition through full range with the requisite quality. It is important to consider that body weight will affect the comparison of one patient to another. Monitor for symptoms, notably in the plantar heel. Normal is estimated at greater than 25 repetitions.

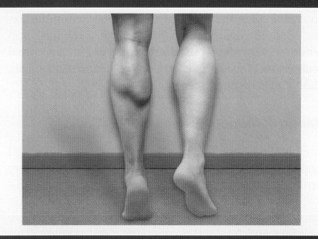

Fat pad (special test)

Provocation: Grasp the calcaneus and apply rotational and torsional movement to the fat pad while stabilizing the calcaneus (not shown here) and observe for symptoms indicating sensitivity in the fat pad.

Alleviation (Sequestration): If tenderness is along the plantar surface of the heel, first get a baseline of pain to palpation with a consistent force. Next, cup the fat pad on the lateral, medial and posterior borders forming a plump mass. Finally, repeat palpation and look for a reduction of symptoms. A positive test indicates possible fat pad atrophy or inadequate fat pad function and may benefit from taping/orthotics to sequester the pad.

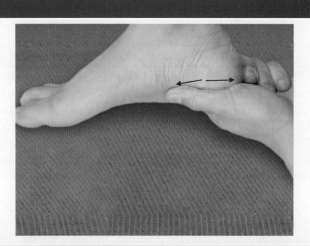

Dorsiflexion-eversion (special test)[3]

In supine, passively evert the foot, dorsiflex the ankle and extend the toes for several seconds. If neurological or painful symptoms are not generated, tap over the tarsal tunnel (posterior and inferior to the medial malleolus) looking for local or distal symptoms in the heel or foot. Further sensitization can be generated by taking up the slack in the sciatic nerve (hip flexion/adduction/internal rotation and knee extension).

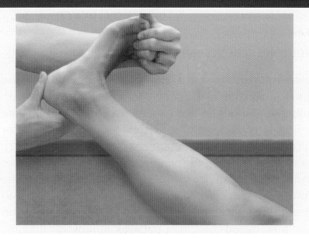

heel may be reduced during the fat pad sequestration test, which indicates possible fat pad atrophy/degeneration as a contributor (Table 3). At a minimum, palpation should include the intrinsic and extrinsic musculature, the deltoid ligament, tarsal tunnel, Achilles and tendons of the deep posterior compartment. Abnormal temperature, swelling, enlargement, texture and spasm should also be noted.

Range of Motion (ROM)

Examination should include the quantity, quality and symptoms for physiologic (osteokinematic) and accessory (arthrokinematic) motion of the ankle, subtalar, tarsals, metatarsals and phalanges. Non-weight bearing ankle dorsiflexion/plantar flexion and inversion/eversion (rearfoot and forefoot) goniometric measurement have reasonable intrarater and fair interrater reliability.[45-47] However, these tests continue to suffer from controversial validity issues based on considerations across disparate studies using a variety of forces, joint positions, axes of motion, among other variables. There is some evidence that closed chain dorsiflexion may have more reliability and may serve as a potential option or a supplement to open chain ROM measurements (Table 3).[48,49] Gathering ROM data should be comprehensive, it is often helpful to look for patterns of tightness during the data gathering process. For example, a patient with excessive pronation may present with a pattern of limited mobility in the superficial posterior compartment, peroneals, ADM, lateral hamstrings and hip internal rotators. A patient with inadequate pronation may present with a pattern of limited mobility in the deep posterior compartment, AH, medial hamstrings and the hip external rotators.

Neurological Screening

A neurological screen is important to fully understand the entire picture of the individual as well as to assist with ruling in and out certain conditions. This would include neural tension testing, a sensory exam to screen for dermatomal and peripheral nerve dysfunction (Fig. 12), motor testing to include peripheral nerves and myotomes and assessment of deep tendon reflexes. Stress tests to the lumbar spine, pelvis, knee and hip may be indicated to clear these joints for pain referral if an index of suspicion has been raised. Common patterns to look for include, but are not limited to: L5-S1 radiculopathy, dural or sciatic entrapment, tibial nerve entrapment and plantar nerve entrapment. If the nerve to the ADM is compressed,

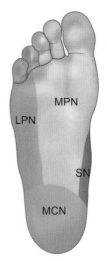

LPN, lateral plantar nerve; MCN, medial calcaneal nerve; MPN, medial plantar nerve; SN, saphenous.

FIG. 12: Sensory distribution of the plantar surface of the foot
Source: Reproduced with permission of Churchill Livingstone.

typically under the plantar fascia, the patient will have weakness of abduction of the 5th toe.[50]

■ PHYSICAL THERAPY TREATMENT

Patient Education

Modifiable risk factors for plantar heel pain have direct implications on rehabilitation. The patient should understand that there are a number of treatment options available and treatment decisions are collaborative.[59] For example, the therapist and patient may need to collaborate on various ways to reduce biomechanical stressors such as shoe-wear habits, training errors, excessive time with weight bearing activities, utilization of external supports, therapeutic exercise regimens and weight loss or fitness programs. Finally, it is critical that realistic expectations be established for this condition and any maladaptive behaviors are addressed such as fear avoidance, kinesiophobia, catastrophization and lack of motivation and self-efficacy. Such maladaptive behaviors may contribute to more expensive and protracted care, dependency on health care providers, and contribute to disability and/or chronic pain.[60,61]

Ligamentous tissue healing persists for several months after injury and this structure may never regain its original tensile strength, which may explain the typical duration of a plantar fasciosis episode being 6–12 months. Function may be delayed after ligamentous tissue injury because the size, organization and type of collagen are still not normalized 1 year after injury, potentially contributing to many cases of plantar fasciosis becoming recalcitrant and/or recurrent.[62] Despite these realities, plantar heel pain of musculoskeletal origin can be efficiently and effectively treated through shared decision making, and by customizing the intervention to the patient's unique risk factors, individual preferences and clinical presentation.

Manual Therapy and Stretching (Mobility Impairments)

Mobility-directed treatments, such as joint mobilization, soft tissue mobilization, neural mobilization and stretching, should be considered as a first line treatment strategy for plantar heel pain if examination findings identify relevant involvement (Tables 4 and 5). Muscle, tendon, ligament and nervous tissue all have different healing rates and loading properties which should be considered when loading the plantar heel structures under pathological and/or non-pathological situations in order to promote a healing response through stimulating collagen turnover.[63] Viscoelastic properties of ligamentous and fascial tissue can be influenced by a number of factors that a clinician must consider when designing a plan of care that include: age (e.g. reduced tissue elasticity with age), sensitivity to hormones (e.g. females estrogen receptors are more responsive than males), proprioceptive function (e.g. peripheral neuropathy), vascular perfusion (e.g. diabetes), history of collagen disease, water concentrations (e.g. dehydration or poor blood pressure control) and fiber density (e.g.

TABLE 4: Soft tissue mobilization

Soft tissue mobilization for the gastrocnemius (GN)—superficial posterior compartment[10]	
Allow slight plantar flexion and knee flexion to slacken the GN and soleus (S) as you clear superficial adhesions via skin rolling, scar mobilization, and/or instrument-assisted scraping of the skin prior to deeper mobilization. Lift the GN firmly away from the S and tibia and separate the medial and lateral tendons of the hamstring (HS) from the medial and lateral GN heads. Split the superficial posterior compartment and the lateral compartments of the leg by tracing along the fibula. Consider mobilizing the Achilles tendon and its paratenon. Add knee extension, ankle dorsiflexion and/or pronatory/supinatory movements actively or passively to further engage the GN.	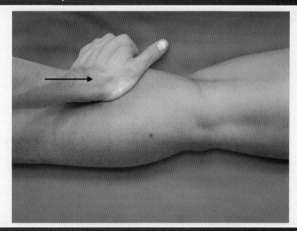
Soft tissue mobilization for the soleus (S)—superficial posterior compartment	
The S can be easily accessed along the medial border of the tibia. While pinning down the S, utilize ankle dorsiflexion/plantar flexion (DF/PF) to separate the S from the GN with the knee straight and flexed as well as toe flexion/extension to separate the S from the flexor hallucis longus (FHL) and the flexor digitorum longus (FDL). While continuing to pin down the soleus, utilize pronation/supination to separate the S from the peroneus longus (PL), peroneus brevis (PB) and posterior tibialis (PT).	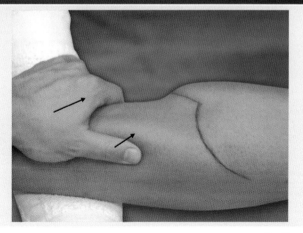

Continued

Continued

Soft tissue mobilization for the deep posterior (FHL, FDL, PT) and lateral compartment (PL, PB)

To address the muscle bellies of the FDL, FHL and PT, pin each muscle belly against the tibia, fibula and/or the interosseous membrane while facilitating gross pronation/supination, toe movements and/or ankle movements. If indicated, consider these same strategies as you address the lateral compartment of the leg starting at the fibular head and following the PB to the 5th ray and the PL through the cuboid tunnel toward the 1st ray.

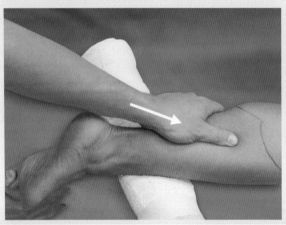
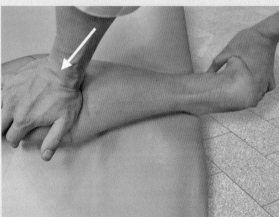

Soft tissue mobilization to plantar soft tissue[10,50,68,70,73,74,81]

Trace the AH along the medial border of the PF from the calcaneus through the 1st MTP and ease between the AH and PF into the FDB and continue to sink toward the deeper layers where the QP resides. It is important to be aware of the plantar nerves and artery which lies directly under the plantar fascia. Mobilize lateral to the central band of the PF with pressure along the ADM and separate this tissue from the PF. Consider including active and passive movements of the toes in isolation and as a group during the mobilization. To further separate the plantar intrinsic muscles from the tendons of the leg add gross pronation/supination of the entire ankle/foot. To further influence the neurological structures in this region, tension the sciatic and tibial nerves as outlined in Table 5 as you trace on, or around, the plantar nerves.

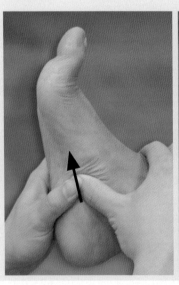
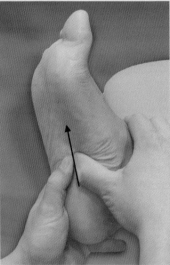
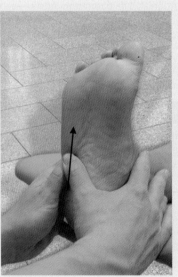

TABLE 5: Stretching and neural mobilization

Gastrocnemius (GN), soleus(S), and posterior tibialis (PT)

GN: Have the patient internally rotate their limb until the toes are pointing directly anterior. While keeping a firmly straight, but not hyperextended knee, encourage ankle dorsiflexion until a springy barrier is felt and a stretch is felt in the GN. Slight adjustments to the position of the limb to ensure that the stretch involves the medial and lateral heads is important as the triceps surae can function medial and lateral to the subtalar joint axis.[46]

S: To target the soleus, follow the same procedures above but with the knee slightly flexed. The stretch should be felt in the posterior leg and/or Achilles but not in the GN.

PT: Follow the same procedure as the soleus, but encourage midtarsal joint pronation via drop of the navicular and the medial longitudinal arch and forefoot abduction.

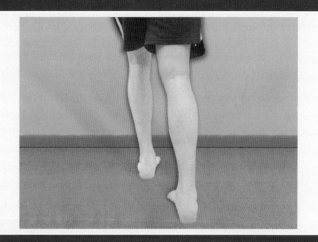

Plantar fascia, intrinsics and extrinsic toe flexors (FHL, FDL)[47]

Non-weight bearing: Add maximum toe and ankle dorsiflexion of all the toes. Use 1st MTP DF to bias the FHL and DF through toes 2–5 for the FDL. To bias the abductor hallucis, remove ankle DF and add a DF and adductor force to the 1st MTP. To further direct forces to specific tissue add force (e.g. thumb) to the specific tissue you are targeting (plantar fascia shown in top image). Adding oscillatory movements to the toes may also help to address the multiplanar fiber orientation of the tissue in this region.

Weight bearing: Have the patient maximally dorsiflex their ankle and place this on the wall with their forefoot and MTP joints in maximum dorsiflexion. Instruct the patient to drive their slightly flexed knee into the wall allowing slight tibial internal rotation and pronation of the foot.

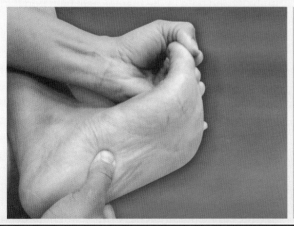 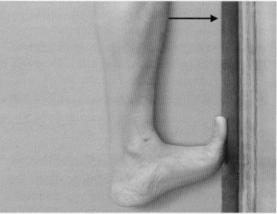

Neural tension testing and neural mobilization[72]

Supine: Perform a straight leg raise during full dorsiflexion and eversion of the ankle and foot. Look for symptom reproduction/elimination with the alteration of hip flexion/extension, hip adduction/abduction, ankle dorsiflexion/plantar flexion, eversion/inversion of the entire foot, toe dorsiflexion/plantar flexion and toe abduction/adduction until maximum tissue tension is engaged in the plantar heel and/or associated region(s). Spinal movements can be added here, but are often easier to add in the slump position.

Slump: Follow the procedures above in a sitting posture. Further sensitization can be engaged in this posture via spinal flexion (notably full cervical flexion), side-bending and/or rotation until maximum tissue tension is engaged in the plantar heel and/or associated regions.

Continued

Continued

Tips: Engage the tissue barrier via isolated head movements and/or isolated lower extremity movements. Perform gentle oscillatory movements to the symptom and/or tissue barrier and progress intensity based on signs of improved movement quantity, quality or symptoms. Further details on neurodynamics and treatment can be found elsewhere.[82]

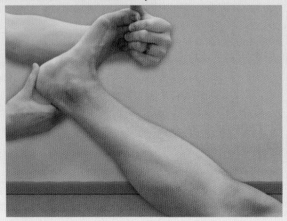 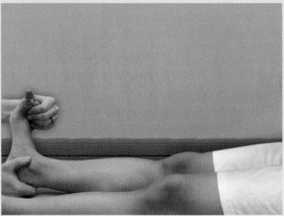

reduced density with fasciosis).[62] The viscoelastic tissue property of creep leads to exponential stress relaxation and deformation under a constant load, such as sustained stretching/positioning, and may also lead to reduced muscle activity in the region.[62] Furthermore, hysteresis leads to a progressive loss of potential energy with consistent and repeated load. For example, stretching ligamentous tissue such as the plantar fascia 5% beyond its non-loaded length can lead to non-recoverable damage, necrosis, and ultimately, laxity or rupture.[62,64] It should also be considered that ligamentous tissue may not return to its normal resting length quickly after end range loads.[62,65,66] Therefore, when implementing a therapeutic exercise program, signs of tissue tolerance should be monitored closely and dosage should be adjusted accordingly for each individual.[67]

Despite the lack of current evidence addressing specific joint mobility in this patient population, if joint mobility deficits, or symptoms that are identified with accessory (arthrokinematic) and/or physiologic (osteokinematic) joint testing, joint mobilization may be required to restore proper translation and/or rotation of the associated synovial joint(s) to include, but not limited to the talocrural, subtalar, midtarsal, tarsometatarsal joints and the MTP joints. There is moderate evidence to support soft tissue mobilization as a tool to augment treatment of plantar heel pain.[3,68-71] The direct fascial connection between the Achilles tendon, intrinsic muscles of the foot and the plantar fascia are significant and should be considered when designing a mobility based therapeutic regimen.[9,10] There is preliminary

evidence that trigger point therapy and/or deep massage combined with stretching may have superior efficacy than stretching alone.[68,71] There is also mounting evidence that interventions directed at the nervous tissue in this region (sciatic, tibial and plantar nerves) may improve functional mobility and pain in the plantar heel pain population.[71,72]

Soft tissue mobilization requires a level of specificity to optimize outcome and safety. The anatomy in this region requires tactile, visual and verbal skills to monitor patient response, tissue tone and pliability, temperature, and color. Commonly prescribed non-specific approaches (e.g. foam roll) should be issued to patients with caution. The following tissues demand particular caution: tibial nerve near the center of the popliteal crease; the superficial peroneal and sural nerves near the superior aspect of the lateral compartment; the sural cutaneous nerve, which is superficial to the GN, the tibial nerve in and around the tarsal tunnel and along the plantar fascia; and the cutaneous branches of the saphenous nerve which travels along the medial border of the tibia. However, if nervous tissue is implicated, manual mobilization of these structures from origin to insertion and on or around these nerves may be indicated. Anatomy software may be helpful for the manual therapy practitioner to orient themselves to relevant neurovascular and myofascial structures in three dimensions.

Begin soft tissue mobilization by addressing superficial restrictions and next proceed into deeper tissues by mobilizing the lower leg and foot musculature from origin to insertion ensuring adequate compartment separation (superficial, deep and lateral) and plantar layer mobility by kneading and stroking. The clinician can then proceed gently into the hard to reach deep posterior compartment and the deeper layers of the plantar aspect of the foot while paying particular attention to trigger points that may refer into the heel. Although substantial force may be required in this region, if patient guarding occurs, then efforts to reach the deeper layers will be both uncomfortable and potentially ineffective. The clinician may need to make alterations to the depth, direction and angle of force being used if the results prove insufficient. Soft tissue mobilization techniques, such as contract-relax, mobilization with movement and weight bearing positions (e.g. squatting), may be helpful when passive techniques are not effective. However, if the main impediment to recovery is recalcitrant soft-tissue healing, cross friction massage may be indicated to assist with collagen remodeling (i.e. targeting plantar fascia and plantar intrinsic muscles).[73,74] Once a manual therapy sequence is complete, notably if the target tissues were adequately addressed, the patient should experience reduced pain and should be primed for active therapeutic exercise from a neurological, psychological and biomechanical perspective.

Substantial evidence supports that direct stretching to the plantar fascia tissue is likely superior to Achilles-directed stretching alone in the plantar heel pain population.[3,75-79] Some studies have established that a stretching dosage of 2–3 minutes, 2–5 times per day has shown to improve function and pain in the plantar fasciitis population.[7,80] However, stretching targets and dosage should be based on clinical judgment and factors such as the location and severity of the restriction, stage of healing, symptom response and improvement in function upon reassessment. A home soft tissue mobilization and stretching program should be prescribed by the treating clinician as needed until maximum medical improvement is reached, and should be maintained as necessary for prevention of reinjury.

Motor Function (Strength, Coordination and Endurance Impairments)

There is a paucity of research directed at motor-related therapeutic exercise interventions in the plantar heel pain population, although there is a reasonable level of biomechanical research that addresses potential stressors to the plantar heel structures with some of these studies highlighted below. Additionally, biomechanical comorbidities at the level of the foot and above need to be considered when designing a therapeutic exercise

program for this patient population. For example, those with non-severe hallux abductovalgus may need to bias the AH (toe spreading) and ensure that the adductor hallucis is not overactive to allow for proper sagittal plane function of the intrinsic muscles and the plantar fascia.[83] Those with lateral ankle instability may need to bias the evertors as necessary, without generating excessive pronation, while also being cautious with orthotics or shoes that have a varus wedge. Those with posterior tibialis and/or spring ligament insufficiency (e.g. pes planus) may need to initially, or permanently, perform therapeutic exercise with an orthotic and/or appropriate shoe gear. Additionally, those with fat pad atrophy should bear weight cautiously through the heel during closed chain exercise and may need an orthotic with a heel cup or fat pad taping during exercise. For those with severe and/or permanent loss of ankle dorsiflexion, exercises may need to be performed in slight plantar flexion (e.g. shoes with elevated heel) to prevent compensations during activities such as squatting. Patients with hallux rigidus, MTP capsulitis, sesamoiditis, interdigital neuroma, and/or other forefoot disorders, may have difficulty loading their forefoot and MTP joints through a full range and/or under full body weight load, and therapeutic exercise must be adjusted accordingly. The individual tissue state, the biomechanical comorbidities, as well as tissue loading principles must be carefully dosed and monitored for each individual.

Strengthening of the Intrinsic and Extrinsic Muscles of the Leg and Foot

Encouraging complete muscle failure should rarely be used when initially designing a strengthening program for a patient with a painful plantar heel, notably if instability is already a factor in their symptoms. The initial focus is complex multi-joint motor control, body awareness and establishing tissue tolerance. Open chain exercises will not be the focus of this chapter and, in most cases, should be temporarily used or avoided, if the patient has the ability to bias the different muscular structures of the leg with training in functional weight bearing positions (Table 6). Most exercises should begin in partial or full bilateral weight bearing on a relatively firm surface, with bare feet to enhance the visualization by the patient and the therapist. Once the patient demonstrates conscious competence to perform these exercises with sufficient quality, it may be deemed appropriate to utilize shoes, socks and/or orthotics during exercise to promote skill transfer under realistic scenarios.

TABLE 6: Motor interventions (strength, coordination and endurance)

Intrinsic coordination

In sitting, facilitate MTP joint plantar flexion with the cues "pull your toes toward your heels" and/or "cramp your arch muscles". Ensure that the foot shortens a few millimeters while the medial longitudinal arch raises a few millimeters. Ensure that the long toe flexors do not engage excessively via the cue "don't curl your toe nails and keep your calf as relaxed as you can" while discouraging DIP flexion. Next, ensure that the intrinsic great toe flexors can function independently of the other toes by DF toes 2–5 while pressing down at the 1st toe (top image). Additionally, ensure that the ADM and FDB can function independently by elevating the great toe while pressing down with toes 2–5 (middle image). Finally, perform a "toe spreading" exercise to facilitate AH and ADM contraction via 1st and 5th MTP flexion and slight abduction force (bottom image). Begin with isometric holds and then progress to controlled transitions between the three variations described above.

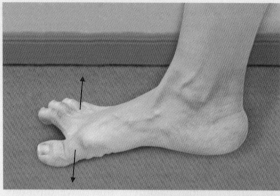 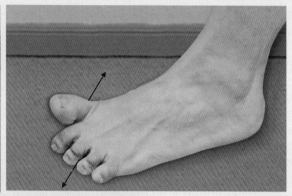

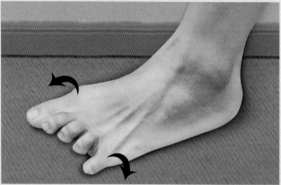

Intrinsic strengthening

Go through the sequence above in a standing position. Progress to surfaces that generate a challenge in postural sway. A foam pad will recruit the intrinsic better than a hard surfaced wobble or rocker board, as the variable surface itself adds local instability to all toes, versus global instability of a wobble or rocker board. Furthermore, placing a foam pad on top of a rocker or wobble board is an excellent way to address various postural challenges and muscle groups simultaneously for the higher level patient. Next, progress to single leg stance. To maximally recruit the intrinsic, curl the toes over the top of a half foam roll and perform isometric holds and progress to heel raises.

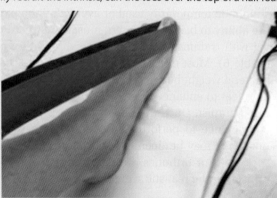 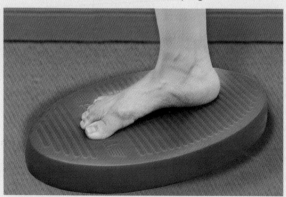

Continued

Continued

Plantar flexion strengthening (GN, S, PL, PT, FHL, FDL)

This exercise can be done on a flat surface or off the edge of a step starting at end range ankle dorsiflexion if possible. If the patient uses the edge of a step, ensure the patient has a thick shoe midsole so as not to create excessive compression of the plantar fascia and other plantar soft tissues. For the GN, ensure the knee remains straight and maintain a relatively balanced load on the forefoot via all five metatarsal heads and relatively relaxed toes. Follow the same procedure as the GN with slight knee flexion for the S. For the FHL, encourage 1st MTP weight bearing, firm great toe flexion and supination at the mid and rearfoot. To bias the PL, follow the procedure for the FHL but do not facilitate 1st MTP PF and consider foot position to create an inversion moment. For the FDL, follow the FHL procedure except encourage weight bearing and plantar flexion through toes 2–5. Finally, to encourage PT activation, follow the same procedure as the S but relax the long toe flexors and consider adding a more aggressive pronatory load such that may occur with a balance pad. If optimal muscle fatigue does not occur in the target tissue, consider using elastic resistance bands in open chain or machines in closed chain to isolate the target tissue as a supplement to a closed chain program.

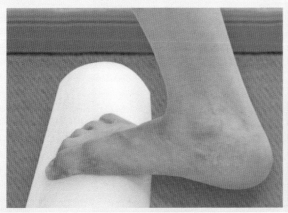
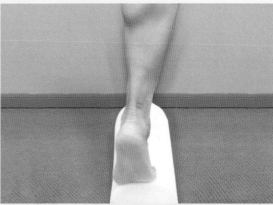

Squatting progression (double leg)

Ensure that the patient's unique anatomy is respected as you facilitate a neutral spine, hip, knee and ankle alignment with emphasis on facilitating nearly sagittal plane dorsiflexion movement, and slight pronation and tibial internal rotation during the squat. A sit to stand movement or a wall slide is a good place to start. Ensure that the intrinsic and extrinsic toe muscles and the plantar flexors are active through the eccentric and concentric phases. Progress to performance primarily on toes to strengthen plantar flexors and perform primarily on heels to strengthen dorsiflexors. Progress to performance on a foam pad to challenge plantar sensory feedback and intrinsic strength and then a wobble board to challenge more global joint stability. Progressing the squat with a variety of positions such as wide based squat (e.g. sumo squat with kettle bell in two hands), narrow based squat (e.g. suitcase squat with weight in one extremity) or even a more heavily loaded standard squat can be used and should match the impairments, ability and functional demands of the patient.

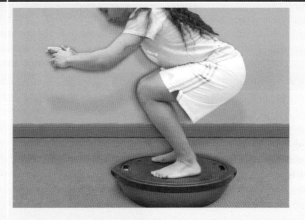

Single leg balance progression

In standing, bring the feet close together and then engage the intrinsic muscles of the stance limb and remove one foot. Do not allow the pelvis to shift more than 1–3 cm if possible, keeping the COM over the foot while maintaining an upright position of the trunk and hip. Attempt to stabilize the leg while performing hip motions with or without a band. Progress to performing this on an unstable surface such as a foam pad. When pulling into hip adduction, do not allow the stance foot to pronate via intrinsic and posterior compartment activation, or the limb to internally rotate or adduct via gluteal activation. When pushing into hip abduction,

Continued

Continued

do not allow the stance foot to supinate or the 1st ray to come off the ground, and firmly recruit the lateral hip muscles (gluteus medius) and the lateral leg muscles, notably the PL.

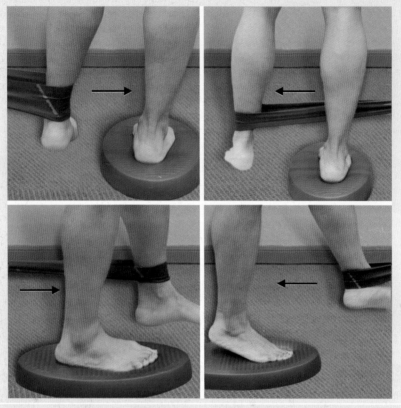

When pushing into hip extension, encourage activation of the plantar flexors in the stance foot via weight bearing primarily on the forefoot. During hip flexion, encourage stance leg ankle dorsiflexors via weight bearing primarily through the heel. Adjust the cadence of the movement to optimally match the functional demands and capabilities of the patient.

Single leg squatting progression

Once the patient has mastered the appropriate double leg squat and single leg balance progression, it is important that a single leg squat sequence ensues for many patients. To optimize training specificity, match the foot position, cadence and ROM needs to the unique needs of that individual (e.g. stair climbing, running). Many patients may benefit from a star excursion, where the non-weight-bearing limb reaches in various directions (e.g. posterolateral, posteromedial, anterior, posterior). Further progression examples include single leg sit/stand, step up/down, stair master, lunge, Romanian split squat, etc. Many of these exercises should be initiated with some upper extremity support until stability is mastered.

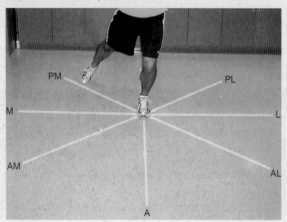

Continued

Continued

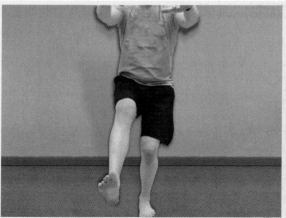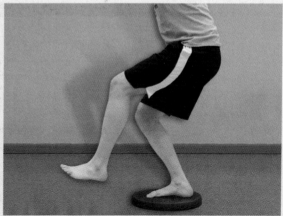

Plyometric progression

To promote skill transfer to sport, plyometrics should be considered in the therapeutic exercise program for an active population that jumps or runs, even if short distances such as to cross a street or up a flight of stairs. First, ensure the patient has mastered a controlled brisk narrow based squat and progress this via small jumps. Ensure the patient lands evenly on all metatarsal heads and with flat well-balanced phalanges and generates a forceful contraction of all antigravity muscles (e.g. trunk, hip, knee extensors). For this patient population, pay particular attention to ensuring the patient utilizes most of their available ankle dorsiflexion without inappropriate compensations. Adjust the hopping height and cadence to simulate their functional needs.

This can easily be paced with a metronome. Once a double leg hopping sequence has been mastered, the program should be adjusted to simulate the true environment the individual functions within such as complexity (e.g. catching a ball), surfaces, shoe gear, fatigue levels, unexpected perturbations and cutting/pivoting.

Strengthening the intrinsic muscles of the foot has been shown to increase the cross sectional area of the intrinsic muscles and reduce navicular drop during static single limb stance and multi-planar dynamic single leg reaching tasks.[84,85] Furthermore, there is evidence that the intrinsic muscles are important in posture, balance, single leg stance and plyometric loading which indicates that intrinsic motor performance should be considered when designing a therapeutic exercise program.[28,84,86]

Enhancing Motor Control

Ruffini endings, Pacinian corpuscles, Golgi tendon organs and free nerve endings have been shown to reside in the plantar fascia, ligaments of the ankle, short/long plantar ligaments and the spring ligament.[10] These mechanoreceptors contribute to the spinal reflex arc, which bypasses the CNS and is involved in complex tasks such as walking, squatting and maintaining upright stance. In addition, there is proposed to be a ligamentous-supraspinal connection which may stimulate the somatosensory cortex and generate descending cerebral motor control during foot loading, further contributing to motor control and body awareness through mechanical and sensory means.[62] It has been shown that 6 weeks of 3 and 12 minutes sessions of cognitive and motor based balance training has the ability to make significant improvements in joint position sense, performance on a dynamic balance excursion test, as well as enhanced motoneuron pool excitability and reflex response in the soleus in a chronic ankle instability population.[87] There are many ways to assess motor control during balance challenges such as single leg stance, which are listed below in Table 7, and may help the clinician select optimal intervention tactics. Many activities are single leg dominant, such as walking, stair climbing and running, which highlight the validity of using single leg stance during the intervention process. Besides removing a limb, adding surface challenges, attentional demand challenges (i.e. cognitive tasks such as counting backward), altering visual cues and/or adding vestibular challenges may all be ways to simulate the needs of the patient. Motor control principles should be considered in the design of a therapeutic exercise program to enhance a training response and skill transfer to daily function.

TABLE 7: Postural and motor control pearls[88,89]

Postural control variables	Description
Time to stability	Monitor the time it takes the foot and the whole person to get stable from a two to one foot transition, or from sitting to standing, or other related task
Postural sway velocity	Slow postural corrections may be viewed as disadvantageous and should be noted when assessing balance. However, quick and accurate corrections may be viewed as advantageous
Postural sway excursion	The gross amount of ROM that the navicular, ankle, knee, pelvis or spine travel should be noted during balance challenges
Frequency of postural corrections	Visible postural corrections can be noted within a designated timeframe, such as errors in a 30-second period. High frequency corrections should be viewed as disadvantageous
Postural strategy variability	Humans should be able to use a variety of balance strategies (trunk, knee and ankle) as well as medial/lateral foot weight bearing or forefoot/rearfoot weight bearing while balancing. Encourage a variety of different strategies, notably if a patient defaults to one strategy

Gait and Running

Gait assessment and training may be an important treatment strategy for all patients with dysfunctional gait/running cycles, even if adequate ROM and/or strength are available. Analyzing gait is becoming democratized by the availability of inexpensive video analysis technology. For example, some cell phones and tablets have, or will soon have, the ability to capture slow motion video at 120 fps to 240 fps (frames per second) and motion analysis applications are increasingly affordable, with many of the software applications designed for easy reviewing and sharing with the patient. Components of the gait/running cycle may be viewed in slow motion to enhance the accuracy of assessment, and ultimately, the intervention itself. Table 8 below outlines critical gait events and abnormal patterns which may help to guide intervention.

Restricted ankle dorsiflexion is often considered as a risk factor for developing foot pathology because it may lead to a variety of gait compensations such as early heel off and increased hip and knee flexion, knee hyperextension, overpronation at the midfoot, early and excessive loading of the 1st MTP and excessive tibial internal rotation.[90] However, it has been shown that restoring ankle dorsiflexion through surgical lengthening of the GN may not restore functional use of ankle dorsiflexion 3 months postoperatively highlighting the potential importance of gait retraining.[91] Fat pad atrophy and/or a heel spur may present with a variety of compensatory patterns such as absent or reduced heel strike during initial contact and may need to be addressed with external supports. It has been shown that those suffering from moderate intensity plantar fasciitis may have a significantly reduced contact time and vertical ground reaction force in the rearfoot

TABLE 8: Critical gait events for the foot and ankle region in the plantar heel pain population

Critical event	Abnormal pattern(s)
Initial contact	Absent heel strike, inadequate inversion, heavy/loud landing
Timing of pronation	Early or late pronation
Pronation quantity	Increased or inadequate pronation
Heel off (ankle dorsiflexion)	Heel whip and/or excessive pronation at end range dorsiflexion
Preswing (MTP dorsiflexion)	Heel whip and/or excessive and/or late pronation
Preswing (rearfoot supination)	Inadequate or delayed supination and/or reduced height of heel off
Terminal stance	Shortened time on forefoot, inadequate push off through great toe

during self-selected gait speed, which may need to be addressed with gait training.[92]

The patient's gait speed may significantly alter gait mechanics, and varying speeds during gait assessment may be important to consider.[93] For example, a fast gait speed has been shown to increase the 1st MTP dorsiflexion angle and thus plantar fascia strain.[18] Those with instability or pain during forefoot loading may present with an abnormal preswing phase of the gait cycle. Assuming the patient has achieved adequate strength of the ankle and toe plantar flexors (intrinsic and extrinsic), proper weight shifting through the metatarsal heads from mid to terminal stance may need to be facilitated, notably the 1st MTP. It is important to note that during the gait cycle, foot musculature in the posterior and lateral compartments as well as the intrinsic muscles are increasingly active during mid to terminal stance. Peak activation occurs during the late stance phase, as loads are shifted to the forefoot, and this phenomenon should be considered during gait retraining, as well as during strength program design.

When working with the running population, the considerations cited above for gait analysis remain pertinent, despite some noticeable differences in running mechanics. Mobility, strength and motor control demands may be exaggerated with the increased speed and load of running. Proximal influences such as poor knee flexion wave, lumbopelvic and hip instability, trunk asymmetry, abnormal arm swing, among others, must be addressed to resolve asymmetric and/or excessive loading that may contribute to foot disorders such as plantar heel pain. The skilled clinician must be able to identify local and global factors and design interventions to address existing problems with the gait/running cycle, as well as anticipate problems to prevent future movement related injury.

Modalities

No clear evidence has been found to support the use of ultrasound in the treatment of plantar heel pain, although it is still commonly used in current treatment regimens

for this patient population.[69,71] Iontophoresis using dexamethasone (4%) and acetic acid (5%) has moderate levels of evidence to provide short-term relief in the plantar heel pain population.[69,75,94]

External Supports (Shoes, Orthotics, Splinting and Taping)

Shoe wear modification should be considered as a first line treatment for plantar heel pain as there is strong evidence that biomechanics in multiple dimensions are influenced by shoe gear.[17,95-98] There are many components of a shoe that have clinical relevance and a selection of these are highlighted in Table 9 and Figure 13. Therapeutic considerations while selecting shoe gear for this patient population include: aligning the foot, influencing foot pronation and supination, providing global shock attenuation, influencing the windlass mechanism, reducing transverse plane skin and fat pad shearing and compression, among others.

Footwear may dramatically alter heel loads, as reported in a study of barefoot versus shod walking, where fat pad compression was nearly double in the barefoot group.[99] Minimalist and barefoot style shoes typically have thin midsoles which may reduce protection to the

TABLE 9: Typical shoe components

Shoe component	Description
Midsole	A single density midsole is typical of most shoes, but some shoes will have increased density on the medial side of the rearfoot, in the arch area or both. A dual or triple density midsole is often differentiated by color. Some "stability" shoes will include a varus posting in the shoe itself and is designed to control pronation. Minimalist/barefoot style shoes typically have thin midsoles. Anything above the midsole is part of the upper
Thermal plastic unit	Another option to consider is that some manufacturers will utilize a thermal plastic unit in the midsole, typically in the shank to add stability and pronatory control
Outsole	The density of the outsole should match the needs of the surface of use such as managing roots, pebbles or other obstructions. Some outsoles have flex grooves, which enhance mobility and should be placed optimally for the patient. For example, a patient with unstable MTP extension and a shoe with a flex groove under the MTP may not be ideal. Additionally, the outsole is usually made of carbon rubber, which is more durable but less flexible than blown rubber
Sock liner and socks	The sock interface should not create a slippery environment when dry or wet. Thick socks may help prevent blisters, but impair proprioception. Thick sock liners may feel more comfortable but may also add instability
Last shape (straight, curved, semi-curved) and compliance (board, slip, combo)	Those with severe pes planus (e.g. forefoot abducted) may need a straight last, or those with severe pes cavus may need a curved last (e.g. forefoot adducted). The majority of shoes are semi-curved. A board last is made of stiff fiberboard and is designed to reduce motion. Slip lasted shoes are made without a supporting board and are ideal for increasing motion and/or shock attenuation. A combo last may have a board in the rearfoot for motion control and more cushioning in the forefoot. Ensure that the seam of the last bisects the heel and the $2^{nd}/3^{rd}$ metatarsal
Toe box (vamp)	This should not be so wide to allow for forefoot shearing, but not so narrow to create compression of the 1st and/or 5th metatarsal heads

Continued

Continued

Shoe component	Description
Heel counter, foxing and Achilles tendon protector	This adds stability to the calcaneus and cushions and presumably aligns the Achilles tendon so the line of pull is relatively vertical. Most heel counters are made of plastic but vary in size and should match the stability needs of the rearfoot
Shoe laces	They should be tied as high as possible to the talus and should be snug to prevent the upper of the shoe from being unstable and facilitating transverse plane shearing of the entire foot
Toe spring	The toe spring can be present secondary to the shoe molding process or can be designed as a metatarsal rocker with increased midsole density or thickness around the metatarsal heads allowing for a rocker type motion, and thus less 1st MTP dorsiflexion demand
Heel width (lateral flare)	A shoe that has excessive width lateral to the calcaneus will actually increase the lever for pronation and may need to be cautiously used for the overpronator or could be used intentionally for the underpronator
Drop (rearfoot to forefoot differential)	High heels and cowboy boots have the highest drop and barefoot type shoes have the smallest. Some shoes actually have been designed with a negative drop. The higher the drop, the less ankle dorsiflexion is needed but this may shift load to the forefoot and may increase the dorsiflexion demands of the forefoot and MTP joints. A classic running shoe has a 12 mm drop, but newer running shoes are often broken down into 0, 4, 8, and 12 mm drop categories

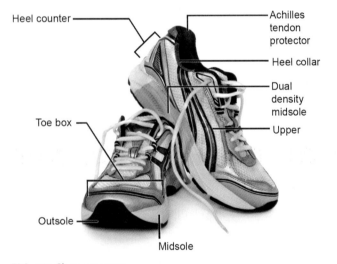

FIG. 13: Shoe anatomy

plantar structures of the foot. However, minimalist and barefoot running may reduce impact loading at the knee, although this is not consistent across natural barefoot runners.[98] Minimalist and barefoot running may lead to a more forefoot (versus rearfoot) striking pattern, which may increase dorsiflexion excursion and velocity of the ankle and MTP joints, as well as pronation excursion and velocity of the foot.[98] This may lead to increased speed and quantity of loading to the deep and superficial compartments of the leg, the intrinsic musculature as well as the noncontractile elements of the foot, including the osseous structures of the forefoot.[98] Therefore,

utilization of barefoot/minimalist shoe gear may increase injury potential for those persons not conditioned for these forces, notably structures in the plantar heel. It has been shown in multiple studies that higher density midsoles reduce postural sway more effectively in the elderly, notably under impaired visual conditions (i.e. eyes closed).[100] This evidence should be considered in the context of the individual when determining the density of the midsole and supportive nature of the shoe itself.

These clinically relevant principles can be extrapolated to casual, dress or other types of athletic shoes. With the ever-changing landscape of shoe manufacturing, it is difficult for the busy clinician to stay abreast of specific shoe brands and designs. Clinicians may benefit from building relationships with local specialty shoe stores that have knowledgeable staff and that carry a variety of brands, sizes and styles in stock. Many clinicians create shoe prescription forms designed for shoe store staff as a way to outline the components of a shoe that are recommended based on the patient examination.

Orthotics

Using orthotics in the treatment of plantar heel pain has received a grade of strong evidence in support for custom or prefabricated orthotics for short-term pain relief (3 months) per recently published clinical practice guidelines.[3] Multilayered and three dimensional plastic orthotics have shown promise in treating the plantar heel pain population over thin and non-supportive orthotics or soft foam based orthotics.[101] There is a reasonable body of literature to support this intervention at a generic level, but sub-classifications of foot type have not been well established, and future studies are indicated before clear recommendations can be made on ideal patient selection criteria and orthotic components.[102-106] Evidence of the correlation between abnormal foot posture and plantar fasciosis is inconclusive, making it unlikely that orthoses intended to address posture alone will be sufficient. Orthotics are thought to impact the lower extremity in several ways aside from foot posture, which include: altering proprioception and contact pressures, slowing down or accelerating speed and excursion of motion and altering muscle firing patterns of the lower extremity (e.g. muscle fatigue). In the absence of specific evidence-based guidelines, clinical reasoning must dominate the decision making process and should be applied at the patient level. Variables, such as shoe gear, casting method, shell and posting material, thickness, shape and cutouts/reliefs, may dramatically influence foot function and should be prescribed with specific risks and benefits in mind, and in close collaboration with the patient and the orthotics manufacturer. The reader is encouraged to explore other resources when deciding if, when and how to prescribe orthotics for specific patient scenarios.

Taping and Splinting

Night splints or socks should be considered as an intervention for plantar heel pain, especially when chronic and recalcitrant to other treatments.[3,6] Best outcomes have been shown for those with greater than 6 months of symptom duration, although many patients do have a positive response to this intervention regardless of chronicity. Treatment duration with splinting may need to persist for 1–3 months. The type of splint has not shown to be as important (e.g. Strassburg sock, hard splint), but it is important that the patient be provided a splint that is comfortable to enhance compliance and effectiveness.

Taping can significantly reduce navicular drop, control pronation and reduce plantar pressures.[107-110] Studies report taping to be an effective treatment tool when combined with other interventions for this patient population.[3,7,111,112] Taping should be considered on the first visit as it has been shown to provide immediate short-term relief for 7–10 days.[94] It may be helpful to consider taping a patient in one or multiple ways simultaneously (Fig. 13). It is important to consider skin integrity, allergies to adhesives and skin irritation. Skin hygiene strategies must be considered and taping should

rarely be considered as a long-term treatment strategy secondary to possible skin breakdown. It is ideal to remove the tape gently on a nightly basis. Moistening the skin before removal may be necessary, as well as cleaning and moisturizing the skin before bed. The patient is instructed to shower and gently remove all residual lotion through firm cleaning of the foot and lower leg and thorough drying before reapplying tape in the morning. If signs of an allergic reaction (contact dermatitis) are present, a thin layer of a basic solution can be used on the skin such as milk of magnesia to counteract the effects of the acidic allergens in tape.[113] The milk of magnesia will dry in a matter of seconds and will be ready for the tape application. Two different types of tape work well to protect skin integrity while also providing firm support. The base layer of tape should be somewhat flexible and include a low allergy adhesive. The top layer should be of firm tensile strength with a stronger adhesive. Some common taping techniques are described and illustrated in Figures 14A to C. Fat Pad taping (Fig. 14A) is designed to sequester the fat pad and stabilize it under the calcaneus and can be taped laterally to medially, or medially to laterally depending on the direction of fat pad displacement. Sometimes it is helpful to pull the fat pad from posterior to anterior as well. The navicular lift taping (Fig. 14B) should originate on the lateral border of the calcaneus, and sweep around the talonavicular joint, along the medial head of the talus and spiral around to the posterior aspect of the leg to give tension to stabilize the rearfoot and midfoot into supination in the transverse and frontal planes. The general arch taping (Fig. 14C) holds the rearfoot and midfoot into a slightly supinated position relative to the forefoot. The tension should be applied in the transverse plane to approximate the rearfoot and forefoot (slight horizontal adduction). Taping in the frontal plane should originate on the lateral side and be pulled into supination toward the medial side of the foot. The three taping options described here can be performed in isolation or combination and should provide instant pain relief with weight bearing if implemented properly in the correct patient population.

Medical, Surgical and Alternative Interventions

There is some evidence that nonsteroidal anti-inflammatory drugs can affect plantar heel pain symptoms.[114] Steroid injections have been shown to provide short-term pain relief.[6,115,116] However, fascial rupture is rated to be as low as 2.4% and as high as 36% after injection, and fascial rupture is correlated with a poor long-term

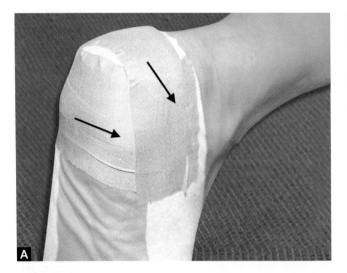

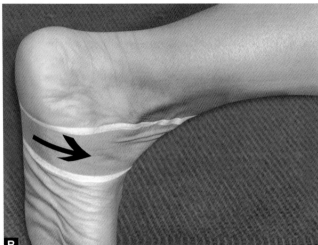

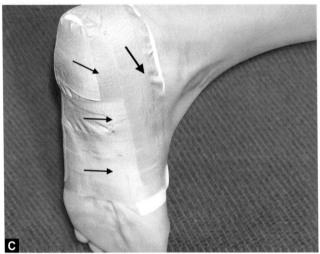

FIGS 14A TO C: Taping techniques of the foot: (A) fat pad taping; (B) navicular lift taping; (C) general arch taping

prognosis.[115,116-118] Platelet-rich plasma is an intriguing and possible treatment option for this condition with inadequate, although steadily mounting, evidence for its support.[115,119-122] Other medical intervention such as prolotherapy, botox, sensory nerve percutaneous ablation, hyaluronic acid injection and extracorporeal shock wave therapy have all shown some promise, but have yet to be included in any clinical practice guidelines to date. For this reason, these interventions may be best reserved for the most recalcitrant of cases at this time. Of course, all of these treatments will likely not address biomechanical, psychosocial and environmental causes of this condition and should never be selected in isolation when considering the patient as a whole.

There are also surgical options (endoscopic and open) that include partial or full release of the plantar

fascia, debridement, calcaneal spur excision, as well as surgical release of the GN, with or without combined surgical release of the plantar fascia. Some studies report long-term success rates with these procedures for symptom relief, although outcomes are unclear and mixed. Therefore these invasive approaches should be considered only in chronic and recalcitrant cases that have failed extensive conservative care.[6,123] Complications post-release can lead to increased strain on the contractile and non-contractile elements that support the arch, as well as injury to the tibial nerve and its branches, and/or the joints of the midfoot and forefoot.[13] For example, a full release leads to 52% increased load on the long plantar ligament and a 94% increase on the spring ligament in cadaver specimens.[14]

CONCLUSION

A close collaboration with the patient, therapist and within an interdisciplinary team is often necessary to navigate the vast number of treatment options available to patients suffering from plantar heel pain. There is a significant and growing body of knowledge that outlines successful and evidence-based treatment conservative care options. However, evidence-based intervention must balance the best scientific evidence with a collaborative reasoning process that leverages the clinician's expertise with the patient's values and expectations. Clinicians should emphasize patient education to address modifiable risk factors, as outlined in sections above. Furthermore, it is important that clinicians realize that there are many different structures that generate plantar heel pain, and many different factors that contribute to plantar heel pain. Specific interventions directed at these unique structures and factors will likely dictate outcomes. Thankfully, this common condition is not typically correlated with severe disability. Unfortunately, 10–20% of individuals will experience a recurrence of symptoms. For these patients, medical, alternative and surgical intervention such as injections and surgery are available and do have some evidence to support their use but should not be used in lieu of evidence-based and patient-centric conservative care.

For the physical therapist, passive modalities appear to have a dwindling role in the current treatment of plantar heel pain, while active approaches such as stretching, manual therapy and neural mobilization are proving to have an increasing role. Additionally, tools such as orthotics, shoes, taping and splinting may serve as potential adjuncts to care that are safe, evidence-based and relatively inexpensive to use. Motor system directed therapeutic exercise (e.g. strengthening, coordination and endurance) has strong promise in this patient population despite a lack of existing translational research. However, existing basic science and foundational evidence prove that dynamic function can be positively influenced with therapeutic exercise at the level of the foot and a person's entire movement system. Further research is warranted to clarify the role of the interdisciplinary team in managing plantar heel pain in a diverse patient population. Research emphasis should be placed on both foundational, basic science research as well as translational research, with a particular emphasis placed on comparative effectiveness studies due to the plethora of treatment options available at this time.

REFERENCES

1. Lemont H, Ammirati KM, Usen N. Plantar fasciitis: a degenerative process (fasciosis) without inflammation. J Am Podiatr Med Assoc. 2003;93(3):234-7.
2. Thomas JL, Christensen JC, Kravitz SR, Mendicino RW, Schuberth JM, Vanore JV, et al. The diagnosis and treatment of heel pain: a clinical practice guideline-revision 2010. J Foot Ankle Surg. 2010;49(3 Suppl):S1-19.
3. McPoil TG, Martin RL, Cornwall MW, Wukich DK, Irrgang JJ, Godges JJ. Heel pain—plantar fasciitis: clinical practice guidelines linked to the international classification of function, disability, and health from the orthopaedic section of the American Physical Therapy Association. J Orthop Sports Phys Ther. 2008;38(4):A1-18.
4. Al Fischer Associates, Inc. 2002 Podiatric Practice Survey. Statistical results. J Am Podiatr Med Assoc. 2003;93(1):67-86.
5. McNally EG, Shetty S. Plantar fascia: imaging diagnosis and guided treatment. Semin Musculoskelet Radiol. 2010;14(3):334-43.
6. Neufeld SK, Cerrato R. Plantar fasciitis: evaluation and treatment. J Am Acad Orthop Surg. 2008;16(6):338-46.
7. Hyland MR, Webber-Gaffney A, Cohen L, Lichtman PTSW. Randomized controlled trial of calcaneal taping, sham taping, and plantar fascia stretching for the short-term management of plantar heel pain. J Orthop Sports Phys Ther. 2006;36(6):364-71.
8. Lopes AD, Hespanhol Júnior LC, Yeung SS, Costa LOP. What are the main running-related musculoskeletal injuries? A systematic review. Sports Med. 2012;42(10):891-905.
9. Carlson RE, Fleming LL, Hutton WC. The biomechanical relationship between the tendoachilles, plantar fascia and metatarsophalangeal joint dorsiflexion angle. Foot ankle Int/Am Orthop Foot Ankle Soc and Swiss Foot Ankle Soc. 2000;21(1):18-25.
10. Stecco C, Corradin M, Macchi V, Morra A, Porzionato A, Biz C, et al. Plantar fascia anatomy and its relationship with Achilles tendon and paratenon. J Anat. 2013;223(6):665-76.
11. Gefen A, Megido-Ravid M, Itzchak Y. In vivo biomechanical behavior of the human heel pad during the stance phase of gait. J Biomech. 2001;34:1661-5.
12. Tweed JL, Barnes MR, Allen MJ, Campbell JA. Biomechanical consequences of total plantar fasciotomy: a review of the literature. J Am Podiatr Med Assoc. 2009;99(5):422-30.
13. Cheung JTM, An KN, Zhang M. Consequences of partial and total plantar fascia release: a finite element study. Foot ankle Int/Am Orthop Foot Ankle Soc and Swiss Foot Ankle Soc. 2006;27(2):125-32.
14. Crary JL, Hollis JM, Manoli A. The effect of plantar fascia release on strain in the spring and long plantar ligaments. Foot ankle Int/Am Orthop Foot Ankle Soc and Swiss Foot Ankle Soc. 2003;24(3):245-50.
15. Ribbans WJ, Garde A. Tibialis posterior tendon and deltoid and spring ligament injuries in the elite athlete. Foot Ankle Clin. 2013;18(2):255-91.
16. Golanó P, Vega J, de Leeuw PA, Malagelada F, Manzanares MC, Götzens V, et al. Anatomy of the ankle ligaments: a pictorial essay. Knee Surg Sports Traumatol Arthrosc. 2010;18(5):557-69.
17. Lin SC, Chen CPC, Tang SFT, Wong AMK, Hsieh JH, Chen WP. Changes in windlass effect in response to different shoe and insole designs during walking. Gait Posture. 2013;37(2):235-41.
18. Caravaggi P, Pataky T, Günther M, Savage R, Crompton R. Dynamics of longitudinal arch support in relation to walking speed: contribution of the plantar aponeurosis. J Anat. 2010;217(3):254-61.
19. Headlee DL, Leonard JL, Hart JM, Ingersoll CD, Hertel J. Fatigue of the plantar intrinsic foot muscles increases navicular drop. J Electromyogr Kinesiol. 2008;18(3):420-5.

20. Chang R, Kent-Braun JA, Hamill J. Use of MRI for volume estimation of tibialis posterior and plantar intrinsic foot muscles in healthy and chronic plantar fasciitis limbs. Clin Biomech (Bristol, Avon). 2012;27(5):500-5.

21. Soysa A, Hiller C, Refshauge K, Burns J. Importance and challenges of measuring intrinsic foot muscle strength. J Foot Ankle Res. 2012;5(1):29.

22. Piazza SJ. Mechanics of the subtalar joint and its function during walking. Foot Ankle Clin. 2005;10(3):425-42.

23. Wang R, Gutierrez-Farewik EM. The effect of subtalar inversion/eversion on the dynamic function of the tibialis anterior, soleus, and gastrocnemius during the stance phase of gait. Gait Posture. 2011;34(1):29-35.

24. Lunsford BR, Perry J. The standing heel-rise test for ankle plantar flexion: criterion for normal. Phys Ther. 1995;75(8):694-8.

25. Hlavackova P, Vuillerme N. Do somatosensory conditions from the foot and ankle affect postural responses to plantar-flexor muscles fatigue during bipedal quiet stance? Gait Posture. 2012;36(1):16-9.

26. Lee SP, Powers C. Fatigue of the hip abductors results in increased medial-lateral center of pressure excursion and altered peroneus longus activation during a unipedal landing task. Clin Biomech (Bristol, Avon). 2013;28(5):524-9.

27. Bisson EJ, McEwen D, Lajoie Y, Bilodeau M. Effects of ankle and hip muscle fatigue on postural sway and attentional demands during unipedal stance. Gait Posture. 2011;33(1):83-7.

28. Kelly LA, Kuitunen S, Racinais S, Cresswell AG. Recruitment of the plantar intrinsic foot muscles with increasing postural demand. Clin Biomech (Bristol, Avon). 2012;27(1):46-51.

29. Alshami AM, Souvlis T, Coppieters MW. A review of plantar heel pain of neural origin: differential diagnosis and management. Man Ther. 2008;13(2):103-11.

30. Chang CW, Wang YC, Hou WH, Lee XX, Chang KF. Medial calcaneal neuropathy is associated with plantar fasciitis. Clin Neurophysiol. 2007;118(1):119-23.

31. Antle DM, Côté JN. Relationships between lower limb and trunk discomfort and vascular, muscular and kinetic outcomes during stationary standing work. Gait Posture. 2013;37(4):615-9.

32. Rome K, Howe T, Haslock I. Risk factors associated with the development of plantar heel pain in athletes. Foot. 2001;11(3):119-25.

33. Riddle DL, Pulisic M, Pidcoe P, Johnson RE. Risk factors for plantar fasciitis: a matched case-control study. J Bone Joint Surg Am. 2003;85-A(5):872-7.

34. Irving DB, Cook JL, Menz HB. Factors associated with chronic plantar heel pain: a systematic review. J Sci Med Sport. 2006;9(1-2):11-22; discussion 23-4.

35. Aranda Y, Munuera PV. Plantar fasciitis and its relationship with hallux limitus. J Am Podiatr Med Assoc. 2014;104(3):263-8.

36. Pohl MB, Hamill J, Davis IS. Biomechanical and anatomic factors associated with a history of plantar fasciitis in female runners. Clin J Sport Med. 2009;19(5):372-6.

37. Wearing SC, Smeathers JE, Yates B, Sullivan PM, Urry SR, Dubois P. Sagittal movement of the medial longitudinal arch is unchanged in plantar fasciitis. Med Sci Sport Exerc. 2004;36(10):1761-7.

38. Tong JWK, Kong PW. Association between foot type and lower extremity injuries: systematic literature review with meta-analysis. J Orthop Sports Phys Ther. 2013;43(10):700-14.

39. Cornwall MW, McPoil TG. Relationship between static foot posture and foot mobility. J Foot Ankle Res. 2011;4:4.

40. Goffar SL, Reber RJ, Christiansen BC, Miller RB, Naylor JA, Rodriguez BM, et al. Changes in dynamic plantar pressure during loaded gait. Phys Ther. 2013;93(9):1175-84.

41. Johal KS, Milner SA. Plantar fasciitis and the calcaneal spur: fact or fiction? Foot Ankle Surg. 2012;18(1):39-41.

42. Duval K, Lam T, Sanderson D. The mechanical relationship between the rearfoot, pelvis and low-back. Gait Posture. 2010;32(4):637-40.

43. Angın S, Ilçin N, Ye ilyaprak SS, Sim ek IE. Prediction of postural sway velocity by foot posture index, foot size and plantar pressure values in unilateral stance. Eklem Hast Cerrahisi and Jt Dis Relat Surg. 2013;24(3):144-8.

44. Cowley E, Marsden J. The effects of prolonged running on foot posture: a repeated measures study of half marathon runners using the foot posture index and navicular height. J Foot Ankle Res. 2013;6(1):20.

45. Gatt A, Chockalingam N. Clinical assessment of ankle joint dorsiflexion: a review of measurement techniques. J Am Podiatr Med Assoc. 2011;101(1):59-69.

46. Johanson M, Baer J, Hovermale H, Phouthavong P. Subtalar joint position during gastrocnemius stretching and ankle dorsiflexion range of motion. J Athl Train. 2008;43(2):172-8.

47. Flanigan RM, Nawoczenski DA, Chen L, Wu H, DiGiovanni BF. The influence of foot position on stretching of the plantar fascia. Foot Ankle Int. 2007;28(7):815-22.

48. Munteanu SE, Strawhorn AB, Landorf KB, Bird AR, Murley GS. A weightbearing technique for the measurement of ankle joint dorsiflexion with the knee extended is reliable. J Sci Med Sport. 2009;12(1):54-9.

49. Chisholm MD, Birmingham TB, Brown J, Macdermid J, Chesworth BM. Reliability and validity of a weight-bearing measure of ankle dorsiflexion range of motion. Physiother Can. 2012;64(4):347-55.

50. Sol M Del, Olave E, Gabrielli C, Mandiola E, Prates J. Innervation of the abductor digiti minimi muscle of the human foot: anatomical basis of the entrapment of the abductor digiti minimi nerve. Surg Radiol Anat. 2002;24(1):18-22.

51. Souza TR, Pinto RZ, Trede RG, Kirkwood RN, Fonseca ST. Temporal couplings between rearfoot-shank complex and hip joint during walking. Clin Biomech (Bristol, Avon). 2010;25(7):745-8.

52. Pohl MB, Buckley JG. Changes in foot and shank coupling due to alterations in foot strike pattern during running. Clin Biomech (Bristol, Avon). 2008;23(3):334-41.

53. O'Shea S, Grafton K. The intra and inter-rater reliability of a modified weight-bearing lunge measure of ankle dorsiflexion. Man Ther. 2013;18(3):264-8.

54. Alshami AM, Babri AS, Souvlis T, Coppieters MW. Biomechanical evaluation of two clinical tests for plantar heel pain: the dorsiflexion-eversion test for tarsal tunnel syndrome and the windlass test for plantar fasciitis. Foot Ankle Int. 2007;28(4):499-505..

55. Rathleff MS, Nielsen RG, Simonsen O, Olesen CG, Kersting UG. Perspectives for clinical measures of dynamic foot function-reference data and methodological considerations. Gait Posture. 2010;31(2):191-6.

56. Power V, Clifford AM. The effects of rearfoot position on lower limb kinematics during bilateral squatting in asymptomatic individuals with a pronated foot type. J Hum Kinet. 2012;31:5-15.

57. Cornwall MW, McPoil TG. Relative movement of the navicular bone during normal walking. Foot Ankle Int. 1999;20(8):507-12.

58. Carcia CR, Martin RL, Houck J, Wukich DK. Achilles pain, stiffness, and muscle power deficits: achilles tendinitis. Clinical practice guidelines linked to the International Classification of Functioning, Disability, and Health from the orthopaedic section of the American Physical Therapy Associat. J Orthop Sports Phys Ther. 2010;40(9):A1-26.

59. Coylewright M, Montori V, Ting HH. Patient-centered shared decision-making: a public imperative. Am J Med. 2012;125(6):545-7.

60. Nicholas MK, Linton SJ, Watson PJ, Main CJ. Early identification and management of psychological risk factors ("yellow flags") in patients with low back pain: a reappraisal. Phys Ther. 2011;91(5):737-53.

61. Leeuw M, Goossens MEJB, Linton SJ, Crombez G, Boersma K, Vlaeyen JWS. The fear-avoidance model of musculoskeletal pain: current state of scientific evidence. J Behav Med. 2007;30(1):77-94.

62. O'Donnell M. Education and Intervention for Musculoskeletal Injuries A Biomechanics Approach. APTA Orthop Sect Indep Study Course Ser. 2012;22.1(22.1.1).

63. Wright DG, Rennels DC. A study of the elastic properties of plantar fascia. J Bone Joint Surg Am. 1964;46:482-92.

64. Lareau CR, Sawyer GA, Wang JH, DiGiovanni CW. Plantar and medial heel pain: diagnosis and management. J Am Acad Orthop Surg. 2014;22(6):372-80.

65. Riley G. The pathogenesis of tendinopathy. A molecular perspective. Rheumatology. 2004;43(2):131-42.

66. Ackermann PW, Renström P. Tendinopathy in sport. Sports Health. 2012;4(3):193-201.

67. Cheung JTM, Zhang M, An KN. Effect of Achilles tendon loading on plantar fascia tension in the standing foot. Clin Biomech (Bristol, Avon). 2006;21(2):194-203.

68. Renan-Ordine R, Alburquerque-Sendín F, de Souza DPR, Cleland JA, Fernández-de-Las-Peñas C. Effectiveness of myofascial trigger point manual therapy combined with a self-stretching protocol for the management of plantar heel pain: a randomized controlled trial. J Orthop Sports Phys Ther. 2011;41(2):43-50.

69. Cleland JA, Abbott JH, Kidd MO, Stockwell S, Cheney S, Gerrard DF, et al. Manual physical therapy and exercise versus electrophysical agents and exercise in the management of plantar heel pain: a multicenter randomized clinical trial. J Orthop Sports Phys Ther. 2009;39(8):573-85.

70. Looney B, Srokose T, Fernández-de-las-Peñas C, Cleland JA. Graston instrument soft tissue mobilization and home stretching for the management of plantar heel pain: a case series. J Manipulative Physiol Ther. 2011;34(2):138-42.

71. Saban B, Deutscher D, Ziv T. Deep massage to posterior calf muscles in combination with neural mobilization exercises as a treatment for heel pain: a pilot randomized clinical trial. Man Ther. 2014;19(2):102-8.

72. Meyer J, Kulig K, Landel R. Differential diagnosis and treatment of subcalcaneal heel pain: a case report. J Orthop Sports Phys Ther. 2002;32(3):114-22; discussion 122-4.

73. Loghmani MT, Warden SJ. Instrument-assisted cross fiber massage increases tissue perfusion and alters microvascular morphology in the vicinity of healing knee ligaments. BMC Complement Altern Med. 2013;13(1):240.

74. Loghmani MT, Warden SJ. Instrument-assisted cross-fiber massage accelerates knee ligament healing. J Orthop Sports Phys Ther. 2009;39(7):506-14.

75. Gudeman SD, Eisele SA, Heidt RS, Colosimo AJ, Stroupe AL. Treatment of plantar fasciitis by iontophoresis of 0.4% dexamethasone. A randomized, double-blind, placebo-controlled study. Am J Sports Med. 1997;25(3):312-6.

76. Rose M. "Our hands will know": the development of tactile diagnostic skill: teaching, learning, and situated cognition in a physical therapy program. Anthropol Educ Q. 1999;30(2):133-60.

77. Digiovanni BF, Nawoczenski DA, Malay DP, Graci PA, Williams TT, Wilding GE, et al. Plantar fascia-specific stretching exercise improves outcomes in patients with chronic plantar fasciitis. A prospective clinical trial with two-year follow-up. J Bone Joint Surg Am. 2006;88(8):1775-81.

78. DiGiovanni BF, Nawoczenski DA, Lintal ME, Moore EA, Murray JC, Wilding GE, et al. Tissue-specific plantar fascia-stretching exercise enhances outcomes in patients with chronic heel pain. A prospective, randomized study. J Bone Joint Surg Am. 2003;85-A(7):1270-7.

79. Garrett T, Neibert PJ. The effectiveness of a gastrocnemius/soleus stretching program as a therapeutic treatment of plantar fasciitis. J Sport Rehabil. 2013:308-12.

80. Drake M, Bittenbender C, Boyles RE. The short-term effects of treating plantar fasciitis with a temporary custom foot orthosis and stretching. J Orthop Sports Phys Ther. 2011;41(4):221-31.

81. Cotchett MP, Landorf KB, Munteanu SE, Raspovic A. Effectiveness of trigger point dry needling for plantar heel pain: study protocol for a randomised controlled trial. J Foot Ankle Res. 2011;4(1):5.

82. Butler D. The Sensitive Nervous System, 1st edition. Adelaide Australia: Noigroup Publications; 2000.

83. Kim MH, Kwon OY, Kim SH, Jung DY. Comparison of muscle activities of abductor hallucis and adductor hallucis between the short foot and toe-spread-out exercises in subjects with mild hallux valgus. J Back Musculoskelet Rehabil. 2013;26(2):163-8.

84. Mulligan EP, Cook PG. Effect of plantar intrinsic muscle training on medial longitudinal arch morphology and dynamic function. Man Ther. 2013;18(5):425-30.

85. Jung DY, Koh EK, Kwon OY. Effect of foot orthoses and short-foot exercise on the cross-sectional area of the abductor hallucis muscle in subjects with pes planus: a randomized controlled trial. J Back Musculoskelet Rehabil. 2011;24(4):225-31.

86. Tosovic D, Ghebremedhin E, Glen C, Gorelick M, Mark Brown J. The architecture and contraction time of intrinsic foot muscles. J Electromyogr Kinesiol. 2012;22(6):930-8.

87. Sefton JM, Yarar C, Hicks-Little CA, Berry JW, Cordova ML. Six weeks of balance training improves sensorimotor function in individuals with chronic ankle instability. J Orthop Sports Phys Ther. 2011;41(2):81-9.

88. Dingenen B, Staes FF, Janssens L. A new method to analyze postural stability during a transition task from double-leg stance to single-leg stance. J Biomech. 2013;46(13):2213-9.

89. Levin O, Van Nevel A, Malone C, Van Deun S, Duysens J, Staes F. Sway activity and muscle recruitment order during transition from double to single-leg stance in subjects with chronic ankle instability. Gait Posture. 2012;36(3):546-51.

90. You JY, Lee HM, Luo HJ, Leu CC, Cheng PG, Wu SK. Gastrocnemius tightness on joint angle and work of lower extremity during gait. Clin Biomech (Bristol, Avon). 2009;24(9):744-50.

91. Chimera NJ, Castro M, Davis I, Manal K. The effect of isolated gastrocnemius contracture and gastrocnemius recession on lower extremity kinematics and kinetics during stance. Clin Biomech (Bristol, Avon). 2012;27(9):917-23.

92. Wearing SC, Smeathers JE, Urry SR. The effect of plantar fasciitis on vertical foot-ground reaction force. Clin Orthop Relat Res. 2003;(409):175-85.

93. Spears IR, Miller-Young JE, Sharma J, Ker RF, Smith FW. The potential influence of the heel counter on internal stress during static standing: a combined finite element and positional MRI investigation. J Biomech. 2007;40(12):2774-80.

94. Osborne HR, Allison GT. Treatment of plantar fasciitis by LowDye taping and iontophoresis: short term results of a double blinded, randomised, placebo controlled clinical trial of dexamethasone and acetic acid. Br J Sports Med. 2006;40(6):545-9;discussion 549.

95. Cheung RTH, Ng GYF. Efficacy of motion control shoes for reducing excessive rearfoot motion in fatigued runners. Phys Ther Sport. 2007;8(2):75-81.

96. Cheung RT, Ng GYF. Motion control shoe delays fatigue of shank muscles in runners with overpronating feet. Am J Sports Med. 2010;38(3):486-91.

97. Cheung RTH, Ng GYF. Influence of different footwear on force of landing during running. Phys Ther. 2008;88(5):620-8.

98. Lieberman DE, Venkadesan M, Werbel WA, Daoud AI, D'Andrea S, Davis IS, et al. Foot strike patterns and collision forces in habitually barefoot versus shod runners. Nature. 2010;463(7280):531-5.

99. Wearing SC, Smeathers JE, Yates B, Urry SR, Dubois P. Bulk compressive properties of the heel fat pad during walking : a pilot investigation in plantar heel pain. Clin Biomech. 2009;24(4):397-402.

100. Losa Iglesias ME, Becerro de Bengoa Vallejo R, Palacios Peña D. Impact of soft and hard insole density on postural stability in older adults. Geriatr Nurs. 2012;33(4):264-71.

101. Walther M, Kratschmer B, Verschl J, Volkering C, Altenberger S, Kriegelstein S, et al. Effect of different orthotic concepts as first line treatment of plantar fasciitis. Foot Ankle Surg. 2013;19(2):103-7.

102. Anderson J, Stanek J. Effect of foot orthoses as treatment for plantar fasciitis or heel pain. J Sport Rehabil. 2013;22(2):130-6.

103. Pfeffer G, Bacchetti P, Deland J, Lewis A, Anderson R, Davis W, et al. Comparison of custom and prefabricated orthoses in the initial treatment of proximal plantar fasciitis. Foot Ankle Int. 1999;20(4):214-21.

104. Hawke F, Burns J, Ja R, Toit V. Custom-made foot orthoses for the treatment of foot pain (Review). Cochrane Collab. 2008;(3):CD006801.

105. Lee SY, McKeon P, Hertel J. Does the use of orthoses improve self-reported pain and function measures in patients with plantar fasciitis? A meta-analysis. Phys Ther Sport. 2009;10(1):12-8.

106. Landorf KB, Keenan A, Herbert RD. Effectiveness of foot orthoses to treat plantar fasciitis: a randomized trial. Arch Intern Med. 2006;166(12):1305-10.

107. Van Lunen B, Cortes N, Andrus T, Walker M, Pasquale M, Onate J. Immediate effects of a heel-pain orthosis and an augmented low-dye taping on plantar pressures and pain in subjects with plantar fasciitis. Clin J Sport Med. 2011;21(6):474-9.

108. Radford JA, Burns J, Buchbinder R, Landorf KB, Cook C. The effect of low-Dye taping on kinematic, kinetic, and electromyographic variables: a systematic review. J Orthop Sports Phys Ther. 2006;36(4):232-41.

109. O'Sullivan K, Kennedy N, O'Neill E, Ni Mhainin U. The effect of low-dye taping on rearfoot motion and plantar pressure during the stance phase of gait. BMC Musculoskelet Disord. 2008;9:111.

110. Cheung RTH, Chung RCK, Ng GYF. Efficacies of different external controls for excessive foot pronation: a meta-analysis. Br J Sports Med. 2011;45(9):743-51.

111. Van de Water ATM, Speksnijder CM. Efficacy of taping for the treatment of plantar fasciosis: a systematic review of controlled trials. J Am Podiatr Med Assoc. 2010;100(1):41-51.

112. Podolsky R, Kalichman L. Taping for plantar fasciitis. J Back Musculoskelet Rehabil. 2014.

113. Corazza M, Minghetti S, Benetti S, Marchetti N, Borghi A, Virgili A. Allergic contact dermatitis in a volleyball player due to protective adhesive taping. Eur J Dermatol. 2011;21(3):430-1.

114. Donley BG, Moore T, Sferra J, Gozdanovic J, Smith R. The efficacy of oral nonsteroidal anti-inflammatory medication (NSAID) in the treatment of plantar fasciitis: a randomized, prospective, placebo-controlled study. Foot Ankle Int. 2007;28(1):20-3.

115. Ak ahin E, Do ruyol D, Yüksel HY, Hapa O, Do an O, Celebi L, et al. The comparison of the effect of corticosteroids and platelet-rich plasma (PRP) for the treatment of plantar fasciitis. Arch Orthop Trauma Surg. 2012;132(6):781-5.

116. Chen CM, Chen JS, Tsai WC, Hsu HC, Chen KH, Lin CH. Effectiveness of device-assisted ultrasound-guided steroid injection for treating plantar fasciitis. Am J Phys Med Rehabil. 2013;92(7):597-605.

117. Acevedo JI, Beskin JL. Complications of plantar fascia rupture associated with corticosteroid injection. Foot ankle Int/Am Orthop Foot Ankle Soc and Swiss Foot Ankle Soc. 1998;19:91-7.

118. Genc H, Saracoglu M, Nacir B, Erdem HR, Kacar M. Long-term ultrasonographic follow-up of plantar fasciitis patients treated with steroid injection. Joint Bone Spine. 2005;72(1):61-5. doi:10.1016/j.jbspin.2004.03.006.

119. De Vos RJ, Weir A, van Schie HT, Bierma-Zeinstra SM, Verhaar JA, Weinans H, et al. Platelet-rich plasma injection for chronic Achilles tendinopathy: a randomized controlled trial. J Am Med Assoc. 2010;303(2):144-9.

120. De Vos RJ, van Veldhoven PL, Moen MH, Weir A, Tol JL, Maffulli N. Autologous growth factor injections in chronic tendinopathy: a systematic review. Br Med Bull. 2010;95:63-77.

121. Lyras DN, Kazakos K, Verettas D, Polychronidis A, Tryfonidis M, Botaitis S, et al. The influence of platelet-rich plasma on angiogenesis during the early phase of tendon healing. Foot Ankle Int/Am Orthop Foot Ankle Soc and Swiss Foot Ankle Soc. 2009;30(11):1101-6.

122. Kumar V, Millar T, Murphy PN, Clough T. The treatment of intractable plantar fasciitis with platelet-rich plasma injection. Foot (Edinb). 2013:15-18.

123. League AC. Current concepts review: plantar fasciitis. Foot Ankle Int. 2008;29(3):358-66.

124. Chen DW, Li B, Aubeeluck A, Yang YF, Huang YG, Zhou JQ, et al. Anatomy and biomechanical properties of the plantar aponeurosis: a cadaveric study. PLoS One. 2014;9(1):e84347.

125. Hossain M, Makwana N. "Not plantar fasciitis": the differential diagnosis and management of heel pain syndrome. Orthop Trauma. 2011;25(3):198-206.

126. Michaud T. Human locomotion: the conservative management of gait related disorders. Newton, Massachusetts: Netwon Biomechanics; 2011.

CHAPTER 16

First Metatarsophalangeal Sprain

Joseph M Miller

ABSTRACT

The first metatarsophalangeal (1st MTP) joint is an important weight-bearing joint. During ambulation, the foot is the first part of the body to make contact with the ground. The 1st MTP bears the most weight and is important in propulsion during gait. The joint also plays a pivotal role in balance. Because of the importance of the great toe for propulsion and balance, injuries to this area may greatly affect activities of daily living, occupational demands and athletic participation. Conservative treatment of 1st MTP injuries has been researched as the first-line treatment. Restoring mobility and the strength to control that mobility are the primary objectives of conservative care. However, in many cases, permanent orthotics may be required for functional recovery. Attention not only to the great toe but also to the kinetic chain as a whole contributes to minimizing recurrence and maximizing recovery.

INTRODUCTION

The first metatarsophalangeal (1st MTP) joint is an important weight-bearing joint. The 1st MTP joint bears twice the load compared to the other toes, and around 40–60% of the body weight during stance phase of normal gait.[1,2] During jogging and running, the 1st MTP endures two to three times and up to eight times the body weight, respectively.[1] Management and treatment of 1st MTP injuries can be varied, but conservative care is considered primary. If treated and managed effectively, injuries to this area may not lead to long-term disability and foot biomechanical dysfunction.

Anatomy

The 1st MTP joint is inherently unstable due to the shallow bony surface of the proximal phalanx.[3-6] The capsule, ligaments and sesamoid grouping provide the majority of the stability. The medial and lateral sesamoids provide a bony influence on the joint and lie within the conjoined flexor tendon, providing an increased mechanical advantage for the flexor group (Fig. 1). The other noncontractile structures include the joint capsule, collateral ligament, plantar ligament (plate), plantar fascia and deep transverse ligament. The collateral ligaments provide strong medial and lateral support to the joint, limiting varus and valgus movement. The plantar ligament (plate) provides a point of adhesion for the sesamoids as well as the primary support during extension (Fig. 1). The sesamoids act as a force multiplier for the 1st MTP flexors. The deep transverse ligament runs between the metatarsal heads providing support to the distal forefoot. Biomechanically, the series of joints just proximal and distal to the 1st MTP are often relevant and described as a unit: the first ray. The first ray is the area from the base of the first metatarsal to the hallux.

Contractile structures that affect the joint are both intrinsic and extrinsic to the foot. The contractile structures' primary function is joint mobility, but they also contribute to dynamic joint stability. Extrinsic contractile structures include the flexor hallucis longus (FHL) and the extensor hallucis longus (EHL). The intrinsic contractile structures include abductor hallucis (AbH), adductor hallucis (AdH), flexor hallucis brevis (FHB) and extensor hallucis brevis (EHB). The FHL and FHB both act to flex the hallux, while the EHL and EHB both act to extend the hallux. The AdH has two heads that act to pull the hallux laterally and in a slightly plantar direction. The AbH acts to stabilize the 1st MTP and pull the hallux medially.

Etiology and Epidemiology

First MTP joint pain is a common foot complaint associated with osteoarthritis in more than 20% of people over the age of 40 years.[8] There are two main areas of injury, the MTP joint and the sesamoid. These injuries range in severity from sprain to fracture and dislocations. The most common injury is a 1st MTP hyperextension sprain.[4]

The 1st MTP hyperextension sprain is a sprain or tear of the capsular ligamentous structure of the joint. Originally described by Bower and Martin in 1976, they found an average of 5.4 1st MTP hyperextension sprain injuries per football season in one college team over the course of a single season.[5,6] Because the injuries occurred on an artificial turf surface, the injury was called "turf toe".[5,6,9] The typical mechanism of a turf toe injury is an axial load to a forefoot fixed to the ground while the great toe is in extension.[6,9] Turf toe occurs mostly with sporting or recreational activities played on surfaces that have an

increased coefficient of friction, or with shoes that allow increased flexibility. Rodeo et al. found as early as 1990 that 83% of American National Football League (NFL) turf toe injuries occurred on artificial surfaces.[9] Contact sports have a higher incidence of this type of injury versus non-contact sports.[6,9] The incidence seems to increase particularly with the use of artificial surfaces for sport training and competition.[5,6] A recent study of American collegiate football players revealed that artificial surfaces and game time specifically, more so than practice, were risk factors for turf toe injuries.[10]

■ CLINICAL PRESENTATION

Individuals presenting with turf toe will complain of different pain level intensities. Swelling, ecchymosis and range of motion (ROM) restriction (specifically hallux extension) quantity usually correlate with severity of injury. Clinical classification of the severity of 1st MTP sprains is described in Table 1.

Antalgic gait, or refusal to bear full weight, may be present, necessitating the need for an assistive device, modified footwear and/or activity modification.[5,6,11,12] The common gait compensation is a lack of push-off in terminal stance due to the increased requirement to extend the hallux during this phase of gait. However, any gait deviation may occur, such as hip circumduction, an external rotated hip, or a flat foot gait pattern. Walking uphill will be more difficult and painful because of the greater demand for hallux extension compared to level surfaces. Additionally, the ability to cut or change direction

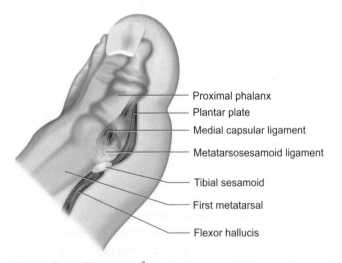
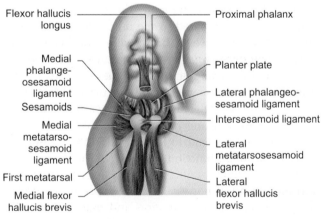

FIG. 1: First MTP anatomy[7]

TABLE 1: Clinical classification of turf toe injuries[15]

Grade	Findings
I	• Localize plantar or medial tenderness • Minimal swelling • No ecchymosis
II	• More diffuse and intense tenderness • Mild to moderate swelling • Mild to moderate ecchymosis • Painful and limited ROM
III	• Severe and diffuse tenderness • Marked swelling • Moderate to severe ecchymosis • Painful and limited ROM

Source: Adapted from Anderson RB. Great Toe Disorders, with permission from Elsevier Health Sciences.

TABLE 2: Grading of hallux rigidus based on radiographs and clinical findings[16]

Grade	Radiological findings	Clinical findings
I	Plantar subluxation of proximal phalanx with no radiographic evidence of degenerative joint disease	Pain at end of passive ROM
II	Dorsal spurring, subchondral degeneration, sclerosis and possible development of osteochondral defects	Limited passive ROM
III	Subchondral bone cyst, severe flattening of joint, severe spurring, asymmetrical space loss, articular cartilage loss	Grade II plus joint crepitation and pain with joint ROM
IV	Obliteration of joint space Intra-articular loose bodies	Grade III plus less than 10 degrees 1st MTP ROM, possible total ankylosis

Source: Adapted from Shurnas PS. Hallux Rigidus, with permission from Elsevier Health Science.

will be difficult and painful. In the case of chronic injury, decreased ROM and increased force across the 1st MTP have been shown to occur in NFL players with a history of turf toe versus similar players without this injury history.[13]

Swelling and ecchymosis will most likely be present; however, the amount usually correlates with the severity and may vary between individual patients. The swelling will be localized to the 1st MTP joint. Along with the swelling, tenderness may be present both on the plantar and dorsal aspect of the 1st MTP.

Depending on the grade of injury, ROM will be restricted. The greatest restrictions occur in extension of the 1st MTP. However, there may also be restriction in the ankle joint and first ray itself.[14]

Differential Diagnosis

Due to the location of the sesamoid bones, simultaneous injury and associated symptoms of a sesamoid injury may also be present with turf toe. Additionally, axial loading can occur with a valgus or varus load, causing a subsequent deviation of the hallux into varus or valgus. This deviation can cause injury to the medial and lateral structures of the 1st MTP. Turf toe can progress to hallux limitus once the acute injury has subsided.

Hallux limitus is as a limitation in ROM (typically, with little to no pain) usually because of repetitive injury or previous trauma (e.g. the later sequela from a turf toe injury). If not treated, this condition progresses to greater limitation in motion and pain called hallux rigidus. Individuals with a longer first metatarsal may be more prone to developing hallux rigidus.[1] Hallux rigidus is commonly present in individuals suffering from rheumatoid arthritis.[1,16] Family history of 1st MTP arthritis or hallux valgus correlated to 80% incidence of bilateral disease.[16] Additionally, females show a higher incidence of hallux rigidus versus males.[16] Both hallux limitus and rigidus symptoms include 1st MTP joint pain, swelling and stiffness—predominantly restricted extension. Pain with this condition is initially located dorsally. Eventually, the entire 1st MTP joint may become painful. Initially, pain may only be present without wearing footwear, but ultimately progress to both with and without footwear. Severity of hallux limitus is graded using plain film radiography (Table 2).

Hallux valgus is one of the most common chronic foot conditions, characterized by lateral deviation of the first phalanx and decreased ROM.[4,17] If hallux valgus progresses, an osseous prominence can form on the medial side of the 1st MTP, which is commonly referred to as a bunion (Fig. 2). This condition occurs from a variety of factors, the two most common being poor fitting shoes and genetic predisposition.[4,18] Biomechanical instability and neuromuscular issues also contribute to this condition. Prevalence of hallux valgus is estimated at 23% for adults aged 18–65 years and 35.7% for the elderly.[19] Females also demonstrate a higher prevalence than males (30% vs 13%, respectively).[19] The hallmark of hallux valgus is the medial protuberance, or bunion. Pain is mostly located medially at the protuberance but can progress to the whole joint. The bunion may appear

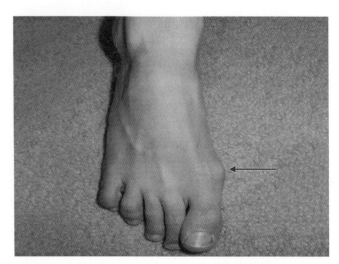

FIG. 2: Hallux valgus with the hallmark protuberance

TABLE 3: Classification of hallux valgus[17]

Angle	Normal	Mild	Moderate	Severe
Hallux valgus (degree)	<15	<20	20–40	>40
Intermetatarsal (degree)	<9	<11	<16	≥16

Source: Adapted from Hecht and Lin. Hallux Valgus, with permission from Elsevier Health Science.

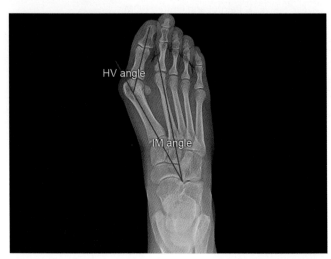

FIG. 3: Hallux valgus measurements. Hallux valgus (HV) represents the angle formed by the shaft of the first metatarsal and the first phalanx at the MTP. IM is the angle formed by the intersection of the first and second metatarsals

without discoloration, or as a red protuberance. Shoes with narrow toe boxes tend to aggravate this condition. Higher heeled shoes also displace more force toward the forefoot and cause aggravation.[4] ROM restriction increases with progression of this condition, especially abduction, flexion and extension ranges. Progression is associated with increased medial deviation of the hallux. Hallux valgus grading is based on the angle between the proximal phalanx and the first metatarsal bones, measured on plain film radiography and known as the metatarsal angle (Table 3 and Fig. 3). Antalgic gait, or refusal to bear full weight, may necessitate the use of assistive device, modified footwear or orthotics.

The sesamoid bones are important structures for proper ambulation because they help to lengthen the first ray during gait and facilitate lateral to medial weight transfer.[6,20] A bipartite or multipartite sesamoid is present in 5–33% of the population. These sesamoidal anomalies may or may not be symptomatic: acute symptoms associated with these radiographs provide the differential diagnosis for sesamoid fractures.[6,20] The most common sesamoid injuries are caused by overuse during weight bearing: stress fracture (occurring 40%) and sesamoiditis—also known as chondromalacia (occurring 30%).[20] Fractures and osteoarthritis have the same occurrence rate as one another of approximately 10%.[20] The medial sesamoid is the larger of the two bones and exposed to greater weight-bearing. The medial sesamoid has the higher incidence of injury, with occurrence of injury to the lateral sesamoid being rare.[20] Individuals with sesamoid injuries will complain of pain on plantar aspect of the foot, most often localized to the medial plantar aspect of the foot.[20] Passive ROM of the 1st MTP

may be painless, but weight-bearing ROM is often painful. Swelling is often present and may be associated with enlargement of the bursa on the plantar aspect of the foot.[1,20] Antalgic gait or refusal to bear full weight may necessitate the use of assistive device, modified footwear or orthotics.

CLINICAL EXAMINATION

Clinical examination of turf toe consists of taking a thorough history and administering a comprehensive objective examination. The history and objective examination should be complemented by a global functional assessment.

The history must include the type of activities the individual regularly performs both for work and for leisure. Establishing a mechanism of injury is especially important with turf toe because the typical mechanism is long axis compression with the dorsiflexed foot.[5,6,9] This mechanism can also cause a sesamoid injury; however, the more typical mechanism for acute sesamoid injury is direct impact. In contrast, chronic sesamoid injuries, hallux limitus and hallux valgus tend to have an insidious onset. Assessing ROM, joint stability, swelling, strength and gait are elements of the objective examination. Visual inspection of swelling and ecchymosis should be conducted initially. Careful and systematic palpation of the joint and associated capsuloligamentous structures should occur next. The plantar aspect of the hallux will be most painful. Normal ROM for the 1st MTP has been reported as 65–70 degrees of extension and 40–45 degrees of flexion.[3] There is very little adduction or abduction motion in the joint comparatively to flexion and extension.[11] For joint stability, a dorsoplantar drawer test (similar to the Lachman test of the knee),[21] and varus and valgus tests should be performed.[5,6] If there is no instability present, then accessory motion assessment occurs next.

Assessing the motion of the entire first ray is necessary to decrease stress and dysfunction of the 1st MTP in relation to the kinetic chain. A grading system exists for assessment of first ray mobility (Table 4).[3] Additionally, comparing 1st MTP mobility of the affected side to unaffected side is critical. Joint anteroposterior (AP), posteroanterior (PA), medial to lateral, lateral to medial play and rotational play of the subtalar and talocrural joints compared to unaffected side identifies manual therapy interventions that may be indicated.

Strength testing should be conducted for the entire kinetic chain. Gait deviations, pain and swelling can inhibit muscle activity. Hip, knee and ankle strength should be tested as long as pain does not limit the test. Ankle and toe strength testing may not be feasible for an acute injury due to severe pain and the need to protect the soft tissues while healing. Once pain and swelling is no longer present, great toe flexion and extension can be tested. Strength assessment may be conducted with manual muscle testing or with a handheld dynamometer. Initially, isometric strength of the great toe may be safely

conducted, while isotonic assessment of the ankle, knee and hip is appropriate. Differences from the injured to noninjured side should be noted.

Beyond local assessment of the injured joint, evaluation of lower extremity biomechanics, including; gait, strength of lower extremity, ROM of lower extremity and integrated motion can prove helpful in the design of a comprehensive rehabilitation program.

Kinetic Chain Assessment

There is evidence to support dysfunctional lumbopelvic muscular activity correlates with lower extremity injury.[22,23] Additionally, decrease in ROM in any part of the kinetic chain may result in compensatory changes in other areas. In order to help mitigate future injury, assessing and addressing any identified dysfunctions in the kinetic chain has recently shown to be helpful.[22,24-26] For this reason comprehensive rehabilitation for 1st MTP injuries should include the entire kinetic chain. Due to the functional relationship between the ankle, foot and toes, assessment of ankle motion, stability and proprioception should occur as well. There is growing evidence that functional movement deficits contribute to injury.[24,25,27] There are many ways to assess the kinetic chain but evidence exists for several specific clinical assessments.[22-25,27] Single leg squatting, double leg squatting, step-ups, step-downs (multidirectional) and the Y-Balance™ (Star Excursion Balance Test)[28,29] are well-researched assessment tools.

Single leg squatting is an appropriate assessment for many sporting and daily activities that require a running type cadence or single limb support. The single leg squat is compared side-to-side. This test is quick and easy to do and allows for a side-to-side comparison. It is also a very functional assessment. The disadvantage of this test is that requires uniplanar motion only. The single leg squat should be viewed from multiple angles (front, sides and rear) in order to view deviations in every plane of motion.

Double leg squatting allows for visualization of both limbs simultaneously and the movement forms the basis for many activities. However, most sports or recreational activities usually involve single leg demands. As with the single leg squat, the double leg squat should be viewed from multiple positions (front, sides and rear).

Step-ups and step-downs have the advantage of challenging the kinetic chain multiple planes. The balance and control requirements are higher than a double leg squat and single leg squat on flat ground due to inherent weight shift from one limb to another,

TABLE 4: First ray mobility classification[3]

Grades	Criterion
Hypomobile	If dorsiflexion motion of the first metatarsal head does not translate equal to the sagittal plane of the lesser metatarsal heads
Normal	If dorsiflexion motion is equal to the sagittal plane of the lesser metatarsal heads
Hypermobile	If dorsiflexion motion of the first metatarsal head clearly rises above the dorsal aspect of the lesser metatarsal heads

and greater excursion of the patient's center of mass. It is important to assess the step-up and step-down in multiple directions (front, back and both sides) to assess multiplane mechanics.

The Y-Balance Test™, which is a condensed version of the Star Excursion Balance Test, enables the detection of dynamic postural control deficits in the lower extremity.[29] The test consists of standing on one leg and moving the non-weight-bearing leg in three directions (anterior, posteromedial and posterolateral). The test may be normalized for the individual by reporting the results in a manner proportionate to the size of the subject. For example, if the sum of the maximal reach in each direction is divided by three times the length of the tested limb, the results will be reported proportionate to lower extremity limb length, which can account for approximately 20% of the measured reach.[28]

■ PHYSICAL THERAPY TREATMENT

Physical therapy treatment of turf toe varies depending on the stage of the condition. The specific treatments selected also depend on the individual patient's presentation. While there are protocols for conservative rehabilitation,[1,4,5,9,15,17-20] tailoring the treatment based on the examination and goals of the individual patient is best. Additionally, the level of athletic participation to which the patient is attempting to return should be considered. Limited evidence for conservative care for 1st MTP injures exists,[3,4,12,30-32] most of the research has analyzed operative measures and rehabilitation after

surgery.[1,3-6,20,30,31] Despite the sparse research, evidence exists for manual therapy, taping, exercise and modalities in the management of 1st MTP injuries.[3,4,11,22-25] The three phases of healing with soft tissue injury are inflammatory, proliferative and maturation stages. With rehabilitation, interventions should follow the stages of healing. It is imperative that during recovery, the patient is educated that pain is a warning to the body, but that gentle, graded motion and activity with discomfort—not necessarily pain—is necessary for functional recovery.

Inflammatory Stage Rehabilitation

Protection, control of pain and control of swelling are the goals of rehabilitation during the inflammatory stage. The duration of this stage lasts up to 6 days.[33]

Modalities, such as cryotherapy with or without compression, help to decrease inflammation and control pain for turf toe injuries, while bracing and/or padding help to decrease pain.[34,35] Therapeutic ultrasound has been utilized for swelling; however, a systematic review found no effect for therapeutic ultrasound on swelling for acute ankle injuries.[36] Electrical stimulation, especially high volt, can be effective for swelling management.[37] Kinesiology tape provides flexibility and rebound in one or multiple directions, depending on the type of tape. This tape can be applied for support and swelling control (Fig. 4).[38,39]

A walking boot or hard-soled shoes may decrease pain and stress to the 1st MTP. The objective of these devices is to limit forced great toe extension. Gentle motion from

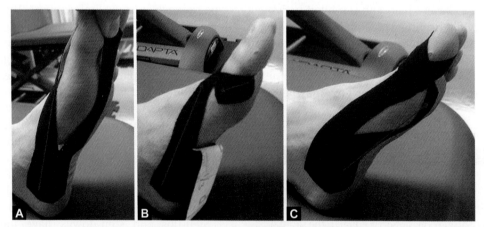

FIGS 4A TO C: Kinesiotape™ application for turf toe support. (A) Y-strip is cut with the uncut end anchored (without tension) at the plantar medial heel; (B) With 50–75% tension (clinician will see wavy lines in material) and the great toe extended as much as possible, the most medial strip of the tape is applied to the dorsum of the 1st MTP, wrapping around the medial aspect of the first phalanx to finish anchored on itself; (C) The remaining strip is placed with the same tensioning procedure, but applied along the plantar surface of the foot, crossing the volar aspect of the 1st MTP, wrapping around the first phalanx to anchor on itself

neutral to tolerable flexion may begin immediately as long as it is not contraindicated by fracture or more severe injury. To avoid further strain or tearing of injured plantar structures, minimizing extension early on is essential for recovery.

If no contraindications exist, gentle manual therapies that do not increase pain are indicated (Tables 5 and 6). The sesamoids influence the 1st MTP joint in a way analogous to how the patella influences the knee joint. Therefore, assessing and facilitating mobility of the sesamoids while the 1st MTP motion is limited will help to prevent possible sesamoid and capsule adhesion.[6] Grade I–II joint mobilization, in anatomical and accessory motion, are the grades employed at this stage, as the objective is pain management (Tables 5 and 6). The mobilizations should be conducted with the MTP joint in a neutral or plantar flexed position (Table 6).

Low impact cardiovascular activity, such as upper body ergometer or pool therapy, can be attempted. The toe should be splinted for protection during cardiovascular activities, if necessary to avoid pain, with a splint that restricts extension.

Assessing and addressing the proximal chain should be conducted early in the rehabilitation. Since direct intervention to the 1st MTP may be limited, focusing on deficient mobility and on control proximally will decrease the need for compensation. Hip and ankle mobility and control (strength and activation) are essential for weight-

TABLE 5: Grades of joint mobilization[43]

Grades	Purpose	Motion
I	Decrease pain / Decrease pain with motion	Small amplitude within available ROM not near end-range
II	Decrease pain / Decrease pain with motion	Large amplitude within available ROM not near end-range
III	Improve motion / Decrease pain with motion	Large amplitude mid- to end-ROM
IV	Improve motion / Decrease pain with motion	Small amplitude mid- to end-ROM

TABLE 6: Mobilizations of the foot and ankle

Mobilization	Hand placement	Action (distraction or compression may be helpful to reduce discomfort)	Purpose
Anteroposterior 1st MTP		AP glide with the distal thumb and index finger while proximal hand stabilizes	To increase inferior glide and roll to facilitate extension
Posteroanterior 1st MTP		PA glide with the distal thumb and index finger while proximal hand stabilizes	To increased superior glide and roll to facilitate flexion

419

Continued

Continued

Mobilization	Hand placement	Action (distraction or compression may be helpful to reduce discomfort)	Purpose
Medial glide 1st MTP		Medial glide through distal thumb and index while the proximal hand stabilizes	To increase medial glide to facilitate abduction
Lateral glide 1st MTP		Lateral glide through distal thumb and index finger with the proximal hand stabilizes	To increase lateral glide to facilitate adduction
Flexion		Distal thumb and index finger induce flexion while proximal hand stabilizes	To facilitate flexion
Extension		Distal thumb and index finger induce extension while proximal hand stabilizes	To facilitate extension

Continued

Continued

Mobilization	Hand placement	Action (distraction or compression may be helpful to reduce discomfort)	Purpose
Abduction		Distal thumb and index finger induce abduction while proximal hand stabilizes	To facilitate abduction
Adduction		Distal thumb and index finger induce adduction while proximal hand stabilizes	To facilitate adduction
Sesamoid proximal to distal and distal to proximal		Pinching sesamoid or sesamoids between thumb and index finger and induce proximal to distal and distal to proximal motion	Proximal to distal motion facilitates extension Distal to proximal facilitates flexion
Sesamoid medial to lateral and lateral to medial		Pinching sesamoid or sesamoids between thumb and index finger and induce medial to lateral and lateral to medial motion	Medial to lateral facilitates adduction Lateral to medial facilitates abduction

Continued

Continued

Mobilization	Hand placement	Action (distraction or compression may be helpful to reduce discomfort)	Purpose
Ankle AP		With the patient lying supine, the distal hand induces an AP force while the proximal hand stabilizes	To increase posterior glide and roll that facilitates ankle dorsiflexion
Ankle PA		With the patient lying prone, the distal hand induces PA force while the proximal hand stabilizes	To increase anterior glide and roll that facilitates ankle plantar flexion
Ankle 4-way (plantar flexion, dorsiflexion, inversion, and eversion)		With the patient lying prone and knee bent to 90 degrees both hands in induce anatomical motion	To increase multi-planar motion

bearing activities, particularly running.[40,41] Addressing hip and ankle motion and control in all three planes of motion is essential.[30,31] If there are hypomobility issues, then hip mobilizations and/or stretching may be appropriate. AP, caudal and PA mobilizations, hands-on or self-directed, may be beneficial. Stretching the hip flexor in supine off the edge of the table, the quadriceps in side lying and the hip external rotators in supine are typical stretches employed for hip tightness. Clamshells, hip abduction, hip extension and hip adduction should be employed initially to increase hip muscle activation

and ability to generate resistance.[41,42] Typical ankle mobilizations to address ankle hypomobility include AP, PA and four-way (Table 6). Four-way ankle strengthening with a resistance band can be utilized as long as painful pressure is not applied to the 1st MTP.

Proliferation Stage Rehabilitation

This stage begins at the termination of the inflammatory stage and lasts approximately 4 weeks.[33] During this time, the objective is to add graded activities based on the individual's presentation. Treatment of turf toe during this stage focuses on return of motion, progressive strengthening and progressive normalization of activities based on the grade of the injury. Manual therapy techniques will progress to grade III–IV to promote restoration of motion (Tables 5 and 6). Initiation of gentle ROM is indicated if there is no fracture nor any other severe injury (e.g. Grade III sprain).[5,6] Motion may begin into extension, within pain tolerance. This motion can be active or active-assisted, with the patient or clinician providing assistance with their hands.

Progression of mobilizations from Grade I–II to III–IV is appropriate based on pain and stability of the joint. Mobilizations can be conducted at different angles of flexion and extension as pain allows. Both anatomical and accessory motion may be beneficial. The patient should be instructed to comment on any pain during the mobilizations as well if the pain increases or decreases during the ensuing treatment. If the pain is moderate to high, the grade of mobilization should be reduced. Many of the 1st MTP mobilizations can be taught to the patient for more frequent implementation and long-term maintenance as needed.

At this time, cardiovascular activities such as stationary biking or elliptical are safe.

Initiation of isometric strengthening of the 1st MTP occurs at this point and progressed as tolerated. Exercises at this stage include: isometrics in all directions of motion for the 1st MTP, pebble or marble pickup, towel toe crunches and pushes, active-assisted toe flexion and extension and seated rising on toes and lowering. Progression of these exercises should be based on severity of injury and other concomitant injuries.

For grade I sprains, return to athletic competition can occur with an orthotic and/or taping when the patient is pain-free and demonstrates at least 50–60 degrees of painless passive extension at the 1st MTP.[5,6] For Grade II sprains, return to athletic competition with an orthotic and/or taping usually will not occur earlier than 2 weeks postinjury.[5,6]

Protection of the toe with taping in flexion will help to limit motion and provide compression. The main purpose of taping for turf toe is to provide support while not restricting motion completely. Athletic tape and leukotape-more rigid tapes than the previously mentioned kinesiology tape-provide more support (Fig. 5). The figure of eight techniques is the most common for this injury.

For turf toe injuries, an orthotic with carbon fiber support is typically utilized (Fig. 6). The purpose of the orthotic is to provide support for this relatively unstable

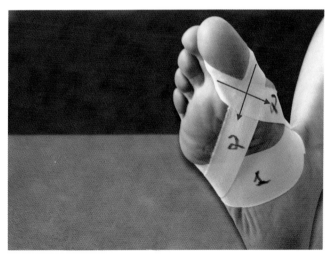

FIG. 5: Turf toe taping with athletic tape. Tape 1 is the anchor placed mid foot. Tape 2 is placed on the dorsal aspect of the first phalanx and pulled volarly, both medially and laterally, providing a plantar force that limits extension. Typically, three strips of tape, each overlapping by ½ their width, will be placed in the Tape 2 orientation; and a second strip, applied in the same manner as Tape 1, will cover the loose ends of the prior strips.

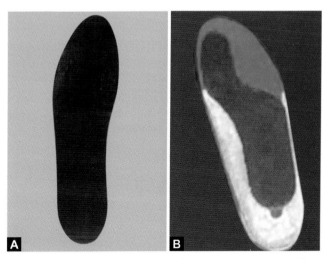

FIGS 6A AND B: Typical orthotics for turf toe. (A) Carbon fiber full-length shank insert; (B) Three-quarter length insert with hallux extension[44]

Source: Reproduced with permission from Elsevier Health Science.

joint in order to avoid reinjury or aggravation. If the injury progresses to hallux rigidus or limitus, a first ray cutout or dancer pad (Fig. 7) is effective in off-loading pressure, and allowing flexion of the first ray, thus reducing the 1st MTP extension needed. If the temporary pad or cutout is beneficial, a more permanent solution may be to add the cutout or padding to a more permanent orthotic device.

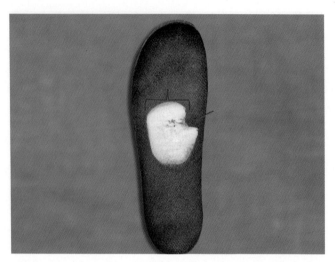

FIG. 7: Dancer pad placed on top the shoe's factory inserts. The arrow represents where the plantar first metatarsal head will be. The bracket is where the 2nd through 5th metatarsal heads will sit.

Maturation Stage Rehabilitation

Progressive endurance and functional activities are the goal of this stage. Table 7 provides examples of specific exercise progressions for the maturation stage, many of which can be initiated in the acute inflammatory stage, with the precautions discussed earlier. The maturation stage occurs after 6 weeks but may be delayed in cases of fracture or severe injury. For example, a grade III turf toe may require immobilization for up to 8 weeks, with full recovery as late as 6 months.[5,6] For all injuries, maximizing function is essential. Manual therapies may need to be continued in cases where limited mobility persists or recurs, and training patients to perform self-mobilizations can be useful in mitigating future issues and allowing for timely discharge. Agility training, plyometrics and weight training are emphasized prior to full athletic and recreational participation. Some individuals may require

TABLE 7: Exercise progression

Initial exercise	Progression			
Isometric great toe flexion into other foot	Marble pick up	Towel curls	Toes raises seated	Toe raises standing
Isometric great toe extension one foot on top of the other	Towel push away	Resistance band		
Four-way ankle isometrics	Four-way ankle resistance with band or ankle isolator	Standing leg swings	Standing leg swings with resistance	
Ankle circles or alphabet	BAPS™ board motion seated	BAPS™ board motion standing	Single leg clock reach, Star Excursion Balance Test or Y-Balance	
Hip abduction side-lying	Gluteal bridging with resisted abduction supine	Standing resisted abduction	Side stepping with band resistance	
Clamshells	Fire hydrants or hip circles quadruped	Hip rotation standing with band resistance		
Hip extension prone	Gluteal bridging supine	Quadruped hip extension	Hip extension standing with band resistance	Romanian deadlift or single leg
Leg press double leg	Leg press single leg	Double leg squat	Lunge	Single leg squat
Progress to the below exercises once able to do weight-bearing activities above				
Shuttle MVP™ or Total Gym™ double leg hop	Shuttle MVP™ or Total Gym single leg hop	Standing double leg uniplanar hop back and forth	Standing single leg uniplanar hop back and forth	Uniplanar ladder drills

Continued

Continued

Initial exercise	Progression	
Walking S-turns, M agility, W agility, figure 8's	Jogging S-turns, M agility, W agility, figure 8's	Increased speed S-turns, M agility, W agility, figure 8's

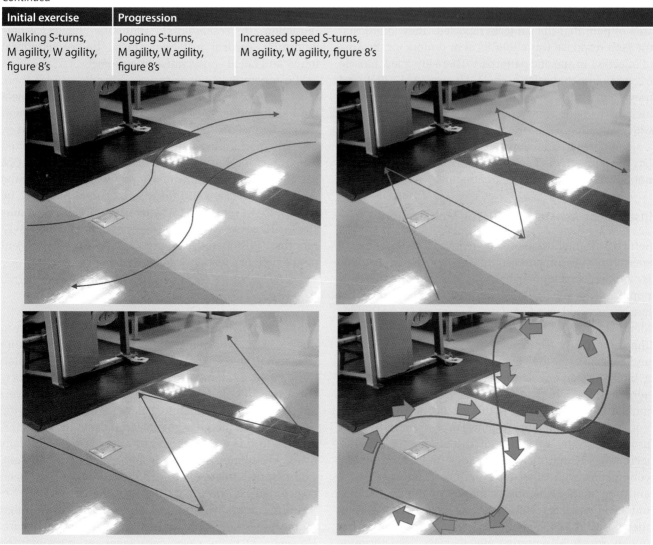

more permanent orthoses for successful resumption of prior activity levels without injury recurrence. Many of the strategies employed in the temporary orthoses during the protected motion phase of healing can be incorporated into permanent devices, if needed. However, specific recommendations for orthoses prescription are beyond the scope of this chapter.

Alternative Therapies and Medical Interventions

Patients pursuing physical therapy intervention may seek complimentary interventions concurrently, or may resort to other treatments if they fail to gain satisfactory resolution with traditional physical therapy alone.

Dry Needling

Another therapy that may facilitate recovery is trigger point dry needling (intramuscular manual therapy). While there is limited research for dry needling, the evidence is emerging as to the efficacy of this treatment.[45,46] Trigger point dry needling is the utilization of acupuncture type needles with the intent of inserting the needle into an area of irritability. These areas of irritability are called trigger points. Simons and Travell mapped out these trigger points by injecting saline solution into specific areas in thousands of subjects.[47] Simons and Travell recorded the area of pain that the subjects reported. They found that the pain response was either local or remote for the area of injection in specific patterns.[47] There are a few muscle trigger points that refer to the MTP area (AbH, FHL and brevis and tibialis posterior). Assessment of trigger points includes palpation and reporting of symptom provocation with palpation. The treatment should be based on assessment of dysfunction and subsequent reassessment. Dry needling should be combined with rehabilitation and not utilized as a standalone treatment.

Instrument-Assisted Soft Tissue Mobilization

Soft tissue mobilization augmented by the use of specialized instruments, commonly known as scraping, is another technique that has become increasingly popular. Scraping has origins in Eastern medicine, but of late has evolved as a popular intervention for conditions identified in Western medicine as soft tissue in nature. There are many techniques (e.g. Graston™, ASTYM™ and Guasha), but the common aim of each is the use of a blunt instrument to increase mobility by disrupting adhesions of soft tissue that has lost some degree of mobility. Additionally, it is theorized that the scraping initiates an inflammatory response to promote the healing process.[48,49] The weakness of the studies in scraping techniques is that the methodology utilizes scraping in conjunction with other interventions (such as exercise and other manual therapy techniques) without separating out the immediate results of each of the treatments. Thus, there are limited high quality studies, but some low quality research, reporting effectiveness.[48,49] Utilization of this technique should be like any manual therapy; if there is no response in two to three treatments, then other interventions should be pursued.

Injections

Injections can provide relief from pain and help to reduce swelling. However, injectable steroids have been shown to breakdown connective tissue. With turf toe, it is not advisable to perform injections for this condition.[50]

Surgery

Turf toe injuries seldom require surgical intervention. However, there exist relative indications for surgery for related pathologies: larger capsular avulsion with unstable joint, diastasis of bipartite sesamoid or fracture, retraction of sesamoid(s), traumatic hallux valgus deformity, vertical instability, loose bodies, chondral injury and failed conservative treatment.[50]

Postoperative management is difficult because there must be a balance between immobilization to protect the repair and early ROM. Early on, excessive extension should be avoided and protective splint should be worn when not performing gentle ROM.[50] At 4 weeks, protected weight bearing can begin in a walking boot. Active ROM can begin at this point with symptoms of pain being the guide. At 8 weeks, a turf toe insert, or rigid plate can be utilized to prevent 1st MTP hyperextension. Running may start at 12 weeks with full recovery at approximately 6–12 months.[50] Postoperative progression should be dependent on the patient's response and the surgeon's restrictions.

CONCLUSION

During ambulation, the foot is the first part of the body to make contact with the ground. The 1st MTP bears more weight than any other MTP and is important in propulsion during gait. The joint also plays a pivotal role in balance. Great toe immobilization has been shown to negatively affect static and dynamic balance.[51] Because of the importance of the great toe for propulsion and balance, injuries to this area may greatly affect activities of daily living, occupational demands and athletic participation. Conservative treatment of 1st MTP injuries has been researched as the first line treatment.[1,3-6,12,18,20,30-32] Restoring mobility and the strength to control that mobility are the primary objectives of conservative care. However, in many cases permanent orthotics may be required for functional recovery.[6,50] Attention not only to the great toe but also to the kinetic chain as a whole contributes to minimizing recurrence and maximizing recovery. Each individual presents differently. Examining and treating the individual will allow for greater success with any level of function and mitigation of potential future disability. Conservative care for turf toe injuries is considered the first line of treatment and has been shown to be very effective. However, there is a lack of research when it comes to prevention of turf toe injuries, except with regard to surface and footwear. There is little research looking into movement dysfunction that may contribute to this injury and its severity. Future research should focus on prevention especially with the increasing popularity of sports for children and adults.

REFERENCES

1. Nihal A, Trepman E, Nag D. First ray disorders in athletes. Sports Med Arthrosc Rev. 2009;17(3):160-6. doi:10.1097/JSA.0b013e3181a5cb1f.
2. Stokes IA, Hutton WC, Scott JR. Forces acting on the metatarsals during normal walking. J Anat. 1979;129(3):579-90.
3. Albers D, Agnone M, Isear J. Rehabilitation and taping techniques in the athlete: hallux and first ray problems. Tech Foot Ankle Surg. 2003;2(1): 61-72. doi:10.1097/00132587-200303000-00010.
4. Hart E, deAsla R, Grottkau B. Current concepts in the treatment of hallux valgus. Orthop Nurs. 2008;27(5):274-80. doi:10.1097/01.NOR.0000337276.17552.1f.
5. McCormick J, Anderson R. Turf Toe: anatomy, diagnosis, and treatment. Sports Heal Multidiscip Approach. 2010;2(6):487-94. doi:10.1177/1941738110386681.
6. McCormick J, Anderson R. The great toe: failed turf toe, chronic turf toe, and complicated sesamoid injuries. Foot Ankle Clin North Am. 2009;14:135-50. doi:10.1016/j.fcl.2009.01.001.
7. Ohlson B. (2012). Turf Toe. [online] Available from http://emedicine.medscape.com/article/1236962-overview. [Accessed April 1, 2014].
8. Welsh B, Redmond A, Chockalingam N, Keenan AM. A case-series to explore the efficacy of foot orthoses in treating first metatarsophalangeal joint pain. J Foot Ankle Res. 2010;3(17):1-9. doi:10.1186/1757-1146-3-17.
9. Rodeo S, O'Brien S, Warren R, Barnes R, Wickiewicz T, Dillingham M. Turf-toe: an analysis of metatarsophalangeal joint sprains in professional football players. Am J Sports Med. 1990;18(3):280-5.
10. George E, Harris A, Dragoo J, Hunt K. Incidence and Risk Factors for Turf Toe Injuries in Intercollegiate Football: Data From the National Collegiate Athletic Association Injury Surveillance System. Foot Ankle Int. 2014;35(2):108-15. doi:10.1177/1071100713514038.
11. Mullen J, O'Malley M. Sprains-residual instability of subtalar, Lisfranc joints, and turf toe. Clin Sports Med. 2004;23:97-121. doi:10.1016/S0278-5919(03)00089-9.
12. Chinn L, Hertel J. Rehabilitation of ankle and foot injuries in athletes. Clin Sports Med. 2010;29(1):157-67. doi:10.1016/j.csm.2009.09.006.
13. Brophy R, Gamradt S, Ellis S, Barnes RP, Rodeo SA, Warren RF, et al. Effect of turf toe on foot contact pressures in professional american football players. Foot Ankle Int. 2009;30(5):405-9. doi:10.3113/FAI.2009.0405.
14. Hudson Z. Rehabilitation and return to play after foot and ankle injuries in athletes. Sports Med Arthrosc Rev. 2009;17(3):203-7. doi:10.1097/JSA.0b013e3181a5ce96.
15. Anderson, Robert. Great toe disorders. In: Porter DA, Schon LC (Eds). Baxter's the Foot and Ankle in Sport, 2nd edition. Philadelphia, PA: Elsevier Health Sciences; 2007. pp. 423-4.
16. Shurnas PS. Hallux rigidus: etiology, biomechanics, and nonoperative treatment. Foot Ankle Clin North Am. 2009;14:1-8. doi:10.1016/j.fcl.2008.11.001.
17. Hecht PJ, Lin TJ. Hallux valgus. Med Clin North Am. 2014;98:227-32. doi:10.1016/j.mcna.2013.10.007.
18. Glasoe W, Nuckley D, Ludewig P. Hallux valgus and the first metatarsal arch segment: a theoretical biomechanical perspective. Phys Ther. 2010;90(1):110-20. doi:10.2522/ptj.20080298.
19. Nix S, Smith M, Vicenzino B. Prevalence of hallux valgus in the general population: a systematic review and meta-analysis. J Foot Ankle Res. 2010;3(21):1-9. doi:10.1186/1757-1146-3-21.
20. Cohen B. Hallux sesamoid disorders. Foot Ankle Clin North Am. 2009;14:91-104. doi:10.1016/j.fcl.2008.11.003.
21. Wheeless CR. (2012). Lachman Test. Duke Orthop. Presents Wheel. Textb Orthop. [online] Available from http://www.wheelessonline.com/ortho/lachman_test. [Accessed June, 2014].
22. Huxel Bliven KC, Anderson BE. Core stability training for injury prevention. Sports Heal Multidiscip Approach. 2013;5(6):514-22. doi:10.1177/1941738113481200.
23. Leetun D, Ireland ML, Wilson JD, Ballantine BT, Davis IM. Core stability measures as risk factors for lower extremity injury in athletes. Med Sci Sports Exerc. 2004;36(6):926-34.
24. O'Conner FG, Deuster PA, Davis J, Pappas CG, Knapik JJ. Functional movement screening: predicting injuries in officer candidates. Med Sci Sports Exerc. 2011;43(12):2224-30. doi:10.1249/MSS.0b013e318223522d.
25. Kiesel K, Plisky P, Voight ML. Can serious injury in professional football be predicted by a preseason functional movement screen? North Am J Sport Phys Ther. 2007;2(3):147-58.
26. Letafatkar A, Hadadnezhad M, Shojaedin S, Mohamadi E. Relationship between functional movement screening score and history of injury. Int J Sports Phys Ther. 2014;9(1):21-27. doi:PMC3924605.
27. Chorba RS, Chorba DJ, Bouillon LE, Overmeyer CA, Landis JA. Use of a functional movement screening tool to determine injury risk in female collegiate athletes. North Am J Sport Phys Ther. 2010;5(2):47-54. doi:PMC2953387.
28. Functional Movement Systems. (2013). What Is Balance Test. [online] Available from http://www.ybalancetest.com/what/. [Accessed May 3, 2014].
29. Gribble P, Hertel J, Plisky P. Using the star excursion balance test to assess dynamic postural-control deficits and outcomes in lower extremity injury: a literature review. J Athl Train. 2012;47(3):339-57. doi:10.4085/1062-6050-47.3.08.
31. Kindred J, Trubey C, Simons S. Foot injuries in runners. Curr Sports Med Rep. 2011;10(5):249-54. doi:10.1249/JSR.0b013e31822d3ea4.
32. Shamus J, Shamus E, Gugel RN, Brucker BS, Skaruppa C. The effect of sesamoid mobilization, flexor hallucis strengthening, and gait training on reducing pain and restoring function in individuals with hallux limitus: a clinical trial. J Orthop Sports Phys Ther. 2004;34(7):368-76. doi:10.2519/jospt.2004.34.7.368.
33. Mercandetti M. (2013). Wound Healing and Repair. [online] Available from http://emedicine.medscape.com/article/1298129-overview#a1. [Accessed April 27, 2014].
34. Bleakley C, Domhall M. Chapter 11: What is the role of ice in soft-tissue injury management? Evid Based Sports Med. 2007;1:204. doi:10.1002/9780470988732.ch11.
35. Hubbard T, Denegar C. Does cryotherapy improve outcomes with soft tissue injury? J Athl Train. 2004;39(3):278-9. doi:PMC522152.
36. Van der Windt D, Van der Heijden G, Van den Berg A, Bouter L, ter Riet G, van den Bekerom M. Ultrasound therapy for acute ankle sprains. Cochrane Database Syst Rev. 2002;1:CD001250. doi:10.1002/14651858.CD001250.
37. Snyder A, Perotti A, Lam K, Bay R. The influence of high-voltage electrical stimulation on the edema formation after acute injury: a systematic review. J Sports Rehabil. 2010;19(4):436-51. doi:PMID: 21116012.
38. Boguszewski D, Tomaszewski I, Adamczyk J, Bialoszewski D. Evaluation of effectiveness of kinesiology taping as an adjunct to rehabilitation following anterior cruciate ligament reconstruction. Preliminary report. Ortop Traumatol Rehabil. 2013;15(5):469-78. doi:10.5604/15093492.1084361.
39. Bialoszewski D, Wozniak W, Zarek S. Clinical efficacy of kinesiology taping in reducing edema of the lower limbs in patients treated with the ilizarov method—preliminary report. Ortop Traumatol Rehabil. 2009;11(1):46-54.
40. Ferber R, Hreljac A, Kendall KD. Suspected mechanisms in the cause of overuse running injuries: a clinical review. Sports Heal Multidiscip Approach. 2009;1(3):242-6. doi:PMC3445255.
41. Snyder KR, Earl JE, O'Connor KM, Ebersole KT. Resistance training is accompanied by increases in hip strength and changes in lower

extremity biomechanics during running. Clin Biomech. 2009;24(1):26-34. doi:10.1016/j.clinbiomech.2008.09.009.

42. Boren K, Conrey C, Le Coguic J, Paprocki L, Voight ML, Robinson T. Electromyographic analysis of gluteus medius and gluteus maximus during rehabilitation exercises. Int J Sports Phys Ther. 2011;6(3):206-23. doi:PMC3201064.

43. Hengevled E, Banks K. Musculoskeletal foot and ankle disorders. Maitland's Peripheral Manipulation, vol 2, 5th edition. New York: Churchill Livingstone Elsevier; 2014. pp. 516-57.

44. McCormick J, Anderson R. Rehabilitation following turf toe injury and plantar plate repair. Clin Sports Med. 2010;29:313-23. doi:10.1016/j.csm.2009.12.010.

45. Dommerholt J, Fernandez-de-las-Penas C. Trigger Point Dry Needling: An Evidence and Clinical-Based Approach. New York: Churchill Livingstone Elsevier; 2013.

46. Kietrys DM, Palombaro KM, Azzaretto E, et al. Effectiveness of dry needling for upper-quarter myofascial pain: a systematic review and meta-analysis. J Orthop Sports Phys Ther. 2013;43(9):620-34. doi:10.2519/jospt.2013.4668.

47. Simons DG, Travell JG, Simons LS, Cummings BD. Travell & Simons' Myofascial Pain and Dysfunction: The Trigger Point Manual, 2nd edition. Baltimore, MD: Lippincott Williams & Wilkins; 1998.

48. Looney B, Srokose T, Fernandez-de-las-Penas C, Cleland J. Graston instrument soft tissue mobilization and home stretching for the management of plantar heel pain: a case series. J Manipulative Physiol Ther. 2011;34(2):138-42. doi:10.1016/j.jmpt.2010.12.003.

49. Slaven E, Mathers J. Management of chronic ankle pain using joint mobilization and ASTYM treatment: a case report. J Man Manip Ther. 2011;19(2):108-12. doi:10.1179/2042618611Y.0000000004.

50. McCormick J, Anderson R. Surgical correction of the recalcitrant turf toe. Tech Foot Ankle Surg. 2013;12(1):29-38. doi:10.1097/BTF.0b013e318282ee8d.

51. Chou SW, Chen KHY, Chen JH, Ju YY, Wong AMK. The role of the great toe in balance performance. J Orthop Res. 2009;27(4):549-54.

Appendices

Throwers Ten Exercises

▓ THROWER'S TEN EXERCISE LIST

1A. D2 extension
1B. D2 flexion
2A. External rotation (ER) at 0° abduction
2B. Internal rotation (IR) at 0° abduction
2C. ER at 90° abduction
2D. IR at 90° abduction
3.   Abduction to 90°
4.   Scaption ER
5.   Side-lying ER
6A. Prone horizontal abduction (Neutral)
6B. Prone horizontal abduction (Full ER, 100° abduction)
6C. Prone rowing
6D. Prone rowing into ER
7.   Press ups
8.   Push-ups
9A. Elbow flexion
9B. Elbow extension
10A. Wrist flexion
10B. Wrist extension
10C. Supination
10D. Pronation

Patient-Specific Functional Scale

▨ INITIAL ASSESSMENT

Patient-specific functional scale (PSFS): "I am going to ask you to please identify up to three important activities that you are unable to do or are having difficulty with as a result of your _____ problem." "Please rate your *ability* to perform these activities on a scale from 0 to 10, where 0 equals completely unable to perform the activity, and 10 equals fully able (or 100% able)." (Clinician: Show scale to patient and have the patient rate each activity).

▨ FOLLOW-UP ASSESSMENTS

PSFS: "When I assessed you on (state previous assessment date), you told me that you had difficulty with (read all activities from list). Please rate your *ability* to perform these activities today on a scale from 0 to 10, where 0 equals completely unable to perform the activity, and 10 equals fully able (or 100% able)." (Read and have patient score each item in the list one at a time).

PSFS scoring scheme (Point to one number)										
0	1	2	3	4	5	6	7	8	9	10
Unable to perform activity										*Able* to perform activity at the same level as before injury or problem

Date	Initial	6th visit	Discharge
PSFS 1.			
PSFS 2.			
PSFS 3.			
PSFS 4. Optional			
PSFS 5. Optional			

Numeric Pain Rating Scale

▨ INITIAL ASSESSMENT

Numeric pain rating scale (NPRS): "I am going to ask you to rate your _____ pain on a scale from 0 to 10, where 0 equals no pain, and 10 equals the worst imaginable pain (or worst possible pain). Please rate your level of pain: right now...; .at its worst in the last 24 hours...; at its best in the last 24 hours."

▨ FOLLOW-UP ASSESSMENTS

Same as above

NPRS Scoring Scheme (Point to One Number)

0	1	2	3	4	5	6	7	8	9	10
No Pain										Worst Possible pain

NPRS pain scale score:	Current			
	Worst in last 24 hours			
	Best in last 24 hours			

Pain Beliefs Screening Instrument

1. How much pain have you experienced on average in the last week? (*Mark ONE*)

O	O	O	O	O	O	O	O	O	O	O
0	1	2	3	4	5	6	7	8	9	10

No pain   Worst
                                                                        pain possible

2. To what extent have you managed activities related to the home and family? (*Mark ONE*)

O	O	O	O	O	O	O	O	O	O	O
0	1	2	3	4	5	6	7	8	9	10

Not at all   To a high
                                                                        degree

3. Simply being careful that I do not make any unnecessary movements is the safest thing I can do to prevent my pain from worsening. Agree or disagree? (*Mark ONE*)

O	O	O	O	O	O	O	O	O	O	O
0	1	2	3	4	5	6	7	8	9	10

No, I strongly   Yes, I strongly
disagree   agree

4. My body is telling me I have something dangerously wrong. Agree or disagree? (*Mark ONE*)

O	O	O	O	O	O	O	O	O	O	O
0	1	2	3	4	5	6	7	8	9	10

No, I strongly   Yes, I strongly
disagree   agree

5. My pain is awful and it overwhelms me. Agree or disagree? (*Mark ONE*)

O	O	O	O	O	O	O	O	O	O	O
0	1	2	3	4	5	6	7	8	9	10

No, I strongly
disagree

Yes, I strongly
agree

6. How confident are you in your ability to go to a movie? (*Mark ONE*)

O	O	O	O	O	O	O	O	O	O	O
0	1	2	3	4	5	6	7	8	9	10

Not at all
confident

Very
confident

7. How confident are you in your ability to go shopping? (*Mark ONE*)

O	O	O	O	O	O	O	O	O	O	O
0	1	2	3	4	5	6	7	8	9	10

Not at all
confident

Very
confident

Running Simulation Program

1. Standing pronation/ supination with dots at shin and 2nd metatarsal

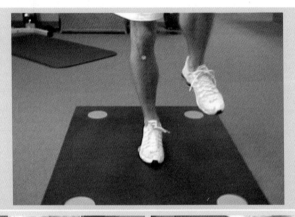

2a. Single leg standing pronation
2b. Single leg stance supination

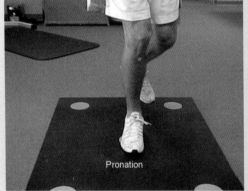
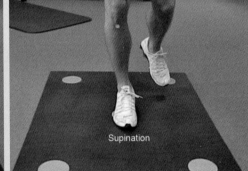

3. Single leg standing and maintaining balance, swing arms to simulate running

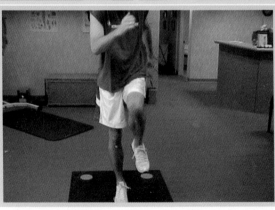

Continued

Return to Running Progression

GUIDELINES

The following guidelines need to be followed to ensure an optimal outcome of the progressive running program.
1. Initially, you will start with a run/walk program and then progress to a running only program.
2. Cross-train with non-impact activities on the "off-days".
3. *REST* 1–2 days per week.
4. Integrate *core strengthening* exercises into your running program.
5. Initially, start running approximately 1–2 minutes/mile then your preinjury pace without losing proper form.
6. *LISTEN TO YOUR BODY!* If you have pain, stop for that day. At your next schedule run, return *back* to the last "successful" run that you had without pain.

Day (weeks 1 and 2)	Walk (minutes)	Run (minutes)	Repeat	Total time
1	10	5	2x	30
2	8	4	3x	36
3	5	5	3x	30
4	4	6	3x	30
5	3	7	3x	30
6	2	8	3x	30
7	2	10	3x	36

Day (weeks 3 and 4)	Run (minutes)	Walk (minutes)	Run (minutes)	Total time
1	15	2	15	32
2	18	2	12	32
3	20	2	10	32
4	20	5	10	35
5	25	-	-	25
6	25	5	5	35
7	25	-	-	25

Week ↓/Day →	1	2	3	4	5	6	7
5	30	–	30	–	30	–	35
6	–	30	–	35	–	35	–
7	35	–	30	–	35	–	35
8	–	35	–	40	–	35	–

At this point, increase your distance by increasing either *intensity* or *time*
- Intensity increase: Repeat weeks 5–8. Increase pace by 15–20 sec/mile every other week.
- Time increase: Progress to weeks 9–12.

Week ↓/Day →	1	2	3	4	5	6	7
9	35	–	40	–	40	35	–
10	–	40	35	–	40	–	40
11	–	45	30	–	40	–	45
12	–	45	–	40	–	45	35

Source: Used with permission and Courtesy of Thomas Goodwin, D.O./Mary Vajgrt, M.D.

Victorian Institute of
Sport Assessment Scale

Name:
Age:
Date:

Victorian Institute of Sport Assessment Scale

1. For how many minutes can you sit pain-free?

Points ☐

0 mins | 0 1 2 3 4 5 6 7 8 9 10 | 10 mins

2. Do you have pain walking downstairs with a normal gait cycle?

Points ☐

Severe | 0 1 2 3 4 5 6 7 8 9 10 | None

3. Do you have pain at the knee with full active non-weight bearing knee extension?

Points ☐

Severe | 0 1 2 3 4 5 6 7 8 9 10 | None

4. Do you have pain when doing a full weight-bearing lunge?

Points ☐

Severe | 0 1 2 3 4 5 6 7 8 9 10 | None

5. Do you have problems squatting?

Points ☐

Unable | 0 1 2 3 4 5 6 7 8 9 10 | None

6. Do you have pain during or immediately after doing 10 single leg hops?

Points ☐

Severe/Unable | 0 1 2 3 4 5 6 7 8 9 10 | None

7. Are you currently undertaking sport or other physical activity?

Points ☐

0 ☐ Not at all

4 ☐ Modified training ± modified competition

7 ☐ Full training ± competition but not at the same level as when symptoms began

10 ☐ Competing at the same or higher level when symptoms began

8. Please complete EITHER A, B or C in this question.
- If you have *no pain* while undertaking sport please complete *Q8a only*
- If you have *pain while undertaking sport but it does not stop you* from completing the activity, please complete *Q8b only*
- If you *have pain that stops you from completing sporting activities,* please complete *Q8 c only*

8a. If you have no pain while undertaking sport, for how long can you train/practice?

Points ☐

NIL	0–5 mins	5–10 mins	11–15 mins	>15 mins
☐	☐	☐	☐	☐
0	**7**	**14**	**21**	**30**

or

8b. If you have some pain while undertaking sport, but it does not stop you from completing your training/practice, for how long can you train/practice?

Points ☐

NIL	0–5 mins	5–10 mins	11–15 mins	>15 mins
☐	☐	☐	☐	☐
0	**4**	**10**	**14**	**20**

or

8c. If you have pain that stops you from completing your training/practice, for how long can you train/practice?

Points ☐

NIL	0–5 mins	5–10 mins	11–15 mins	>15 mins
☐	☐	☐	☐	☐
0	**2**	**5**	**7**	**10**

TOTAL VISA SCORE _____

Foot Posture Index Datasheet

FACTOR		PLANE	SCORE 1 Date_____ Comment_____		SCORE 2 Date_____ Comment_____		SCORE 3 Date_____ Comment_____	
			Left (-2 to +2)	Right (-2 to +2)	Left (-2 to +2)	Right (-2 to +2)	Left (-2 to +2)	Right (-2 to +2)
Rearfoot	Talar head palpation	Transverse						
	Curves above and below lateral malleoli	Frontal/ trans						
	Inversion/eversion of the calcaneus	Frontal						
Forefoot	Bulge in the region of the TNJ	Transverse						
	Congruence of the medial longitudinal arch	Sagittal						
	Abd/adduction of forefoot on rearfoot (too-many-toes)	Transverse						
	TOTAL							

Reference values
Normal = 0 to +5
Pronated = +6 to +9, Highly pronated 10+
Supinated = -1 to –4, Highly supinated –5 to -12

©Anthony Redmond 1998. (May be copied for clinical use, and adapted with the permission of the copyright holder)
Available at: http://www.leeds.ac.uk/medicine/FASTER/fpi.htm

FACTOR		PLANE	SCORE 1 Date_____ Comment_____		SCORE 2 Date_____ Comment_____		SCORE 3 Date_____ Comment_____	
			Left (-2 to +2)	Right (-2 to +2)	Left (-2 to +2)	Right (-2 to +2)	Left (-2 to +2)	Right (-2 to +2)
Rearfoot	Talar head palpation	Transverse						
	Curves above and below lateral malleoli	Frontal/ trans						
	Inversion/eversion of the calcaneus	Frontal						
Forefoot	Bulge in the region of the TNJ	Transverse						
	Congruence of the medial longitudinal arch	Sagittal						
	Abd/adduction of forefoot rear foot (too-many-toes)	Transverse						
	TOTAL							

Reference values
Normal = 0 to +5
Pronated = +6 to +9, Severely pronated 10+
Supinated = -1 to –4, Severely supinated –5 to -12

©Anthony Redmond 1998. (May be copied for clinical use, and adapted with the permission of the copyright holder)
Available at: http://www.leeds.ac.uk/medicine/FASTER/fpi.htm

Index

Page numbers followed by '*f*', '*t*', and '*b*' indicate figures, tables, and boxes, respectively.